THE HANDBOOK OF
AUGMENTATIVE AND
ALTERNATIVE COMMUNICATION

THE HANDBOOK OF AUGMENTATIVE AND ALTERNATIVE COMMUNICATION

Sharon L. Glennen, Ph.D.

and

Denise C. DeCoste, Ed.D.

With Contributions

DELMAR
CENGAGE Learning

Australia Canada Mexico Singapore Spain United Kingdom United States

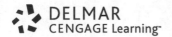

Handbook of Augmentative and Alternative Communication
Sharon L. Glennen

Denise C. DeCoste

For product information and technology assistance, contact us at
Cengage Learning Customer & Sales Support, 1-800-354-9706

For permission to use material from this text or product, submit all requests online at **cengage.com/permissions** Further permissions questions can be emailed to **permissionrequest@cengage.com**

Library of Congress Control Number: 96-28455

ISBN-13: 978-1-5659-3684-3

ISBN-10: 1-5659-3684-1

Delmar Cengage Learning
5 Maxwell Drive
Clifton Park, NY 12065-2919
USA

Cengage Learning products are represented in Canada by Nelson Education, Ltd.

For your lifelong learning solutions, visit **delmar.cengage.com**

Visit our corporate website at **www.cengage.com**

Notice to the Reader
Publisher does not warrant or guarantee any of the products described herein or perform any independent analysis in connection with any of the product information contained herein. Publisher does not assume, and expressly disclaims, any obligation to obtain and include information other than that provided to it by the manufacturer. The reader is expressly warned to consider and adopt all safety precautions that might be indicated by the activities described herein and to avoid all potential hazards. By following the instructions contained herein, the reader willingly assumes all risks in connection with such instructions. The publisher makes no representations or warranties of any kind, including but not limited to, the warranties of fitness for particular purpose or merchantability, nor are any such representations implied with respect to the material set forth herein, and the publisher takes no responsibility with respect to such material. The publisher shall not be liable for any special, consequential, or exemplary damages resulting, in whole or part, from the readers' use of, or reliance upon, this material.

Printed in the United States of America
13 14 15 16 17 XX 12 11 10 09

CONTENTS

PREFACE

Augmentative and alternative communication (AAC) is a unique area of clinical practice. The nonspeaking population encompasses a wide range of diverse individuals whose only common link is the inability to communicate vocally. Although the field of AAC is viewed as a cohesive area of practice, in reality AAC is an intervention technique that is applied across a wide variety of medical and developmental disorders. Underlying causes for nonspeaking conditions vary widely, from young children with developmental language disorders, to individuals with severe physical disabilities such as cerebral palsy, to senior citizens who have had strokes. This diversity makes it difficult to write a textbook that encompasses AAC in its entirety. Nevertheless, that is what we have endeavored to do.

The underlying philosophy of *The Handbook of Augmentative and Alternative Communication* was to develop a practical text written by professionals with direct clinical experience in the field of AAC. The goal was to write a text that would combine AAC theory and research with clinical practice and case studies. The main authors have AAC experiences dating back to the beginnings of the field, providing a broad perspective of where AAC has come from, the current state-of-the-art of the field, and future directions for AAC. The contributing authors also bring a wealth of direct clinical experiences from diverse settings including schools, rehabilitation hospitals, universities, acute care hospitals, community outreach programs and regional assistive technology centers. The contributing authors also add diversity by applying AAC concepts across a wide variety of disability populations in their clinical practices. Finally, the authors represent the multidisciplinary nature of AAC. Chapters are written by speech-language pathologists, special educators, occupational therapists, and physical therapists, with each profession bringing its unique background and perspective to the topic.

The book was organized to provide both breadth and depth of information about AAC. The first section of the book provides a broad overview written to introduce the topic to professionals and students who are approaching the field for the first time. The chapters in Section 1 contain basic material that is typically covered in introductory AAC courses at the university level. Sections 2 and 3 of the book provide depth of information. Section 2, which focuses on specific disabilities and AAC, reviews AAC as it applies to various disability populations. Section 3, AAC in specific environments, discusses differences in implementation strategies across various settings. Sections 2 and 3 were written for the professional who needs in-depth information to apply AAC to specific individuals and situations, and for use in advanced AAC university classes. Each of the chapters in Sections 2 and 3 is followed by a case study. In an attempt to make the case studies come alive, we expanded them into "AAC Life Stories" and provide detailed information to make the process of clinical decision-making as realistic as possible. The case studies are written to complement main points in the accompanying chapters, but are detailed enough to stand alone.

The first section of the book, Overview of Augmentative and Alternative Communication, contains nine chapters that provide a broad overview of AAC. Chapter 1, Introduction to Augmentative and Alternative Communication, written by Sharon Glennen, provides an historical perspective for the field while simultaneously introducing basic terminology. Chapter 2, Service Delivery in AAC, written by Kristen Swengel and Judith Marquette, discusses AAC team members and their roles, and reviews various models of providing AAC services. Sharon Glennen is the author of Chapter 3, Augmentative and Alternative Communication Systems. This chapter reviews aided AAC devices and equipment, providing a conceptual model for categorizing AAC technology. Chapter 4, Symbol Systems and Vocabulary Selection Strategies, is written by Cindy Millikin. This chapter reviews both aided and unaided language systems and the important topic of selecting and organizing AAC vocabulary. Chapters 5, 6, and 7 form the AAC assessment trilogy. Sharon Glennen is the author of Chapter 5, Augmentative and Alternative Communication Assessment Strategies. This chapter presents an overview of the entire assessment process, then provides detailed information on the linguistic and cognitive aspects of an AAC evaluation. Chapter 6 by Ulrika Radell continues the topic of Augmentative and Alternative Communication Assessment Strategies, with a focus on Seating and Positioning for individuals with physical disabilities. Finally, Denise DeCoste in Chapter 7 writes on the topic of Augmentative and Alternative Communication Assessment Strategies: Motor and Visual Considerations. This chapter reviews the process of evaluating motor abilities and visual skills as they apply to AAC. Section 1 then continues with Chapter 8, The Role of Lit-

eracy in Augmentative and Alternative Communication, by Denise DeCoste. This chapter discusses the importance of literacy for individuals who are nonspeaking and provides evaluation and remediation strategies for use with AAC consumers. Section 1 concludes with Chapter 9 by Patricia Ourand and Sylvia Gray. Funding and Legal Issues in Augmentative and Alternative Communication discusses federal laws that govern the funding process along with guidelines for accessing funding resources.

Section 2 of the *Handbook of Augmentative and Alternative Communication*, Specific Disabilities and AAC, begins the process of providing the reader with in-depth information on specific AAC topics. Chapter 10, AAC and Individuals with Physical Disabilities, by Denise DeCoste, discusses the use of AAC with persons with cerebral palsy, ataxia, and childhood neurodegenerative disorders, among others. Chapter 11 is authored by Cynthia Weitz, Mark Dexter, and Jacquelyn Moore. This chapter, entitled AAC and Children with Developmental Disabilities, focuses on the topic from the generic perspective of children with severe expressive language disorders, using AAC in children with severe apraxia of speech, and autism. Stephen Calculator is the author of Chapter 12, AAC and Individuals with Severe to Profound Disabilities. This chapter reviews the concept of AAC and inclusion for individuals with severe disabilities. It also discusses unique assessment and intervention strategies for the population. Chapter 13, AAC and Adults with Acquired Disabilities, by Patricia Pyatak Fletcher provides information about the use of AAC with adults recovering from traumatic brain injury and stroke. It also reviews the use of AAC for adults with neurodegenerative diseases such as multiple sclerosis, and amyotrophic lateral sclerosis.

The final section of the book, AAC in Specific Environments, is predicated on the recognition that AAC implementation strategies are different across different user environments. With this perspective, separate chapters were written to discuss the unique aspects of various AAC implementation settings. Chapter 14, AAC in the Family and Home, by Dianne Angelo reviews existing research regarding family perspectives relating to AAC. Family-friendly service delivery models are discussed along with introductory information regarding multiculturalism and AAC. Sylvia Gray is the author of Chapter 15, AAC in the Educational Setting. The process of developing a school-based AAC assessment and implementation model is discussed, and strategies for implementing AAC in the classroom are reviewed.

In chapter 16, AAC in the Hospital Setting, Sharon Glennen discusses the fast-paced nature of providing AAC services in the acute care hospital setting and reviews AAC strategies for individuals with tracheotomies who have intact oral motor abilities. Section 3 concludes with Chapter 17 by Elizabeth Delsandro. Augmentative and Alternative Communication for Adults with Developmental Disabilities discusses AAC implementation strategies in adult community living, supported employment, and sheltered employment settings.

At the end of the book, readers will find four appendixes and a glossary of terms. Appendix A is a product directory with detailed descriptions of AAC devices, related computer hardware and software, switches, and other AAC products. Appendix B provides addresses, telephone numbers, and internet world wide web site information for the product vendors mentioned in Appendix A. Appendix C is a listing of AAC organizations with brief descriptions of each organization and contact information. Finally, Appendix D lists traditional and nontraditional information resources. AAC journals and newsletters are listed, along with internet resources such as world wide web sites, usenet newsgroups, and electronic journals. The Glossary provides definitions of terms found in this text which are pertinent to AAC.

The *Handbook of Augmentative and Alternative Communication* is the culmination of more than 100 years of combined author experience. It was written to be a comprehensive yet practical text for both novice and experienced practitioners. By providing both breadth and depth on the topic of AAC, readers will be able to discern practice patterns that apply across the spectrum of AAC users, as well as unusual aspects of AAC implementation relevant to specific populations and settings.

The process of writing this book began one evening at the Closing The Gap Conference. After sharing a bottle of wine that resulted in a late night personal and professional discussion, we decided to collaborate on a new AAC book. Although the beginnings of this book were deceivingly simple, the process of completing the text required the assistance of many individuals and 3 years of hard work. We would like to thank the officers and members of the Maryland Augmentative Communication Association for their professional networking support throughout this project. Many of them are contributing authors for the text, and others contributed indirectly by sharing professional stories and strategies. Support was also provided by many individuals at the Kennedy Krieger Institute and the Johns Hopkins University Center for Technology in Education. We specifically would like to thank Bougie Hopkins for fielding phone calls, faxing messages, copying chapters, and keeping the world at bay during writing deadlines. We would also like to extend heartfelt thanks to Sam Gutter for his layman's perspective and editorial help. Finally, we would like to thank each of the contributing authors for taking the time to write chapters and case studies. This book would not have been the same without their professional expertise.

AUTHORS

Sharon L. Glennen, Ph.D., CCC-SLP
Director, Department of Assistive Technology
Kennedy Krieger Institute
Instructor, Department of Otolaryngology
Johns Hopkins University School of Medicine
Baltimore, Maryland

Denise C. DeCoste, Ed.D., OTR
Team Leader, InterACT
Interdisciplinary Augmentative Communication
and Technology Team
Montgomery County Public Schools
Rockville, Maryland

CONTRIBUTING AUTHORS

Dianne H. Angelo, Ph.D., CCC-SLP
Professor, Department of Communication
Disorders and Special Education
Bloomsburg University
Bloomsburg, Pennsylvania

Stephen N. Calculator, Ph.D., CCC-SLP
Chair, Department of Communication Disorders
University of New Hampshire
Durham, New Hampshire

Elizabeth M. DelSandro, M.S., CCC-SLP
Speech-Language Pathologist
Department of Assistive Technology
Kennedy Krieger Institute
Baltimore, Maryland

Mark E. Dexter, M.A., CCC-SLP
Speech-Language Pathologist
Interdisciplinary Augmentative Communication
and Technology Team
Montgomery County Public Schools
Rockville, Maryland

Patricia Pyatak Fletcher M.S., CCC-SLP
Senior Speech Language Pathologist
Coordinator of the Augmentative Alternative
Communication Clinic
National Rehabilitation Hospital
Washington, D C

Sylvia Gray, M.S.
Assistive Technology Specialist
Region 18 Education Service Center
Midland, Texas

Nancy Larson Horne, M.S., CCC-SLP
Assistive Technology Specialist
Anne Arundel County Public Schools
Annapolis, Maryland

Judith S. Marquette, M.S. Ed
Educational Consultant
PennTech
Harrisburg, Pennsylvania

Cindy C. Millikin, Ph.D., CCC-SLP
Augmentative Communication and Assistive
Technology Specialist
Prince Georges County Public Schools
Upper Marlboro, Maryland

Jacquelyn R. Moore, M.S., CCC-SLP
Speech-Language Pathologist
Interdisciplinary Augmentative Communication
and Technology Team
Montgomery County Public Schools
Rockville, Maryland

Patricia R. Ourand, M.A., CCC-SLP
Speech-Language Pathologist
Rehab Networking
Baltimore, Maryland

Ulrika Radell, B.S., PT
Senior Physical Therapist
Department of Assistive Technology
Kennedy Kreiger Institute
Baltimore, Maryland

Beth Reckord, M.S., CCC-SLP
Director of Speech-Language Pathology
Chesapeake Assessment and Treatment Center
Westminster, Maryland

Kristen E. Swengel, M.S., CCC-SLP
Educational Consultant
Penn Tech
Harrisburg, Pennsylvania

Nancy D. Underhill, M.A., CCC-SLP
Speech-Language Pathologist
Anne Arundel County Public Schools
Annapolis, Maryland

Cynthia R. Weitz, M.S., CCC-SLP
Speech-Language Pathologist
Interdisciplinary Augmentative Communication
and Technology Team
Montgomery County Public Schools
Rockville, Maryland

In memory of Christina Albert and to the many families and individuals who sought our professional advice yet taught us more than we can ever return.

To our continued professional and personal friendship.

To Wayne who has always supported my endeavors; to Matthew who keeps me laughing with his pragmatic first-grade outlook on the world; and to the latest addition, Kevin Vladimir, the Russian toddler prince who keeps me blissfully exhausted. You are the roots and wings that keep me grounded yet let me soar.

To my parents, Mamie and Francis DeCoste for their love and friendship. To my wonderful husband, Sam, whose unflagging support made this endeavor possible, and to my daughters, Rachel and Bess, for their patience throughout.

Section 1

OVERVIEW OF AUGMENTATIVE AND ALTERNATIVE COMMUNICATION

Chapter 1

INTRODUCTION TO AUGMENTATIVE AND ALTERNATIVE COMMUNICATION

Sharon L. Glennen

The ability to communicate is often taken for granted. A thought is formed, translated into a sequence of words, and transferred into motor signals to the laryngeal and oral muscles which then move in a coordinated manner to produce speech. For most people, the entire process occurs instantly and without effort. Communication is used to exchange information, make requests, socialize, and interact with others. These interactions form the social bonds that bind people to each other, their communities, and their culture. According to the American Speech-Language-Hearing Association, "communication is the essence of human life" (1991, p. 9).

There are many individuals who are unable to use speech as their primary method of communication. The American Speech-Language-Hearing Association (1991) estimated that there were more than 2 million individuals in the United States who were unable to communicate using speech or had severe communication impairments. Results of surveys indicate that ap-

proximately 0.3% to 1% of school-aged children are identified as nonspeaking (Matas, Mathy-Laikko, Beukelman, & Legresley, 1985). These individuals need to use other methods of communication in order to interact with their environment. The term *augmentative and alternative communication* (AAC) is used to define these other communication methods. AAC ranges from use of gestures, sign languages, and facial expressions, to the use of alphabet or picture symbol boards, and even sophisticated computer systems with synthesized speech.

AAC is now integrated into the mainstream of communication options for individuals with severe speech impairments (ASHA, 1991; Zangari, Lloyd, & Vicker, 1994). However, it wasn't long ago that many nonspeaking individuals were not given access to AAC. Professionals and families were often unaware of the existence of AAC techniques. As early information about AAC was disseminated, the use of AAC was viewed by some as detrimental to the development of speech, which was seen as the primary goal for communication professionals and their clients. Up through the 1970s and early 1980s, AAC was typically recommended only after traditional speech therapy options had failed (Zangari et al., 1994).

Imagine not being able to speak, yet being denied the opportunity to communicate using other methods. Until a few years ago, this was the situation for many nonspeaking individuals. "Bill" is an example of an individual who was placed in this dilemma. Bill was born in 1957 with severe cerebral palsy. As a preschooler, he lived at home and was able to attend therapies at a children's hospital. Early efforts were focused on teaching him to walk and talk. As Bill approached school age, the public schools would not let him attend. When he was 6, his parents made the difficult decision to send him to a residential school for individuals with cerebral palsy. He describes this early separation from his family as an emotionally upsetting experience. During his stay at the residential school, Bill spent years in speech therapy with limited results. As a child, he felt that his lack of progress was his own fault. He saw other children improve their speech and wondered what he was doing wrong. When Bill was 11, he came home permanently to live with his family. His communication consisted of nodding yes or no in response to questions, saying a few single words that his family could understand, and pointing to things that he wanted.

Bill remembers learning to read at his residential school when he was 8 or 9 years old. As his reading skills improved, the school began looking for methods to teach him spelling. Because he couldn't write using paper and pencil, the school provided him with an alphabet board, and also tried to have him use a typewriter. Bill began to learn to spell words, then phrases, and sentences. Throughout this period, writing with the alphabet board was viewed by his teachers as an educational tool, not a method of communication.

When Bill tried to use the alphabet board to communicate, he was urged to "use your speech." When Bill returned home to live, his school sent the alphabet board to his new teachers to use for educational purposes.

Bill's family was the first to realize that he could use the alphabet board to communicate. They began leaving the alphabet board on his wheelchair tray all the time. At school, Bill continued to work on improving his speech in therapy; but at home he relied on the alphabet board. This continued throughout his childhood and adolescence until he graduated from school. Speech therapy sessions thankfully ended at that time. Bill describes the support of his family as crucial to his development as a communicator. With their acceptance of the alphabet board, he was finally able to convey his thoughts freely.

During the late 1970s, a family member heard about a communication board combining the alphabet and whole written words that was distributed free through the Shriners. Bill obtained one of these boards and to this day still uses it as his primary method of communication. Using this board, he describes his early years of being unable to communicate as extremely frustrating. Bill states that even he did not initially recognize that the alphabet board, introduced to him for spelling, could also be used for communication. He had been led to believe that if he worked hard, his speech would ultimately improve. As a child, he never had the opportunity to communicate complex thoughts to others. He recalls being upset every time he was separated from his parents to go back to the residential school, yet was unable to communicate his fears or feelings to others except by crying. He stated that, at the time, he accepted this as "normal" because many of his friends at the residential school were in the same situation.

Bill now works part-time at the same children's hospital that he attended so many years ago. He is able to see firsthand how differently nonspeaking children with cerebral palsy are treated today. AAC methods are now viewed by professionals at the hospital as a primary communication option. Children with severe physical disabilities are often provided with AAC systems before they are expected to learn to talk. AAC is sometimes implemented in combination with traditional speech and language therapy methods, and other times is implemented alone. The underlying philosophy is that all children have the right to communicate, regardless of their method of communication. Bill's experiences provide a good chronology for the evolution of AAC over the past 30 years. AAC has grown from nonexistence, to emergence, to acceptance during Bill's lifetime. The next two sections of this chapter will review how the AAC field grew and developed.

DEVELOPMENT OF AAC TERMINOLOGY

All new fields of study go through a period of establishing common terms and definitions. Over the years, AAC has struggled to develop standards for terminology (Zangari et al., 1994). One of the first terms to evolve over time was the name for the field. Initially, the terms Nonverbal, Non-vocal, Non-oral, and Non-Speech Communication were widely used. Although these terms were popular in their day, they have since been abandoned because they did not describe the skills of many individuals using AAC who were able to vocalize, had an oral mechanism, and in many cases had some limited speech abilities. In 1985, Lloyd reviewed existing terminology in the field and proposed to standardize the use of augmentative and alternative communication. This term had already been adopted within the name of the International Society for Augmentative and Alternative Communication (ISAAC), which was formed in 1983. *Augmentative* was defined as the process of augmenting existing speech abilities, *alternative* was defined as the process of providing a substitute for speech (Lloyd, 1985). Given our cultural propensity for creating acronyms out of lengthy terminology, augmentative and alternative communication was quickly shortened to AAC, which remains the standard descriptor for the field today (Lloyd & Kangas, 1988).

Use of the term AAC is still debated from time to time. Zangari et al. (1994) argued that professionals are not merely augmenting or providing alternatives to an individual's *speech*, but instead are working to improve an individual's *communication*. This perspective views all attempts at improving communication as attempts to augment existing communication abilities. They proposed the possibility of revising the name of the field to augmentative communication. Despite these debates, the term AAC has become entrenched in the professional literature and will likely be used for some years to come.

Descriptors of the population of individuals who require AAC have also changed over the years. In the past, the terms nonverbal, non-vocal, and non-speaking were used to describe the population. All of these terms have limitations. Lloyd and Kangas (1988) stated that the term nonverbal implied that the individual had no symbolic language skills (either spoken or unspoken), and thus should be avoided. The terms non-vocal and non-speaking are problematic because many individuals using AAC are able to vocalize and some of them are able to speak. The term paravocal has been used intermittently in the field but has not been adopted widely. The terms AAC users, AAC consumer, and augmentative communicators have also been used, but do not adequately describe individuals who have severe communication impairments but have not yet been exposed to AAC options (Lloyd &

Kangas, 1988). At this time, there is no consensus on terminology to define the population. Throughout this text, readers will see the terms *nonspeaking, AAC user,* and *AAC consumer.* Whenever possible, chapter authors have tried to avoid unnecessary labels and have referred to users of AAC systems simply as individuals, students, children, and persons.

Terminology to classify various AAC methods has also undergone changes over the years. Initially there was confusion over what to call graphic pictures, sign languages, and other communication methods, including speech. Lloyd and Fuller (1986) developed a taxonomy of symbol descriptions that has been adopted widely by professionals in the field. Symbols are defined broadly as representing "objects, actions, and relationships, etc., and can be spoken, graphic, or manual . . . spoken symbols are conveyed through the auditory-vocal modality, graphic and manual symbols are conveyed through the visual modality" (Fristoe & Lloyd, 1979, p. 402). Thus, the term *symbol* can refer to spoken words, sign languages, picture symbols, and written words, among others.

Symbols are then classified into the subcategories of unaided and aided. "*Unaided symbols* refer to symbols that do not require any aids or devices for production" (Lloyd & Fuller, 1986, p. 168). The communicator's body (i.e., face, hands, head, larynx, etc.) is the only communication tool necessary for unaided symbols. Speech, manual sign languages, gestures, and facial expressions are all examples of unaided communication. *Aided symbols* require devices or equipment in addition to the communicator's body. Writing words on a piece of paper is an aided method of communication, as is the use of picture communication boards, eye gaze boards, head pointing mechanisms, and computers with synthesized speech options, among

others. Chapter 4 in this text reviews more information regarding symbols and their classifications.

During the last decade, the study of AAC has begun to merge together with the overall field of *assistive technology.* Assistive technology is broadly defined as using aided tools to improve the skills, abilities, lifestyle, and independence of individuals with disabilities. Using this broad definition, assistive technology encompasses the use of eyeglasses, hearing aids, enlarged handles on kitchen utensils, braille codes on elevator buttons, switch-activated light switches, close-caption televisions, grab bars on bathroom walls, wheelchairs, adapted computers, and aided augmentative communication devices, among others. Users of AAC systems often require other types of assistive technology to increase their overall ability to function within their communities.

There are many other AAC terms and definitions. Some are widely used and appear frequently in the literature; others have emerged recently as new developments have occurred in the field. Readers who are new to AAC are encouraged to review the glossary for an overview of terminology.

HISTORY OF AAC

Within the past decade, the practice and study of AAC have entered the professional mainstream. Conferences on the topic of AAC are held at local, regional, national, and international levels. Special interest groups for professionals, families, and users have been formed (e.g., The United States Augmentative and Alternative Communication Association; Hear Our Voices). There are specific journals and newsletters devoted to AAC, severe communication impairments, and assistive technology issues (e.g., *Augmentative and Alternative Communication; Augmentative Communi-*

cation News; Assistive Technology; The Journal of the Association for the Severely Handicapped). Assistive technology trade shows such as Closing the Gap, CSUN, or RESNA have hundreds of vendors demonstrating products for individuals in need of AAC. Finally, legislation has been enacted to ensure that individuals have access to AAC technology and related services for implementing technology (e.g., Individuals with Disabilities Education Act [IDEA, reauthorization of P.L. 94-142]; and the Technology Related Assistance for Individuals with Disabilities Act [Tech Act, P.L. 100-407]).

With the emergence of AAC into the mainstream of disability issues, it is easy to forget how far the field of AAC has progressed. Bill's AAC history is a compelling example of just how far we have come. Professionals, families, and AAC communicators need to have knowledge of the history of AAC. This awareness helps place current issues into their proper perspective, and helps to avoid attempts to "reinvent the wheel" as new practitioners and users join the AAC ranks. Zangari et al. (1994) recently provided the field with an extensive review of the history of AAC. Readers are encouraged to refer to their article for more in-depth information.

Ancient History

The use of alternative methods of communication for individuals who are deaf can be traced back to classical Rome (Levinson, 1967, as cited in Zangari et al., 1994). Manual languages for individuals who were deaf were documented in European cultures during the sixteenth through eighteenth centuries. Manual languages were also used by Native Americans, who used a system of gestures to interact with members of other tribes. Indian Hand Talk evolved into a complex method of communicating information between speakers of multiple languages (Skelly, 1979).

Pioneer Days

The 1950s can be considered the beginning of AAC as it is currently known. Early pioneers in the field were professionals and individuals with severe communication impairments who developed communication boards using seat-of-the-pants intuition. Christy Brown's autobiography *My Left Foot* (1954) described his childhood struggle to develop a method of communication that could be understood by others. Michael Williams, an AAC user with cerebral palsy, described his own personal process of developing an AAC system in the following excerpt:

Before I learned to read and write, I used a system of grunts and hand signals my parents and I developed for expressing my everyday needs and desires. The fact that nobody outside my immediate family could understand this communication system didn't bother me in the least. As I became literate, I started to communicate by spelling words in the air, and this greatly increased my ability to communicate with people outside my family.

I used air writing to communicate with people outside my family until I was well out of college. All this changed very dramatically one day when I was working at my job as a volunteer news writer for a radio station in Los Angeles. One of my coworkers became extremely irritated with my mode of communication. He found it extremely slow and tedious. He walked in the next day and threw a checkbook cover at me. I opened it and found the letters of the alphabet pasted inside. My friend had given me what all these professionals I had seen over the years had not given me: an alternative means of communication. This simple piece of low-tech assistive technology opened up a whole new world of communication for me. Thinking back on this incident over thirty years later, I realize it is one of the watershed events of my life. Had this fellow not been frustrated enough with my communication techniques to actually do something about them, I hate to think where I would be today. (1995, p. 3)

Professionally, AAC was sometimes considered for individuals following laryngectomy or glossectomy surgery. These individuals were provided with electrolarynges, or were urged to use writing for communication. There was no thought to using AAC with patients who had intact oral and laryngeal anatomy (Zangari et al., 1994). As the decade progressed, more children began surviving the effects of premature birth, and more adults survived the results of stroke, disease, or trauma. The population of individuals with cerebral palsy, other motor impairments, or paralysis increased. Many of these individuals were unable to communicate using speech. A few individuals went against the professional tide and began using AAC with persons with severe communication impairments. These early efforts were presented as case studies in professional journals. AAC was documented with nonspeaking persons with aphasia (Goldstein & Cameron, 1952; Sklar & Bennett, 1956) and with individuals with cerebral palsy (Feallock, 1958; Goldberg & Fenton, 1960).

Manual languages were widely used and proliferated naturally within the deaf community. However, professionals who worked with the deaf rarely promoted the use of manual language. The notion that speaking abilities were related to intelligence was prevalent. Nonspeaking deaf individuals were referred to as "deaf and dumb," or "deaf mute." Sign languages were viewed as inferior methods of communication by most educators of hearing-impaired persons. The majority of schools for the deaf that were founded in the United States maintained an "oral" approach which discouraged the use of sign language.

Early Growth

During the 1960s and early 1970s, public and governmental awareness of disabilities gradually increased (Zangari et al., 1994). This change in perceptions led to the beginning of wider acceptance of AAC.

The deaf community began their process of empowerment during the 1960s. Many hearing-impaired individuals pursued their civil right to be educated using American Sign Language (ASL). Stokoe (1960) published *Sign Language Structure* which was the first academic text to consider ASL as a fully formed language with syntactic and semantic rules. The philosophy of total communication for the deaf (use of all communication modalities) was developed in the 1960s and was implemented during the 1970s (Evans, 1982).

During the late 1960s, some children with multiple disabilities began to receive educational services. Many of these children had hearing and cognitive impairments. The use of manual signs with this subset of the hearing-impaired population began to become accepted practice (Hall & Talkington, 1970; Hoffmeister & Farmer, 1972). In 1969, Gardner and Gardner presented their efforts to teach sign language to Washoe, a chimpanzee. This led to a new area of primate research which focused on teaching sign languages, and graphic visual languages to apes (Gardner & Gardner, 1979; Premack & Premack, 1974). This research planted the idea of using alternative methods of communication with individuals who had severe cognitive disabilities yet were not hearing impaired. Based on this work, manual signs and graphic symbol systems were taught using highly structured behavioral teaching programs with individuals with mental retardation (Carrier, 1976; Woolman, 1980), and autism (Alpert, 1980; Kopchick & Lloyd, 1976; Premack & Premack, 1974). The implication of generalizing teaching techniques from apes to nonspeaking cognitively impaired individuals would understandably raise many eyebrows and questions in today's society. However, many early texts in AAC included chapters discussing primate communication research and its application to individuals with severe communication impairments (Carrier, 1976; Premack & Premack, 1974).

The use of AAC was also more prevalent for individuals with neuromotor impairments. The field of speech-language pathology began extensively studying oral motor patterns of persons with dysarthria. It was concluded that some individuals with severe neuromotor disabilities were at risk for never developing intelligible speech (Hixson & Hardy, 1964). Case studies documenting use of communication boards or Morse code with individuals with cerebral palsy and amyotrophic lateral sclerosis (ALS) were published (Clement, 1961; Dixon, 1965; Sayre, 1963). The Non-Oral Communication Systems Project was initiated at the University Hospital in Iowa City, Iowa, in 1964 (Vicker, 1974). This 10-year project followed more than 20 children with cerebral palsy who were provided with AAC. It was the first program in the United States to document AAC use across a wide number of individuals with neuromotor disabilities.

An awareness of using technology to circumvent communication impairments was also developing. Case studies reported using typewriters as alternative communication methods (Jones, 1961; Miller & Carpenter, 1964). In 1963 Maling and Clarkson developed POSSUM, the first piece of technology specifically designed as a communication tool for individuals with severe physical disabilities. POSSUM integrated a typewriter with a switch-controlled scanning device. Several variations of POSSUM were developed over the years and were still available for purchase into the late 1970s (Vanderheiden & Grilley, 1976). From that beginning, rehabilitation specialists began developing other AAC systems.

Many of the early AAC devices relied on alphabet spelling and were only applicable for nonspeaking individuals who had literacy skills. Many of these early systems were shown in photographs and described in detail by Vanderheiden and Grilley (1976). They were often large, heavy pieces of equipment which had limited use for nonspeaking individuals in the real world.

Vanderheiden and his colleagues at the Trace Center at the University of Wisconsin were instrumental in introducing the notion of using technology for individuals with severe communication impairments in the United States. The Trace Center developed many early AAC systems, and conducted workshops introducing professionals to AAC technology. Even now, the Trace Center continues to focus on rehabilitation engineering and assistive technology for individuals with disabilities.

AAC Moves into the Mainstream

Towards the end of the 1970s, AAC began to be viewed as a legitimate method of communication (Zangari et al., 1994). This change in perception was due in part to legislation in 1975 that mandated a free and appropriate education for all children (P.L. 94-142), and the Rehabilitation Act of 1973 which prohibited discrimination against individuals with disabilities within any program receiving federal money. Federal laws helped to move nonspeaking individuals who were previously left out of the mainstream of American life into the educational and work community.

As AAC moved to the forefront, much of the debate focused on determining if use of AAC was detrimental to the development of speech. Many professionals felt that children would opt for the easy (i.e., lazy) method of communication and would not push themselves to learn speech once AAC was provided. Several lines of theoretical and applied research began to merge at this time to turn the tide around. In the field of linguistics and language development, researchers began studying the function of language rather than focusing on the form of language (Bates, 1976; Dore, 1978). This view of language broadened the scope of professionals from viewing *speech* as the end product to viewing communication as the goal. Silverman (1980) beautifully summarized the issue by stating,

Speech pathologists would best serve their clients if their orientation were that of a communication pathologist rather than a speech pathologist. From the speech orientation, the ultimate goal of therapy is either normal speech or speech that is adequate for the client's communicative purposes. The emphasis in therapy is on improving speech. Improving speech tends to be regarded as an end in itself rather than as a means to an end. From the communication orientation, on the other hand, the ultimate goal of therapy would be developing the ability to communicate to a level adequate to meet communication needs. (pp. 15 & 16)

Anecdotal evidence from case studies also began to emerge at this time that documented the continued development of speech in AAC users. In a review of the published and unpublished literature, Silverman (1980) stated that "Teaching a person to use a nonspeech communication mode does not appear to reduce his or her motivation for speech" (p. 39). He then reviewed the possibility that AAC could facilitate further speech development. Based on anecdotal case study evidence, he stated "intervention with nonspeech communication modes can be rationalized for the purpose of speech facilitation" (p. 45). Despite this anecdotal evidence, many early AAC decision-making processes were oriented toward implementing AAC only after traditional forms of speech therapy had failed (Shane & Bashir, 1980). This author's first job in 1980 was at a residential school for children with multiple handicaps where use of AAC with a student had to first receive the approval of a committee.

Another factor in the development of AAC as a mainstream field was the emergence of graphic picture symbols for persons who were unable to use the alphabet for communication. *Blissymbols* was the first graphic symbol system to be adopted for widespread use in AAC. Silverman, McNaughton, and Kates (1978) published a thorough clinical review of the application of this symbol set with individuals seen at

the Ontario Crippled Children's Center. Through the efforts of Shirley McNaughton, the Blissymbolics Communication Institute was formed to promote professional training in the use of Blissymbols in AAC. Hundreds of professionals from around the world came to Toronto and elsewhere for training, and hundreds more purchased symbol materials from the foundation. The Blissymbolics Communication Institute was instrumental in providing training in AAC for many professionals at a time when knowledge in the field was limited. For many years, the use of Blissymbol communication boards was widespread among individuals who were unable to communicate verbally. Based on clinical experiences with Blissymbols, other comprehensive graphic symbol sets emerged. Although use of Blissymbols has diminished in the United States, this symbol system is still widely used internationally. Chapter 4 in this text reviews Blissymbols and other symbol systems in detail.

By the beginning of the 1980s, AAC had emerged as an area of professional specialization. Articles and textbooks on the topic of AAC were published, and newsletters for professionals were distributed. The first international conferences on AAC were held in Toronto in 1980 and 1982. At those conferences, the idea for ISAAC, the International Society for Augmentative and Alternative Communication, was formed. ISAAC was established in 1983 and has since expanded over the years to encompass 2,500 members from over 47 nations (Kraat, 1993).

As more professionals began to learn about and implement AAC, professional organizations and universities began to respond. The American Speech-Language-Hearing Association (1981) published a position paper stating that AAC was an area of practice for speech-language pathologists and suggested that specific competencies were needed to provide these services. In 1978, Purdue University was one of the first universities to offer a course on the topic of AAC. Reflecting the multidisciplinary nature of the field, the course was a combined offering of both the Special Education Department and the Audiology and Speech Department. Today over 100 universities offer AAC courses, and a limited number of universities offer more than one course on AAC (Ratcliff & Beukelman, 1995).

Where Are We Now?

During the past 10 years, the growth in AAC as a profession has been breathtakingly rapid. Millions of individuals with severe communication impairments are now using AAC across all segments of society and around the world. As the number of individuals using AAC has increased, acceptance of AAC as a standard method of clinical practice has strengthened. During the past decade, the profession has moved away from debates regarding candidacy for AAC, toward an interest in a variety of research issues (Zangari et al., 1994). Strands of expertise are emerging in the field across a multitude of topics. Current areas of research and interest include vocabulary selection (Beukelman, McGinnis, & Morrow, 1991; Fried-Oken & More, 1992); communication competence and interaction (Light, 1988); demographics (Murphy, Markova, Moodie, Scott, & Boa, 1995); synthesizer intelligibility (Mirenda & Beukelman, 1990); literacy and AAC (DeCoste, 1993; Koppenhaver, 1991); symbol research (Lloyd, Karlan & Nail, 1991); AAC and educational inclusion (Calculator & Jorgensen, 1991); relationships between graphic symbol or manual sign comprehension versus expression (Remington & Clarke, 1993; Romski, Sevcik, & Pate, 1988); decreasing problem behaviors through the use of AAC (Vaughn & Horner, 1995); and rate enhancement strategies (Venkatagiri, 1993).

This increase in use of AAC across a wide variety of populations has also resulted in an explosion of new technology for individuals with severe communication impairments. In 1978, Trace Center published the first *Non-vocal Communication Resource Book*, which was a page-by-page listing of AAC devices and equipment with accompanying photographs (Vanderheiden, 1978). The original intent was to update the book annually with a few new pages inserted into its notebook format. As changes in the microcomputer industry brought about improvements in AAC technology, the number and variety of devices available mushroomed. Trace Center gave up on the notebook format and developed the first software database of assistive technology, known as Abledata, which is available on CD-ROM or accessible through the Internet. In 1990, Abledata contained over 16,000 references from 2,200 manufacturers for AAC and other assistive technology products (Enders & Hall, 1990). Abledata is updated monthly, and can be searched by type of product, product name, or manufacturer's name.

The sheer number of AAC products available on the market has made it difficult for professionals who do not practice AAC full-time to keep up with changes in technology. There is now a multitude of hardware, software, and accessory options which have to be individually coordinated into a comprehensive AAC system package. In addition, individuals with severe physical disabilities often need to integrate use of an AAC system with other types of assistive technology, such as computers for education and work, power wheelchairs, and environmental controls. In an effort to keep professionals abreast of the latest improvements in technology, conferences that focus on hands-on applications of AAC and other assistive technology devices have proliferated. These include Closing the Gap, the California State University Northridge (CSUN) Conference, and the Communication Aids Manufacturers Association (CAMA) conferences. Chapter 3 in this text provides a comprehensive review of currently available AAC technologies.

As AAC emerged as an area of specialization, the American Speech-Language-Hearing Association (ASHA) realized that professionals who wished to provide AAC services needed competency in skills specific to AAC. A multidisciplinary committee developed a listing of these competencies which were approved by ASHA in 1988 (ASHA, 1989). These roles and responsibilities were further defined by another AAC committee which developed a report on the role of the AAC professional (ASHA, 1991; see Table 1–1). Because AAC is a specialty that has grown in a bottom-up process, many specialists who currently provide AAC services are not speech-language pathologists by training. Special ed-

ucators, occupational therapists, and rehabilitation engineers, among others, are all interested in AAC and actively provide services within the field. Their varied professional backgrounds and experiences have allowed AAC to evolve into a true transdisciplinary area of interest (Zangari et al., 1994).

Recent legislation has also brought about changes in perspective regarding AAC. The Technology Related Assistance for Individuals with Disabilities Act (Tech Act, P.L. 100-407), and Americans with Disabilities Act (ADA, P.L. 101-336) were implemented in 1988 and 1990, respectively. These enactments occurred simultaneously with the re-enactment of the Individuals with Disabilities Education Act (IDEA, P.L. 101-476) in 1990. These statutes emphasize the importance of disseminating information about assistive technology including AAC, use of AAC as a civil right, and use of AAC as an educational tool.

Table 1–1. Roles and responsibilities for AAC professionals.

- Identification of persons who might benefit from AAC intervention.

- Determination of specific AAC components and the strategies needed to maximize functional communication.

- Development of an intervention plan to achieve maximal functional communication between individuals who use AAC components and their communication partners.

- Implementation of an intervention plan to achieve maximal functional communication.

- Evaluation of the functional communication outcomes of the intervention plan.

- Evaluation and application of evolving AAC aids, techniques, symbols, and strategies in AAC.

- Advocacy for increased attention from community, regional, government, and education agencies to the communication and funding needs of persons with severe speech and language impairments.

- Consultation with the individual using AAC, family, caregivers, and allied personnel regarding communication status and AAC needs and intervention approaches.

- Provision of inservice education for medical and allied health personnel, other health and education professionals, and consumers on the communication needs and AAC potential of individuals with AAC needs.

- Coordination of AAC services.

- Development of follow-up procedures to evaluate the effectiveness of an individual's AAC system.

- Development of procedures to disseminate clinical, educational, and research information in AAC.

- Recognition of the need for and promotion of basic and applied research in the field of AAC.

Source: From "Report: Augmentative and Alternative Communication," by the American Speech-Language-Hearing Association, 1991, ASHA, 33(Suppl. 5), 9-12. Adapted from the text with permission.

Although legislation has produced increased governmental awareness and commitment to AAC, subsequent funding for individual consumers who require AAC technology and services has not significantly increased. This has led to frustration on the part of consumers who are more aware of AAC options, yet are forced to fight for AAC within an inequitable system of service delivery. For example, IDEA has specifically mandated that students who require AAC should receive equipment and services as part of their free and appropriate public education if it is required as part of their educational program. In theory, this legislation is necessary and forward thinking. Yet state and local school systems have not been allocated any additional funding resources to meet this need. In reality, the ability to fund AAC devices and services for all children ages 0 to 21 within existing school budgets is difficult. Some school systems have responded to the law by developing AAC teams and providing the necessary technology. Other schools have quibbled over the definition of "appropriate public education," and have provided AAC services and equipment at a level that may be minimally appropriate, but is certainly not optimal for the language or communication development of the child. Still other schools have refused to allocate any special services or equipment in hopes that the problem (or student) will simply go away. This unevenness in service delivery in the educational setting has led many parents to form advocacy groups and to seek legal advice to resolve the issue. Chapters 9 and 15 in this text review legislative and other issues related to providing AAC.

The issue of inclusion as an educational practice has also caused many changes in the delivery of AAC services (Calculator & Jorgensen, 1991). Inclusion is the process of educating students with disabilities as included members within regular education classrooms (Stainback & Stainback, 1990). Prior to the adoption of inclusionary educational practices, individuals with severe communication impairments were clustered together in separate special classrooms, often within a separate special school. Teachers and other professionals in the special classroom setting typically have AAC experience, and have received specific training in the area of AAC. In the inclusionary school setting, students who are nonspeaking are mainstreamed into the regular education classroom. The student may be the only child in the classroom or entire school using AAC. As a result, students are often taught by regular education teachers and speech-language pathologists who have little to no experience with AAC. These professionals have typically not received any training on the topic of AAC, communication disabilities, or educational issues with nonspeaking populations.

In response to the inclusion movement, AAC professionals have moved away from the expert model, which relied heavily on key personnel trained to implement AAC. Instead, a model that views the AAC user's entire community as a support for AAC has developed. The AAC expert still serves as a collaborative consultant to the community of supports, but relies on the community to provide ongoing AAC services (Phillips & McCullough, 1990).

As the notion of inclusion has spread, inclusionary practices are also being applied to adult vocational and community settings. Supported employment and assisted community living places nonspeaking persons in contact with typical community members. These individuals all become the community of AAC support for the adult who uses AAC. Chapter 2 of this text discusses general service delivery issues in AAC. In addition, the third section of this book (Chapters 14 through 17) reviews service delivery issues specific to home, educational, hospital, and adult community settings.

The move toward inclusion combined with acceptance of AAC as a valid method of communication has made professionals, community members, families, and legislators more aware of the communication potential of individuals with severe communication impairments. Despite this growing awareness, many individuals who are unable to communicate using speech are not consistently empowered to make decisions. In 1992, the National Joint Committee for the Communication Needs of Persons with Severe Disabilities developed guidelines to meet the communication needs of persons with severe disabilities. As part of the guidelines, a Communication Bill of Rights was developed which is presented in Table 1–2. Under the guidelines, individuals with severe communication impairments have the right to use AAC at all times; have the right to be given information and choices and to communicate preferences between choices; have the right to interact with others and to participate in those interactions as a full partner; and have the right to interact in a dignified yet meaningful manner. Readers of this text are encouraged to review the Communication Bill of Rights and to keep its tenets in mind when interacting with individuals who have severe communication disabilities.

CONCLUSION

This chapter began with a description of Bill's life as an AAC user. He provided a real-life example of how an individual of his generation was limited by early knowledge and attitudes toward AAC. In contrast to Bill's life, "Susan" is a teenager who has grown up in a time when AAC is an accepted method of communication. Susan is a 17-year-old with cerebral palsy who uses a power wheelchair and AAC.

Her mother and the professionals at the same children's hospital that Bill attended provided her with picture communication boards when she was 2 years old. At the age of 7, she received a Touch Talker AAC system which provided her with synthesized voice output. She also received her first power chair that year. She describes the independence that both pieces of technology gave her as "liberating." Susan was introduced to reading and writing activities by her mother at an early age. She acquired an Apple IIe computer for writing in elementary school, and in middle school received a switch-activated page turning system so that she could read independently. Susan now communicates using a Liberator communication system and completes her school work using the Liberator as the keyboard to operate a Macintosh Power Book computer.

Although Susan's AAC experiences have been much more positive than Bill's, there were still many difficulties encountered along the way. One of the biggest hurdles was funding the technology that allowed Susan to become an independent communicator. During her early years, neither Susan's health insurance nor her school would fund her AAC or computer equipment. The Touch Talker and Apple IIe computer were bought by her family with charity assistance. A few years later, when Susan was transferring from middle school to high school, she required many new pieces of technology to make the transition. Once again, funding remained a crucial issue. The public school system obtained the Macintosh computer for her after a year of testimony from outside professionals and several meetings. Her health insurance paid for a new power wheelchair. However, her Liberator was not covered by health insurance, nor by the school system; both stated that the Touch Talker (which by now was on its last legs) was adequate to meet her needs. Once again, the AAC system was funded through charity

Table 1–2. A communication bill of rights.

All persons, regardless of the extent or severity of their disabilities, have a basic right to affect, through communication, the conditions of their own existence. Beyond this general right, a number of specific communication rights should be ensured in all daily interactions and interventions involving persons who have severe disabilities. These basic communication rights are as follows:

1. The right to request desired objects, actions, events, and persons, and to express personal preferences, or feelings.

2. The right to be offered choices and alternatives.

3. The right to reject or refuse undesired objects, events, or actions, including the right to decline or request all proffered choices.

4. The right to request, and be given, attention from and interaction with another person.

5. The right to request feedback or information about a state, an object, a person, or an event of interest.

6. The right to active treatment and intervention efforts to enable people with severe disabilities to communicate messages in whatever modes and as effectively and efficiently as their specific abilities will allow.

7. The right to have communicative acts acknowledged and responded to, even when the intent of these acts cannot be fulfilled by the responder.

8. The right to have access at all times to any needed augmentative and alternative communication devices and other assistive devices, and to have those devices in good working order.

9. The right to environmental contexts, interactions, and opportunities that expect and encourage persons with disabilities to participate as full communicative partners with other people, including peers.

10. The right to be informed about people, things, and events in one's immediate environment.

11. The right to be communicated with in a manner that recognizes and acknowledges the inherent dignity of the person being addressed, including the right to be part of communication exchanges about individuals that are conducted in his or her presence.

12. The right to be communicated with in ways that are meaningful, understandable, and culturally and linguistically appropriate.

Source: The National Joint Committee for the Communication Needs of Persons with Severe Disabilities. (1992). Guidelines for meeting the communication needs of persons with severe disabilities. *ASHA*, 34(Suppl. 7), 1–8. Reprinted with permission.

sources, and from her parents' savings. As stated previously in this chapter, federal legislation has increased awareness of the need for AAC, but has not added any funding for users, school systems, or other third party payers to purchase equipment. Although much has changed over the years, there is still a long way to go.

Susan also had difficulty obtaining an inclusive mainstreamed education. She remained to some degree in "special" classes through middle school. Her mother worked hard to have her teachers focus on grade level reading, writing, and math through elementary and middle school. Because Susan did not have access to a computer at school, much of her written work and homework was completed at home during the evening. There were many times when Susan's teachers did not believe that the homework being turned in was her own work.

When Susan entered high school, she was still tracked into "special" classes. During her freshman year, she was not provided with a computer to complete writing assignments in the majority of her classes. In the two classes where computers were available, they were desktop models, which were incompatible with her home computer. Susan could begin an assignment in class, but was unable to complete it later at home. Susan had to complete many of her assignments using the notebook features of the Liberator communication system. Because the Liberator uses pictures to encode words, many of her teachers felt that her writing was below grade level, since it wasn't spelled letter by letter. One teacher stated, "She has to learn to spell correctly to pass her examinations."

By the spring of Susan's freshman year, she stopped trying to complete any assignments or written work at school. She stopped communicating with the Liberator unless specifically required to do so; even then, her answers were short responses. She spent most of her time with her head down waiting to go home. She privately informed me that it was useless to try, as she was never given the opportunity to do her best. The head of special services at her high school felt that Susan's performance was due to her inability to meet the school's curriculum. A series of meetings was held to determine if Susan should continue in an academic track, headed for a regular high school diploma, or whether she should opt out for a "certificate," which is awarded to students who cannot meet normal graduation standards. By this point, Susan and her family decided that if the special education experts didn't have anything better to offer, they had nothing to lose by asking to attend Susan's neighborhood high school. This demand was accompanied with a request for the Macintosh Powerbook laptop computer and intensive AAC services over the summer to work on her communication and writing skills using the Liberator combined with the computer.

Susan worked hard over the summer to improve her skills. Videotapes of her communication and writing abilities using the Liberator and Macintosh Powerbook were made so that staff at her new school could see what she was capable of doing independently. Videotapes were also made to show her new teachers how best to communicate with Susan. The staff at Susan's new high school worked equally hard to welcome her. Staff attended training to learn about the Liberator before the first day of school, contacted outside professionals to obtain additional information and training, and made curriculum accommodations to use the laptop computer combined with the Liberator for the majority of Susan's assignments. As a sophomore at her new school, she was fully included with other peers in an academic track. The only concession to her physical disability was a lighter course load each semester. At the time this book was written, Susan had passed all of the achievement examinations required for a regular high school diploma and will graduate with her peers next spring. Susan's future plans are already under consideration. She plans to attend the local community college next year, and like most high school seniors, changes her career goals on a daily basis.

It would be nice to end this chapter on a high note. Only a few years ago Susan's achievements would have been impossible. During the past 20 years, changes in attitudes toward AAC, changes in technology, and changes in inclusive educational practices have made it possible for Susan to graduate from high school as a "regular" student. Yet for every Susan that I am privileged to encounter, there are hundreds of other individuals with severe communication impairments who do not have access to adequate AAC services or technology, do not have the chance to interact within mainstreamed educational and community settings, and do not have the opportunity to achieve independence in their lives. Michael Williams, an AAC user with cerebral palsy, stated "If people expect nothing from you because they think you are too disabled to do anything, and you do almost anything at all, people will be impressed. And if you reach a little higher and do something interesting with your life, people will be amazed" (Williams, 1995, p. 4). The purpose of *The Handbook of Augmentative and Alternative Communication* is to ensure that during the next decade Susan's successes become the norm and not the amazing exception for AAC users.

REFERENCES

Alpert, C. (1980). A presymbolic training program. In R. L. Schiefelbusch (Ed.), *Nonspeech language and communication: Analysis and intervention* (pp. 389–420). Baltimore, MD: University Park Press.

American Speech-Language-Hearing Association. (1981). Position statement on nonspeech communication. *ASHA, 23,* 577–581.

American Speech-Language-Hearing Association. (1989). Competencies for speech language pathologists providing services in augmentative communication. *ASHA, 31,* 107–110.

American Speech-Language-Hearing Association. (1991). Report: Augmentative and alternative communication. *ASHA, 33*(Suppl. 5), 9–12.

Bates, E. (1976). *Language and context: The acquisition of pragmatics.* New York: Academic Press.

Beukelman, D., McGinnis, J., & Morrow, D. (1991). Vocabulary selection in augmentative and alternative communication. *Augmentative and Alternative Communication, 7,* 865–875.

Brown, C. (1954). *My left foot.* London: Secker & Warburg.

Calculator, S. N., & Jorgensen, C. (1991). Integrating AAC instruction into regular education settings: Expounding on best practices. *Augmentative and Alternative Communication, 7,* 204–214.

Carrier, J. K. (1976). Application of a nonspeech language system with the severely language handicapped. In L. L. Lloyd (Ed.), *Communication assessment and intervention strategies* (pp. 523–548). Baltimore, MD: University Park Press.

Clement, M. (1961). Morse code method of communication for the severely handicapped cerebral palsied child. *Cerebral Palsy Review,* 15–16.

DeCoste, D. (1993). Effects of intervention on the writing and spelling skill of elementary school students with severe speech and physical impairments. Unpublished doctoral dissertation, Georgetown University, Washington, DC.

Dixon, C. (1965). Some thoughts on communication boards. *Cerebral Palsy Journal, 26,* 12–13.

Dore, J. (1978). Requestive systems in nursery school conversations: Analysis of talk in its social context. In R. Campbell & P. Smith (Eds.), *Recent advances in the psychology of language: Language development and mother-child interaction.* (pp. 271–292). New York, NY: Plenum Press.

Enders, A., & Hall, M. (1990). *Assistive technology sourcebook.* Washington, DC: Resna Press.

Evans, L. (1982). *Total communication: Structure and strategy.* Washington, DC: Gallaudet College Press.

Feallock, B. (1958). Communication for the nonvocal individual. *American Journal of Occupational Therapy, 12,* 60–63.

Fried-Oken, M., & More, L. (1992). An initial vocabulary for nonspeaking preschool children based on developmental and environmental language sources. Augmentative and *Alternative Communication, 8,* 41–56.

Fristoe, M., & Lloyd, L. L. (1979). Nonspeech communication. In N. R. Ellis (Ed.), *Handbook of mental deficiency: Psychological theory and research* (2nd ed.). (pp. 401–430). New York: Lawrence Erlbaum Associates.

Fuller, D. R., Lloyd, L. L., & Schlosser, R. W. (1992). Further development of an augmentative and alternative communication symbol taxonomy. *Augmentative and Alternative Communication, 8,* 67–74.

Gardner, R. A., & Gardner, B. T. (1979). Teaching sign language to a chimpanzee. In R. L. Schiefelbusch & J. S. Hollis (Eds.), *Language intervention from ape to child* (pp. 171–204). Baltimore: University Park Press. (Reprinted from Science, 1969, *165,* 664–672).

Goldberg, H. R., & Fenton, J. (1960). *Aphonic communication for those with cerebral palsy: Guide for the development and use of a communication board.* New York: United Cerebral Palsy of New York State.

Goldstein, H., & Cameron, H. (1952). New method of communication for the aphasic patient. *Arizona Medicine, 8*, 17–21.

Hall, S., & Talkington, L. (1970). Evaluation of a manual approach to programming for deaf retarded. *American Journal on Mental Deficiency, 75*, 378–380.

Hixson, J., & Hardy, J. (1964). Restricted mobility of the speech articulators in cerebral palsy. *Journal of Speech and Hearing Disorders, 29*, 293–306.

Hoffmeister, R., & Farmer, A. (1972). The development of manual sign language in mentally retarded deaf individuals. *Journal of Rehabilitation of the Deaf, 6*, 19–26.

Jones, M. (1961). Electrical communication devices. *American Journal of Occupational Therapy, 15*, 110–111.

Kopchick, G., & Lloyd, L. L. (1976). Total communication programming for the severely language impaired: A 24 hour approach. In L. L. Lloyd (Ed.), *Communication assessment and intervention strategies* (pp. 501–521). Baltimore: University Park Press.

Koppenhaver, D. A. (1991). The implications of emergent literacy research for children with developmental disabilities. *American Journal of Speech Language Pathology, 1*, 38–44.

Kraat, A. (1993). ISAAC's voices grow louder and stronger. *The ISAAC Bulletin, 29*, 10–11.

Levinson, R. (1967). A Plato reader. Boston: Houghton-Mifflin.

Light, J. (1988). Interaction involving individuals using augmentative and alternative communication systems: State of the art and future directions. *Augmentative and Alternative Communication, 2*, 66–82.

Lloyd, L. L. (1985). Comments on terminology. *Augmentative and Alternative Communication, 1*, 95–97.

Lloyd, L. L., & Fuller, D. R. (1986). Toward an augmentative and alternative communication symbol taxonomy: A proposed superordinate classification. *Augmentative and Alternative Communication, 2*, 165–171.

Lloyd, L. L., & Kangas, K. A. (1988). AAC terminology and policy issues. *Augmentative and Alternative Communication, 4*, 54–57.

Lloyd, L. L., Karlan, G., & Nail, B. (1991). Translucency values of 910 Blissymbols. Unpublished manuscript. Purdue University, West Lafayette, IN.

Matas, J., Mathy-Laikko, P., Beukelman, D., & Legresley, K. (1985). Identifying the nonspeaking population: A demographic study. *Augmentative and Alternative Communication, 1*, 17–31.

Miller, J., & Carpenter, C. (1964). Electronics for communication: Approaches to the problem of communication in children with severe cerebral palsy. *American Journal of Occupational Therapy, 18*, 20–23.

Mirenda, P., & Beukelman, D. (1990). A comparison of intelligibility among the natural speech and seven speech synthesizers with listeners from three age groups. *Augmentative and Alternative Communication, 6*, 61–68.

Murphy, J., Markova, I., Moodie, E., Scott, J., & Boa, S. (1995). AAC systems used by people with cerebral palsy in Scotland: A demographic study. *Augmentative and Alternative Communication, 11*, 26–36.

National Joint Committee for the Communication Needs of Persons with Severe Disabilities. (1992). Guidelines for meeting the communication needs of persons with severe disabilities. *ASHA, 34*(Suppl. 7), 1–8.

Phillips, V., & McCullough, L. (1990). Consultation-based programming: Instituting the collaboration ethic in schools. *Exceptional Children, 56*, 291–304.

Premack, D., & Premack, A. (1974). Teaching visual language to apes and language deficient persons. In R. L. Schiefelbusch & L. L. Lloyd, (Eds.), *Language perspectives: Acquisition, retardation, and intervention.* (pp. 347–375). Baltimore: University Park Press.

Ratcliff, A., & Beukelman, D. (1995). Preprofessional preparation in augmentative and alternative communication: State-of-the-art report. *Augmentative and Alternative Communication, 11*, 61–73.

Remington, B., & Clarke, S. (1993). Simultaneous communication and speech comprehension, part I: Comparison of two methods of teaching expressive signing and speech comprehension. *Augmentative and Alternative Communication, 9*, 36–48.

Romski, M., Sevcik, R., & Pate, J. (1988). The establishment of symbolic communication in persons with severe mental retardation. *Journal of Speech and Hearing Disorders, 53*, 97–107.

Sayre, J. (1963). Communication for the non-verbal cerebral palsied. *Cerebral Palsy Review, 24,* 3–8.

Shane, H., & Bashir, A. S. (1980). Election criteria for the adoption of an augmentative communication system: Preliminary considerations. *Journal of Speech and Hearing Disorders, 45,* 408–414.

Silverman, F. (1980). *Communication for the speechless.* Englewood Cliffs, NJ: Prentice-Hall.

Silverman, F., McNaughton, S., & Kates, B. (1978). *Handbook of Blissymbolics.* Toronto: Blissymbolics Communication Institute.

Skelly, M. (1979). *Amer-Ind gestural code based on universal American Indian Hand Talk.* New York: Elsevier.

Sklar, M., & Bennett, D. (1956). Initial communication chart for aphasics. *Journal of the Association of Physical and Mental Rehabilitation, 10,* 43–53.

Stainback, W., & Stainback, S. (1990). *Supportive networks for inclusive schooling: Interdependent integrated education.* Baltimore: Paul H. Brookes.

Stokoe, W. (1960). *Sign language structure: An outline of the visual communication system of the American deaf.* Washington, DC: Gallaudet College.

Vanderheiden, G. C. (1978). *Non-vocal communication resource book.* Baltimore: University Park Press.

Vanderheiden, G. C., & Grilley, K. (1976). *Nonvocal communication techniques and aids for the severely physically handicapped.* Austin, TX: Pro-Ed.

Vaughn, B., & Horner, R. (1995). Effects of concrete versus verbal choice systems on problem behavior. *Augmentative and Alternative Communication, 11,* 89–92.

Venkatagiri, H. S. (1993). Efficiency of lexical prediction as a communication acceleration technique. *Augmentative and Alternative Communication, 9,* 161–167.

Vicker, B. (Ed.). (1974). *Nonoral communication system project 1964–1973.* Iowa City, IA: Campus Stores.

Williams, M. B. (1995). Transitions and transformations. *Ninth Annual Minspeak Conference Proceedings.* Wooster, OH: Prentke-Romich.

Woolman, D. H. (1980). A presymbolic training program. In R. L. Schiefelbusch (Ed.), *Nonspeech language and communication: Analysis and intervention.* (pp. 325–356). Baltimore, MD: University Park Press.

Zangari, C., Lloyd, L. L., & Vicker, B. (1994). Augmentative and alternative communication: An historic perspective. *Augmentative and Alternative Communication, 10,* 27–59.

Chapter 2

SERVICE DELIVERY IN AAC

Kristen E. Swengel and Judith S. Marquette

Augmentative and alternative communication (AAC) is a field with multiple service delivery issues that affect the quality of care provided to AAC users and their families. Service delivery traditionally has been viewed as the process of providing AAC assessment and treatment. Over time the service delivery process has expanded to include increasing consumer and family awareness of AAC options, pursuing AAC funding strategies, providing technical support for AAC and other assistive technologies, and assisting in the integration of AAC into the community setting. These changes in AAC service delivery mechanisms have evolved gradually as AAC has moved from the outreaches into the mainstream of disability issues.

Increasing support for AAC through public policy at the federal level has helped to promote systems change at state and local service delivery levels. Individuals with disabilities of all ages now have basic legislative policy support within many different public laws to guarantee the provision of assistive technology services, including AAC. Public law 99-457, which was an amendment to the reauthorization of the Education of the Handi-

capped Act (P.L. 94-142), is the structure for the provision of assistive technology for infants and toddlers. The Individuals with Disabilities Education Act (IDEA, P.L. 101-476) is the foundation for students with disabilities in the public schools to receive the assistive technology services and devices they need to meet their educational curriculum in the least restrictive environment. Amendments to the Rehabilitation Act of 1973 reprioritized assistive technology services for individuals with vocational needs. Under the provisions of these amendments, those with the most severe disabilities are to be the first served. The Technology-Related Assistance for Individuals with Disabilities Act of 1988 (Tech-Act, P.L. 100-407) provided states with the means to establish projects focused on systems change and to increase consumer access to assistive technology devices and services. These frameworks of legal policy provide parameters to define and refine service delivery within the field of AAC.

Although changes in public policy have significantly impacted service delivery in AAC, there is still a need for further change. In order to develop goals for systems change, the service delivery mechanisms that have already been developed to provide AAC services and devices to individuals with disabilities will be examined in this chapter. The knowledge gained from this process will ensure the establishment of more consumer-responsive mechanisms for individuals to access AAC services. With the individual consumer as the core of the AAC process, this chapter focuses on service delivery systems and models that are currently available for consumers in need of AAC services and devices. As teams are the foundation for provision of these services, team composition, structure, and building are discussed with a focus on a collaborative team approach. As part of the service delivery process, 10 critical areas of support for the AAC consumer are discussed (PennTech, 1994). Finally, service delivery settings in AAC are explored. Service delivery issues unique to each setting are presented for consideration.

AAC SERVICES

When entering the arena of service delivery in AAC, the first question to ask is "What is needed for a person to receive comprehensive AAC services?" AAC services and the ways in which they are delivered vary widely. In order to fully access the scope of benefits available through the delivery of AAC services, there are a variety of supports that need to be considered. It is essential that the team working with an individual who needs AAC carefully plans to provide all of these necessary supports. The Tech Act of 1988 (P.L. 100-407) provides a basic foundation to look at the range of assistive technology evaluation and intervention services that are needed for a person to receive AAC support. These assessment and treatment services are defined and listed in Table 2-1. Tech Act services include the provision of assistive technology evaluation services; funding equipment; fitting, customization, and repair of equipment; coordinating interventions; training the AAC consumer or family; and training other professionals. Two important support components that are missing from the Tech Act specifications are family involvement and team development. These two components are essential in the provision

Table 2-1. Assistive technology services.

... any services that directly assist an individual with a disability in the selection, acquisition, or use of an assistive technology device:

1. Evaluating the needs of an individual with a disability including a functional evaluation of the individual in the individual's customary environment.

2. Purchasing, leasing or otherwise providing for the acquisition of assistive technology devices for use by individuals with disabilities.

3. Selecting, designing, fitting, customizing, adapting, applying, retaining, repairing or replacing assistive technology devices.

4. Coordinating and using other therapies, interventions or services with assistive technology devices, such as those associated with existing education and rehabilitation plans and programs.

5. Training or technical assistance for an individual with a disability or, if appropriate, that individual's family.

6. Training or technical assistance for professionals (including individuals promoting education and rehabilitation services), employers or other individuals who provide services to, employ or are otherwise substantially involved in the major life functions of individuals with disabilities.

Source: Public Law 100-407, Section 3, 1988.

of comprehensive services that promote the development of a life-long support system for the AAC user.

This expanded definition of the Tech Act can be used as a framework for focusing on services that are essential for successful implementation of AAC systems, and the ways that AAC services can be delivered. The challenge in meeting the consumer's AAC goals is to ensure that all of these components are available, easily accessible, and of quality content to meet the needs of each individual. This is the responsibility of AAC consumers and the teams that support them.

THE TEAM PROCESS

A team can be defined as a group of people who are invested in working together to reach a common goal. In the area of AAC, the team would consist of people who are invested in the individual and collaboratively provide various supports to enable the individual to become and remain a competent communicator. Although the concept of using a team to deliver AAC services is not new to most service providers, in many instances the benefits of using a team approach have not been fully realized.

Team Structures

To begin looking at the benefits of the team approach in the area of AAC, it is first necessary to examine the three primary team structures that have been used to provide a variety of services to persons with disabilities. Reviewing the evolution of those three primary team structures will clarify the team organization that is required for a person needing and using AAC. The three primary structures, multidisciplinary, interdisciplinary, and transdisciplinary differ in team member interactions and in the way services are delivered (Bagnato & Neisworth, 1991).

Multidisciplinary

With this type of team structure, the team consists of many different specialists from multiple disciplines or areas of expertise who provide services in isolation from each other, performing only those tasks that are specific to their respective discipline. Communication and problem solving occurs only within the specific discipline and the team member is only informed of discipline-specific goals (Sheldon & Craig, 1994). Figure 2–1 illustrates the multidisciplinary model. The multidisciplinary team approach developed from a medical model that recognized the important contributions of each discipline and the need for team members from multiple disciplines to be involved with the individual. This model has many weaknesses. Communication between team members is limited, and in many situations nonexistent. With this lack of communication, the activities of one specialist do not directly impact the actions of another. As a result of team members working separately in their own areas of expertise and in an independent manner, results, recommendations, and interventions are reported and implemented separately, leading to fragmented, repetitive, and sometimes confusing information and services (Bagnato & Neisworth, 1991).

Interdisciplinary

This type of team structure also consists of specialists from many different disciplines who perform only those tasks that are specific to their respective discipline. Figure 2–1 illustrates the interdisciplinary model. The interdisciplinary team structure is more interactive than the multidisciplinary team. Team members share information with each other and attempt to unify their findings (Musselwhite & St. Louis, 1988). This greater level of communication between team members provides

TEAM STRUCTURES

Multidisciplinary

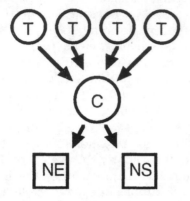

Interdisciplinary

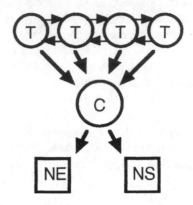

Transdisciplinary

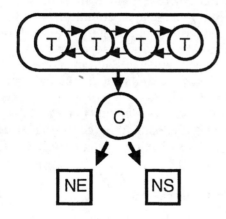

Collaborative

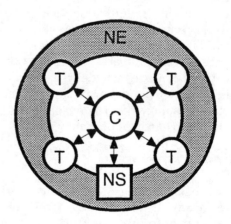

T   = Team members
C   = Consumer, including the AAC user and Family
NS = Natural Supports
NE = Natural Environments

Figure 2–1. Team Structures.

the opportunity to jointly plan for the individual, and allows the team to link information for more practical programs and interventions (Bagnato & Neisworth, 1991). With the interdisciplinary team structure, specialists share responsibilities, but are only concerned with goals within their respective disciplines. Even though team members interact with one another, the focus of each specialist is still limited to the narrow view of one aspect of the individual's life. Services provided with this narrow view may result in fragmented communication skills that do not transfer to all areas of the individual's life.

Transdisciplinary

The transdisciplinary team structure also consists of members from many different disciplines but involves a much greater degree of collaboration than the multidisciplinary or interdisciplinary team models. Figure 2-1 illustrates the transdisciplinary model. The transdisciplinary team structure emerged from the recognition that people do not perform isolated skills irrespective of functional and environmental demands (Rainforth, York, & Macdonald, 1992). With this type of structure, team members are focused on holistic goals for the individual instead of on discipline-specific goals. When team members collaborate, information and skills are transferred between disciplines, creating an integrated approach to service delivery. This integration encourages specialists to cross the traditional disciplinary boundaries and assimilate knowledge and skills from other areas and disciplines (Lerner, Mardell-Czudnowski, & Goldenberg, 1987). Crossing disciplinary boundaries, or role release, is the defining characteristic of the transdisciplinary team. Role release is the process of transferring information and skills traditionally associated with one discipline to team members

of other disciplines, including sharing general information, informational skills, and performance competencies (Lyon & Lyon, 1980; Patterson et al., 1976; Rainforth et al., 1992). Transferring information between disciplines enables team members to share responsibility for delivering quality services.

Comparisons of Team Models

There are elements that overlap among the three major models as well as elements that make them distinctly different. The primary similarity between the three structures is that the teams are all composed of specialists from multiple disciplines. Another similarity prevalent in each of the three structures is the type of interaction with the consumer, which includes the individual as well as the family. Although interaction patterns between team members are the primary difference between the three team models, the consumer, even when considered a member, is interacted with from outside the team unit. In addition, across all three models natural supports and consideration of the natural environment remain outside of the team parameters.

In reality, it is questionable whether any team exists that truly follows the three primary team models in their purest forms. Teams within any area of service delivery take on the personalities of the members who compose the team, often resulting in a team structure that follows the philosophies that its members embrace.

Collaborative Team Model

When reviewing traditional team models, three crucial elements of service delivery are clearly missing. These elements are (1) focusing on the individual and family as central to the service delivery process; (2) integrating the participation of other natural supports (i.e., teachers, employers, professional staff, friends); and (3) providing service delivery within the individual's natural environment. In order for an AAC user to become a competent communicator, it is crucial for the team to work within a structure that involves these three crucial elements.

Although the transdisciplinary team comes the closest to meeting these needs because of the collaborative interaction between disciplines, these three crucial elements are missing in each of the three primary team structures previously discussed. It is for this reason that the collaborative team structure is evolving to further address the needs of AAC users. Figure 2–1 illustrates the collaborative team structure. A collaborative team structure involves all of the critical points of the transdisciplinary team, including holistic goals, transferring information and skills between team members, and role release. In addition to these critical points, the collaborative team works within the context of natural environments, considers the individual and family as central to the process, and integrates natural supports, including friends, community members, and other relevant persons, as fully participating members of the team. Essentially, the collaborative team is not limited to specialists from various disciplines, but includes those disciplines in addition to people in the individual's life who can provide natural supports. Most importantly, with the collaborative team structure, the individual is the foundation of the team and is included as a fully interactive member of the team.

As depicted in Figure 2–1, the collaborative team works within the natural environment, and the flow of interaction and supports collaboratively involve the consumer, natural supports, and individuals from various disciplines. In the remainder of this chapter, when a team or team of supports is mentioned a collaborative team structure is implied.

The Collaborative Team Approach

There is a wealth of information, knowledge, and skills that can be obtained by using multiple team members with varying backgrounds, diverse areas of expertise, and experiences from various aspects of the individual's life. When providing quality AAC services and support, intervention strategies are developed using a broad range of information from many different aspects of an individual's life. A sampling of the information that is required would include the cognitive, language, sensory, and motor capabilities of the individual. In addition, information is needed regarding the operational, linguistic, social, and strategic competence of the individual's current communication. Information about current and future communicative contexts is important, as is information about the support system available to the potential AAC user (Beukelman & Mirenda, 1992). It would be impossible for one or even two people to access quality information in all of these areas. In the collaborative team approach, it is assumed that no one person or profession has an adequate knowledge base or sufficient expertise to execute all of the functions associated with providing services. As a result, team members are involved with the entire AAC process and thus share joint ownership and responsibility (Blackstone, 1992).

Another issue that supports the use of a collaborative team approach is the need for different perspectives to provide a well-rounded intervention. The process of developing creative solutions can be enhanced by gaining different perspectives on the problem. Each individual needing or using AAC presents a unique set of situations, needs, and challenges. The old adage of "two heads are better than one" can be used here, in that brainstorming for creative solutions is more successful when a variety of people are involved. In addition to bringing varied ideas and perspectives to the team, many of the creative solutions that are found require a time commitment that would be impossible for less than a team of people to accomplish. The fact that most AAC users require life-long support, coupled with the many time-consuming responsibilities that are necessary for any AAC system, further advocates for the use of a team approach to service delivery.

Team Members

The composition of the team is variable, and is dependent upon a number of factors. The availability of qualified service providers may be a factor that influences team composition (Langton, 1990). The setting that the team is originating from may influence potential team makeup. For example, in the educational setting it is common to find educators, speech-language pathologists, and occupational therapists, among others. However, it is not common to find rehabilitation engineers in educational settings. Similarly, rehabilitation hospitals seldom employ educators,

yet often have rehabilitation engineers on staff. The most important factor to keep in mind with regard to team composition is that each team may look different depending upon the individuals needs, goals, and existing circle of support. Teams should include those people affected by the decisions made by the team and those who have information or skills to help the team make informed decisions (Thousand & Villa, 1992).

The Consumer

In the collaborative model, there are two members that are the foundation of every team, the AAC user and his or her family. These are the team members who are the consumers of the AAC service delivery system. Their feedback will let the rest of the team know if the process is meeting their needs. The individual and the family have invaluable skills and information to contribute to the team process, as indicated in Table 2–2.

The preferences and goals of the AAC user and his or her family should be validated and regarded with the utmost re-

Table 2–2. Input from consumers.

Individual	Family
• dreams/goals for oneself	• desired outcomes for family members
• abilities, needs, and expectations	• relevant family history
• input, processing, and output needs	• communication targets
• personal preferences	• communication effectiveness at home
• motivating activities for communication	• technology preferences
• challenges in communication	• previous AAC experience
• technology preferences	• environmental needs
• experience with AAC options	• educational and vocational expectations
• expected outcomes	• anticipated life transitions
• ongoing and changing needs	• needs in the community
• environmental needs	• interaction with family members
• educational/vocational needs	

spect. It is the individual and the family who will be living with the outcomes of the team's decisions. By listening to the individual and family members, the team can gain a more complete understanding of the individual's total life (Giangreco, Cloninger, & Iverson, 1993). For example, Sean's school AAC team selected a communication system for Sean without any input from him or his family. After Sean experienced frustration with the AAC system, a meeting was requested which included the therapists, Sean, and his family. At this meeting it was discovered that Sean's home life revolved around the family's landscaping business. The AAC system did not provide the portability or the features that he needed to participate in business activities. Sean also was not comfortable with the voice quality of the system, therefore he did not like using it. As a result, the newly formed collaborative team realized that the recommended AAC system was not meeting his communication needs and different AAC methods were explored.

The role of AAC service providers is to provide information, opportunity, and access to AAC devices and services. The final decision as to whether or not to use AAC devices and services, and the types of services needed, lies in the hands of the individual and the family. These persons are centered at the core of the collaborative team model.

Other Team Members

Determining all of the potential members of the AAC team is dependent on the needs of the individual, the type of information that is needed, the setting of the team, and the supports that are needed. Table 2–3 lists just a few of the possible team members that may be a part of the AAC team and some of the possible contributions that each of these team members can bring to the team. AAC team members can include

administrators, therapists, educators, medical personnel, AAC manufacturers, and community members, among others.

A wide range of team members can exchange valuable information, and can provide much needed support to each other throughout the AAC process. For potential team members to become invested in the AAC system, they must be included in the decision-making processes of the team. Therapists and educators often forget the family when making these team decisions. Conversely, some families have also forgotten to include other team members. Tom's parents were enthusiastic about the possibility of AAC for their son. They worked hard to acquire a communication device that would be in place when Tom entered school the next year. Although supportive of the AAC system, school staff were not involved in the process and were not invested in the implementation of the system. Tom's family became solely responsible for selecting vocabulary, programming messages, and general maintenance of the system. As a result, the frustrated family became terribly overwhelmed, and felt that they were not getting support from school staff. A meeting was requested to develop a plan for AAC implementation that would involve all members of the team, including the family and school, sharing responsibilities for the AAC system.

Skills of Team Members

The skill levels of AAC team members vary greatly from member to member and from team to team. Many times crucial skills are acquired by the team during service delivery as team members face a given challenge. Along with bringing different perspectives to the team, different members bring different areas of expertise and skills. Possible team member contributions are listed in Table 2–3. When developing an AAC system for an individual, it is essential that the team is composed of members

Table 2–3. Team member contributions.

Team Members	Potential Contributions
Administrator:	Program mission, legal compliance information, funding resource for AAC devices and services.
AAC Consultant:	AAC resources, available AAC systems, effective practices, AAC training information.
Educator:	Curriculum needs, classroom communication needs, functional skills, script messages, develop overlays, program device.
Friends:	Individual's preferences, age-appropriate needs, message selection ideas, motivating communication targets, programming AAC device.
Hearing Consultant:	Auditory skills and needs.
Manufacturer's Representative:	Technical assistance, feature match, funding options.
Occupational Therapist:	Physical access issues, mounting, positioning.
Paraprofessionals:	Assist with manipulation of system in the environment, develop overlays, program device.
Personal Attendant:	Environmental issues, script messages, program device.
Physical Therapist:	Physical access issues, mounting, positioning.
Physician/Nurse:	Relevant medical needs.
Psychologist:	Cognitive/linguistic skills.
Rehabilitation Engineers:	Customization, design, ongoing technical assistance.
Residential Program Staff:	Identify and prioritize activities, target activities, ensure system access, program device.
School Principal:	Staff release for training, coordinate team process.
Service Coordinator/Case Manager:	Interagency coordination, available resources, funding options.
Speech-Language Pathologist:	Language development, communication skills, support implementation of system, script messages, develop and organize overlays.
Vision Consultant:	Visual acuity, visual perception, symbol selection.
Vocational Counselor:	Vocational evaluations, transition planning, funding options.

who possess skills that would fall within each of the 10 support components that are discussed later in this chapter.

Probably the most important skill for team members to possess is that of accessing resources. This is a valuable skill because each AAC user presents a different set of situations and challenges, and because the field of assistive technology continues to change and grow rapidly.

No one person or team can possess all of the skills needed for every AAC consumer. Therefore, the key is to face the challenge and access resources to acquire the skills. Team members need to know what resources are available and how to access resources that are needed, when they are needed. The Appendixes of this textbook provide information about AAC resources.

Building the Team

Identifying potential team members is one of the initial steps to build a team. All potential team members need to realize at the onset that being a member of a team involves more than attending periodic meetings. Being a member of the team also involves sharing various responsibilities as they are designated by the team and being committed to achieving a common goal, which, in the area of AAC is to enable an individual to become and remain a competent communicator.

A team is not just a group of people who have come together, but a group of people who must work collaboratively with the common goal remaining foremost. Merely bringing together many people does not ensure that the group will function as a team (Giangreco et al., 1993). Teams do not automatically happen, they must be built and nurtured (Bagnato & Neisworth, 1991). To successfully build a team, each team member must have a commitment to the AAC user as well as a commitment to the team as a whole. In essence, the team not only needs to develop a plan of action for AAC services, but also to develop an action plan to build the team.

In building a team it is important that all team members clearly understand their roles and responsibilities at the onset of the process. Because communication and interaction among team members is crucial, it is important to examine three basic strategies that team members historically have used to interact. These three strategies are individualistic, competitive, and cooperative. They are summarized in Table 2–4.

Individualistic

Within this type of interaction, people work independently from other team members. The outcome of one individual's efforts has no effect on and is not affected by the actions of another person (Rainforth et al., 1992). When using this type of structure, successes may occur in isolated settings for isolated periods of time, but it is unlikely that successes will be transferred to all areas of the individual's life.

Competitive

Within this type of interaction, for one member of the team to achieve his of her goal another team member must fail, creating win or lose situations (Rainforth et al., 1992). For example, in the rehabilitation hospital setting, when speech therapy time conflicts with a physician's bedside

Table 2–4. Team member interaction.

Individualistic	Competitive	Cooperative
work independently of one another	creates win or lose situations	help and support each other
individual members work toward separate goals	individual members work toward separate goals	all members work toward a common goal
outcomes are not related	promotes separate outcomes	all members share rewards of outcomes
creates isolated successes	often creates frustration	more likely to create success
lack of transfer to all areas of consumer's life	lack of tranfer to all areas of consumer's life	more likely to transfer to all areas of consumer's life

consult, the therapist and doctor are in competition for the patient's time. Or, when one member of the team is adamant that one AAC device is appropriate, and another member insists on a different device, they have competitive goals. Having a competitive goal structure promotes individual team member goals, instead of maintaining the overall goal of the team foremost. Although very difficult to avoid, this type of structure frequently causes frustration at the expense of the consumer and the team.

Cooperative

Within this type of interaction, members of the team help and support each other. Cooperative goal structures occur when all members of the team commit themselves and their respective talents to achieving a mutually agreed-on goal and divide tasks in an efficient, fair, and agreed upon manner. When the team works cooperatively, each team member equally shares the rewards and feelings of accomplishment for the work done by the team (Rainforth et al., 1992). A team working cooperatively is more likely to succeed as a team, and thus more likely to provide the total supports that the individual needs throughout all areas of his or her life.

Effective Teams

In addition to understanding the dynamics of interaction between team members, it is important to explore elements that are characteristic of effective teams. According to Giangreco et al. (1993), effective teams have members who possess skills that can serve different functions. For example, the speech-language pathologist might encompass traditional roles of the profession, yet also be experienced in case management and integrating AAC systems with environmental control units. Effective teams also develop a shared

framework and set of goals, and engage in collaborative activities to achieve those goals. As part of the process, team members collectively evaluate and offer feedback to each other. Finally, effective teams judge successes or failures by the group's performance, rather than by each individual's contribution.

Team Strategies

As a team is building to support the AAC user, various strategies need to be developed to work through teaming issues or challenges. Time constraints are an issue that is prevalent in almost every team. Service providers are frequently booked to the limit, and adding additional time for teaming seems impossible. In some cases team members are on more than one team, which can create difficulties scheduling meetings and maintaining realistic time expectations to participate in the responsibilities of the team. The team needs to directly address time issues and develop creative time management strategies. This may be the time to involve an administrator in the process to support the provision of time for teaming when scheduling. It is beneficial to involve administrators from the beginning and throughout the entire process so that they are at least aware of time allocations needed.

When a team consists of many members the question of cost-effective use of staff time is another issue often raised by administrators. Considering the large amounts of staff time involved, using a collaborative team approach may initially appear to be very costly. However, the initial investment for release of staff for collaborative meetings and trainings will ultimately be more cost-effective. By providing staff time to collaboratively address issues as they arise, the team is better able to avoid time-consuming frustrations once AAC is implemented. For example, Brice was an adult who lived in a group home residential setting. Following his initial assessment, arrangements were made to rent an AAC system for a 1-month trial. When the rental device arrived, the agency supervising the group home only allowed one staff member to be released for training. This staff member worked the 7:00 to 3:00 shift. Brice's usual morning routine was to catch a van to work at 7:30 each morning. He did not return from work until 3:30. Since Brice and the trained staff person only interacted together for 30 minutes each morning, the AAC system was not adequately implemented in the home setting. Because a collaborative team approach was not used, Brice's group home supervisor was unable to determine if the rented AAC system was effective in the residential setting. Additional funds had to be spent to extend the rental period and to provide additional training for staff before a final decision could be made.

The number of people on a team is another issue that has an effect on the team process. Theoretically, involving more people with the process provides more diverse information and areas of expertise. However, the more people involved, the greater the difficulty in coordinating schedules and enabling team members to have access to one another (Rainforth et al., 1992). Including all potential team members may create a team so large that it has difficulty functioning. Strategies to address large group sizes involve different types of team organization. For example, the small group of people who interact with an individual on a daily basis is sometimes referred to as the core team. An extended team includes all of the core team members, plus those who interact with the individual on a less frequent basis, but who have specific skills and information to add to the team. The core team would naturally need to devote more time to the service delivery process than the entire extended team. In order to maintain a reasonable group size and to use team member time efficiently, subteams formed by any logical combination of team members may be continually created and dissolved to address specific individual AAC needs (Giangreco et al., 1993; Skrtic, 1991; Thousand & Villa, 1990). For example, to address the needs of a particular individual, the core team may consist of the individual, the family, a paraprofessional, a classroom teacher and a speech-language pathologist. When addressing access and mounting issues a subteam including the occupational and physical therapist could be formed to work with part of the core team. A subteam to address funding issues could include administrators and a social worker. As the need arises to address training issues, the administrator and a computer specialist could be involved in another subteam. The core team remains constant throughout the process and subteams are formed as needed. Some subteam members can serve on more than one subteam. As illustrated in Figure 2–2, an extended AAC team consists of all members of the core team in addition to members of the subteams.

In summary, building an effective team requires an action plan to elicit and sustain a commitment from team members to work collaboratively to share both responsibilities and rewards in attaining a common goal. This can be achieved by defining the group goal, promoting open communication among team members, developing strategies for conflict resolution, equally distributing power and influence throughout the group, and placing emphasis on reaching group consensus for decisions made by the team (Johnson & Johnson, 1975).

AAC SUPPORT PROCESS COMPONENTS

Although a wide variety of AAC technologies have been developed to address the

AAC TEAMING STRATEGY

Core Team + Subteams = Extended AAC Team

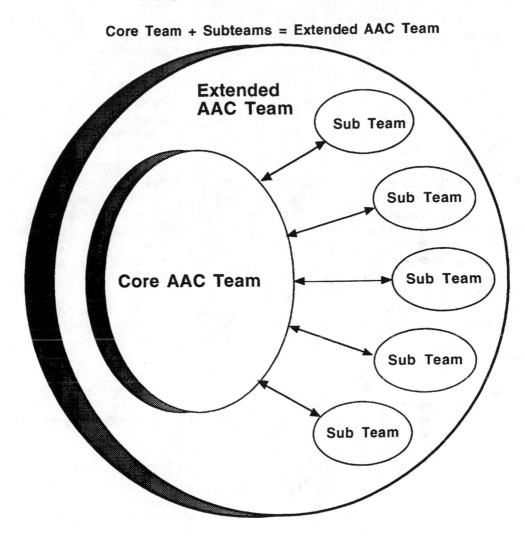

Figure 2–2. AAC Teaming Strategy.

diverse needs of people with disabilities, many people have been unable to fully access or make full use of their AAC systems because of inadequate supports. The provision of any type of support is contingent, in part, on mutual understanding of the expected outcomes provided by the support (Stainback & Stainback, 1992). In the area of AAC, support exists when (a) the consumer perceives that he or she is being helped; (b) the responsibility for achieving desired outcomes is shared among team members; (c) the goal of meeting the diverse needs of the consumer is better accomplished as a team; (d) the effort required for collaboration is worth the outcome; and (e) priority outcomes for the consumer in all environments are achieved (Stainback & Stainback, 1992). Thus, providing AAC supports is a process that requires team planning, develops over time, and cannot be achieved in isolation.

Accessing programs of service delivery that are responsive to the individual is essential for any human service activity, including AAC. Effective AAC services depend on active involvement of the consumer throughout the entire process. AAC consumers can be involved in a variety of ways including planning and advisory capacities, volunteer support efforts, user-to-user information networks, and technical consultation for designing and using AAC systems (Langton, 1990).

For individuals of all ages to receive adequate technology supports, it is imperative that support be provided in all areas of the technology process. By focusing on the definition of assistive technology services, 10 components have been identified as essential supports for effective AAC implementation (PennTech, 1994). The team supporting an individual using augmentative communication technologies will need varying levels of support in each of these areas of the process; however, for successful implementation, it is essential that each of the 10 support components

listed in Table 2–5 be addressed (Penn-Tech, 1994).

Awareness of Available Assistive Technology

In order for the team supporting an individual to make informed choices about the AAC system that will work best for that person, it is necessary for team members to be aware of the ever-changing, variety of technologies that are available and the different features that each piece possesses (PennTech, 1994). Chapter 3 reviews AAC device options and categorizing features. Additional information is available in the Appendix.

Assessment

Assessment is a flexible, collaborative decision-making process in which teams of families, professionals, and friends repeatedly revise their decisions and reach consensus about the ever-changing abilities, needs, and expectations of the person with a disability (Bagnato & Neisworth, 1991). Planning for this ongoing process

Table 2–5. AAC support components.

1. Awareness of available assistive technology

2. Assessment

3. Funding and device acquisition mechanisms

4. Technical assistance for customization

5. Training

6. Interagency service coordination

7. Application of AAC systems

8. Transitional services

9. Ongoing technical assistance

10. AAC system maintenance

Source: Assistive Technology Statewide Support Initiative: Service Delivery, PennTech, 1994. Adapted with permission.

should ensure that assessment occurs in natural environments, with the majority of input coming from the individual and persons who are most closely associated with the individual.

Assessment for AAC systems should focus on the needs of the individual in multiple environments and the features of different augmentative communication devices that will enable the individual to accomplish communication goals. When looking at features of AAC systems, the issues that should be addressed include system input methods, type of symbol processing, and types of output that the individual desires (PennTech, 1994). Chapters 5, 6, and 7 in this text review the AAC assessment process more thoroughly.

Funding and System Acquisition Mechanisms

A variety of funding streams for both AAC services and equipment are available for individuals in need of augmentative communication systems. Frequently, the funding stream available for an individual may guide other areas of the process, such as where and when services can be provided, what types of services are accessible, and the availability of funding support for AAC systems. Therefore, funding sources should be discussed and explored at the onset of the process. Chapter 9 provides more information on funding.

Technical Assistance for Customization

Customization of the system can involve many different issues such as device mounting and positioning, ongoing symbol display development, and ongoing vocabulary selection and scripting. Because of the wide range of technical issues that require attention, this area often needs to involve several members of the AAC support team.

Training

Training is twofold in that training needs to occur for both the individual using AAC and the team members supporting the individual.

Training for the Individual

Training an individual to competently communicate with an augmentative communication system involves thorough planning by the AAC support team. Training should focus on establishing competencies in the linguistic, operational, social, and strategic aspects of communication (Light, 1989). Training tends to be more effective and more easily generalized by the user when it occurs in natural environments and through participation in natural activities (PennTech, 1994). This emphasis on natural language training activities is well known to most communication specialists, but other members of the AAC support team may not be as familiar with natural language strategies.

Training for the Support System

It is essential that training be directed at both sides of the communication dyad to facilitate involvement and empowerment (PennTech, 1994). Different members of the AAC support team require varying levels of training regarding the implementation of AAC devices and strategies. The support team should discuss who from the team should receive training, how much training each of those team members should receive, who is going to provide the training, and a realistic timeline for training support team members. The team should also plan for ongoing training of team members keeping in mind that support team members are subject to change over time (PennTech, 1994).

Interagency Service Coordination

Typically, the individual who needs support with the implementation of an AAC system is involved with or has access to numerous different service provision agencies and organizations (PennTech, 1994). Examples of these service providers include private therapists, school programs, family supports, physicians, rehabilitation and hospital facilities, work settings, and social service agencies.

Each of these agencies has a focus in a specific area of the individual's life, and many of these services overlap with one another. The augmentative communication system that an individual uses will have an impact upon most of the other services that the individual accesses, and those services could have an impact on AAC technology supports. Therefore, coordination of these services with technology support is beneficial in providing a seamless system of supports and services.

Application of AAC Systems

The application of an AAC system involves enabling the individual to become a competent communicator. Using an AAC system to support competent communication requires a variety of supports, ranging from integrating the system into the individual's life to daily setup and preparation for use (PennTech, 1994). As an individual grows communicatively, the AAC system must also grow, requiring ongoing support in this area.

Transitional Services

There are many different types of transitions that people encounter in life, including transitions from home to school, preschool to elementary school, home to community, grade level to grade level, classroom to classroom, school to workplace, workplace to workplace, and living situation to living situation. Adult AAC users with acquired disabilities have transitions between hospital settings, from hospital to home, and from home to com-

munity. For someone who is using augmentative communication, success in these transitions requires additional planning and support to ensure access and availability of the AAC system when and where it is needed (PennTech, 1994). Many times the team of support also changes with the transition. It is important to prepare not only the individual making the transition, but also new team members.

Issues that arise when transitioning to a new situation can include different positioning, mounting, and transportation of the AAC system; the programming of new vocabulary that may be needed in the new environment; and additional or different AAC system features that the individual needs. Many AAC users will need to be reevaluated prior to transitioning into the new environment. For example, Will was a young adult with mental retardation who successfully used a Macaw for several years at school. At the age of 21, he graduated and began attending an adult day program with employment in a supported work setting three mornings each week. Prior to graduation, his AAC needs were evaluated in his new environments. At the day program, he was employed packing boxes in a large warehouse with a metal roof and concrete floor. The noise in the warehouse was so loud that his Macaw could not be heard. His supported work employment was to wash dishes at a local restaurant. Needless to say, an electronic AAC system was not feasible in that setting either. With the assistance from staff in his new environments, a wallet-sized picture communication book was developed which attached to his pants with a keychain. Will continued to use his Macaw at home, but used his new AAC communication wallet at work.

Ongoing Technical Assistance

Many equipment manufacturers provide valuable free technical assistance over the phone and on site for their specific products. However, many AAC consumers use a variety of products from more than one manufacturer which must be pieced together to develop a completely integrated system. When considering various multiple applications of technology and the unique configurations that may be involved in an individual's system, there may be a need for assistance that surpasses what is available through a single manufacturer (PennTech, 1994). Additionally, as an individual encounters new communication opportunities, different operational features of the AAC system may need to be accessed.

In addition to getting technical assistance from specific manufacturers, this type of technical assistance can also be efficiently accessed through members of the local team of support, including computer teachers and coordinators, local technology businesses, engineering and technology departments within local universities, information systems and engineering staff in hospitals, and local volunteer groups.

AAC System Maintenance

The need for maintenance and repair of an AAC system is an inevitable fact in the implementation of technology. Mechanisms for maintenance and repair need to be put in place to reduce "down time" and to ensure uninterrupted use of the equipment. These mechanisms need to be put in place the first day the user receives AAC equipment. For example, Clarissa was a 6-year-old who received an *Alpha Talker* in January. A collaborative process was used during initial trainings which involved her family, teacher, school speech-language pathologist, equipment vendor, and the school system's AAC team. In February, the charger for the Alpha Talker was lost. For several weeks, Clarissa's family and teacher blamed each other for the missing charger and failed to pursue options to obtain a new one. When the school system's

AAC team returned in March to document Clarissa's progress, the device was sitting in a box, and the vocabulary that had been stored into the system was erased because the batteries had not been charged in 2 months. Clarissa lost 2 months of training and AAC device use due to a simple maintenance issue.

Summary of AAC Support Components

In today's environment, successful AAC service delivery must be comprehensive, in that multiple lifelong AAC needs of the individual have to be considered. In order to address these needs across various disabilities, settings, and cultures, a wide range of services need to be readily accessible and coordinated (Brandt & Rice, 1990). Failure to address any one of the 10 AAC support components can result in unmet service delivery needs for the AAC user. When this occurs, the individual is in danger of not developing to his or her full potential to become a dynamic, competent AAC communicator (PennTech, 1994).

SERVICE DELIVERY MODELS

Numerous types of service delivery programs have come into existence to address supports that are needed for the implementation of AAC systems. Proponents of each service delivery program embrace their own beliefs concerning the methods in which services are delivered. Frequently these beliefs are driven by the administrative plan and service delivery guidelines of the program and by the skills and strengths of individual staff members within the program.

Each AAC service delivery model has its own features and personality with characteristic strengths and weaknesses. It is clear that there is a need for each type of AAC service delivery model, and probably a need for many more. The advantages and disadvantages related to each provide some suggestions as to which model is preferable in given situations and environments (Enders & Hall, 1990). In discussing the various service delivery models and the strengths of each, it is essential that provisions for the 10 AAC support components discussed in the previous section are given primary consideration .

Service delivery models for AAC programs have developed through a variety of methods. Some agencies that were already providing other services for people with disabilities have enhanced their programs by adding AAC services. With this type of program, AAC services are typically delivered following the model of service delivery that was already in place. Other programs are developed to provide a wide variety of assistive technology services including AAC, and still others have been developed for the sole purpose of providing AAC services. In the delivery of AAC services each program has a primary focus which is based on the overall mission or goal of the program itself. Table 2–6 lists areas in which AAC programs typically focus. Readers will realize that many of the 10 AAC support components are contained within this listing.

Using the listing of AAC service areas as a guide, service delivery can be categorized into seven primary models. Figure 2–3 provides an outline that lists the seven models of AAC service delivery and the areas that each of the service delivery models typically include.

The following is a general discussion of the seven primary models of service delivery that provide supports to individuals needing AAC systems. Keep in mind that there are many other types of service delivery models, and the following discussion is by no means comprehensive. In addition, readers should remember that these proposed service delivery mechanisms are models, not actual programs. Each AAC program is unique and may or may not adhere closely to the service delivery models. Many programs providing AAC services combine features of more than one type of service delivery model.

Comprehensive Team

The comprehensive team model ideally involves team members from all aspects of the individual's life. These team members provide all of the needed supports and address all 10 of the AAC support components previously discussed in this chapter (see Figure 2–3). The true comprehensive team provides AAC support across all natural environments and across all transitions in the individual's life. In reality, a true comprehensive team model is a utopian dream and is basically nonexistent at

Table 2-6. Focus of AAC programs.

1. Coordination of various AAC and assistive technology services
2. Direct AAC services including individual therapies and instruction
3. Short- and long-term loans of AAC equipment
4. Providing AAC information and resources
5. Referral to other agencies and professionals
6. AAC systems change
7. Training and in-servicing local AAC teams
8. Funding equipment and services

Focus of AAC Service Delivery Models

Focus of Programs	AAC Service Delivery Model						
	Compre-hensive Team	Center Based	Consulta-tive	Mobile	Regional Service Center	Specialist	Statewide Program
Coordination of Services	X		X		X		X
Direct Service	X	X		X		X	
Equipment Loans	X	X		X	X		X
Information & Resource	X	X	X	X	X	X	X
Referral	X		X				
Systems Change	X				X		X
Training & Inservicing	X		X	X	X	X	X
Funding	X						X

Figure 2–3. Focus of AAC Service Delivery Models.

this time. However, various programs in existence see the value in addressing all 10 AAC support components and are striving to develop more comprehensive team approaches to service delivery.

Center-Based

Accessing supports in a center-based model involves a visit to the facility in which is the center is housed. Center-based programs are typically associated with either a medical or rehabilitation facility, or private clinics. Some school systems operate center-based programs where students are brought to a central location within the district for AAC assessment. With this type of model, professionals from various disciplines, (i.e., speech-language pathologists, occupational therapists, physical therapists) are typically available to provide direct services and to work collaboratively to provide supports. Frequently, center-based programs have AAC equipment available for individuals to try, and possibly even to borrow for long or short periods of time. Center-based programs can help to facilitate the coordination of services within the center, but cannot easily coordinate services in the natural environment.

Consultative

In a consultative model, a consultant, or team of consultants, assists the individual to access AAC supports. The consultant primarily achieves this by coordinating members of the local team. Generally, the consultant's main goal is to enable the local AAC team to make informed decisions about the needs of the individual. In addition to coordinating necessary AAC supports, a consultant provides information to the team by (a) explaining the types of resources that are available and how to access them; (b) providing AAC ideas and suggestions; (c) providing guidance and direction; or (d) by providing trainings, workshops, and in-services. Areas of focus for the consultative model are noted in Figure 2–3.

Mobile

There are two different types of mobile AAC service delivery models. The first involves a mobile team, the second involves a mobile facility. A mobile model is beneficial in rural areas where services are less geographically accessible, or in situations where it is virtually impossible for the individual to leave the home or local area. Figure 2–3 illustrates focus areas of mobile service delivery.

Mobile Team

A mobile team typically involves a multidisciplinary team of various professionals who travel as a group to an individual's residence or other local site to provide supports. The mobile team typically coordinates members of the local AAC support team and integrates with the local team to provide services. The mobile team usually provides evaluative and consultative training services. The local support team is trained by the mobile team to provide daily ongoing training and support for the AAC user.

Mobile Facility

A mobile AAC facility involves a multidisciplinary team that travels to the individual's residence or local site with equipment. The equipment can include AAC devices, a computer lab, equipment loan library, or machine shop, in some type of van or truck. With this type of model, staff members provide supports when they are scheduled to be at that individual's particular site. Having the center "on wheels" allows the staff to provide limited direct support by demonstrating basic systems, providing training, providing equipment for trials, lending equipment, repairing equipment, constructing modifications, and providing resources conveniently on site.

Regional Service Center

Many areas are developing programs that address a variety of independent living skills, including augmentative communication. A regional service center typically serves individuals within a specific county, counties, or region. These programs typically employ staff members from a variety of disciplines to provide integrated supports in the individual's residence, community, and workplace. Typical focus areas of regional service centers are represented in Figure 2–3. The primary focus of these programs is to coordinate AAC services, to provide training to local AAC specialists in the region, and to promote systems change within the region. Systems change can involve AAC support training or assistance with funding equipment. Direct services are rarely provided by regional service center programs.

Specialist

An AAC specialist typically has valuable expertise in AAC. Usually the specialist works in isolation from other possible support team members, however, many specialists confer with other team members when providing direct service and training, as referred to in Figure 2–3. Most specialists are private therapists contracted by the family or AAC user to provide evaluative or direct treatment services. The specialist model differs from the consultative model in that the consultant rarely provides direct service. Some specialists take on the broader role of a consultant and provide both types of AAC service.

Statewide Program

Many states have developed statewide programs to coordinate AAC supports for individuals. Many statewide programs focus on systems change to provide a seamless system of AAC supports. While addressing systems change, the statewide program considers the most effective practices in the field, and promotes those practices throughout various programs in the state. A statewide program is in a prime position to coordinate services across many different programs, and is typically able to elicit support from various areas of the individual's life. Many statewide programs are also more likely to support and be working toward a comprehensive model of supports (see Figure 2–3). Similar to the regional model, the statewide program typically does not provide AAC services directly. Instead, the focus is on developing direct service delivery mechanisms at regional or local levels.

Summary of AAC Service Delivery Models

Individuals seeking AAC supports may have difficulty accessing coordinated, comprehensive services. Across the country there are many agencies and programs, yet they operate in relative isolation. Shortages of skilled service providers and limited funding for AAC present challenging obstacles. The AAC needs of many individuals may exceed the resources and capabilities of a single agency (Langton, 1990). When searching for AAC supports for an individual, it may be necessary to access needed services through multiple programs. Regardless of the service delivery model available, it is essential that all AAC support issues be addressed.

There are many essential program components that need to be considered when selecting AAC services. These are listed in Table 2–7. Ideal programs should provide consumer-oriented services which are delivered within the natural environment whenever possible. The 10 AAC support components previously discussed in this chapter need to be addressed by the program. In order to achieve this goal, it is often necessary to simultaneously coordinate multiple programs into a unique service delivery system for each AAC user.

SETTINGS FOR AAC SERVICE DELIVERY

There are a wide range of settings where augmentative communication service delivery occurs. These settings include home, community, educational, vocational, transitional, and medical environments (see Table 2–8). Service delivery settings are different from the AAC program models that were previously discussed. These are the environments where AAC consumers interact and receive services on a

Table 2–7. Issues to address when accessing AAC services.

- Services should be consumer-responsive.
- Service providers should encourage involvement of the individual and the family during all phases of the process.
- Services should be available in natural environments whenever possible.
- Services provided must address support across all of the 10 support components.
- To access all needed supports, the individual may need to access services through multiple programs.
- A firm foundation of support persons should be established.
- AAC supports should be coordinated with other services that the individual receives.
- Services should be geographically accessible.
- Service delivery models accessed should consider the individual's and the family's philosophical beliefs in decision-making processes.

Table 2–8. AAC service delivery settings.

1. Home
   (a) Individual Home
   (b) Group Home
   (c) Residential/Extended Care Facility

2. Community
   (a) Child Day Care
   (b) Adult Day Care
   (c) Respite Care
   (d) Community Resources

3. Educational
   (a) Self-Contained Classroom
   (b) Inclusive Classroom
   (c) Combination

4. Transitional and Vocational
   (a) Vocational Training Setting
   (b) Employment Setting

5. Medical
   (a) Intensive and Acute Care Facilities
   (b) Inpatient and Outpatient Rehabilitation Facilities

regular basis. AAC service delivery is a blend between the AAC program providing services and the need to provide intervention within the individual's typical communicative setting. For example, a regional AAC service center might provide services to individuals in the local school setting. A rehabilitation program might begin by providing services to hospital inpatients, then follow individuals through outreach programs providing AAC service delivery in the home and on the job. Each service delivery setting brings unique issues that influence the provision of augmentative communication services. These setting-specific issues will be reviewed at a general level in this chapter. More information regarding service provision in specific settings is available Section III of this book.

Home Settings

The communicative setting that is a part of everyone's life is the home. There are many advantages for service providers to go into the home environment to deliver AAC services (Donahue-Kilburg, 1992). There are many different types of homes. Home living environments include the individual's family home, group homes, and residential or extended care facilities. Each type of home environment has factors that play into the challenge of delivering effective AAC services. These factors include issues such as the desired level of communicative independence for the individual, as perceived by themselves and by their family; the actual makeup and dynamics of the family system; the level of interaction that the AAC service provider has with the family; environmental factors; and daily demands of the natural environment.

Individual's Family Home

The opportunity to provide augmentative communication services in the home promotes the building of solid relationships between the AAC team and the family. The team is able to work with a family's level of knowledge and comfort in terms of issues related to disabilities, communication, and augmentative communication in the home. If the individual receiving AAC services is a young child, the team often needs to work together through issues related to the disability grieving process (Todis & Singer, 1991). During the early years, parents are frequently bombarded with information related to their child's medical status, future medical needs, and predictions

from the medical and educational community regarding what their child "will or will not be able to do" in the future. During these times families may not always be receptive to exploring AAC options. A tightly knit team will be able to work together and move forward when the family is ready to consider AAC options for their child.

One advantage of providing AAC services in the home is seeing firsthand the desired level of communicative independence and perceived outcomes for the individual. The AAC user and the family may have expectations that are in synchrony with one another and the rest of the team, or they may be very different. These life expectations will have a direct impact on the perceived need for AAC systems and the role AAC systems play in meeting these outcomes. For example, Kevin was a bright 9-year-old child with cerebral palsy who was raised by parents who wished to shelter him. Across a 6-month evaluation period, Kevin's parents rejected every high tech AAC system that was loaned or recommended for his use. The family was finally informed that they had exhausted all potential technology options. During further discussions, it was apparent that Kevin's family was having difficulty dealing with independence issues. They were reluctant to let go of their role as "communication intermediaries" between Kevin and others in his environment. The AAC team began providing services in the home and community environment to assist Kevin's parents in resolving this issue. In addition, support was also established between Kevin's parents and other families who had children using AAC systems.

A significant benefit to providing AAC services in the family home is the opportunity to identify and integrate ethnic and cultural issues into AAC implementation. Communication and disability issues are viewed differently by different cultures (Blackstone, 1994). For example, Tom was a first-generation Korean who sustained a significant head injury and was unable to speak. His parents initially rejected the use of an AAC system in the belief that Tom would rely on the device and never learn to speak again. It took several months of rehabilitation before Tom's family would even consider the use of AAC. Even then, he was only allowed to use his device at the rehabilitation program. At home, he was still expected to use his limited vocalizations. The family had the same rules for Tom's wheelchair, keeping it in the garage when he was home. An Asian social worker was finally assigned to Tom's team. She worked with the AAC team to assist them in understanding the cultural basis for the family's decisions. A team approach including the social worker was then implemented in the home environment. Tom's family finally agreed to allow him to use his AAC system in the home. However, they still believed that his speech skills could improve. The team agreed to continue providing speech therapy services focused on improving his oral motor skills, along with AAC services.

If multicultural differences are not considered, the AAC system will not reflect an individual's needs (Bender & Baglin, 1992). David was a Hispanic 6-year-old with Down syndrome who had severely delayed expressive language. He used picture communication books for several years, and was being considered for a high-tech AAC system. David was evaluated in the home setting with his parents present. Both parents spoke English, but explained that they had a large extended family, some of whom could only speak Spanish. In addition, the parents often spoke Spanish at home among themselves. It was determined that David's AAC system should have digitized speech features so that messages could be recorded in both English and Spanish.

Intervention in the family home gives the AAC team the chance to provide training to people who live through life's daily communication routines with the individual. Those who are key in the person's life are able to be active participants in the AAC assessment process and implementation planning (Baumgart, Johnson, & Helmstetter, 1990). Although training and involvement of key family supports can occur in other settings, providing training in the home environment ensures that family members are learning to provide AAC support within real-life experiences.

One challenge when providing home-based AAC services is that services are typically provided by one person or discipline at a time. School-age students and adults who receive AAC services at home often receive them from private independent consultants who may or may not communicate with other team members outside of the home setting. The challenge is to establish a mechanism of communication among all AAC team members, not just between the family and the private home-based service provider.

A strength of home-based AAC services is the team's access to information about the individual's physical and communicative environment. The team is able to problem solve within real-life situations. For example, Elaine was observed to go from the first floor to the second floor of her home by crawling up a flight of steps. After watching her, the AAC team decided that she needed a portable lightweight communication system with a carrying strap or handle. In the home setting, the transitions individuals make in their environments and the accommodations that are needed to address their communication needs are seen firsthand. The primary advantage to providing AAC services in an individual's home is that assessment and intervention are occurring where the desired outcomes are expected. The consumer learns to use an AAC system in functional, natural life routines and the home setting is the primary foundation for these daily needs.

Group Home

Another type of home setting for some individuals is a group home. This is typically an environment where several individuals with disabilities are living together. Group homes may be privately owned, run by state social service agencies, or operated using an individual's personal funds. A strength of many group homes is a program focus toward increasing independence and access to community resources. Therefore, there is value in the need for AAC systems. Family involvement or other AAC supports will vary as in any situation. Team planning for the needed supports will help to ensure the use of an AAC communication system in group home environments (Miltich & Rogan, 1992; Parrette, Hourcade, & VanBiervliet, 1993). For example, Joe was a young adult living in a group home. He did not receive consistent support from his family. However, the staff at his group home was very committed to implementing a program that encouraged increased independence and participation in his life activities. Joe and his group home staff were very interested in pursuing augmentative communication options. Joe's AAC circle of support became the group home staff, with minimal involvement from his natural family.

One challenge in providing AAC services in this environment is identifying key personnel who have a history of personal interactions with the AAC user. There is often frequent staff turnover in group homes making AAC training difficult. Many staff members may not have had any post high school training. Therefore their experience with individuals with disabilities and AAC systems may be limited. There is often a program manager or house supervisor who has been employed by the agency for a longer period of time. These individuals usually have some secondary education and are more experienced.

Program managers are more likely to be invested in the selection and use of AAC systems and should be members of the home AAC support team. Another issue for consideration in group home settings is whether there are individuals who are effective communicators and can serve as peer models for the individuals using AAC systems.

A strength related to providing AAC services in the group home environment is that it is one of the primary settings where communication outcomes are expected to occur. This is the individual's natural environment for AAC assessment and intervention. Therefore, the selection and use of AAC systems will be more likely to reflect the individual's actual communication needs. Chapter 17 in this text provides additional information regarding services for adults in the group home setting.

Residential or Long-term Care Facility

There are many individuals who have AAC systems or are in need of them that reside in larger residential facilities specifically designed for people with disabilities. These residential facilities are run by state agencies or are privately owned and operated. Another type of residential facility setting is the long-term care facility, such as a retirement community or nursing home. These settings bring different challenges to the team process when delivering AAC services to individuals.

Individuals residing in residential settings are in these environments because their family or support system is no longer able to meet their daily needs. This may be due to the need for physical care, medical intervention, or behavioral issues. As we see in other home settings, family involvement varies. For example, Jeff's family made the decision to place him in a residential program based on behavioral issues and family needs. Even though Jeff did not reside with his family, they were still very active in the AAC team process. They attended all evaluations and provided suggestions for motivating AAC system vocabulary. Jeff's parents also monitored ongoing use of the AAC system to make sure that staff were implementing the device appropriately. When the family is not living with the individual on a day-to-day basis, their ability to provide AAC support is different than in a situation where the family and the individual reside together. Some residential programs may only provide partial-year residence, so the individual may have two home environments, the residential facility and the family home.

The expectation for individuals in these settings is often set by the facilities' attitudes regarding the potential for independence and ability to care for individuals with disabilities. A challenge for the team may be developing the positive attitudes that are needed to provide effective AAC services. These positive attitudes are those that promote a sense of value for communication. The team needs to look at the individual's circle of support and see what the commitment for support looks like for a person with AAC needs. Some individuals or their families may be able to advocate for themselves, but many individuals with disabilities in these facilities are not able to do this. Another factor to consider when delivering AAC services is to see if there is a plan for increased independence and if the individual and their team have a vision for increasing interaction with others in their environment.

A challenging issue to address in a residential care facility is staff consistency and commitment. Staff members of the facility are the people who can ensure that an AAC system is available for a person's use throughout the day. Residential facilities are often short-staffed, which limits the time available to dedicate to AAC selection and use for an individual with unmet communication needs. The team needs to look at staff makeup, availability for training, level of experience and knowledge in the areas of communication and

AAC systems, and issues related to staff turnover. Related service providers such as speech-language pathologists, physical therapists, and occupational therapists may only have limited time with each individual, so they need to be creative in terms of providing team support and commitment.

One administrator at a state residential facility was interested in providing AAC options for many of the facility's clients and requested services from the AAC program in his region. When the local assistive technology consultant met with direct care staff at the facility, it was clearly evident that staff members were more concerned about issues such as staffing shortages, toileting schedules, and whose responsibility it was to clean up the residents after feeding. Communication for the residents was clearly not a priority for the facility staff. It was determined that the value of communication first needed to be realized by direct care staff and identified by them as an unmet need for residents at the facility. A series of trainings emphasizing the importance of communication and simple methods of providing choice making within the environment was implemented for the staff. The trainings were held before any direct AAC intervention was attempted.

A final strength of a residential facility is that the daily environment is highly structured and predictable. For AAC teams, this framework of daily routines provides an opportunity to select and implement AAC strategies in a more structured way because the individual's interactive environment and communicative choices are limited.

Community

The second setting where AAC services are delivered is in the community. This setting can be included as a component of service delivery in conjunction with other settings. For example, some educational programs provide community-based instruction as preparation for adult life and independent living skills (Rainforth & York, 1987). There is an endless list of locations in the community setting where AAC services can be delivered. The most common include short-term care facilities and community resources.

Short-term Care Facility

Short-term care facilities include options such as child day care, respite care for children and adults, and adult day care agencies (Bender & Baglin, 1992). Many of these community service providers are "for profit" agencies. Because of the for profit nature of these programs, it is sometimes difficult to get release time for staff members to receive training to support use of an AAC system. There may be frequent changeovers of staff at these care facilities, which means an ongoing need to educate staff about the communication needs of the individual. The team that is providing AAC support will need to address these issues in the assessment and implementation planning process.

Child Day Care. A major strength in providing AAC services in the child day care setting is that the individual is with other children from the home community, as opposed to receiving services in a therapeutic child care setting. For example, Cameron is a preschool child who uses a voice output augmentative communication device. He uses his AAC system at the day care center with children from his local community. This provides an opportunity for the family to build a lifetime AAC support system within the community. Children who are in public child care settings have many peer models around them for communicating, learning, and playing.

Adult Day Programs. When adults are in day programs, it is typically because they are unable to be left alone at home. This may be due to physical, medical, or safety issues. A drawback to an adult day program is that it is not representative of the community as a whole. Service providers will need to identify if there are effective, functional peer models for communication. This setting also brings the challenges of staff turnover and the need for ongoing training to support the individual using the AAC system.

Community Resources

Additional community settings for AAC service delivery include neighborhood resources such as stores, restaurants, banks, and churches. Community-based instruction can be provided on a daily, weekly, or biweekly basis (Rainforth & York, 1987). Community settings provide opportunities for communication exchanges with both familiar and unfamiliar communication partners. For example, Frannie's team incorporated community-based AAC instruction into her independent living plan. She had a variety of different community settings that were used to implement her AAC program, including the grocery store and local restaurants. The team could evaluate firsthand the effectiveness of Frannie's AAC system in these daily community routines.

A challenge to service providers is to train communication partners within the community environment, so the AAC system can be used on a regular basis. These settings may be among the most challenging because of the inability to control what might occur in a given situation. One method of providing structure is to discuss use of the AAC system with community members prior to the actual community outing. Frannie's group home supervisor provided this structure by calling the manager of the local fast food restaurant to discuss Frannie's AAC system. The manager was informed of the time of the visit and arranged to have a specific trained employee available to take Frannie's order.

By providing AAC intervention in community settings, networks of support can be built to include community volunteers who will assist with custom fabrication of AAC materials, technical support, educating other community members, and sometimes funding support. These "people resources" in an individual's local community are invaluable to the AAC process. These are the persons who will interact with the AAC user for life.

Educational Settings

Public policy is the foundation for the provision of AAC service delivery in most educational settings. Public policy for early intervention, preschool, and school-aged children who receive public educational programming details the provision of assistive technology services. Individuals receiving educational programming in a private school setting are not protected by these mandates. Readers are referred to Chapters 9 and 15 for more information regarding these policies.

Educational settings in the twentieth century can be categorized on the basis of inclusive practices (Simon, Karasoff, Smith, Haloorsen, & Neary, 1992). Public education agencies operate their programs for individuals with disabilities using the following three models: (1) self-contained educational environments, (2) inclusive educational environments, or (3) a combination of self-contained and inclusive environments. Other educational settings to consider are those settings available following the completion of high school, such as trade school and college. Each type of setting raises issues to consider in the provision of AAC services.

Self-contained Classroom Settings

Self-contained classroom settings are seen in early intervention programs, preschool programs, and school-aged programs. These types of classroom environments are designed to provide learning opportunities specifically for children with disabilities. One issue in considering this setting for AAC service delivery is to determine the overall vision for children with disabilities, specifically the expected educational and communicative outcomes. In some self-contained classrooms there are low expectations for children with disabilities, while other self-contained classroom environments strive to foster communicative independence and growth. These positively oriented classrooms place greater emphasis on interaction and the use of AAC systems.

One concern regarding self-contained classrooms is that students with disabilities are not with their community friends. They are in classrooms with other children with disabilities who are often brought in by bus over great distances to participate in educational programs. They are not learning, playing, or communicating with their local group of friends and building a community support system for use of their AAC system. The family may not be in a situation to build a local network of parents and children in their community. The value of a local community support system for the selection and use of assistive technology cannot be emphasized enough.

Self-contained educational settings vary in terms of the type of parent partnerships they foster. Early intervention programs often include parents in the classroom where they are active participants in educational programming. As children move into elementary and secondary settings, the educational environment may not encourage as much day-to-day parent participation. However, many teachers of self-contained classrooms try to keep the lines of communication open with families through the use of communication notebooks and parent meetings. Mrs. Fonner was a teacher in a self-contained classroom in an elementary school. She encouraged communication with families by writing a monthly newsletter, keeping communication notebooks for all of the students, and planning regular social gatherings for student families and their children. Regular communication and joint planning between educational staff and families is essential to successful AAC service delivery.

In a self-contained classroom, related service staff such as the occupational therapist, the physical therapist, and the speech therapist frequently provide services to children in the classroom itself. A strength to providing support in this setting is their familiarity with the educational curriculum, which is the foundation for educational activities and classroom communication needs (Graden, Zins, & Curtis, 1988). Because all of the children in the class have special needs, the classroom teacher and paraprofessionals often have prior experience working with students who use AAC systems. There may also be other students using AAC systems who can serve as language models. These can be effective supports for a student using AAC.

One challenge with self-contained classrooms is providing a curriculum that is reflective of functional life outcomes. This is often difficult given that the individuals in the classroom are not representative of people in the students' home community. These classrooms may not have any other students who can model functional and effective communication skills. Classroom activities are often simulations of real life routines, instead of actually providing intervention in the environment where the outcome is expected. When intervention does not occur in natural environments, the issue of carryover of AAC systems into natural routines will need to be addressed.

Many service providers feel that self-contained classrooms provide a structured, predictable daily routine for students. This structured schedule can be used as the foundation for determining a specific child's AAC needs. This type of classroom does provide a predictable environment and consistent communication partners for the child, which can initially enhance learning in that setting. However, communication within this setting may not facilitate the child's potential to communicate in other educational or community environments.

Inclusive Classroom Settings

With the ongoing interpretation and implementation of the concept of least restrictive environment, more AAC students are now receiving their education in inclusive classroom settings. A strength is that the primary focus of these classrooms is students, not disabilities. Local educational agencies are developing programs and adapting curriculums to meet the needs of all students with disabilities in the regular classroom. This type of service delivery setting has brought new issues to the field of AAC service delivery.

Family participation in inclusive settings may be different from that in self-contained classrooms. Families may spend time in the student's classroom, but the focus is not on disability issues for the student with AAC needs. The focus is on learning the educational curriculum in the regular classroom. The family may spend time in the classroom educating classroom staff and other students about AAC and how it supports their child's life. Parents are able to build a support network with other parents in their local community because their child is being educated with neighborhood children.

The child receiving AAC services in an inclusive setting may be the only child in the school or school district with a disability and AAC needs. One challenge in inclusive classroom settings is ensuring that the student's team receives training to address augmentative communication needs.

This includes training on the selection of AAC systems, the operational use of different types of communication systems, and the implementation of AAC systems into real life routines. A local educational agency may not recognize the need to release staff for multiple days of training for a single student. Creative planning may be needed to provide essential training for key members of the team. One method is to provide duplicate trainings with only a few team members at a time. Team training needs should be built into educational plans to ensure that the direct service team, including the family, is comfortable in the implementation of an AAC system.

Staff in inclusive classroom settings need to be provided with training before students using AAC begin attending classes. When Sheree was transitioning from a self-contained preschool to an inclusive kindergarten classroom, her preschool team made it a priority to share information with her new team. They made videotapes of Sheree using her light tech and high tech AAC systems in the preschool. The vendor for the high tech AAC system was brought in to train the new school team how to program the device. Arrangements were made for Sheree's preschool speech-language pathologist to provide consultative services during the first 3 months in her new classroom. Sheree's transition went well, and within a few weeks her teacher viewed her as "just another student" in the class. When children are in inclusive settings at an early age, they begin to build a lifetime support network for the use and implementation of their AAC systems.

The challenges of providing AAC training increase when students enter inclusive classrooms in middle school and high school. Students often have multiple teachers providing their educational programming. The local team must decide what type of training is needed to implement the AAC system and who on the team

needs training. The team may want to identify individuals that are consistent throughout the student's educational program within the school. In addition to staff, other resources available for AAC system support include parent volunteers and student peers. School friends are wonderful resources for support (Stainback & Stainback, 1992). Older student peers can often assume responsibility for the programming of the system. Younger student peers can provide input into communication message selection, assist with system portability, and be a general support for the individual using the augmentative communication system. Stephen uses a high tech AAC device in many of his environments. His communication needs change rapidly and his team needed a way to program all of his communication messages. Their solution was to have students in his fifth-grade classroom program the system. This set up an ongoing support system to move with Stephen as he progressed through school. Given the time constraints that most teams are under, using students as a resource should not be overlooked as an option in inclusionary school settings. An additional outcome to having students as a support system for the AAC system is that lifetime bonds and friendships can develop (Stainback, Stainback, & Forest, 1989).

The provision of related services for AAC in inclusive settings is driven by the model of service delivery. Related service personnel such as speech therapists, occupational therapists, and physical therapists can choose to provide pullout services where they meet one on one with the student. They can provide integrated therapy services where they provide supports in the child's natural environments. They can also provide consultative services where they spend time sharing intervention information with the staff who works with the individual on a regular basis (Jenkins & Heinen, 1989).

Bob's educational team struggled with how to provide the necessary supports for the implementation of his AAC system. They initially decided to provide only consultative support to the classroom teacher and paraprofessionals. After a period of time, the team determined that Bob needed short-term one on one instruction to gain familiarity with the location of new communication messages on his device. He was seen for individual pull-out therapy two times weekly. With this additional support, he was able to successfully and efficiently communicate in the classroom during functional activities. Bob's assistive technology consultant used the analogy of learning to play a musical instrument. Sometimes we need to practice alone before we can play with the band. Ideally, AAC users should have therapy programs that combine consultative, integrated, and individual pull-out methods of service delivery. The model of service delivery that is selected will determine the types of team issues that need to be addressed to ensure that AAC intervention is approached in a comprehensive manner.

The primary benefit for young children receiving AAC intervention in inclusive settings is that they are in the school environment where natural outcomes are expected. They have the opportunity to use the AAC system in real life situations with other students who communicate effectively. They experience the routines of daily life and ever-changing communication needs that are a part of interaction. They have these experiences with the children in their community that they live with, work with, and play with, their AAC support network for life.

Combination Classroom Settings

The final classroom environment splits students between inclusive and self-contained settings. Students spend varied amounts of time in different classrooms depending upon the needs identified in the individual's educational plan. This pre-sents numerous challenges for consideration. The student is receiving support in multiple classrooms which means there are distinctly different environments where the individual is expected to use an AAC system. For example, James spent part of his day in a self-contained classroom and 2 hours each day in the regular third-grade classroom. His teacher in the inclusive classroom sometimes adjusted the class schedule without notifying his other teachers. James was often brought into the class in the middle of a lesson, meaning that he had missed the introduction to the activity. This made it difficult for him to have clear expectations about what kind of communication was needed during the class lesson. Students who attend combinations of classrooms also have to adjust to different styles of teaching across multiple teachers and have different sets of friends across class settings.

Transitional and Vocational Settings

One setting that is starting to receive more attention is the transitional vocational environment. As assistive technology options and philosophies have evolved for individuals with disabilities, there are greater opportunities to access in terms of postsecondary training and employment (Enders & Hall, 1990). Transitional environments include those settings where individuals receive vocational training and additional education. This includes on-the-job training in high school, continuing education at a trade or technical school, or attendance at a community college or university. Vocational settings can include supported employment situations or independent employment (Gardner & Chapman, 1993). The field of AAC is looking at these settings to determine the types of supports that are necessary for individuals who use augmentative communication.

Vocational Training Setting

Vocational preparation begins when students are in elementary school and high school (Sowers & Powers, 1991). As AAC users enter into vocational preparation environments, the most important point to address is the establishment of a support team. This is often difficult in employment education and training environments. AAC consumers need supports for technical assistance and implementation of the AAC system within everyday routines in these settings. Many postsecondary settings have student services departments to assist in setting up necessary supports for individuals with disabilities attending their facility.

One accommodation made for some individuals in these settings has been to have a personal assistant. This assistant can provide physical support to the individual using the AAC system, as well as valuable technical assistance with the AAC system itself. Pamela is a sophomore at a state university majoring in computer science. She has a personal assistant to support her in the everyday management of her educational materials, as well as the technical support for her communication system and computer. The issue of training for the support system must also be addressed. As part of the support process, Pamela's personal assistant received training about the AAC system and the computer. Other enrolled students can also serve as an AAC support system in these environments

A key component to build into the individual's implementation plan is a mechanism to monitor ongoing needs. As the individual's communication needs change and as assistive technology continues to evolve, there will be a need to continually reassess the effectiveness of the AAC system. By building this component into the action plan, AAC consumers will have their communication needs assessed on an ongoing basis.

Employment Settings

The transition into a work environment for an individual who uses an AAC system involves intensive planning on the part of the team. Individuals may be able to get support from public vocational agencies to assist in transition planning and to secure needed AAC systems and services. This planning should begin early to ensure a smooth and successful transition into the work setting. The issues to address in the transition plan will be addressed in this section.

AAC communication needs and requirements in the job setting need to be determined. The team studies the job environment and the responsibilities of the job to identify the types of communication that are required. The individual may need to communicate one-on-one, in small groups, in large groups, via telephone, or using the computer. Identifying daily communication situations that the individual will encounter will ensure that the AAC system meets these needs.

An issue to address is employee training in the areas of disabilities and augmentative communication. Some co-workers may not have experience interacting with an individual with a disability. Basic awareness of disability issues will need to be trained. Co-workers also need basic knowledge of how an augmentative communication system serves as a tool for effective communication interaction. Part of the planning process for use of an AAC system in the work environment is to develop a circle of support within the work setting. This circle of support may be able to provide technical assistance as needs arise with the augmentative communication system. The individuals in this support system, as well as others in the work setting, may need training on how to interact with AAC consumers. Partner training with co-workers may decrease the potential for stress as AAC consumers enter the work environment.

A key component to include in the implementation plan for individuals who use AAC systems on the job is to make sure there are provisions for ongoing assessment of communication needs. For example, Scott is an employee at a graphics company. His employer uses the computer for the production of graphic materials. When the company updated their computer system, Scott's team addressed issues related to integrating his AAC device with the new computer system. He needed additional software to fully access the new computer system through his high tech communication device. Given that technology is ever-changing, communication needs should be continually reassessed to determine the most effective and efficient means of interaction.

Medical Service Delivery Settings

The final setting for consideration in AAC service delivery is the medical setting. Medical settings include intensive or acute care facilities, and inpatient and outpatient rehabilitation programs. These settings are typically temporary settings for the AAC consumer. Each medical setting presents unique issues in the delivery of AAC services. Chapters 13 and 16 provide the reader with more details regarding these settings.

Intensive and Acute Care Facilities

Intensive and acute care hospitals are difficult settings for providing AAC services. The primary concern in these settings is meeting the individual's medical needs rather than communication. Speed of intervention is also an issue. Once medical needs are stabilized and the individual is ready for AAC intervention, the individual is immediately transferred out to a rehabilitation hospital or home. Almost all nonspeaking individuals in acute care and intensive care hospitals previously had normal speech and communication skills. The loss of existing communication skills adds another dimension to service delivery in this setting. Daniel was a young man in intensive care as a result of a lesion in his brain from a bacterial infection. Daniel was unable to breath independently, phonate, or mouth words. Although the primary concern was Daniel's medical condition, his AAC team needed to provide him with potential options for communication during his hospital stay. After an initial bedside assessment, it was decided that Daniel could use eye gaze, gestures, and head nods to communicate. His family and friends were interviewed to obtain information about Daniel's past communication style and interaction preferences. These communication strategies were taught to hospital staff, family, and friends. As in all settings, the choices made by individuals and their families need to be respected (Blackstone, 1994).

When an individual is in the acute care hospital, there may be minimal time to address unmet communication needs. However, the hospital team needs to establish an acceptable means for interaction, so the individual is able to express medical and functional needs, along with thoughts and desires. As the person's medical status changes, communication needs and abilities may also change. The AAC team needs to identify and meet these changing needs during the intensive and acute care hospital stay.

Inpatient and Outpatient Rehabilitation Facilities

AAC services can also be offered by inpatient and outpatient rehabilitation facilities. An advantage to these settings is they can offer additional professional services that may not be available in other settings. There is typically access to a wide range of professionals, such as physicians, psychologists, and rehabilitation engineers. Access to specialty medical personnel can provide the AAC team with valuable information that may not be available in other settings.

Teams in rehabilitation facilities can provide AAC services on a one-to-one basis, in a co-treatment program where two or more therapists provide services simultaneously, or provide outreach services in the individual's home or community. When services are provided in an isolated therapeutic setting, the therapy provided may not match the individuals everyday communication needs in the real world (Blackstone, 1989). Individual therapy does not provide opportunities for other disciplines to have integrated goals and implementation plans. Co-treatment and outreach services provide an opportunity for more natural goal setting.

Community-based rehabilitation services are an ideal way for AAC services to be provided where the person lives, works, and plays. This is the environment where the augmentative communication system is really needed. In order to achieve community-based services, the team from the rehabilitation facility needs to provide AAC supports to the individual's local team. It is this local team that will implement the AAC action plan and work with the individual on a daily basis. This type of AAC service delivery is likely to provide the necessary supports to ensure successful selection of an AAC system. The implementation plan will also reflect natural communication situations that occur on a daily basis.

AAC Settings: Transitions and Other Issues

This section of the chapter addressed issues related to AAC service delivery in a variety of different communicative settings. One issue that is a challenge in providing AAC services across all settings is the process of transition; addressing individual needs as consumers move from one setting to another. Transitions can involve complete changes in settings, such as a move from an elementary school to a high school. Transitions can also occur daily, as users move from their home environment to the educational or work setting. Because the AAC support team often changes across settings, transitions are a key source of breakdowns in service delivery. Transitions frequently do not receive adequate attention to ensure smooth service delivery for AAC consumers.

Several strategies can increase the likelihood of successful transitions. The primary effective strategy is planning in advance. A new AAC team should be identified before the individual transitions to the new setting. The team can visit the individual and receive AAC training prior to the transition. The individual can also visit the new setting to meet the new team and to see what the new environment will offer. Other strategies that have been successful for some teams is to share videotape clips of the individual using the AAC system in multiple environments. Strategies to ensure smooth transitions can occur with a coordinated system of services (Schoech, Cavalier, & Hoover, 1993).

Additional issues can also effect the delivery of AAC services. Access to AAC services often varies depending on whether someone lives in an urban or a rural setting (American Speech-Language-Hearing Association, 1990). Public policy affects the availability and requirement for the provision of services in specific settings. These policies can vary from state to state and between agencies within a state. Another factor that affects the availability of AAC services is funding streams. Funding sources may drive the service delivery process for a specific environment, setting criteria for the types of individuals who can receive services, and the specific types of services that can be provided. Readers are referred to Chapter 9 which addresses funding issues in depth.

Each setting brings unique strengths and challenges for consideration when providing support to individuals who use AAC systems. Teams need to be aware of these unique issues to ensure that AAC users receive necessary supports to successfully implement augmentative communication strategies.

SUMMARY

This chapter reviewed the provision of augmentative communication services. There are a variety of different service delivery models and service delivery settings for the consumer to consider when seeking AAC supports. The foundation of these supports is the AAC team. Individuals and families will need to determine what supports they need, where they want and need to receive AAC services, and how these services will be provided. The most important issue is that each individual gains access to all 10 components of the AAC service delivery process (see Table 2–5). These components can be accessed in a variety of ways, and frequently require coordination of services across multiple programs, but these components are essential to successful and comprehensive AAC service delivery.

The field of AAC has little information available on the effectiveness of AAC service delivery (DeRuyter, 1992). This is an area that is in need of additional research. As service providers we need to be aware of the outcomes of our service delivery models. As the effectiveness of service delivery models in a variety of different settings is evaluated, information can be obtained to ensure more successful outcomes in AAC. A significant result of additional research in this area will be providing the most efficient and effective AAC services to individuals who use AAC systems. As AAC services improve, individuals will be able to achieve successful communication interactions throughout their lives (Benton, 1994; Blackstone, 1992).

REFERENCES

American Speech-Language-Hearing Association. (1990). The roles of the speech-language pathologists in service delivery to infants, toddlers and their families. *ASHA, 32* (2), 4.

Bagnato, S. J., & Neisworth, J. T. (1991). *Assessment for early intervention: Best practices for professionals.* New York: Guilford Press.

Baumgart, D., Johnson, J., & Helmstetter, E. (1990). *Augmentative and alternative communication systems for persons with moderate and severe disabilities.* Baltimore, MD: Paul H. Brookes Publishing.

Bender, M., & Baglin, C. A. (1992). *Infants and toddlers: A resource guide for practitioners.* San Diego, CA: Singular Publishing Group.

Benton, S. (1994). Assuring quality in assistive technology. *REHAB management, 6–7,* 161–163.

Beukelman, D. R., & Mirenda, P. (1992). *Augmentative and alternative communication: Management of severe communication disorders in children and adults.* Baltimore, MD: Paul H. Brookes Publishing.

Blackstone, S. W. (1989). Augmentative communication services in the schools. *ASHA, 33,* 61–64.

Blackstone, S. W. (1992). Evaluation of AAC service delivery programs: Meanings and methodologies. *ISAAC research symposium proceedings.* McKee City, NJ: CTA.

Blackstone, S. W. (1992). *Technology in the classroom: Communication module.* Rockville, MD: ASHA.

Blackstone, S.W. (1994). Cultural diversity in AAC. *Augmentative Communication News. 7*(6), 1.

Brandt, B., & Rice, D. B. (1990). *The provision of assistive technology services in rehabilitation.* Unpublished paper, Hot Springs, AR: Arkansas Research and Training Center in Vocational Rehabilitation.

DeRuyter, F. (1992). The importance of cost benefit analysis in AAC. *Concensus validation conference: Resource papers.* Washington, DC: The National Institute on Disability and Rehabilitation Research.

Donahue-Kilburg, G. (1992). *Family-centered early intervention for communication disorders: Prevention and treatment.* Gaithersburg, MD: Aspen Publishers.

Enders, A., & Hall, M. (1990). *Assistive technology sourcebook.* Washington, DC: Resna Press.

Gardner, J. F., & Chapman, M. S. (1993). *Developing staff competencies for supporting people with developmental disabilities.* Baltimore, MD: Paul H. Brookes Publishing.

Giangreco, M. F., Cloninger, C. J., & Iverson, V. S. (1993). *Choosing options and accommodations for children* (COACH). Baltimore, MD: Paul H. Brookes Publishing.

Graden, J. L., Zins, J. E., & Curtis, M. J. (1988). *Alternative educational delivery systems: Enhancing instructional options for all students.* Washington, DC: National Association of School Psychologists.

Jenkins, J. R., & Heinen, A. (1989). Students' preferences for service delivery: Pull-out, in-class or integrated models. *Exceptional Children, 55,* 516–523.

Johnson, D. W., & Johnson, F. P. (1975). *Joining together: Group theory and group skill.* Englewood Cliffs, NJ: Prentice-Hall.

Langton, A. J. (1990). *Delivering assistive technology services: Challenges and realities.* Unpublished paper, Columbia, SC: Center for Rehabilitation Technology Services.

Lerner, J., Mardell-Czudnowski, C., & Goldenberg, D. (1987). *Special education for the early childhood years.* Englewood Cliffs, NJ: Prentice-Hall.

Light, J. (1989). Toward a definition of communicative competence for individuals using augmentative and alternative communication systems. *Augmentative and Alternative Communication, 5,* 137–144.

Lyon, S., & Lyon, G. (1980). Team functioning and staff development: A role release approach to providing integrated educational services for severely handicapped students. *Journal of the Association for the Severely Handicapped, 5,* 250–263.

Miltich, S. H., & Rogan, J. M. (1992). *Collaborative consultation as a service delivery model for group homes.* Paper presented at the American Speech-Language-Hearing Association annual convention, San Antonio, TX.

Musselwhite, C. R., & St. Louis, K. W. (1988). *Communication programming for persons with severe handicaps.* Boston, MA: College-Hill Press.

Parrette, H. P., Hourcade, J. J., & VanBiervliet, A. (1993). Selection of appropriate technology for children with disabilities. *Teaching Exceptional Children, 25,* 18–22.

Patterson, E. G., D'Wolff, N., Hutchison, D., Lowry, M., Schilling, M., & Siepp, J. (1976). *Staff development handbook: A resource for the transdisciplinary process.* New York: United Cerebral Palsy Association.

PennTech (1994). *Assistive technology statewide support initiative: Service delivery.* Unpublished paper, Harrisburg, PA: PennTech.

Public Law 100–407 (1988). *Technology Related Assistance for Individuals with Disabilities Act.* Section 3.

Rainforth, B., & York, J. (1987). Integrating related services in community instruction. *Journal of the Association for the Severely Handicapped, 12,* 190–198.

Rainforth, B., York, J., & Macdonald, C. (1992). *Collaborative teams for students with severe disabilities.* Baltimore, MD: Paul H. Brookes Publishing.

Schoech, D., Cavalier, A., & Hoover, B. (1993). A model for integrating technology into a multi-agency community service delivery system. *Assistive Technology, 3,* 11–23.

Sheldon, J., & Craig, H. M. (1994). Building teams. *Advance, 4,* 8.

Simon, M., Karasoff, P., Smith, A., Halvorsen, A., & Neary, T. (1992). Effective practices for inclusive programs: A technical assistance planning guide. *PEERS Project-California Research Institute.* San Francisco, CA: San Francisco State University.

Skrtic, T. M. (1991). *Behind special education: A critical analysis of professional culture and school organization.* Denver, CO: Love Publishing.

Sowers, J., & Powers, L. (1991). *Vocational preparation and employment of students with physical and multiple disabilities.* Baltimore, MD: Paul H. Brookes Publishing.

Stainback, S., & Stainback, W. (1992). *Curriculum considerations in inclusive classrooms.* Baltimore, MD: Paul H. Brookes Publishing.

Stainback, S., Stainback, W., & Forest, M. (1989). *Educating all students in the mainstream of regular education.* Baltimore, MD: Paul H. Brookes Publishing.

Thousand, J. S., & Villa, R. A. (1990). *Support networks for inclusive schooling: Interdependent integrated education.* Baltimore, MD: Paul H. Brookes Publishing.

Thousand, J. S., & Villa, R. A. (1992). *Collaborative teams: A powerful tool in school restructuring.* Baltimore, MD: Paul H. Brookes Publishing.

Todis, B., & Singer, G. (1991). Stress management in families with adopted children who have severe disabilities. *Journal of the Association for the Severely Handicapped, 16*, 3.

Chapter 3

AUGMENTATIVE AND ALTERNATIVE COMMUNICATION SYSTEMS

Sharon L. Glennen

The history of using augmentative and alternative communication (AAC) systems for communication is rather brief. Prior to 1975, there were descriptions of nonspeaking individuals using simple letter boards, picture boards, and typewriters to communicate messages (Goldberg & Fenton, 1960; Goldstein & Cameron, 1952; McDonald & Schultz, 1973; Vicker, 1974). The early use of AAC systems was limited to a few individuals with physical handicaps or aphasia who had the ability to independently point to symbols. Several factors came together in the late 1970s that had a major impact on the development of AAC devices. In 1975, PL 94-142 was implemented, mandating that all handicapped children between 5 and 21 years of age be provided with a free public education. With the implementation of this law, nonspeaking individuals who previously had been excluded from the educational mainstream began receiving the attention of speech-language pathologists and educators.

The development of microcomputer technology was the second factor that im-

pacted the AAC field. Prior to the development of microcomputers, AAC devices were handmade electrical systems, or nonportable computer systems. Vanderheiden and Grilley (1977) offered an overview of electronic AAC devices that were available in the early 1970s. Many of these early AAC systems consisted of adaptations to electric typewriters, or were simplistic electronic scanning devices without printed or spoken output.

The Canon Communicator was one of the first commercially available augmentative communication devices specifically designed for nonspeaking individuals. It was a small device that strapped to the user's wrist. A small touchpad with alphabet letters could be used to spell messages which were printed on a small strip printer. The Canon Communicator could only be used by individuals with sufficient spelling and fine motor abilities. A modified version of the device is still available commercially (see Appendix). The AutoCom was of one of the first computer-based electronic AAC systems that could be adapted for a wide variety of users (Vanderheiden & Grilley, 1976). In its time, the AutoCom was considered to be a sophisticated portable AAC device with 128 symbol areas that could be programmed and customized for the user. It was a whopping 20 by 24 inches in size, and weighed a hefty 17 pounds. The AutoCom provided the user with printed output on a small strip paper printer, and a 32 character LED display. Although the AutoCom provided options for using picture symbols and multiple levels of programming, its use was still limited to individuals who could access the device by directly touching the symbols with a special pointer. Synthesized speech was not an option in most of these early systems.

In 1978, the Phonic Ear HandiVoice 110 and 120 were developed. These two devices were the first portable, commercially available AAC systems with synthesized speech output. Michael Williams, an AAC user with cerebral palsy, was one of the first individuals to use the HandiVoice 120. He describes his use of the system as follows:

It claimed to be a communication device, but what it really was, was a speech synthesizer hooked up to a numeric keypad with some firmware in between. The firmware held the device's very limited vocabulary plus forty-eight phonemes from which the user could construct any word of his choosing, thus allowing the manufacturer to claim that the device had an unlimited vocabulary. Saying something with this device was like chiseling words into a stone tablet. Each vocabulary item or phoneme was accessed by a unique three digit code. One could build up a series of these codes in the device buffer and then push a button to say the assembled linguistic utterance. Does this sound like work? You bet it was! Communicating with my letterboard was much faster, and my friends kept asking me why I was torturing myself with this crude ugly sounding voice synthesizer. I had no answer for them that I could put into words. I only knew that this piece of voice output technology struck a chord so deep inside me it hurt. It

gave me a hint of what it would be like if I had a voice, and it was also a hint of things to come. (Williams, 1995, pp. 3–4)

The HandiVoice devices made professionals and users aware of the communicative potential for portable AAC systems with voice output. With continued advances in microcomputer technology, AAC devices have become more sophisticated and more adaptable for a wide variety of users.

Augmentative and alternative communication strategies can range from using vocalizations and gestures, to the use of picture-based AAC systems, to the use of microcomputers for communication. Although the use of AAC devices tends to be the focus of the assessment and intervention process, research shows AAC users rely on other methods of communication for a large portion of their communicated messages (Glennen, 1989). Therefore, although this chapter will focus on AAC devices and equipment, the use of unaided communication (e.g., vocalizations, gestures, and sign language) which is reviewed in Chapter 4, should not be overlooked.

OVERVIEW OF AAC SYSTEM TERMINOLOGY

Augmentative and alternative communication strategies are categorized as unaided or aided. Unaided methods of communication rely completely on the user's body to convey communicative messages. Vocalizations, gestures, sign language, head nods, and eye gaze are all methods of unaided communication. Aided communication methods require the use of tools or equipment in addition to the user's body. Aided communication methods can range from using paper and pencil to using sophisticated laptop computers with speech synthesizers. In reality, most nonspeaking persons rely on multiple modalities of communication that combine several unaided and aided methods together.

Aided communication systems are typically classified as being lite technolo-gy, or high technology strategies (see Figure 3–1). Most lite technology systems are nonelectronic and typically handmade. Simple picture communication boards, let-

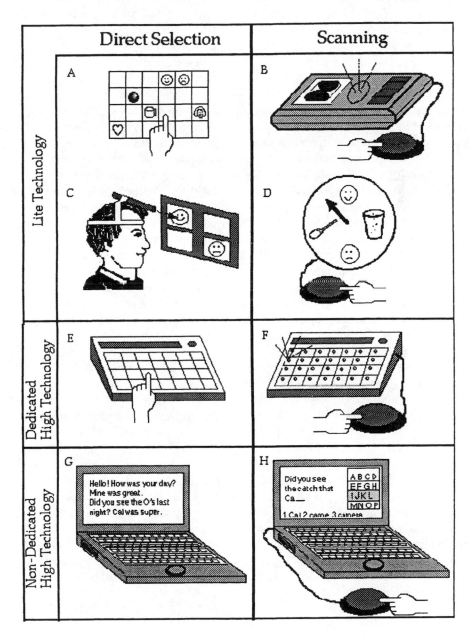

Figure 3–1. Augmentative communication system classification. (A) Picture communication board; (B) Scanning loop tape recorder; (C) Laser light pointer with simple picture communication board; (D) Clock Communicator; (E) Direct selection AAC system; (F) Scanning AAC system; (G) Laptop computer with speech synthesizer; (H) Laptop computer with speech synthesizer and scanning word prediction software.

ter boards, and eye gaze boards are examples of lite technology AAC systems. Other lite technology strategies use electronic components but are not computer-based. A Clock Communicator, which has a battery-operated dial controlled by a switch, is an example of lite AAC technology. Use of Light Pointers with simple communication boards, and switch-activated tape recorders are other examples. High technology AAC systems contain microcomputer components which allow for the storage and retrieval of message information. They almost always have spoken message output, and sometimes printed output.

High technology AAC systems can be further divided into the categories of dedicated devices and nondedicated devices (see Figure 3–1). Dedicated AAC systems are those that were developed for the sole purpose of being an AAC device. The software and hardware of a dedicated AAC device is designed with features essential for communication. Although dedicated systems can often be attached to a computer to serve as an alternative keyboard, their primary stand-alone purpose is to enhance the communication process. Nondedicated AAC systems are devices that were not specifically designed for communication, but through adaptations can be used as AAC systems. Desktop and laptop computers are often used as nondedicated AAC devices. By adding special software, adapted hardware access methods, and a speech synthesizer, the computer can be used as a communication tool, yet can still be used for other functions such as word processing, spreadsheets, educational software, and computer games.

AAC systems can be used with a variety of access methods. The access method determines how the user will select symbols on the AAC device. Users with good physical ability typically access their systems using direct selection methods (see Figure 3–1). When using direct selection, the user is able to point to all possible

symbol choices on the AAC system. Direct selection can be achieved by pointing with fingers and hands, pointing with other body parts, pointing with head sticks, splints, or light pointers, and pointing using eye gaze. The author knows of one AAC user who pointed to letters on a communication board with his nose! Eventually a better method of direct selection was found for this individual.

Users with more limited physical ability often cannot directly access symbols with good accuracy. They need to indirectly select symbol choices by using scanning access methods (see Figure 3–1). Scanning involves the systematic presentation of symbol choices to the user. Once the desired symbol is reached it is selected by the user. Unaided methods of scanning involve a communication partner who asks 20 questions (or more), and waits for a yes/no response after each question. Aided methods of scanning usually require the use of a switch, which is activated when the desired selection is reached on the AAC device.

High technology AAC systems have many different features. The size and weight of AAC systems vary widely, which affects portability. AAC systems vary in the number of key/symbol locations available, the size of the keys, and the configuration of the keys. Feedback given after selecting a key also varies. Some AAC devices have fixed displays, in which the picture or letter symbols never change. Other devices have dynamic displays, in which the screen is constantly changing. A standard computer monitor is an example of a dynamic display. When using dynamic displays for augmentative communication, symbol choices on the screen change based on previous symbol selections. For example, the Dynavox user begins with a page of category symbols. By pressing the category symbol for *Fast Food*, the device then changes to a different page with many symbols for food choices (see Figure 3–2).

The method of storing and retrieving messages also differs across various AAC devices. Message storage is the process of prestoring messages into the AAC system. Message retrieval is the process of using or retrieving the prestored messages. All high technology AAC systems have message storage and retrieval capabilities. The various methods of storing and retreiving messages will be reviewed in greater detail later in this chapter.

ACCESS METHODS

As described previously, there are two basic access methods for using AAC devices, direct selection and scanning. Each of these methods will be reviewed in detail in this section.

Direct Selection Access Methods

Direct Selection Keyboards

Direct selection allows the user access to all possible symbol choices at all times. Many dedicated and nondedicated AAC systems allow the user to directly select choices by pressing a keyboard. Fingers and hands are traditionally used to access these keyboards, but head sticks, adaptive pointers, or other body parts can also be used. Some keyboards use a mechanical system of direct selection in which the keys are physically pushed down by the user. Mechanical key depression is used to operate standard computer keyboards. When the key is depressed a sufficient amount, a signal that the key has been selected is activated. The Delta Talker, Alpha Talker, Canon Communicator, Walker Talker, RealVoice, Light Writer SL30, and Liberator are dedicated devices that rely on mechanical key depression for activation.

Other direct selection keyboards rely on touch membrane or touch screen surfaces. A touch membrane keyboard consists of two electrically conductive flat surfaces separated by nonconductive spacers. Touching the keyboard lightly presses the two surfaces together which sends an electronic signal to the AAC system. Many computer touch screens operate similarly. When using a touch membrane keyboard or touch screen, the user does not feel any physical depression of the surface. The Macaw, Parrot, Digivox, Speak Easy, Say It All, Say it Simply Plus, VOIS Series, Message Mate Series, Voice Pal, Mega Wolf, Voice Mate, Hawk, and Finger Fonicks, among others, are dedicated AAC devices which have touch membranes. Nondedicated adapted computer keyboards that use touch membranes include Intellikeys, TASH Mini Keyboard, and Discover: Board. The DynaVox is a dedicated AAC device with a touch screen surface. It operates similarly to the Touch Window which attaches to microcomputers to provide a touch screen surface. Touch screens can also be added to standard computer monitors through a process available from Troll Technologies, among other companies.

The primary benefit of using a device with mechanically depressed keys is the tactile feedback that the user receives when pressing the keys. Some children and adults demonstrate better access when using devices that provide a physical sensation of movement for each key press. The drawback of using mechanical key depression is that it requires a set minimal force and pressure for the user to physically activate the key. Many individuals with low muscle tone are unable to apply enough pressure. In contrast, touch membrane surfaces require very little pressure for activation. In many cases, touch membrane activation is achieved by using a light touch for a set duration of time. Because touch membrane surfaces

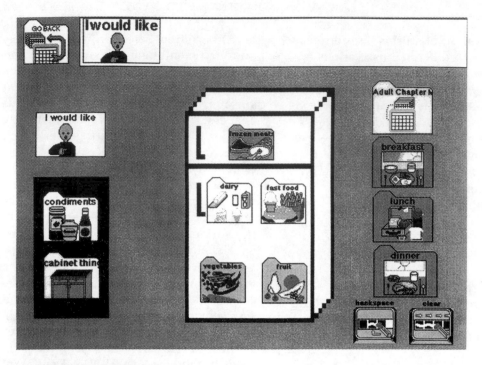

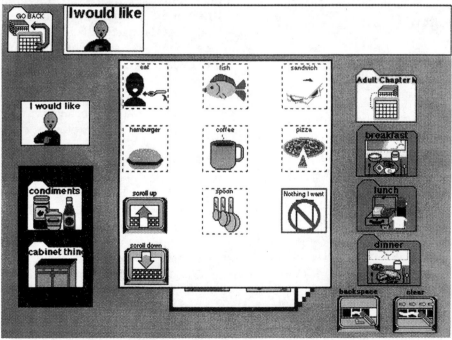

Figure 3–2. Dynavox2C dynamic display pages. Users select from an array of food category symbols (top). Fast Foods is selected. The display on the Dynavox2C changes to an array of fast food menu choices (bottom). The scroll buttons are used to view more selections in the category. After a selection is made, the fast food menu will close and the user will see the display in A once again. (Photo courtesy of Sentient Systems Technology).

do not give any tactile feedback when a key activation occurs, other auditory or visual feedback methods are usually added. Feedback might include an auditory beep, or a blinking symbol.

In addition to dedicated augmentative communication systems, desktop and laptop computers can easily be adapted to perform communication functions through direct selection. These adaptations typically involve adding augmentative communication software and other software and hardware peripherals such as keyguards, speech synthesizers, or adapted keyboards. Talk About , Write Out Loud, Speaking Dynamically, and Intellitalk, are direct selection software programs that can be used for augmentative communication on the Macintosh. EZ Keys, Talking Screen, and Handi Chat are similar programs for IBM operating system platforms.

Switch-Activated Direct Selection Systems

There are several direct selection AAC devices that rely on switches as substitutes for the keyboard (see Figure 3–3). These devices are often called switch-activated input systems. Depending on the device, up to 12 different switches can be plugged into the system. Pressing the switch activates a corresponding message. The Speak Easy, AlphaTalker, Voice Pal, AIPS Wolf, Lynx, and Voice Mate are examples of switch-activated direct selection devices. The benefit of switch-activated systems is that they provide a method of direct selection for individuals who do not have the physical capability to access a more traditional keyboard. Switches can be spaced farther apart than keys on a keyboard. The use of a wide variety of switches gives flexibility in the body part that activates the switch, the amount of pressure required to activate the switch, and the movement required to activate the switch. The drawback to these systems is that the user is limited to accessing fewer than 12 messages at any one time. In addition, the use of multiple switches connected to a device by multiple switch cables can be unwieldy. Switch-activated systems are typically used for nonspeaking individuals with

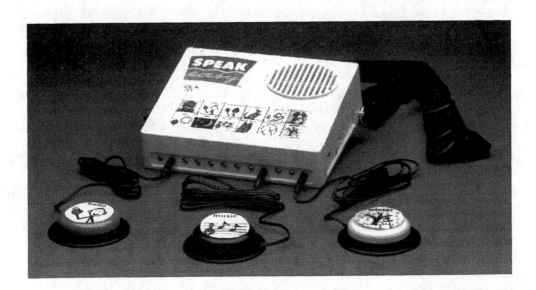

Figure 3–3. Speak Easy AAC system. Photograph courtesy of Ablenet.

limited physical capabilities, who only require a limited number of messages at any one time.

Light and Optical Direct Selection Pointers

There are many methods of accessing direct selection devices through light or optical pointer systems. The most cost-effective method uses a Class II laser light pointer which shines a small focused red beam of light onto the surface of a communication system. The beam is powerful enough to be used across a room to point to persons or objects. Laser light pointers designed for pointing to charts during speeches and presentations can often be purchased for a reasonable price from office supply stores. Laser light pointers can also be obtained with rechargeable battery packs which allow them to be used over longer periods of time. Class II laser light pointers can cause eye injuries if used incorrectly (Salamo & Jakobs, 1996). These light pointers should never be directly pointed at an open eye for more than 1 second. Most individuals will reflexively blink when a laser light pointer is shined into the eye, which provides protection from injury. Nonspeaking light pointer users often do not have the physical ability to independently remove their own light pointers and shine them into their own eyes. However, other individuals in the user's environment might remove the laser light and use it inappropriately. Class IIIa laser light pointers are also commercially available, and can cause eye injury before reflexive blinking occurs. To date, no eye injuries have been medically reported for either type of laser light pointer (Salamo & Jakobs, 1996).

Other light pointers aren't really "lights" at all. The Delta Talker uses a reflective mirror on the pointer, which catches a beam from a red light-emitting-diode (LED) beside each symbol and reflects the beam back to the device to signal a message. When the pointer is aimed between LEDs, there is no visible light signal observable to the user. Other methods of making selections with a pointer involve sonar and infrared technology. The pointer of a sonar device produces a sound signal that cannot be heard by humans. A sensor located on the AAC device reads the location of the sonar pointer. The HeadMaster system works with Macintosh computers and is a sonar pointer system. Infrared signals are similar to those used in TV remote controls. Infrared technology uses imperceptible high frequency light beams emitted by the pointer, which are received by a sensor located near the AAC device. Freewheel, which is an IBM access method, uses infrared pointer technology. The Liberator can also be accessed using an infrared pointer.

Typically light and optical pointers are mounted on a user's head, preferably at midline, but sometimes toward the side. Headbands, hats, and glasses can be used to mount the pointers. Light pointers can also be held in a user's hands. This is a beneficial method of direct selection for individuals with good fine motor control but limited range of movement with their hands. Use of light or optical pointers requires good motor abilities. The user must be able to control small head movements to direct the beam onto a symbol choice, and then must hold the beam steady for a period of time to activate the selection. This need for fine movement and lack of tactile feedback make light and optical pointers more difficult to control than head stick pointers. A head stick gives the user direct physical feedback for each selection, has a pointer that is visible to the user at all times, and allows for more involuntary movement when making selections. However, head sticks are not cosmetically appealing to some users.

Eye Gaze Direct Selection

Direct selection pointing can also be achieved through the use of eye gaze. Eye gaze can be used to point to objects or pictures on lite technology systems. Symbols are arranged onto a clear plexiglass board

called an E-Tran. The E-Tran allows the user and listener to stand on either side of the board, yet follow eye gaze movements clearly. Some E-Tran boards are held stationary, with symbols arranged on the periphery (see Figure 3–4). The user and listener look at symbols while sitting in

Fixed Eyegaze Display

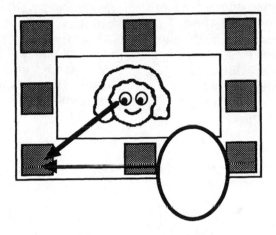

Dynamic Eyegaze Display

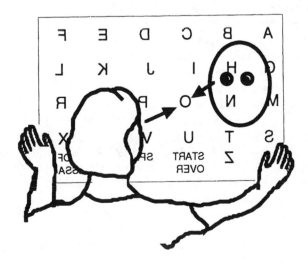

Figure 3–4. Fixed and dynamic eye gaze displays.

stationary positions looking through the board. Another method of using E-Tran boards is to use a dynamic moving eye gaze display. This method requires the listener to hold the board for the user. The user then locks his or her eye gaze on a target and continues to visually track the target while the listener moves the board. The listener looks at the user's eyes while moving the board. When the user's and listener's eye gaze lock together through the E-Tran, the symbol that both are looking at is selected. This method allows for more symbols to be placed onto the E-Tran board. Eye gaze systems can be designed to communicate hundreds of symbols through the use of encoding methods (Goosens & Crain, 1986).

Methods of Adjusting Direct Selection Systems

Many nonspeaking persons require extensive adaptations to direct selection systems to make the AAC device accessible. Most dedicated and nondedicated AAC systems have many points of adjustment that can be made. Key sensitivity can be adjusted by increasing the length of time the key must be held before activation occurs. Individuals with tremor often accidentally produce multiple activations of keys by hitting the same key repeatedly during the activation process. Many AAC systems have a method of setting a time period between key activations. Any activations produced before the time period has ended are ignored.

For users who need to rest their hands or pointers on the surface of the AAC device, systems can sometimes be altered to activate symbols when the pointer is lifted from the surface of the device rather than when the pointer first touches the device. This strategy is called release activation, and it allows users to move their hands across the surface of the system without accidentally activating symbols. Once the

desired symbol is reached, lifting the hand produces the activation.

Some users of optical pointer systems have difficulty keeping the beam focused on a target for a sufficient length of time. The time necessary for activating a key can be reduced, but if it is reduced too much, many accidental key activations will occur. Some AAC devices use an averaging function for direct selection to circumvent this problem. When averaging is used, multiple selections of the same key are added together until a predetermined threshold is hit. At that time, the key activation is triggered. This allows the user to swipe across the target several times before activing the key. Averaging can also be used with other methods of direct selection, but is not as common.

Feedback information provided to the user can also be varied on most AAC devices. Tactile feedback is available on devices with mechanical key activation. Auditory feedback is frequently provided by adding click or beep sounds when keys are selected. Some devices provide auditory feedback by immediately speaking the message associated with the key. Finally, some devices provide visual feedback. For example, Prentke Romich AAC devices have small LED lights next to each symbol. The devices can be set up to blink when keys are activated.

The size of keys can be altered, usually in multiples that divide the surface of the device into smaller areas (e.g., 2, 4, 8, 16, 32, 64, 128 keys). Keys can be spaced by not programming every location, leaving blank keys or dead areas between active keys. Keyguards, which are plastic or plexiglass overlays with holes cut out for each key, can be placed on top of the keyboard of most AAC devices. Keyguards let users stabilize their hands or other pointing mechanisms on top of the keyboard during the pointing process. The users entire hand can rest on the device, yet not activate a symbol until a selection is made by pointing to a key through the keyguard hole. When keyguards are used with small key sizes, they can visually block the user from easily viewing the keys. Clear plastic droolguards are also available for users who require them.

In summary, there are many different methods of using and adapting direct selection AAC devices. The AAC assessment process requires reviewing all potential access methods and adjusting those methods to obtain optimum speed and accuracy for the user. Chapters 5 and 7 in this text reviews these assessment methods in more detail.

Strengths and Limitations of Direct Selection Systems

Direct selection AAC systems are typically faster and more efficient methods of communication than scanning AAC systems. Users of direct selection systems can average speeds of 13 to 43 words per minute when communicating (Foulds, 1980; Szeto, Allen, & Littrell, 1993). Adding encoding or prediction methods designed to reduce keystrokes often speeds up the communication process even more, sometimes reducing the number of keystrokes by 50% (Higginbotham, 1992; Venkatagiri, 1993). However, it should be noted that these communication speeds are still slow when compared to speaking rates for nondisabled individuals (126 to 200 words per minute).

Portability of direct selection AAC systems is an issue for ambulatory individuals. Many children and adults with good ambulation skills cannot reasonably carry an 8 to 10 pound device from location to location. Children and adults who are not steady ambulators, or who require walkers and canes for support, have even more difficulty carrying an AAC device. Several lightweight AAC devices have been designed to address this problem, including the Parrot, Canon Communicator, Walker Talker, Message Mate, Language Master SE, Voice Mate, and Finger Foniks. Manufacturers of AAC devices are aware of porta-

bility issues and have made a concerted effort to design newer systems that are lighter in weight and smaller in size.

Indirect Selection Methods

Many physically disabled individuals do not have the motor abilities necessary for operating direct selection AAC devices. These individuals require devices which are accessed using scanning or other indirect selection methods. As reviewed previously, scanning methods systematically present selections to users, who activate switches or other mechanisms to choose the desired selection. Many dedicated and nondedicated AAC devices can be adapted for scanning. These include the AlphaTalker, Delta Talker, DigiVox, Macaw, DynaVox, Liberator, Real Voice, Voice Pal Plus, Light Writer SL8, and Scan It All. Microcomputers can also be adapted for augmentative communication access through scanning methods. Talking Screen, Speaking Dynamically, Scanning WSKE, Ke:nx, Handi Chat, and Talk About are all software programs that can be configured for scanning users. These devices and software programs can be adapted to use many different methods of scanning which will be reviewed in this section.

Single Switch Scanning Methods

Single switch scanning methods allow individuals to use a simple repetitive motor movement to activate a single switch to control an AAC system. Scanning systems operated with a single switch usually offer several different methods of presenting symbol choices to the user for selection. The simplest methods of scanning are linear and circular scanning. Linear scanning involves presenting symbol choices to the user one at a time in a line-by-line pattern (see Figure 3–5). The user hits a switch when the desired selection is reached. All possible choices are scanned using this

AAC SCANNING PATTERNS

Circular Scanning

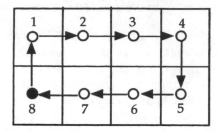

Linear Scanning

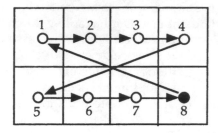

Row Column Scanning

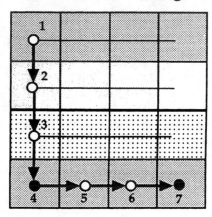

Group Item Scanning

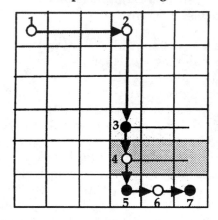

◯ White dots indicate "wait" scanning locations to reach the last display symbol during automatic scanning.

● Black dots indicate switch activation locations to reach the last display symbol during automatic scanning.

Figure 3–5. AAC scanning patterns.

one-at-a-time approach. Circular scanning is similar except that the presentation of symbols follows a circular pattern. A Clock Communicator is a lite technology method of using circular scanning. The clock hand moves in one direction and passes over every symbol on the face of the clock. The user waits for the clock hand to point to the desired symbol, then hits a switch to indicate the choice. Linear and circular scanning are cognitively easy to learn since they only require a one-step switch selection process. However, because the device must individually scan through all possible choices, these methods of scanning are extremely slow and are only recommended for AAC systems with a limited number of symbol choices.

In order to speed up the scanning process, multiple symbol choices have to be simultaneously presented to the user. This is achieved through several different scanning methods. The most commonly used method is row-column scanning. In row-column scanning, an entire row of symbols is presented at once. The rows are scanned through in sequence until a switch activation is made. At that time, the device scans individually through all symbols in the selected row. The user must then make a second switch activation when the desired symbol is reached (see Figure 3–5). The switch activation process for row-column scanning is a two-step task. Some AAC devices use the opposite approach and offer column-row scanning.

Group-item scanning is a variation of row-column scanning that can take many forms. In group-item scanning, large groups of symbols are presented at once. The user activates the switch when the desired group is reached. The symbols within the selected group are then scanned. At this point the AAC system might scan smaller groupings within the originally selected area by row-column methods or by group-area methods. The scanned groups get gradually smaller until the device scans item-by-item through the smallest symbol group (see Figure 3–5). Group-item scanning usually involves at least a three- to four-step scanning process. This scanning method is cognitively the most difficult for users to master, but offers efficiency when many symbols are needed on the AAC system.

Single switch scanning methods also vary in terms of how the switch is used during the scanning process. One technique is known as automatic scanning. During automatic scanning, the AAC device presents symbol choices while the user waits. Once the desired symbol is reached, the switch is pressed once for selection. Directed scanning is the opposite of automatic scanning. During directed scanning, the user presses the switch con-

tinuously to move the AAC device cursor through the scanning choices. Once the desired choice is reached, the user releases the switch. Step scanning is another variation of the switch activation process. Step scanning requires the user to press the switch to move the system cursor to the next symbol choice. The switch is pressed repeatedly to move the cursor through the choices. Once the desired symbol is reached, the user stops pressing the switch.

These three switch selection methods have their own strengths and weaknesses. Automatic scanning requires less physical movement for the user, as the switch only has to be pressed once when a desired choice is reached. However, the user must be able to wait patiently through the scanning process. Many young children do not have the attention span necessary to passively wait for the AAC system to get to the desired symbol choice. Directed and step scanning methods require more physical ability than automatic scanning. This is especially true for step scanning, which requires multiple switch presses, and can be fatiguing for many individuals with physical disabilities. However, these two methods put the user in control of cursor movement, and make scanning a more active cognitive process. Step scanning is especially beneficial for very young children who require immediate feedback that their switch activations are controlling the AAC system.

Joystick and Multiple Switch Scanning Methods

AAC systems can be operated using a combination of two or more switches, or joysticks. Joysticks are used to control the movement of the cursor on the AAC device. A joystick feeds vertical and horizontal movement coordinates to the AAC system to control the direction of the cursor. The speed of cursor movement and starting point for cursor movement can usually be changed to accomodate different user capabilities. Standard joysticks consist of a small stationary box with a moveable control stick (see Figure 3–6). Using a joystick to control an AAC system requires more physical ability than using a single switch. The user must be able to control the directional movement of the joystick, and maintain continuous physical contact on the joystick until the desired symbol is reached. Many physically disabled indi-

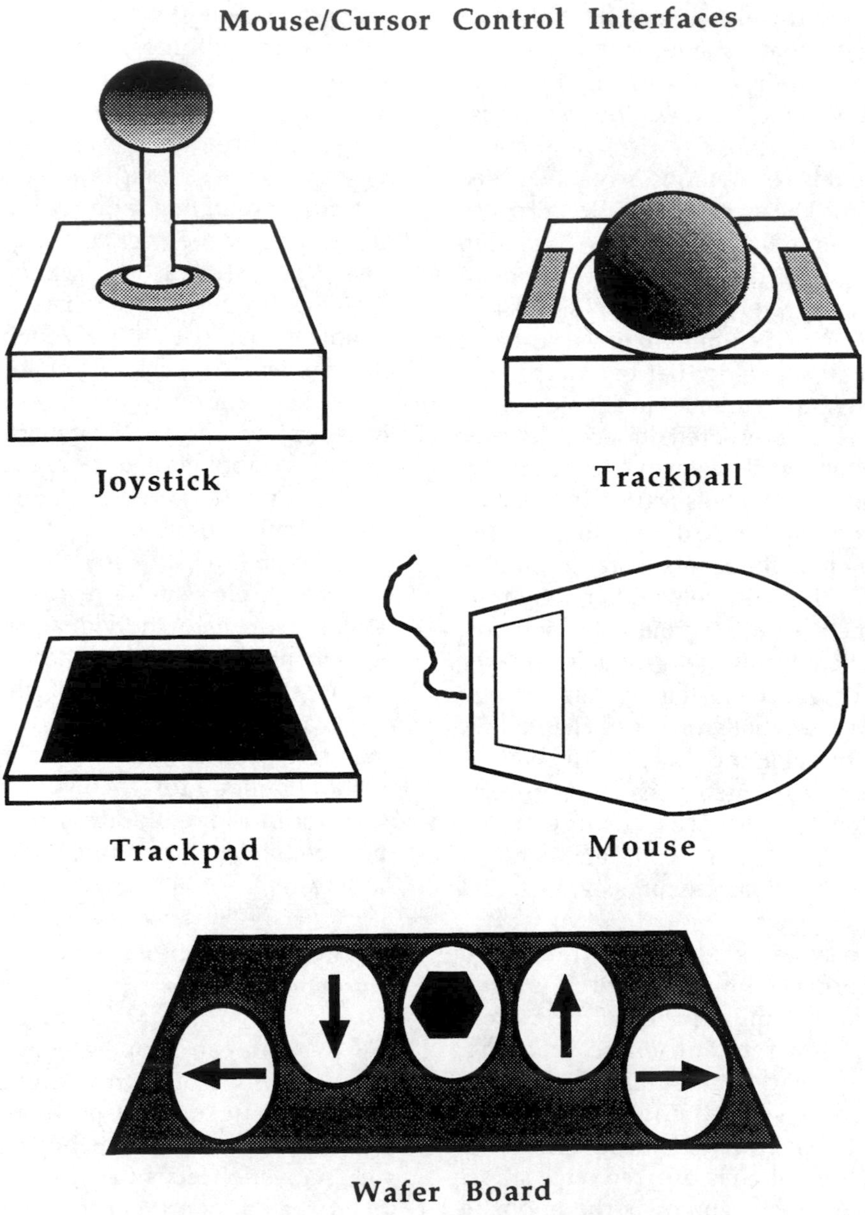

Mouse/Cursor Control Interfaces

Joystick

Trackball

Trackpad

Mouse

Wafer Board

Figure 3–6. Mouse and cursor control interfaces.

viduals who are able to control a joystick on a power chair have difficulty controlling a joystick well enough to operate an AAC system. When using a power chair, the driver usually has room to sway from side to side if an even forward directional pressure cannot be maintained. On a computer screen or AAC system, these changes in direction often produce large jumps as the cursor moves from side to side. Joystick cursor control for AAC devices requires good fine motor abilities.

Joysticks designed to work with computers or AAC systems are known as microswitch joysticks. These joysticks have simple on-off mechanisms to indicate which direction the joystick is pointing. The cursor moves at a preset speed and direction when the joystick is pushed. Proportional joysticks are designed to work with power wheelchairs. Proportional joysticks allow for fine gradations in the speed and angle of movement (Harryman & Warren, 1992). Plugging a proportional joystick directly into an AAC system will usually result in an electrical malfunction, and sometimes will completely short out the device. This causes difficulty for a user who wishes to use a single joystick to control both a power chair and an AAC system. Several power chair companies manufacture environmental control units designed to work with their chairs. The proportional joystick sends signals to the environmental control unit, which then translates the signals into a microswitch form to send to the AAC system or computer.

There are several variations of joysticks that can be used with dedicated and nondedicated AAC devices. Standard joysticks can be used alone, or in combination with a single switch. When using the joystick alone, the user pushes the joystick until the desired symbol is reached; releasing the joystick selects the symbol. Users who might accidently release a joystick can press a single switch once they reach the desired symbol selection. A trackball, trackpad, or mouse can be used instead of a joystick to operate some AAC systems (see Figure 3–6). This is especially true for nondedicated computer-based systems. A trackball is a stationary box with a large or small ball built into the surface. Moving the ball controls directional cursor movements on the screen. Many laptop computers have trackballs built into the keyboard. Trackpads have small touch areas to control cursor movements. The user moves a finger along the touch area in the direction that the cursor needs to move. A mouse can also be used to select choices on a computer-based AAC system. Using a mouse requires more range of motion than either a joystick, trackpad, or trackball.

Multiple switch scanning is a technique used with individuals who have the physical and cognitive capability to progress beyond single switch scanning, but do not have enough physical control to operate a joystick or direct selection system. Multiple switch scanning simulates joystick movements by using several different switches to direct movements of the AAC device cursor. A wafer board is a multiple switch access method (see Figure 3–6). Four switches control directional movement of the cursor, and the fifth switch is used to confirm the selected choice. Individuals with more limited physical abilities might use two-switch scanning processes. In two-switch scanning, one switch controls vertical movements of the cursor, the second switch controls horizontal movements.

More Scanning Variations

The scanning process cognitively requires the nonspeaking user to maintain attention to the AAC system throughout the symbol selection process. For some users, the rate of scanning is so slow that the symbol selection process can take several minutes. One method of reducing the visual attention necessary for using an AAC device is to use auditory scanning. Auditory scanning was initially developed for visually impaired users who could not track the scanning process. During auditory scanning, the user is given an auditory cue as selections are scanned. The cue might be a row/column location (i.e., *Row One, Row Two, Row Three . . .*) or a category cue (i.e., *Things to Eat, Things to Wear, Places to Go . . .*), or a symbol name (i.e., *Hamburger, Hotdog, Chicken Nuggets . . .*). Selecting a symbol choice results in communicating a message that may be the same or different as the auditory scanning cue (i.e., I *want a Big Mac, Get me a hotdog to go,* and *Chicken nuggets would be great*). Dedicated AAC devices that offer auditory scanning features include the Liberator, DynaVox, Whisper Wolf, Lynx, Digivox, and AlphaTalker. Several of these devices allow the use of one "voice" for the auditory cue, and a different "voice" for messages. Auditory scanning combined with visual scanning is useful for very young children who are first learning the scanning process. The auditory cue helps to keep them attuned to the symbol choices despite their limited attention to task.

Predictive scanning is used to speed up the symbol selection process. This scanning method limits the scanned symbols to those that are predicted to be selected next. Devices that use predictive scanning begin by only scanning symbol locations that have message information. Blank locations are not scanned. Once an initial symbol is selected, the device then only scans symbols that are used in sequence with the original selection. Other symbols are not scanned unless the user fails to make a selection from the predicted choices. The Liberator, Dynavox, and AlphaTalker, can be adapted to use predictive scanning methods. While predictive scanning is faster than other scanning methods, it is sometimes difficult for young children to follow as the scanning pattern is different each time a symbol is selected.

Morse Code Switch Systems

Several dedicated and nondedicated AAC systems can be adapted to use Morse code as an input method. These include the Real Voice, Light Talker, Morse Code WSKE, Handi Code, and Ke:nx. Standard Morse code requires that a user combine a series of dots (dits) and dashes (dahs) to communicate letters and punctuation markers. This input method can be adapted to single or two-switch operation modes. For a single switch user, the timing of switch activations is used to convey dots and dashes. Shorter activations are usually dots, longer activations are used to convey dashes. Two-switch users have one switch representing the dot, and the other the dash.

Morse code can also be used as a lite technology system with listeners who know the system well. Mary was a young woman with severe quadriplegia following a stroke. Her family was so adept at interpreting Morse code that they rarely attached her switches to her AAC device. Instead she simply pressed the two switches while her family translated the Morse code for other listeners. Not only was her family skilled at translating the code, they were also skilled interpreters who did not interrupt her messages with their own comments. Over a period of time, her family metamorphized themselves into portable, voice output, switch-activated, biological AAC devices!

Methods of Adjusting Scanning Techniques

Many of the techniques that can be used to adjust AAC devices for different scanning methods have already been mentioned. These include changing the scanning pattern, changing the switch activation method, using multiple switches, and adding auditory or predictive scanning. In addition, other adjustments can also be made. Scanning AAC systems allow for changes in the scanning speed, and changes in the length of time the switch needs to be pressed to trigger activation. In addition, many systems have methods of correcting accidental switch activations. If the user accidentally presses the switch, quickly pressing it a second time will negate the switch activation and start the scanning process over again.

After a symbol selection is made, the response of the AAC system can also vary. Some devices can be configured to automatically continue the scanning process at the point where the last symbol was chosen. Other options include automatically beginning the scanning process at a consistent starting point. Finally, AAC scanning systems can be configured to stop scanning after a symbol is selected. The user needs to hit the switch again to initiate the scanning process.

Strengths and Limitations of the Scanning Process

AAC systems that use scanning as an access method have strengths and limitations that are almost the opposite of direct selection systems. The strength of scanning is its ability to be used as an access method for individuals with limited physical abilities. If a user is able to make a single replicable movement, that movement can usually be adapted for switch access. The major limitation of using scanning approaches is the rate of communication. Users of single switch scanning methods have average communication rates of only 8 to 24 words per minute. Two switch scanning and joystick methods of access are faster, averaging 18 to 26 words per minute. However, direct selection systems are still faster, averaging 13 to 43 words per minute (Szeto et al., 1993).

Because of the slow rates of communication associated with scanning, direct selection AAC systems are usually preferred. However, some users who are physically capable of operating direct selection AAC systems benefit from using scanning systems. Individuals who fatigue easily initially have the strength and ability to operate a direct selection device but sometimes lose that ability after a few minutes. Scanning systems can circumvent these fatigue factors. Sometimes individuals can access direct selection sytems but have extremely slow access times. They can sometimes access a system faster when using scanning at a rapid rate. Finally, some individuals have good range of motion for direct selection, but are unable to accurately select a target symbol within that range. Once again, scanning systems should be considered during the assessment process.

Switches

Switches are required to activate scanning AAC systems. There are a wide variety of switches available commercially. In addition, many how-to books have been written that describe how to make homemade switches (Burkhart, 1982). If a nonspeaking individual is able to move a body part, and can control and replicate the movement, then a switch can usually be used to access an AAC device. Chapter 7 reviews methods of evaluation to determine the best method of switch access.

Switches vary in terms of the body movement necessary to activate the switch, the mechanism that triggers switch activation, and the pressure or length of touch necessary to activate the switch. In addition, switches also vary in terms of the kind of feedback given to the user. Some switches produce a mechanical physical movement that provides tactile feedback. Other switches provide auditory feedback in the form of clicks or tones when the switch is activated. Switches can also be designed to provide visual feedback by using a light that is activated when the switch is pressed.

Pressure switches are designed to be used with persons with high to normal muscle tone using body movement and force to activate the switch. These switches require that the user press or push the switch to produce an activation. The switches vary in the amount of pressure necessary to activate the switch. Switches with higher pressures are extremely durable and are designed to work with individuals with extremely high tone who may not be able to control the strength of their sudden movements. Switches with lower activation pressures are usually less durable, but easier to activate. Pressure switches also vary in the amount of surface area available. The Plate Switch from Toys for Special Children, Square Pad from Tash, and Big Red Switch from Ablenet are three switches that have especially large surface areas for activation. Most manufacturers give information on the amount of pressure necessary to activate the switch and the size of the switch in their catalogues and information brochures. Figure 3–7 from Church and Glennen (1992) illustrates several commercially available pressure switches.

Individuals with lower tone require switches that are sensitive to minimal motor movements. Some pressure switches require minimal force to produce activations. These include Zygo's Leaf Switch and Lever Switch, along with TASH's MicroLight Switch among others (see Figure 3–7). Other switches use a touch membrane surface for activation. A minimal amount of pressure applied to the touch membrane surface for a specified period of time activates the switch. TASH produces a Plate Switch which comes in four different colors with touch membrane surfaces. Finally, some switches use the skin's electroconductive capabilities to activate the switch mechanism. AdapTech manufactures Taction Pads which are flat pliable wires or stickers that can be wrapped around objects. Touching the pads on the objects activates the switch.

Other switches are designed for individuals with spinal cord injuries or other motor disorders which result in paralysis. These switches do not require touch for activation. The Blink Switch from Innocomp uses an infrared light beam (see Figure 3–8). When the light beam is "broken" the switch is activated. This switch is typically used by aiming the infrared beam toward the user's eye. The surface of the eye reflects the beam back to the light source. Blinking the eye causes a break in the light beam's reflection and activates the switch. It can also be used by passing a body part over the beam to break the light source. Sip- and-puff switches are used by individuals with high level spinal cord injuries. These switches use breath inhalations and exhalations for activation. Typically, a sip produces one type of activation, and a puff another. Mercury switches are used with individuals who can move body parts, but do not have sufficient pressure or accuracy to touch a pressure switch. The mercury switch works similar to a carpenter's level. If the switch is held in balance, no activation occurs. Tilting the switch out of balance results in an activation. Because of this movement, mercury switches are often called Tip Switches. Finally, Prentke Romich manufactures a P-Switch which consists of a piezo-electric sensor that is strapped onto the user's body (see Figure 3–8). Any muscle tensing or movement can be picked up by the sensor. The sensor can be strapped onto the forehead, cheek, jaw, or around arm and leg muscles. The sensitivity of the switch sensor can be adjusted.

Most switches are single switches, in that they produce a simple on/off activation signal to control the AAC system. Some switches are dual switches, in that they can perform more than one function. The sip-and-puff switch is a dual switch, as the sip produces one type of activation, and the puff another. The Rocking Lever Switch is another example of a dual pres-

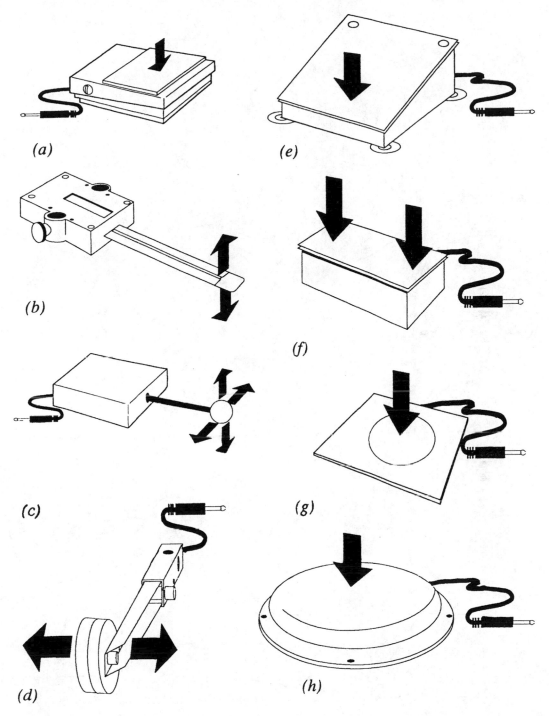

Figure 3–7. Adaptive Switches. (a) Zygo Tread Switch; (b) Zygo Leaf Switch; (c) Toys for Special Children's Ultimate Switch, or Prentke Romich Wobble Switch; (d) Zygo Lever Switch; (e) Toys for Special Children's Plate Switch; (f) Prentke Romich Rocking Lever Switch; (g) TASH Plate Membrane Switch; (h) Able Net Big Red Switch. Note: from G. Church and S. Glennen, (Eds.) 1992. *The Handbook of Assistive Technology*, San Diego: Singular Publishing. Reprinted by permission.

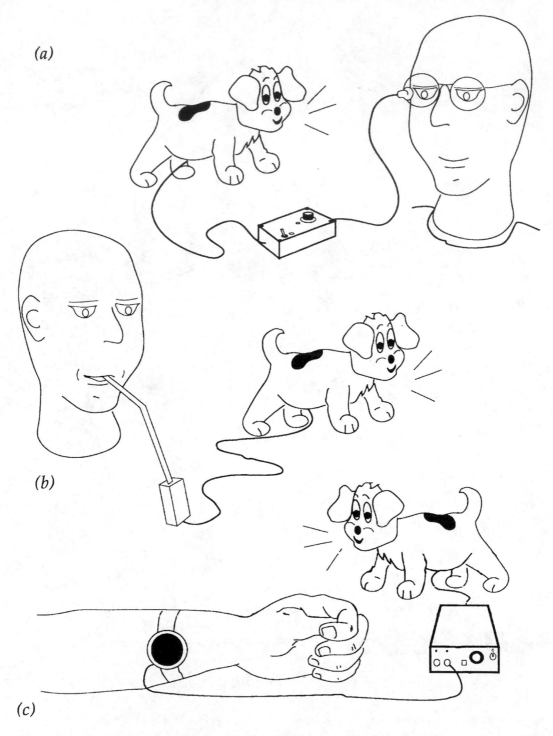

Figure 3–8. Switches for individuals with low tone or paralysis. (a) Blink Switch; (b) Sip and Puff switch; and (c) Prentke Romich's P-Switch. Note: from G. Church and S. Glennen, (Eds.), 1992. *The Handbook of Assistive Technology.* San Diego: Singular Publishing. Reprinted by permission.

sure switch. Pressing one side produces one type of activation, the other side produces a different signal. Dual switches need to be used in AAC devices that are designed to receive both switch signals. Dual switches can be used to perform an on/off control function. That is, one type of activation turns the AAC system on and off, the other controls the scanning process. Dual switches are also used for Morse code, and for two switch scanning.

MESSAGE STORAGE AND RETRIEVAL METHODS

When nonspeaking individuals use picture communication boards to convey messages, each symbol on the board has a single meaning. To produce messages that go beyond the single meaning level, the symbols need to be sequenced together. Pictures can be strung together in sequence to communicate a novel message (i.e., *Boy + Go + Car*), or individual alphabet letters can be sequenced into words and sentences to communicate messages. Although this is an effective form of communication, it is not always efficient. Simple picture communication boards require the user to access a large number of symbols in order to combine them into various communicative messages. Many persons with physical disabilities cannot access a large array of small symbol choices. When spelling, the number of symbols is reduced, but the user is required to make many selections to convey a single thought. For individuals with slow access times, letter spelling is extremely slow and fatiguing. Because of these limitations, high technology AAC systems were developed that use complex message storage and retrieval methods designed to make the communication process more efficient. Message storage and retrieval techniques allow the user to access frequently used messages quickly, to access many messages through a limited symbol

set, and to increase the speed and complexity of communication. The most commonly used message storage and retrieval strategies will be reviewed in this section.

Communication through letter spelling gives a nonspeaking individual the ability to create any novel message at any time. However, this process requires literacy skills that many children and developmentally disabled adults have not acquired. In addition, letter spelling entire messages requires a large number of keystrokes to communicate simple messages such as *Hello how are you?* (14 letters, 1 punctuation marker, 3 spaces, and 1 shift = 19 keystrokes). Some high technology AAC devices get around these difficulties by allowing the user to prestore or preprogram frequently used messages. Prestored messages are useful for communicating routine messages that can be predicted ahead of time. The user simply presses a single key or combination of keys to produce the message. For example, *Hello how are you?* could be stored under a single key with a waving hand picture symbol. Prestored messages can range from lengthy narratives to sentences, phrases, words, and word fragments. There are several different methods for storing and retrieving prestored messages.

The purpose of message storage and retrieval systems is to provide a method for delivering maximum communication with minimum effort. In the previous example (i.e., Waving Hand Symbol = Hello how are you?), an entire message is communicated with minimum effort. However, if each key of the AAC system is capable of communicating only a single message, the goal of maximum communication could not be achieved. By using a 1 key = 1 message approach, the user is limited to communicating a small number of messages. An AAC device with 32 picture symbols would only produce 32 messages. Although this is certainly fine for very young children, or severely cognitively delayed individuals, 32 messages would be extremely limiting to most nonspeaking persons. Considering that speaking children have average vocabularies of 50 words by the age of 18 months, and 150 to 300 words by age 2, the limitations of this method of message retrieval are apparent (Owens, 1988).

One method of increasing the number of available communicative messages is to create different levels or pages of symbols within the AAC system. Each level consists of different picture symbols, with the number of symbols limited by the number of keys available on that level. Several different AAC devices offer the option of levels as a way of increasing communication. These include the DigiVox, Macaw, Wolf, Holly.Com, VOIS 160 and Say It Simply Plus, among others. In addition, devices that use Minspeak operating systems (Alpha Talker, Delta Talker, Walker Talker and Liberator), and the DynaVox can be programmed to create separate levels. Although use of levels increases the total number of messages that can be programmed into the AAC system, the number of messages that can be accessed at any one time is still limited. The use of levels works well for children or adults who have a number of different environments and activities that require a limited number of specialized messages (i.e., circle time, cooking, watching videos, reading books, and playing with dolls). Specific levels, with accompanying pages of picture symbols, can be developed for each activity. Typically, adults in the user's environment have to change AAC device levels for the user and must also change the available picture symbol overlay. This again makes the use of levels limiting for those who have more vocabulary needs.

To give the AAC user constant access to a maximum number of prestored messages, the AAC device must use strategies that provide maximum communication with a minimum number of keystrokes. Currently, two different methods are used

to acheive this goal, acceleration techniques and prediction strategies.

Acceleration Techniques

Acceleration techniques are message storage and retrieval methods that limit the number of keystrokes by encoding all messages into two or three keystroke sequences. Acceleration techniques can be used with picture symbols, letters, written words, and other symbol systems.

Picture-Based Acceleration Techniques

Many different AAC systems use picture-based acceleration techniques. Picture based acceleration involves prestoring messages under a sequence of two or three picture symbols. For example, the message *Hello how are you?* might be encoded using the picture symbol sequence of *Waving Hand + Pointing Finger*. Although this strategy seems simple, it can provide the user with a large number of messages using a minimum number of keys. On a 32 symbol AAC device, if each picture symbol was combined into a sequence with every other symbol, the number of messages that could potentially be accessed would equal 1,024.

Picture symbol sequences can range from simple concrete sequences to those that require abstract associations. A simple concrete sequence is one in which the pictures combine to form a direct referent to the message. For example, *I'm hungry* might be sequenced as *I/Me + Eat*. A more abstract picture sequence might encode the same message as *Eye + Horse*. The language skills of the user often limits the level of abstractness that can be developed into the sequences. Very young children require systems with limited concrete sequences, older children and adults can often learn abstract picture sequences that are based on rhyming, grammatical, or category-based associations. The more abstract the sequences become for the user, the more the individual must rely on memory to recall and use the sequences.

Bruce Baker was the first to develop the concept of sequencing picture symbols together as an encoding system (Baker, 1986). This system was patented under the name Minspeak. AAC devices available from Prentke Romich Company use the Minspeak operating system (AlphaTalker, Delta Talker, Walker Talker, and Liberator). The basic tenet of Minspeak is the concept that a single picture symbol can serve as a referent for many different ideas. For example, the picture symbol *Frog* can be a referent for the concepts of frog, green, jump, water, animal, insects, sore throat, and death (to croak). By linking each picture symbol to all possible referents, a limited set of pictures can be used to communicate a wide variety of messages (i.e., *Rainbow + Frog = Green; Frog + Arrow = Jump; Frog + Cup = Pond*). Other AAC devices also use picture symbols se-

quenced together to encode messages. The Macaw and Digivox among others, are dedicated AAC devices that can be programmed to use picture symbol sequences.

In order to aid vocabulary recall, many of the Minspeak picture systems rely on rule-based orderings to determine the picture symbol sequences. For example, all color words might start with the picture of a Rainbow combined with other pictures that indicate the specific color. Months of the year could start with a *Calendar* picture combined with a symbol referent for the specific month (Bruno, 1988) (see Table 3–1). Minspeak software programs which use rule-based strategies include Unity, Word Strategy, Interaction Education and Play+, Language Learning & Living, and Blissymbol Component Minspeak, among others. Readers are referred to Chapter 4 for further information about Minspeak.

The Dynavox is a dedicated AAC system that also offers picture symbol sequencing. However, instead of using a stat-

Table 3–1. Minspeak rule-based picture symbol sequencing used in the Interaction Education and Play Plus MAP System.

Months Vocabulary	First Symbol	Second Symbol	Rationale
January	Calendar	Baby	New Year's Baby
February	Calendar	Heart	Valentine's Day
March	Calendar	Lamb	March Goes Out Like a Lamb
April	Calendar	Umbrella	April Showers
May	Calendar	Lei	May Flowers
June	Calendar	Outside	Summertime
July	Calendar	Flag	Fourth of July
August	Calendar	Pool	Hot/Go Swimming
September	Calendar	Teacher	Back to School
October	Calendar	Witch	Halloween
November	Calendar	Dinner	Thanksgiving
December	Calendar	Santa Claus	Christmas

Source: "Interaction Education and Play Plus," by Joan Bruno (1988). Wooster, OH: Prentke Romich Company. Adapted with permission.

ic set display of pictures that never change, the Dynavox uses a touch screen with a constantly changing array of picture symbols (see Figure 3–2). The user initially touches a picture symbol on a menu page to indicate the desired message page. The screen automatically changes to a message page displaying different symbols representing the words, phrases, or sentences associated with the page. The user can then go back to the original menu page, or branch off to other associated message pages.

This dynamic display method of symbol sequencing is sometimes easier for individuals who have difficulty making abstract associations with a static set of picture symbols. For example, a child who can only access eight symbols at a time on a static display might request food choices by first selecting a Food symbol, followed by a second symbol related to the food item (see Figure 3–9). The limited number of symbols makes it necessary to rely on highly abstract concepts to retrieve some of the

Food Vocabulary Sequenced on a Static Display Using 8 Symbols

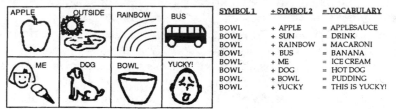

SYMBOL 1	+ SYMBOL 2	= VOCABULARY
BOWL	+ APPLE	= APPLESAUCE
BOWL	+ SUN	= DRINK
BOWL	+ RAINBOW	= MACARONI
BOWL	+ BUS	= BANANA
BOWL	+ ME	= ICE CREAM
BOWL	+ DOG	= HOT DOG
BOWL	+ BOWL	= PUDDING
BOWL	+ YUCKY	= THIS IS YUCKY!

Food Vocabulary Sequenced on a Dynamic Display Using 8 Symbols

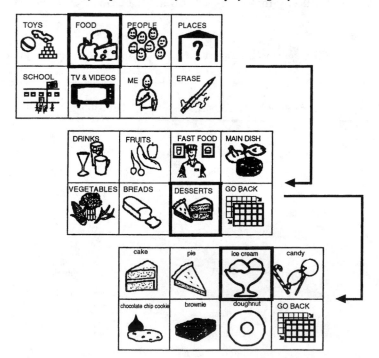

Figure 3–9. Eight location static and dynamic AAC displays. (Made with permission using Boardmaker International Software.)

words. On a dynamic eight symbol display, the child would select a Food symbol, branch to a page of food categories, then branch to a page with concrete pictures of specific foods (see Figure 3–9). The process of communicating with symbols organized into dynamic displays is often initially easier for young children to learn. However, the process still requires that the user comprehend the concepts of categorizing symbols together into word groupings, or functional groupings. Although the concept of categorizing foods into the categories of vegetables, fruits, and desserts is concrete to most adults, to a young 3-year-old the process is still relatively abstract. In addition, because the pictures on a dynamic display are constantly changing, the user must have good visual scanning skills.

There are several software programs for computers that offer variations of the category-based dynamic display picture symbol sequencing concept. These include Speaking Dynamically and Talking Screen. Both of these programs operate similarly to the Dynavox system. In addition, the Dynasyms system, which is the picture-based software used in the Dynavox, is also available for use on the computer.

Alphanumeric Acceleration Methods

The written alphabet and numeral system can also be used as an acceleration system. During the late 1970s Phonic Ear developed the HandiVoice 120 which had several hundred words and phrases encoded by two- and three-digit number sequences. For example, *Hello how are you?* might be encoded as *325*. Needless to say, the process of memorizing hundreds of number codes was a difficult task for most users. Later, several devices began using the alphabet to encode prestored messages. For example, *Hello how are you?* could be encoded as *H + H*. This technique is easier to memorize than number codes, but still requires good literacy and sequencing skills. In addition,

the alphabet codes that are used cannot be letter sequences that would normally occur as a word or within a word. For example, the sentence *I like school* could logically be encoded as *I + S*. However, because this sequence is also a word, every time the user typed the word *is*, the entire prestored message would be recalled. The Real Voice, and Carry Comm are dedicated AAC systems that use letter-based abbreviation expansion strategies. In addition, there are several programs for computers that also offer letter-based abbreviation expansion strategies. These include EZ Keys, Scanning WSKE, Co-Writer, WiVik 2.0, Screen Doors, Handi Word, and Mind Reader.

Some of these systems come from the manufacturer with a core of alphanumeric abbreviations already stored in the system. These factory-installed abbreviations can occasionally cause problems for some users. A youngster whose last name began with the letters *Aq* was set up with a computer-based AAC system using EZ Keys. The first time he tried to use his new system he proudly tried to write his name for his teacher. However, every time he typed *Aq* the word *Albuquerque* popped up on the screen. He would then begin the laborious process of deleting all of the letters in the word, but as soon as he began *Aq* again, the word *Albuquerque* would magically reappear. His teacher and family struggled for several days before calling the center that recommended the system. After a few minutes on the phone, the offending abbreviation was removed from the system and replaced with a new abbreviation that would automatically spell his last name when *Aq* was typed.

Sign Language Acceleration Systems

Sign language is currently being used as an encoding strategy on the VOIS 160 AAC system. The VOIS Shapes method of encoding was developed by Shane and Wilbur (1989). The premise of this encoding strategy is to take signs from American Sign Language and segment them into units that indicate the body location where the sign is made, the handshape used to make the sign, and the movement used to produce the sign. The unit segments are symbolized by various picture symbols on the communication system. By selecting location, handshape, and movement symbols, the device will then produce the encoded word. For example, to produce the word *drink*, the user would press keys representing a mouth location, C handshape, and tilting movement.

Sign language is often used as an unaided AAC strategy. With this in mind, it would appear that using sign language as an encoding method would tap into AAC skills already acquired by users of sign. However, in order to use VOIS Shapes the child must not only learn the original sign, but must be able to segment it into its units of handshape, location, and movement. Young children learning spoken languages typically cannot segment the spoken word into specific phonemic and linguistic units until they are 4 to 6 years of age. The process of segmenting a sign into its cheremic units requires similar levels of linguistic sophistication. This does not mean that young children cannot learn the VOIS Shapes system. However, knowledge of sign language may not be the only prerequisite skill needed to learn to use this acceleration system.

Other Acceleration Encoding Systems

A wide variety of encoding systems for acceleration have been developed for use with AAC devices. There are several strategies that rely on using two- and three-part combinations to convey a specific symbol to the listener. Many of these strategies were originally developed for users of eye gaze E-Tran communication systems. Goossens and Crain (1986) give an overview of many different methods of eye gaze encoding. One of the difficulties of using eye gaze for communication is the limited number of locations that can be looked at by the user. A typical E-Tran arrangement will have eight symbol locations arranged on clear plexiglass (see Figure 3–4). In order to expand beyond eight symbols, the user must use encoding methods.

A simple method of encoding is to place a grid of eight symbols into each of the eight areas of the E-Tran board to achieve a total of 64 symbols (see Figure 3–10). Within the grids, each symbol is colored a different color. Color markers are placed around the rim of the E-Tran. To indicate a specific picture symbol, the user first looks at the grid that contains the picture, then at the color of the picture within the grid. More complex encoding systems expand the number of pictures within the grid, and add additional steps to indicate the pictures. For example, a system might have grids of 16 symbols in each area arranged into four colored rows with four columns in the row. The user looks first at the grid, then at the color for the row, then at a number indicating the column.

Color- and number-based encoding strategies can also be used on electronic AAC systems that prestore messages into picture sequences. One example of a color-based strategy is to use color-coded picture sequences. Each location on the AAC device has four different small pictures with different background colors in the location (see Figure 3–11). The user first selects the location of the symbol group then selects a location representing the color of the picture. This method of sequencing is often beneficial for young children who cannot progress beyond simple concrete symbol choices, yet can match colors together.

Location/Color Encoding Eyegaze Board

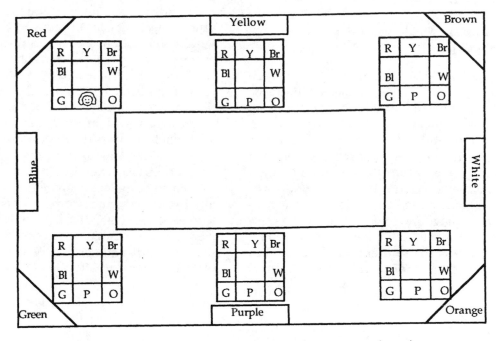

Figure 3-10. Location and color encoding eye gaze board.

Color Symbol Sequencing Using a 24 Location AAC Device

Red	Blue	Red	Blue	Red	Blue	Red	Blue	Red	Blue	**RED**	
Green	Yellow	Green	Yellow	Green	Yellow	Green	Yellow	Green	Yellow		
Red	Blue	Red	Blue	R	B	Red	Blue	Red	Blue	**BLUE**	
Green	Yellow	Green	Yellow	G	Y	Green	Yellow	Green	Yellow		
Red	Blue	Red	Blue	Red	Blue	Red	Blue	Red	Blue	**YELLOW**	
Green	Yellow	Green	Yellow	Green	Yellow	Green	Yellow	Green	Yellow		
Red	Blue	Red	Blue	Red	Blue	Red	Blue	Red	Blue	**GREEN**	
Green	Yellow	Green	Yellow	Green	Yellow	Green	Yellow	Green	Yellow		

Figure 3-11. Color encoded AAC symbol sequencing.

Prediction Strategies

Prediction Strategies Using Written Language

Prediction strategies are another method used to improve the communication speed of AAC devices. Prediction strategies attempt to guess the user's message by displaying choices in a constantly changing array. If the guess is accurate, the user simply selects the intended word or letter from the list of choices. Early AAC devices used prediction strategies simply for letter spelling. The English language is very predictable in using certain letters more frequently than others. Anyone who has watched the television game show *Wheel*

of Fortune knows that the consonants *t, l, n, r,* and *s* occur more frequently than other consonants. In addition, only certain letter combinations can be produced. For example, a word which begins with the letter *T* can only be followed by the letters *a, e, i, o, u, r, w,* and *h*. A letter prediction system presents the user with a constantly changing array of letters based on previously spelled letters (see Figure 3–12). Letter prediction was used in several early computer-based scanning systems.

More sophisticated prediction systems attempt to guess the word a user is trying to spell. These computer programs use semantic and syntactic rules of language to predict word choices. Many words can often be predicted after spelling the first

Letter Prediction for Spelling *THERE*

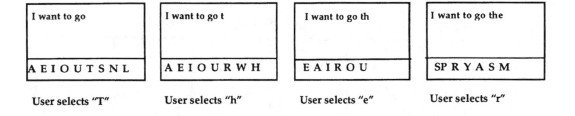

Word Prediction for Spelling *THERE*

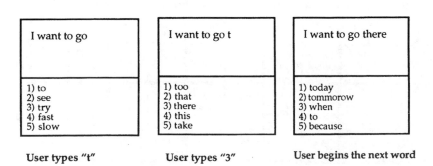

Figure 3–12. Letter and word prediction strategies.

two letters. The user keeps spelling the word until it appears in the prediction list. The user then keys in the number of the desired word to select it (see Figure 3–12). EZ Keys, Co:Writer, Handi Word, Predict It, WiVik 2.0, Screen Doors, PAL, and MindReader are examples of software programs with word prediction features. Use of word prediction software can reduce keystrokes from 44 to 48% (Higginbotham, 1992). However, because the computer display screen is dynamically changing with each new letter typed, the user must be able to visually scan the listed words after each keystroke. Word prediction techniques are beneficial for individuals with slow input rates, but become less beneficial for individuals with faster keystroke rates because the visual scanning process slows them down (Vanderheiden & Lloyd, 1986). Word prediction is also useful for individuals who are poor spellers. If a user is able to make a correct guess for the first two letters of a word, the word prediction program can often finish the spelling process. Newell, Booth, Arnott, and Beattie (1992) provide case study data which indicate that use of word prediction programs improves the writing skills of children over time.

Prediction Strategies Using Picture Symbols Combined with Written Language

Picture symbols can also be incorporated into prediction strategies on AAC systems with dynamic displays. The DynaVox has a picture-based prediction strategy known as DynaWrite which is useful for young children progressing from pictures to written language. This program uses word prediction strategies, but provides the child with picture symbols representing the words in the prediction list. The user begins by typing the initial letter of the desired word. DynaWrite then displays a row of picture symbols which begin with that

letter. As the child continues spelling, the picture symbol choices change until the desired word is located.

Predictive Picture Symbol Sequencing

One difficulty in using AAC systems with static displays designed for picture symbol sequencing is the fact that the user must learn and remember hundreds of picture sequence codes. In an attempt to remove some of the cognitive load from this memory process, Prentke Romich offers predictive symbol sequencing in the Alpha Talker, Delta Talker and Liberator. Each symbol on the device has a small LED light in the upper corner. Initially, only those symbols that can begin a symbol sequence are lighted. Once the initial symbol is selected, the lights change to indicate which symbols are possible sequence choices. For users who operate their devices using scanning, the device can be set up to only scan to predicted choices. Nonpredicted symbols are skipped in the scanning process.

AAC DEVICE OUTPUT METHODS

High technology AAC systems have voice, printed, or combinations of output modes available for the user. The importance of having an intelligible method of communicating messages cannot be underestimated. Glennen (1989) found that when adult listeners interacted with users of low technology AAC systems without any printed or spoken output the listeners increased their use of yes/no and multiple choice questions in an attempt to control the communication situation. When intelligible printed or spoken output was present, the same listeners reduced their attempts to control the conversation by asking fewer questions.

The use of AAC devices with spoken or printed output modes reduces the demands placed on the listener. Without any method of output, the listener must remember every letter or symbol selected, then mentally combine the information into a coherent message. Lack of output also requires the listener to continuously watch the communication system. If the listener momentarily looks away, the message must be repeated. Spoken or printed output also reduces the cognitive load for the user. Young children who are learning how to spell or sequence words together into sentences need constant visual and auditory message feedback. Without this feedback, the child is unable to review his or her work or make corrections to the communication message.

Spoken Output Modes

Almost all of the currently available electronic AAC systems provide the user with the capability of producing spoken messages. There are two basic types of speech output used in AAC systems, digital speech synthesized through waveform coding and digital speech synthesized through parametric coding. This section will provide the reader with a preliminary overview of these two synthesized speech methods. For a comprehensive overview, readers are referred to Venkatagiri and Ramabadran (1995).

Synthesized Speech Using Waveform Coding

Synthesized speech produced through the waveform coding process provides the AAC user with natural sounding human voice. The use of waveform recording is increasing as memory constraints for microcomputers are eliminated. Waveform synthesis works by storing recorded voice information into the AAC system. The process of recording works similarly to operating a tape recorder. The person doing the recording switches the device into a

recording mode, and speaks the message into a microphone attached to the device. When recording is finished, the device is switched back into play mode for the user to access the recorded messages.

On the surface, synthesized speech created through waveform coding works similarly to tape recording. However, the actual process of storing the recorded information is quite different. The synthesizer converts recorded analog information (real time waveform information) into numerical digital representations of the speech formant waveforms. These numerical representations are then stored into the memory of the AAC device. When the appropriate symbol sequence is selected, the digital waveform correlates are retrieved and converted back into analog form to create a spoken message. The process of converting the spoken message from analog to digital form and back again does not require elegant data processing or complex electronics. However, storing the digital waveform information requires large amounts of computer memory. Each second of stored recording requires 4 to 12 kilobytes of memory (Venkatagiri & Ramabadran, 1995). There are a number of AAC devices that have waveform coding synthesized speech capabilities. The reader is referred to the Appendix for a listing of these AAC products.

The primary advantage of using waveform coding to generate synthesized speech is its natural sounding quality. Because the spoken output will sound like the person whose voice is used for recording, matches between the AAC user and the person used as the recording voice can be made. Young children who are nonspeaking can have messages recorded by peers in their environment. Because the voice is natural, emotion and intonation can easily be conveyed in the recording process. The limitation of this method is the fact that all messages must be prerecorded for the user. For young children or adults with significant cognitive disabilities it is easy to predict needed messages and prestore them in the AAC device. However, for older children and adults it is almost impossible to predict every word or phrase that might be needed for communication. In addition, AAC devices that use waveform coding have limited recording time. Early systems limited users to under 2 minutes of recording. As the costs of computer memory components have decreased, manufacturers have been able to increase the recording time limits without significantly increasing AAC device costs. AAC systems with 20 to 30 minutes of recording time are common, with several systems in development that will allow for recording times of 1 hour or more.

Synthesized Speech Using Parametric Coding

Synthesized speech output using parametric coding is used more frequently in AAC systems. The parametric coding process stores part of the numerical waveform correlates for a given word or sound in the memory of the AAC device. Because the system is only storing a partial representation of the spoken waveform, less memory is needed for storing synthesized speech data. Venkatagiri and Ramabadran (1995) estimated that only 2 kilobytes of computer memory are necessary to store 1 second of speech using this process. There are two basic methods of parametric coding, formant coding and linear predictive coding (LPC). They were both developed using the source-filter theory of speech production developed by Fant (Venkatagiri & Ramabadran, 1995).

The process of formant coding involves digitally storing sound waveform parameters to encode the formant frequency and amplitude of the sound. In addition, the features of voicing, frication, aspiration, and resonance are also encoded into digital form. The stored digital signal is sent through a series of multiple filters to create electronically produced versions of naturally occurring sounds. Formant coding requires the use of highly complex electronics and fast computer processors to create spoken output (Venkatagiri & Ramabadran, 1995). Synthesized speech output produced through formant coding is very intelligible but does not sound completely natural as prosody and coarticulation factors cannot yet be reproduced. DecTalk is the most commonly used synthesizer with formant coding capabilities. DecTalk provides users with a choice of 10 different male or female voices, and the capability to create new voices. DecTalk is currently available in the LightWriter, Liberator, DynaVox, and DeltaTalker. Variations of DecTalk have also been developed for use with laptop computers. MultiVoice is a standalone unit that plugs into IBM or Macintosh compatible laptop computers to provide DecTalk quality voice.

Linear predictive coding (LPC) works similarly except that less of the information from the original speech signal source is encoded digitally for use within the system. LPC systems rely on the redundancy of the sound signal to encode information based on time sampling. Each sound is divided into units of time. Within each individual time frame, the sound's characteristics are encoded based on prediction coefficients. Synthesized speech is created when the digital signals are relayed through a single filter that uses prediction coefficients to calculate and produce the sound. Because only a single filter is used, the sound that is created tends to be monotone and robotic sounding. Intelligibility is generally poor when compared with other forms of speech synthesis (Venkatagiri & Ramabadran, 1995). Echo brand synthesizers, which were widely used in early models of AAC devices with speech output, are examples of LPC synthesized speech systems. Macintalk II Pro is an example of a higher quality synthesizer that uses LPC encoding. This synthesizer is widely available in newer models of Macintosh computers.

Text to Speech Synthesis

Users of AAC systems who want to produce novel messages or to access a large number of pre-stored messages require the ability to convert written text-based information into synthesized speech messages. This process is known as text to speech synthesis and can only be achieved through synthesizers with parametric encoding processes. The text to speech process consists of transforming written text into its corresponding phonemes and adding other pronunciation information such as stress, prosody, and segmentation. The information is then used to retrieve stored digital information which corresponds to the required sounds. The digital signals are then converted into analog form (Venkatagiri & Ramabadran, 1995).

The process of converting the written text into a phonetic code relies on using linguistically based rules of pronunciation which are systematically applied to the text. For example, the letter C can be pronounced soft or hard (e.g., circus). These phonemes are stored as two separate sounds. When the letter C is spelled in a word, the synthesizer's software attempts to analyze the word's patterns to select the correct sounds for digital retrieval. Because there are so many pronunciation variations in the English language, the software requires an extensive knowledge of pronunciation exceptions to produce high quality intelligible speech (Venkatagiri & Ramabadran, 1995). Low cost synthesizers such as the Echo brand have few pronunciation exceptions and are less intelligible. Better quality speech synthesizers have more complex rule strategies for determining which sound to retrieve. The DecTalk synthesizer has a pronunciation exception diction-ary of over 6,000 words (Venkatagiri & Ramabadran, 1995).

Printed Output Modes

Many AAC systems provide the user with printed output along with spoken output. The addition of printed output is usually seen on AAC devices that have letter spelling capabilities. AAC systems that are completely picture based rarely provide printed output, assuming that the user does not have literacy skills necessary to read the information. There are several different types of printed output available on commercially available devices.

Paper Printing

AAC devices with paper output typically use small strip printers or adding machine-sized printers. This is done to keep the system small and portable. The Canon Communicator, Real Voice, and Liberator are three dedicated devices with paper output. Messages printed on paper are useful for situations when the user wishes to compose a lengthy text or series of questions for use at a later time. For example, a user might develop a list of questions about an upcoming math assignment. The questions are written ahead of time and printed out. When the user goes to see the teacher, the paper with the printed questions is shown. This method of developing communicative messages ahead of time can greatly enhance the initial rate of communication within an interaction.

Computer-based AAC systems can use standard computer printers to provide users with paper output. There are several small inkjet printers that work with IBM and Macintosh computers. However, the addition of a printer greatly reduces the portability of the system. Many users of laptop computer AAC devices keep their printers in a single location, and simply hook up the printer when they have something to print.

LED and LCD Screens

Printed output can also be provided through the use of light-emitting diode (LED) and liquid crystal display (LCD) screens. LCD screens are more commonly used in AAC devices. These screens are similar to the black and white displays available on most small calculators. They are often difficult to read in bright locations or when the viewing angle is distorted. Prentke Romich Company has added backlighting to its LCD screens which greatly improves readability. LED screens are less commonly used because they require more battery power to keep them going. LED screens provide bright lighted red or blue letters on a black background. LED screens are usually easier to read because the bright letters contrast nicely with the black background. The Light-writer provides a two-way LED screen that can easily be read by listeners from several feet away.

Most dedicated devices with LCD and LED screens provide the user with a small printing area which ranges from one to seven lines of print. As the user communicates, old messages are replaced by new messages. Unlike paper output, these printed messages are only temporary. The addition of LCD or LED printed output screens gives the user immediate feedback about keyboard selections. In addition, they assist listeners who may have missed hearing a message or heard but did not understand a message. Instead of having the user repeat the message again, the listener can simply read the AAC device's display screen.

MOUNTING AND TRANSPORTING AAC DEVICES

Choosing an appropriate AAC system for a given user is only part of the equipment process. In addition to the device itself, the assessment team must also consider how the user will move the AAC system around within his or her environment. For users who spend time in wheelchairs, devices must be mounted onto the chair. For ambulatory users, devices must be made portable for the user. Equipment necessary for transporting AAC devices will be reviewed in this section.

Wheelchair Mounts

When placing an AAC device on a wheelchair, the first consideration is to determine whether the device should be placed on a wheelchair tray or held by a separate wheelchair mounting system. The size and weight of the AAC system is one factor in determining this decision. If the device is small and lightweight, using it on the wheelchair tray surface is often a satisfactory arrangement for many users. Extremely heavy or overly large devices cannot safely sit on a wheelchair tray. If the device can be used on the wheelchair tray, adaptations should be made to stabilize the AAC system on the tray's surface so that it does not accidentally slide around when used or suddenly get thrown off the tray. Velcro and Dycem can be used for this purpose. For users who may try to remove their AAC systems and push them to the floor, custom solutions can be developed in which the device is permanently attached to the tray, or only detaches with some difficulty. Some users may access their AAC devices best when the symbol surface is flush with the surface of the wheelchair tray, or angled slightly into the tray (see Figure 3–13). Adaptations such as these usually need to be custom-made for the individual.

Several companies have developed wheelchair mounts designed to attach AAC or computer equipment to wheelchairs (see Appendix). The mounting systems vary in

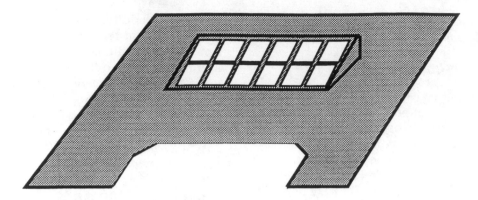

Figure 3–13. AAC system mounted into a wheelchair tray cut-out.

terms of their ability to fold down when not in use, the mechanism for attaching and detaching the AAC system, and the size of the "block" that attaches to the wheelchair (see Figure 3–14). The block is the portion of the mount that is always attached to the wheelchair, usually near the footplate base. Some wheelchair mounts only require 1½ inches of straight wheelchair tubing to attach the block. Other mounts have larger blocks that require more tubing area to attach. When attaching mounts to adult wheelchairs, the size of the block is usually not a problem. However, on pediatric wheelchairs, there is often little room available for attaching the block.

Different wheelchairs use different sizes of tubing, either ¾ inch, ⅞ inch or 1 inch. The block of the wheelchair mount must be sized to fit the wheelchair tubing or it will not safely attach to the chair. During the assessment process, the location that the block will be attached to must be measured to determine clearance, and the size of the wheelchair's tubing at that location must also be measured to get a good fit. Some wheelchair mounts have different parts for right-sided versus left-sided mounting that will need to be specified in the order. Individuals who use more than one wheelchair (i.e., a power and a manual chair) will often require two separate wheelchair mounting

systems. This is because different chair designs make it difficult to attach the mounting block in exactly the same location on both chairs. If a single mount is used across both chairs, the AAC system will be placed in very different positions. For users who access their devices using scanning (and thus do not have to directly touch the device), this is not a problem. However, most direct selection users need to have their devices mounted in the same position across the two chairs. This positioning can only be achieved with two separate mounts.

Many children do not have traditional wheelchairs. Instead, they are transported in lightweight chairs known as strollers (i.e., KidCart, Pogon, and McLaren Stroller). Strollers are lightweight because their tubing is made of aluminum. Standard wheelchair mounts cannot be safely attached to these chairs because the chair tubing will often bend under the weight of the mount and AAC device. In addition, in a stroller the weight of the AAC system and mount are often equal to the weight of the chair. The child's weight is the only stabilizing force preventing the chair from tipping over when the AAC system is attached. If the wheelchair mount is positioned to the side to remove the child from the chair, the chair and system are in danger of tipping over with the child. Lightweight AAC sys-

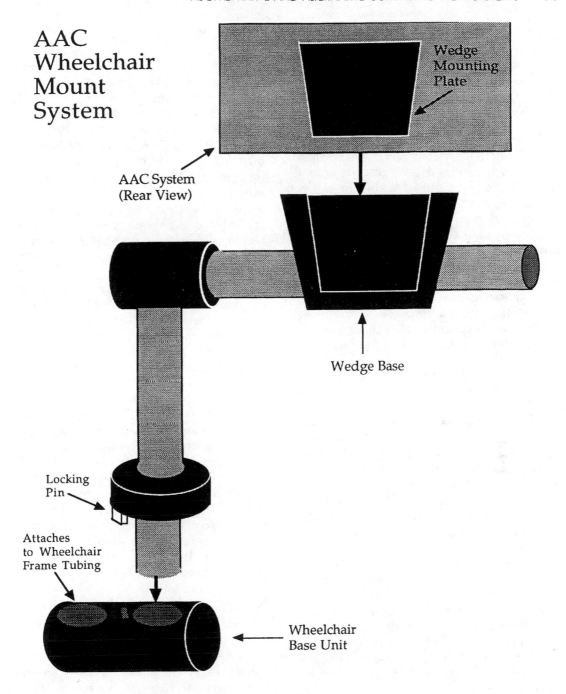

AAC Wheelchair Mount System

Wedge Mounting Plate

AAC System (Rear View)

Wedge Base

Locking Pin

Attaches to Wheelchair Frame Tubing

Wheelchair Base Unit

Figure 3–14. AAC wheelchair mounting system.

tems can be attached to the wheelchair tray of a stroller, or attached to the chair using a switch mount mechanism. Heavier AAC systems will be problematic and should be reconsidered for children seated primarily in strollers.

Other considerations concern whether the wheelchair mount should be rigid or fold down. Rigid mounts cannot be folded and usually provide a sturdier hold for the AAC system. However, rigid mounts are often difficult to transport since they cannot be broken down. Rigid mounts are also not recommended for small children seated in pediatric wheelchairs. Rigid mounts allow for transfers by swinging the mount and AAC device outward 180° from the chair. This changes the distribution of weight and puts the child and chair in danger of tipping over. Folding mounts are sometimes less sturdy because there is an additional angle of play built into the mount. The advantage is the fact that the mount can easily fold down beside the wheelchair which improves portability. Fold down capabilities also make it easier to transfer an individual into and out of the chair without tipping the chair over. Although the AAC device can remain attached when the mount is folded down, it is not a good idea to keep the AAC system in that position because its presence increases the total width of the wheelchair. This makes it difficult to get through tight doorways, and also increases the chance that the wheelchair user might crash the device into the wall when driving. Most users have the AAC system and mount in the upright position when moving in their chairs.

The final consideration when choosing a wheelchair mount is the release mechanism for attaching and detaching the AAC system. Some wheelchair mounts have quick release mechanisms which easily remove the AAC system at the push of a button or lever. Other mounts have large mounting plates which must be permanently attached to the back of the AAC device. Some of these plates make it impossible to remove the device and place it flat on another surface such as a table. If the AAC system is going to be used across multiple positioning situations, a mounting block that will prevent it from sitting flat on another surface will be problematic.

Switch Mounts

There are also several mounts designed to hold single switches in place. Ablenet produces a Jelly Bean Switch Holder which is designed to hold up to four of their Jelly Bean switches in place on a wheelchair tray or table surface. This switch holder is practical for users of switch-activated direct selection AAC devices as it holds the switches in place as a single unit. Similar mounting systems can also be custom-made for other types of switches by attaching the switches with velcro or screws to a single piece of plexiglass or wood to hold them in place.

Several mounts have been developed to position switches in difficult to access locations (usually near the head). Several companies manufacture telescoping switch mounts with several points of rotation for maximum customization. These include the Slim Armstrong, Mighty Mount, and Universal Mounting System (see Appendix). Gooseneck mounts are made of a single flexible piece that can be bent into position. These switch mounts work well for many AAC users. However, if the mount is constantly being removed or repositioned by many individuals in the user's environment, it becomes difficult to reposition the mount back into the exact location over and over again. Some users require a custom-made switch mount that will hold the switch in place with minimal points of positioning.

Portability for Ambulatory AAC Users

Adult AAC users who are steady walkers can usually carry their AAC systems around using carrying cases or backpacks. Most AAC manufacturers make carrying cases for their products. Padded laptop computer carrying cases can also be used to carry AAC systems. These can often be purchased at a lesser cost than the manufacturer's carrying cases through computer supply stores.

Individuals who cannot carry their AAC devices independently while walking will need adaptive equipment to help them transport the device. Small lightweight devices such as the Walker Talker, or Parrot can be attached by a belt or purse strap to the user. Small devices can also be carried in fanny packs belted around the user's waist or onto a walker. Small AAC systems can also be carried in baskets attached to walkers. Larger AAC systems can be transported in portable carts. CJT Technologies makes a wheeled WalkIt cart that is similar to a golf bag cart. The AAC device is placed on the cart and pushed ahead or pulled behind. The Rover Walker is a four-wheeled lightweight walker with a tray available for positioning the AAC system. Any commercially available cart or wagon with four wheels can be used to push an AAC device from location to location. No matter which type of cart or walker is being used, the AAC system must be firmly strapped to the surface of the cart and tested to make sure that the added weight of the AAC device will not tip the cart easily.

CONCLUSION

Considering that sophisticated high technology AAC systems have only been available for the past 20 years, there is now a proliferation of different devices with different features and different strengths and weaknesses. Professionals who work with nonspeaking persons need to constantly update their knowledge as new AAC devices, software, and peripherals are developed. This chapter was an overview of the features and terminology necessary for understanding the wide variety of AAC equipment options available. Appendix A gives a detailed description of all the devices mentioned in this chapter. Appendix B lists vendor resources. Professionals and users who wish to remain up-to-date

in this area are encouraged to contact vendors to request regular mailings and product information, and should attend local or national conferences where AAC products are displayed.

When presented with this vast array of AAC products, the process of determining which device to recommend for a given individual can become an overwhelming experience. When the high cost of AAC systems is added into consideration, it is important that an appropriate device is recommended from the beginning. Most nonspeaking individuals do not have the resources to buy several devices until the "right fit" is found. Culp, Ambriosi, Berninger, and Mitchell (1986) surveyed nonspeaking consumers who were prescribed AAC systems to determine their satisfaction with their devices over a 4-year period. They found that 29% of children and 50% of adults were no longer using their devices for various reasons. In order to decrease this level of rejection, it is essential that nonspeaking individuals be assessed by a team of individuals who have experience with a number of clients using a wide variety of devices before any final decisions are made. Chapters 5, 6, and 7 review this assessment process more thoroughly.

REFERENCES

Baker, B. (1986). Using images to generate speech. *Byte, 3*, 160–168.
Bruno, J. (1988). *Interaction, education and play plus*. Wooster, OH: Prentke Romich Company.
Burkhart, L. (1982). *More homemade battery devices for severely handicapped children with suggested activities.* (Available from the author.)
Church, G., & Glennen, S. (Eds.) (1992). *The handbook of assistive technology*. San Diego, CA: Singular Publishing Group.
Culp, D. M., Ambriosi, D. M., Berninger, T. M., & Mitchell, J. O. (1986). Augmentative communication aid use: A follow-up study. *Augmentative and Alternative Communication, 2*, 19–24.

Foulds, R. (1980). Communication rates for nonspeech expression as a function of manual tasks and linguistic constraints. *Proceeding of the First International Conference on Rehabilitation Engineering*. Toronto, Canada.

Glennen, S. (1989). *The effect of communication aid characteristics on the interaction skills of nonspeaking persons and their adult speaking partners*. Unpublished doctoral dissertation, Pennsylvania State University, State College, PA.

Goldberg, H. R., & Fenton, J. (1960). *Aphonic communication for those with cerebral palsy: Guide for the development and use of a communication board*. New York: United Cerebral Palsy of New York State.

Goldstein, H., & Cameron, H. (1952). New method of communication for the aphasic patient. *Arizona Medicine, 8*, 17–21.

Goosens, C., & Crain, S. (1986). *Augmentative communication intervention resource*. Lake Zurich, IL: Don Johnson Developmental Equipment.

Harryman. S., & Warren, L. (1992). Positioning and power mobility. In G. Church & S. Glennen, (Eds.), *The handbook of assistive technology*. San Diego, CA: Singular Publishing Group.

Higginbotham, D. J. (1992). Evaluation of keystroke savings across five assistive communication technologies. *Augmentative and Alternative Communication, 8*, 258–272.

McDonald, E., & Schultz, A. (1973). Communication boards for cerebral palsied children. *Journal of Speech and Hearing Disorders, 38*, 73-88.

Newell, A. F., Booth, L., Arnott, J. L., & Beattie, W. (1992). Increasing literacy levels through the use of linguistic prediction. *Child Language Teaching and Therapy, 8*, 138–187.

Owens, R. E. (1988). *Language development: An introduction*. Columbus, OH: Merrill Publishing Company.

Salamo, G., & Jakobs, T. (1996). Laser pointers: Are they safe for use by children? *Augmentative and Alternative Communication, 12*, 47–51.

Shane, H., & Wilbur, R. (1989). *A conceptual framework for an AAC strategy based on sign language parameters*. Paper presented at the American Speech Language Hearing Association Annual Meeting, St. Louis, MO.

Szeto, A., Allen, E., & Littrell, M. (1993). Comparison of speed and accuracy for selected electronic communication devices and input methods. *Augmentative and Alternative Communication, 9*, 229–242.

Vanderheiden, G. C., & Grilley, K. (1976). *Nonvocal communication techniques and aids for the severely physically handicapped*. Baltimore, MD: University Park Press.

Vanderheiden G. C., & Lloyd, L. (1986). Communication systems and their components. In S. Blackstone, & D. Ruskin, (Eds.), *Augmentative communication: An introduction*. Rockville, MD: ASHA Press.

Venkatagiri, H. S., (1993). Efficiency of lexical prediction as a communication acceleration technique. *Augmentative and Alternative Communication, 9*, 161-167.

Venkatagiri, H. S., & Ramabadran, T. V., (1995). Digital speech synthesis: Tutorial. *Augmentative and Alternative Communication, 11*, 14–25.

Vicker, B. (1974). *Nonoral Communication System Project 1964–1973*. Iowa City, IA: Campus Stores.

Williams, M. B. (1995). Transitions and transformations. *The Ninth Annual Minspeak Conference Proceedings*. Wooster, OH: Prentke Romich.

Chapter 4

SYMBOL SYSTEMS AND VOCABULARY SELECTION STRATEGIES

Cindy C. Millikin

People use a variety of techniques in order to communicate with one another. Specific message content is typically delivered verbally or symbolically, while other aspects of the same message are delivered nonverbally. Verbal and nonverbal information are often combined together to communicate meaning to the listener. For example, the verbal message "leave me alone" comes across differently depending on the nonverbal signals communicated by the speaker. A speaker can convey the message politely with a brief wave of the hand, or convey the message with an increase in volume and inflection, accompanied by frowning and pushing the listener away. In this example, the message is conveyed verbally through speech, paralinguistically via vocal changes, and gesturally by facial expression and pushing. Thus, communication occurs through multiple modalities (Iacono, Mirenda, & Beukelman, 1993).

Figure 4–1 provides a framework for communication techniques that are typically used when communicating with others. This framework presents communication along two dimensions: (a) whether the messages are verbal or nonverbal, and (b) whether they are vocal or nonvocal.

The term verbal is used to mean "word-based," with specific symbolic word referents. Nonverbal refers to those actions and behaviors that communicate specific messages and intents but may not represent specific word referents.

"Human interaction is characterized by symbolic communication" (Bloomberg, Karlan, & Lloyd, 1990, p. 717). Symbolic communication involves the use of arbitrary symbols which represent ideas, affective states, objects, actions, people, relationships and events (Lloyd & Karlan, 1984; Romski, Sevcik, & Pate, 1988). The use of symbols enables individuals to communicate not only about abstractions, such as ideas and feelings, but also about topics that are temporally and spatially distant (Rowland & Schweigert, 1989). In the normally developing child, this ability develops as the child begins to separate the self from the environment, learns to manipulate objects and people in the environment, and develops associations among objects, people, and events (Stillman & Battle, 1984). Eventually, the child understands the concept that messages can be conveyed in multiple ways (e.g., smiling, whining, body excitation) and that "things" can represent other "things"

STANDARD COMMUNICATION TECHNIQUES

	VOCAL	NONVOCAL
VERBAL	Speech	Written Language
NONVERBAL	Crying Laughter Vocalizations Inflection Variations Volume Changes	Pointing Gestures Facial Expressions Body Language

Figure 4–1. Standard communication techniques.

(e.g., words and pictures represent objects; Bishop, Rankin, & Mirenda, 1994; Wetherby & Prizant, 1993). By 15 months of age the child responds to verbal labels for objects and people in the environment. By 24 months the child sees photographs as symbols for the objects depicted (Mirenda & Locke, 1989). Thus, symbol acquisition gives the child a way to represent the external environment internally and also provides a means to share internal perceptions and feelings with others (Sevcik, Romski, & Wilkinson, 1991).

For individuals without disabilities, the two most common modes of verbal communication are speech, for the provision of vocal messages, and written language, for the delivery of nonvocal messages. For young children, the primary technique is speech (McNaughton, 1993). Speech is the most efficient modality for symbolic communication (Bloomberg et al., 1990). However, speech and written language are not the only methods available for producing symbolic communication. Figure 4–2 provides another frame-work for communication, illustrating a variety of alternative techniques for producing vocal, verbal messages as well as additional techniques for delivering nonvocal, verbal messages that are commonly used in augmentative and alternative communication (AAC). In this framework a new dimension has been added. Communication techniques are divided into the categories of aided and unaided methods.

An aided communication technique involves the presence of an external physical object, whereas unaided communication refers to techniques that do not require external objects (Lloyd & Karlan, 1984; Vanderheiden & Yoder, 1986). Aided communication methods include such items as paper and pencils or computers for written communication, topic picture boards, or electronic AAC devices. There are two unaided verbal techniques illustrated in Figure 4-2: speech and sign language. These techniques rely upon voicing or specific body movements to communicate messages (Lloyd & Karlan, 1984). All verbal communication techniques, whether

STANDARD AND AAC COMMUNICATION TECHNIQUES

	VOCAL	NONVOCAL
VERBAL UNAIDED	Speech	Sign Language
VERBAL AIDED	Language Masters Looptape Systems Computer-Based AAC Aids Dedicated AAC Aids	Written Language Alphanumeric Boards Topic Boards Picture Boards
NONVERBAL	Crying Laughter Vocalizations Inflection Variations Volume Changes	Pointing Gestures Facial Expressions Body Language

Figure 4–2. Standard and AAC communication techniques.

aided or unaided, vocal or nonvocal, have a symbol set or symbol system as their base through which messages are constructed and delivered. Therefore, the decision-making process for the selection of appropriate communication techniques for an individual involves joint consideration of the various techniques as well as their symbolic foundations (Romski & Sevcik, 1988).

OVERVIEW OF SYMBOL FEATURES

Symbolic communication involves the use of arbitrary symbols. Symbols are spoken, graphic, or manual representations of ideas, affective states, objects, actions, people, relationships, and events (Lloyd & Karlan, 1984; Romski, Sevcik, & Pate 1988). Spoken symbols are conveyed vocally, received au-

ditorally, and are temporal in nature (Lloyd & Karlan, 1984). They may also be described as dynamic, due to these transient characteristics. Manual symbols are spatial or spatial-temporal, and received through the visual modality (Lloyd & Karlan, 1984). Like spoken symbols, manual signs are also considered dynamic, due to their changing characteristics and temporary display. Finally, graphic symbols are conveyed and received primarily through the visual modality. Their display is typically permanent or static in nature.

Whether spoken, manual, or graphic, there are certain components necessary for effective communication to occur via symbols (Romski & Sevcik, 1988; Romski et al., 1988). The meanings of symbols must be known to both the sender and the receiver. There should be shared knowledge of the ideas, objects, actions, people, relationships, and events represented by those symbols. The sender needs to understand and perceive the appropriate situations for employing the symbols, and the receiver has to interpret and respond to the symbols as expected by the sender. The "guessability" of symbols to an individual's community of listeners is therefore a primary consideration when determining the symbol set or system for an individual's communication system.

With regard to spoken symbols, this guessability is typically described as the intelligibility of the speaker. The spoken symbol system and rules governing use of the symbols are shared between individuals. However, if the speaker's production of symbols at the phonemic, morphological, or semantic level deviates from the norm, the message can be unintelligible to the listener. Intelligibility is often a major consideration when determining the need for AAC.

With regard to manual and graphic symbol systems, the guessability of symbols is referred to as iconicity, the degree the sign or symbol visually resembles or suggests its referent (Bloomberg et al., 1990; Dunham, 1989; Fuller & Lloyd, 1991; McEwen & Lloyd, 1990; Mizuko, 1987; Orlansky & Bonvillian, 1984; Sevcik et al., 1991). It is helpful to consider iconicity as a continuum, with transparency and opaqueness at each pole and the translucency of symbols occurring somewhere in the middle (Fuller & Lloyd, 1991; Mirenda & Locke, 1989; see Figure 4–3). Transparency refers to those symbols and signs that are considered highly suggestive and therefore readily guessable by the untrained observer without any additional cues (Bloomberg et al., 1990; Dunham, 1989; Granlund, Strom, & Olsson, 1989; Mirenda & Locke, 1989; Mizuko, 1987; Musselwhite & Ruscello, 1984; Sevcik et al., 1991). On the other hand, opaqueness is the term used to describe signs or symbols that show no specific resemblance to their referents and are not readily guessable (Fuller & Lloyd, 1991; Mizuko, 1987; Sevcik et al., 1991). Finally, translucency, which falls somewhere between transparency and opaqueness on the continuum, refers to those signs or symbols that are guessable once the relationships between the signs or symbols and their referents are shown or instructed (Bloomberg et al., 1990; Granlund et al., 1989; Sevcik et al., 1991). These relationships can be semantic, conceptual, or linguistic in nature (Bloomberg et al., 1990). Mizuko described translucency as "an agreement regarding the relationship between a symbol and its referent" (1987, p. 129).

When evaluating symbols for their degree of iconicity, it is important to keep in mind that these judgments are culture-bound, time-bound, and experience-bound (Dunham, 1989; Sevcik et al., 1991). Symbols must be periodically reevaluated for

THE ICONICITY CONTINUUM

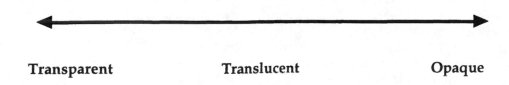

Transparent   Translucent   Opaque

Figure 4–3. The iconicity continuum.

their current relevance and transparency. For example, a picture symbol of an old-fashioned wall telephone with the crank on the side might be transparent to most senior citizens, but opaque to children and adolescents. In a similar fashion, the sign for milk (i.e., pretending to squeeze an udder) may originally have been transparent due to its close imitation to the act of milking a cow; however, dairy farms of today use sophisticated machinery instead of the manual operations of yesterday. Therefore, the relationship between the sign for milk and its referent can be considered more translucent than transparent. This example most likely represents the general rule rather than the exception for children or young adults learning sign language (Orlansky & Bonvillian, 1984). To a preschool child, the printed word would be considered an opaque symbol because it bears no resemblance to the item it represents and the child's experiences have not included the acquisition of reading skills (Sevcik et al., 1991).

Symbol iconicity has to be reviewed from the perspective of both the communicator and the listening partner. A symbol that is transparent to the communicator but not understood by the listener impedes the interaction process. Transparency is particularly important in situations where the AAC communicator will be in regular contact with individuals who are nonreaders and who may be unfamiliar with the symbol set or symbol system (Musselwhite & Ruscello, 1984). For example, if the AAC communicator is a young adult who has regular contact with young children who do not read or know sign language, transparent picture symbols may be needed to facilitate communication between the AAC communicator and his or her young listeners. Whether unaided or aided, the components of a communication system need to reflect consideration of both the communicator and the listener.

UNAIDED COMMUNICATION METHODS

Unaided communication methods include techniques that do not require use of an external object. Primary communication methods in this category include gestures and body language, sign language, vocalizations, and speech. Gestures, body language, and sign language involve manual communication symbols whereas vocalizations and speech are composed of spoken symbols (Lloyd & Karlan, 1984). Gestures, body language, and vocalizations are typically referred to as symbol sets. Symbol sets are finite and lack specific rules regarding the combination of symbols. They are relatively limited with regard to the number of specific messages an individual is able to generate. Sign languages and speech, however, are referred to as symbol systems, with specific rules applying to their sequencing and combination. In addition, they are open and generative systems which expand the repertoire of potential expressions.

Unaided techniques have specific advantages and disadvantages. Unaided methods are "portable" in that they are available to an individual at all times. Messages can be conveyed with speed and efficiency if the individual is communicating to others who are familiar with the unaided symbols. Conventional gestures such as a thumbs up hand signal are particularly efficient for conveying messages to others who culturally understand the signal. Speech and sign language, being generative systems, provide the greatest flexibility with regard to the number and types of different messages that can be conveyed.

There are also certain disadvantages inherent to unaided communication techniques. As noted, naturally occurring gestures, body language, and vocalizations are finite sets that do not offer a wide range of messages. Although sign language offers a great deal of flexibility and depth regarding message generation, the community of listeners is limited to those who are trained and knowledgeable in reading signs. Sign language interpreters are needed to communicate with listeners who do not understand signs. Finally, unaided communication methods require a certain level of physical skill. Many non-speaking individuals have accompanying gross or fine motor disabilities which makes it difficult to produce intelligible communication using unaided methods.

All communication techniques offer certain advantages while also posing disadvantages. Symbols that are effective in one setting or with a specific listener may be ineffective in another situation with different communication partners. Therefore, AAC intervention requires the creation of multimodal communication systems that offer flexibility and applicability across a variety of settings and situations.

Gestures and Body Language

Gestures and body language are manual communication symbols that are not constrained by linguistic rules (Lloyd & Karlan, 1984). Gestures may be conventional or idiosyncratic in nature, contact or distal in production (Wetherby & Prizant, 1992). Conventional gestures are those behavioral postures and movements that are recognized by society as indicative of messages with specific meanings. These meanings tend to be relatively concrete, making them often guessable (Lloyd & Karlan, 1984; Rowland & Schweigert, 1989). Many conventional gestures include a pantomimic component, such as the gesture for sweeping where fisted hands are placed in front of the body and make a sweeping motion back and forth. Other gestures do not include this component but are socially and culturally recognizable (e.g., nodding or shaking the head, thumbs up signals). However, as with all symbol sets and symbol systems, the recognizability of gestures is highly dependent

upon shared cultural experiences (Lloyd & Karlan, 1984). For example, holding up the index and middle fingers in a "V" shape in American culture means "victory" or "peace" depending on the context. However, in other cultures, this gesture communicates very different meanings.

Some gestures do not have a cultural base at all but are specific to particular individuals. Typically, these gestures are opaque to the average observer and are only recognized by individuals who are familiar with the communicator. For example, one mother once described how her son would move his hand in the air in a horizontal, circular fashion over his lap to indicate when he was feeling nauseous. This boy was not physically able to "rub his tummy," a more conventional gesture for nausea. Therefore, he moved his hand in a similar fashion away from his body. However, until the movement was explained, this idiosyncratic gesture was not recognizable to anyone outside of the boy's family.

Finally, for some individuals, aberrant gestural behaviors such as hitting out at others or sweeping items to the floor serve a variety of communicative functions (e.g., requesting attention or assistance, or escaping situations; Reichle, Mirenda, Locke, Piche & Johnston, 1992; Romski & Sevcik, 1988). It is important to analyze these behaviors to determine if they are serving communicative functions. AAC intervention then focuses on replacing undesirable behaviors with more acceptable methods to communicate the same intent. However, it is important that these analyses identify the specific social motivations for the behaviors, or the intervention may be ineffective (Reichle et al., 1992).

Contact gestures are those gestures produced by contact with an object or another individual. For example, tapping someone's arm for attention is a conventional contact gesture in our society. Holding an object toward another person is a showing or giving behavior. Distal gestures, on the other hand, are gestures that communicate messages across distances, such as head nodding, waving, or pointing, with no actu- al contact occurring with objects or people (Wetherby & Prizant, 1992). The develop- ment of gestures in children begins with contact gestures at about 9 months of age, with distal gesturing emerging at about 11 months of age (Wetherby & Prizant, 1992). Finally, body language refers to those pos- tural behaviors and signals that are com- monly recognized and understood as com- municative. For example, leaning toward someone during an interaction to indicate interest is a common communicative be- havior in our society.

Gestures comprise an important com- ponent of everyone's communication sys- tem. Their readily recognizable messages and relatively simple production provide a desirable option for many communica- tors. However, gestures also present very real limitations concerning the number and types of messages that can be con- veyed to others. Messages are limited to the here and now (Rowland & Schweigert, 1989), making it difficult or impossible to refer to ideas, objects, people, and events outside of the current context. In addition, there is a greater responsibility placed on the communicative partner to interpret messages appropriately. Otherwise, com- munication breakdowns occur and the in- teraction partners become frustrated. Communicative exchanges are eventually reduced to a series of yes/no questions, a phenomenon commonly referred to as "twenty questions." This occurs when the listener assumes full responsibility for the communicative exchange and begins a se- ries of yes/no questions with the AAC communicator, trying eventually to nar- row questions to the point where the in- tended message is discovered. Gestural communication may not be feasible for in- dividuals with accompanying severe motor disorders. The individual may not be able to produce gestures accurately, thus reducing their recognizability.

Amer-Ind

One formal gestural system is Amer-Ind, de- veloped by Skelly in 1979 and adapted from American Indian Hand Talk (Lloyd & Karlan, 1984; Skelly & Schinsky, 1979). American Indi- an Hand Talk is a gestural system used among Native Americans. Amer-Ind is based on gestural codes for approximately 250 con- cepts. It is not linguistically based and there- fore does not parallel spoken language. Mus- selwhite and St. Louis (1988) cautioned that this system may be limiting to some individu- als who have lost speech function but have maintained adult-level cognitive functions, such as individuals who have had laryngec- tomies. On the other hand, the gestures have been found to be 80% intelligible to untrained observers (Duncan & Silverman, 1977). Al- though the potential vocabulary may be limit- ed, its use with certain populations or individ- uals may need to be explored further. It may be appropriate to incorporate Amer-Ind as a small part of a larger AAC system.

Sign Languages

Sign languages are conventionalized ges- tures with relatively abstract meanings and specific rules for production (Lloyd & Karlan, 1984). Sign languages are not uni- versal (Orlansky & Bonvillian, 1984; Vander- heiden & Lloyd, 1986). Just as spoken lan- guages differ significantly between coun- tries, sign languages are also different across countries and cultures. To be universal, signs would need to be extremely iconic, al- most pantomimic in nature (Orlansky & Bonvillian, 1984). In essence, they would be reduced to finite gestural systems rather than the generative language systems they currently represent.

Sign languages are not parallel word- for-word equivalents of spoken languages (Vanderheiden & Lloyd, 1986). The only exceptions are those sign languages specifically developed as manual equivalents of the spoken language (e.g., Signing Exact English-SEE II). Systems such as SEE II are considered educational, based on the fact that the rationale for their creation was educationally derived.

Characteristics of Signs

Manual signs are unaided symbols that use the sender's face, head, hands, arms, and other parts of the body to deliver messages to others (Lloyd & Karlan, 1984). They are temporary and dynamic, frequently involving movement or change; they are also described as a symbol system that is primarily visual for the listener (Lloyd & Karlan, 1984; Schuler & Baldwin, 1981). There are three primary components to signs: handshape, location, and movement; these components are referred to as cheremes (Cregan, 1993; DePaul & Yoder, 1986; McEwen & Lloyd, 1990). The orientation of the palm has also been suggested as a fourth sign component (McEwen & Lloyd, 1990). DePaul and Yoder (1986) described cheremes as the minimal units that signify differences in meanings between specific signs. In addition to cheremes, there are several sign features that may affect learnability of the signs (Grove & Walker, 1990). These features include (a) whether there is contact of the hands with each other or with other parts of the body; (b) the number of hands required; (c) the degree of symmetry in the movement (e.g., whether both hands do the same thing); (d) the degree of visibility of the sign to the signer; (e) the need for transition between handshapes; and (f) whether there is repetition of movement within the sign (Granlund et al., 1989; Grove & Walker, 1990; Loeding, Zangari, & Lloyd, 1990; McEwen & Lloyd, 1990).

Although there are a variety of factors that affect the ease of production of signs, children may still successfully communicate with signing even though they do not have precise motor control over all the cheremes involved (Grove & Walker, 1990). Even deaf children 18–24 months old without motor impairments do not produce most of their signs correctly until much later (McEwen & Lloyd, 1990). For example, handshape is the chereme that develops last in signing infants who do not have accompanying motor impairments; it also causes the most problems for individuals with physical and cognitive impairments (McEwen & Lloyd, 1990). Therefore, although it is important to consider the motor requirements of specific signs, it is also important to include other considerations when determining an initial sign language lexicon (e.g., motivation, environment, translucency).

With regard to the physical production of signs, Granlund et al. (1989) summarized their findings concerning the learnability of signs based on the previously described sign features. Signs that involve contact (e.g., *more*) are reported to be easier to learn than signs that do not involve touching (e.g., *play*). In addition, signs that are symmetrical, repetitive, and visible to the signer are easier to learn (e.g., *shoes*). There is some inconsistency regarding the number of hands and ease of learning. Earlier studies reported two-handed signs were easier to learn than one-handed signs; however, Granlund et al. (1989) reported that one-handed signs high in translucency (e.g., *eat, milk*) were easier to produce than two-handed signs. Thus, translucency value appears to have a significant and direct effect on the learnability of signs.

As noted earlier in this chapter, translucency refers to a degree of iconicity, or the guessability of symbols. This guessability is determined by the relationship between a symbol and its referent. An iconic sign "bears a close resemblance to the object, action, or characteristic it represents" (Orlansky & Bonvillian, 1984, p. 287). A sign is described as transparent if it is readily guessable, due to a physical or structural similarity between the sign and its meaning (DePaul & Yoder, 1986; Dunham, 1989). On the other hand, a sign is translucent if the sign is guessable to the observer once the relationship between the sign and its referent is known; in other words, once the meaning of the sign is known (Bloomberg et al., 1990; Granlund et al., 1989; Loeding et al., 1990; Sevcik et al., 1991).

The differentiation between transparency and translucency is more readily understood if specific examples of signs are provided. For example, the sign for *drink* is a transparent sign because its configuration resembles the hand position of holding a cup or glass and the action of the sign mimics the motion of drinking. On the other hand, the sign for *America* is translucent. Once the observer is instructed that the interlocked fingers represent the split-rail fences or log cabins of long ago, the sign is then recognizable. However, before the relationship is known, this sign may be described as opaque or seemingly arbitrary. DePaul and Yoder (1986) pointed out that many signs evolve over time. Their structures or configurations originate with iconic relationships to their referents but become more and more arbitrary as time passes and their original meanings or rationales for construction become lost.

It is logical to assume that if a sign looks or moves like its referent then it would not only be easier to learn but would also be more easily guessed by those observers who are unfamiliar with sign language (DePaul & Yoder, 1986). In addition, one might assume concrete signs are learned before signs that are more arbitrary and opaque. However, research results do not definitively support these assumptions. For example, studies investigating the acquisition and development of sign language in infants and toddlers find that sign vocabularies include fairly equal distributions of signs across all levels or degrees of iconicity (Orlansky & Bonvillian, 1984). In addition, the most frequently used signs of 18-month-old children of deaf parents closely resemble the most frequently used words of children of hearing parents (Orlansky & Bonvillian, 1984). In a study with deaf signers, no differences were found in the recall of signs based on their degree of iconicity (DePaul & Yoder, 1986). Therefore, iconicity does not appear to play a significant role in sign acquisition with deaf children (DePaul & Yoder, 1986). On the other hand, iconicity has been found to have an effect on the learnability of signs by individuals without hearing impairments (Granlund et al., 1989).

Granlund et al. (1989) found a stronger relationship between translucency and the learnability of signs than between transparency and learnability by individuals with normal cognitive abilities. Comprehension of sign meanings was more important than the visual representativeness of the sign. Those individuals who demonstrated good ability to guess the meanings of the signs produced more signs correctly. In addition, signs rated high in translucency were more likely to be symmetrical and visible to the signer; two characteristics of signs found to predict ease of acquisition. It has also been found that adult ratings of the translucency of verb signs were predictive of ease of acquisition of the signs by individuals with moderate cognitive impairments (Bloomberg et al., 1990). Dunham (1989) found verb signs rated higher in translucency than noun signs by children and adults; in addition, she found autistic children acquired verb signs more rapidly than nouns. Therefore, translucency is an important factor to consider when selecting an initial lexicon for individuals with cognitive impairments. Translucency is possibly more important than selecting a lexicon based upon physical characteristics of the signs.

For individuals who have cognitive impairments, the functionality of a sign is an important consideration. Loeding et al.

(1990) defined the functionality of a sign as the degree to which the sign is viewed as useful for communicating with a variety of people in a variety of settings. Teaching signs in their natural environments on a consistent basis will also increase functionality and generalization of use (Goodman & Remington, 1993; Spragale & Micucci, 1990; Watkins, Sprafkin, & Krolikowski, 1993). For example, Goodman and Remington (1993) found signs were more rapidly acquired when taught as requests, with reinforcements specific to the requests provided, than when the signs were taught as labels and reinforcements were nonspecific. Dunham (1989) suggested the production of signs in natural settings may increase their transparency both to the signer and the communication partner.

Sign language, as a component of a multimodal AAC system, offers certain advantages and disadvantages. Although the physical production of signs may involve change and movement, the component handshapes provide static, visual configurations to imitate (Loeding et al., 1990). In addition, an instructor is physically able to shape and mold the learner's hands for correct production. Sign language facilitates language development, providing a medium through which language constructs and communication skills can be taught (Grove & Walker, 1990; Loeding et al., 1990; Schuler & Baldwin, 1981). In addition, if sign and speech are presented simultaneously, signing is hypothesized to facilitate speech acquisition, a position anecdotally supported in research (Schuler & Baldwin, 1981). With its virtually unlimited expressive potential and its constant accessibility, sign language offers a functional and effective means of communication (Schuler & Baldwin, 1981). However, there are certain drawbacks to the use of sign language. The individual learning sign language must have the ability to recall from memory the signs needed to communicate specific messages. In addition, communica-tive partners of the signer must be able to read and comprehend signs. With current movements toward inclusive educational, work, and community settings, the lack of potential communication partners is a major problem. This disadvantage can be overcome if successful training programs are implemented with individuals who frequently interact with the signer. However, other means of communication will be needed for those individuals who are not trained in sign language.

Types of Sign Languages

American Sign Language. American Sign Language (ASL) evolved from French Sign Language and is the primary language system among adults in the deaf community (Lowenbraun & Thompson, 1982; Musselwhite & St. Louis, 1988; Orlansky & Bonvillian, 1984). Consisting of several thousand signs, ASL has its own unique syntax and does not parallel spoken English. Signs may be unilateral or bilateral; bilateral signs may be either symmetrical or asymmetrical (McEwen & Lloyd, 1990). In ASL there are 19 handshapes, 12 locations on the body, and 24 types of movement (Musselwhite & St. Louis, 1988). Meaning is also enhanced and nuances expressed by behavioral changes, body movements, and facial expressions.

Signing Exact English. Signing Exact English (SEE II) and Signed English are educationally derived sign language systems that parallel spoken English. Both are frequently used systems. In Signed English, signs represent meanings and not the sound or spelling of a word. Therefore, a word with two different meanings, such as *land* (i.e., a body of land versus to land a plane), will have two different signs (Musselwhite & St. Louis, 1988). In addition to the 3,100 word signs, there are 14 sign markers to denote morphemes such as verb tense and comparative adjectives. There are many materials and books available in Signed English; storybooks, nursery rhymes, and songbooks provide pictures and/or detailed descriptions of the signs needed for the activities. There are also materials and books available in SEE II, the other frequently used sign system that parallels spoken English. SEE II consists of approximately 4,000 signs, with more than 70 common word endings and markers. This system is more complex than Signed English and places greater motoric and cognitive demands on the signer (Musselwhite & St. Louis, 1988).

Signs Supporting English. Signs Supporting English, or keyword signing, refers to the practice of only signing content-laden words in a message (Grove & Walker, 1990; Loeding et al., 1990). Complete sentences are spoken while content words are simultaneously signed in their spoken word order (Grove & Walker, 1990). The rationale for the selective use of signs is based on the belief that totally mirroring spoken English may potentially result in deletions, distortions, or breakdowns in communication (Grove & Walker, 1990).

Vocalizations and Speech

Vocalizations provide an effective means for quick, general intent to be communicated. When also paired with changes in facial expressions and body language, the meanings of vocalizations can be quite specific. For example, increasing volume while lowering tone, frowning, and pulling toys closer to the body effectively communicates the message that this child is not interested in sharing toys at the moment. On the other hand, a sing-song string of sounds, ending with a slight increase in pitch, presented with low volume, and accompanied by hands in a giving posture with toys in open palms would convey an interest in sharing and interacting. An audible vocalization is also an effective means for gaining the attention of others. These paralinguistic techniques for communication should be encouraged and reinforced in individuals whose speech is functionally ineffective for verbal communication.

Speech is one of the most effective means of unaided communication. It offers a fast, portable, and efficient means of producing verbal messages. Messages can be conveyed across considerable distance with changes in the intensity of production. In addition, as long as the communicative partner is a speaker of the same language, there are few limitations to the number or types of messages that can be produced. It provides the means for an open, generative system for symbolic communication. On the other hand, if there are significant problems with speech production that affect intelligibility, the individual may require an AAC system to supplement spoken communication. Typically, an AAC system will incorporate any residual speech skills an individual communicator possesses due to the heightened efficiency and effectiveness of speech. In addition, the AAC system provides alternative techniques for communicating messages in situations where speech is ineffective or nonfunctional. These alternative techniques include both unaided and aided techniques in order to maximize success in communicating across environments.

AIDED COMMUNICATION SYMBOLS

As noted earlier, aided communication techniques involve the use of physical objects, typically referred to as aids or devices, which are used to communicate messages. Aided techniques may be particularly useful for individuals who have difficulty processing auditory information, such as speech, or who have difficulty with information that is temporal or transient in nature, such as sign language (Mirenda, 1985). Aided symbols provide the means for message formulation with low tech communication boards and are used to represent programmed messages stored in voice output AAC devices. Due to their physical nature, most of these symbols have greater symbol permanency than unaided symbols (Lloyd & Karlan, 1984).

Most AAC aids and devices operate via a symbol set or symbol system. Symbols may be created individually for the AAC communicator or derived from a commercially available set. There are a variety of sources for symbols. Examples of typical symbols include common objects, parts of objects, photographs, line drawings, or printed words. One of the most critical decisions in the design of an AAC system is the selection of the symbol system(s). Research has been conducted on symbols and symbol systems for aided communication and offers important information for designing communication systems and selecting symbol sets. From research conducted thus far an apparent hierarchy has emerged.

The Aided Symbol Hierarchy

Most aided symbols are graphic line drawings, with or without traditional orthography (i.e., printed words); however, aided symbols may also be objects, parts of objects, or even textures. Research studies have compared types of symbols to determine if certain symbols are easier to use than others. In addition, studies have compared some of the various commercially available graphic symbols for their transparency. The effect of word classes on the transparency of symbols has also been investigated. It is important to know what types of symbols are cognitively easier for children to learn. In addition, it is important to know the various types of symbols that can be used for communication, thus ensuring that the best match is made between symbols and individual communicators.

The more iconic the symbol, the easier or faster the symbol is learned (Clark, 1981; Yovetich & Young, 1988). Mirenda and Locke (1989) described the hierarchy for symbol types representing objects, versus actions or modifiers, as fairly predictable and stable (see Figure 4–4). From easiest to hardest, the general hierarchy is reported to be the following: objects, color photographs, black and white pho-

AIDED SYMBOL HIERARCHY (Mirenda & Locke, 1989).

Symbol type	Degree of iconicity
Objects	Most iconic
Color photographs	
Black and white photographs	
Miniature objects	
Black and white line drawings	
Blissymbols	
Traditional orthography	Least iconic

Figure 4–4. Aided symbol hierarchy (Mirenda & Locke, 1989).

tographs, miniature objects, black and white line drawings, Blissymbols, and traditional orthography (i.e., writing) (Mirenda & Locke, 1989; Mirenda & Mathy-Laikko, 1989; Sevcik, et al., 1991; Smith-Lewis, 1994). As expected, transparency decreases as the resemblance between symbols and the objects they represent decreases.

Within these general categories there are ranges of representation. For example, some pictures are exact matches of objects (e.g., pictures of foods from coupons or supermarket ads) whereas other pictures are more symbolic (e.g., pictures from children's books or language kits), thus allowing for and encouraging generalization (Mirenda, 1985). In the category of black and white line drawings, there are significant differences among the various types of symbol sets with regard to transparency or translucency. A hierarchy appears to be developing with these symbol systems based on research studies conducted to compare transparency characteristics. Specific information about the various types of graphic symbol sets, or line drawings, will follow later in this chapter.

The following hierarchy has been determined from studying the representativeness of symbols to objects (from most translucent or transparent to least): Rebus, Picture Communication Symbols (PCS), Picsyms, Blissymbols, Carrier symbols, Lexigrams, Traditional Orthography (Clark, 1981; Ecklund & Reichle, 1987; Mirenda & Locke, 1989; Musselwhite & Ruscello, 1984; Romski, Sevcik, Pate, & Rumbaugh, 1985; Sevcik et al., 1991; Smith-Lewis, 1994). However, other studies have found differences between the symbol sets when comparisons are made based on word classes. Three word classes have been studied with regard to the transparency of symbol sets and systems. These word classes are nouns, verbs, and modifiers. Nouns have been found to be the most translucent category for symbols, specifically for Rebus, PCS, PIC, Pic-

syms, and Blissymbols (Bloomberg et al., 1990; Mizuko, 1987). It is suggested that this is due to nouns generally being a more concrete word class, as well as having features and characteristics that are more easily represented graphically (Bloomberg et al., 1990).

The transparency of Rebus and PCS is considered comparable for nouns. There is a discrepancy between studies, however, regarding the placement of Picsyms in these rankings. Mizuko (1987) found Picsyms to be comparable with PCS for nouns; however, Bloomberg et al. (1990) found Picsyms to be less transparent than either Rebus, PCS, or PIC symbols in the noun word class. Most likely these discrepancies reflect characteristics of the specific symbols selected for study. Later studies have found differences with transparency within symbol sets as well as between symbols sets. Besides this discrepancy, other rankings were found to be consistent between studies.

For verbs, Rebus and PCS do not differ significantly from each other; both are more transparent than PIC, and PIC surpasses Picsyms and Blissymbols, respectively (Mizuko, 1987). With regard to modifiers, Rebus and PCS are more translucent than PIC and Picsyms, which are considered equivalent; and these two symbol sets are more translucent than Blissymbols (Bloomberg et al., 1990; Mirenda & Locke, 1989). Overall, verb symbols are more translucent than modifiers in Rebus, PCS, and PIC. There are no significant differences between verbs and modifiers in Picsyms or Blissymbols (Bloomberg et al., 1990). Figure 4–5 provides a framework of the results organized by word classes.

To summarize translucency studies by word class, Rebus and PCS were the most translucent symbol sets, with Rebus being the most translucent across the three word classes (Mizuko, 1987). However, specific individual symbols in PIC and Picsyms were rated equivalent, or higher, in

TRANSLUCENCY:	NOUNS:	VERBS:	MODIFIERS:
Most translucent	*Rebus - PCS - Picsyms[1]	Rebus - PCS	Rebus - PCS
	PIC	PIC	PIC - Picsyms
	Picsyms[2]	Picsyms	Blissymbols
Least translucent	Blissymbols	Blissymbols	

* Symbol sets listed on the same line indicate no significant differences between the two.

1 Based on Mizuko (1987)

2 Based on Bloomburg, Karlan & Lloyd (1990)

Figure 4–5. Translucency of symbol sets by word class.

translucency than Rebus or PCS. Therefore, in addition to considering the entire symbol set, individual items within the sets must be examined when designing an individual's AAC system.

Objects as Symbols: Real to Miniature

The transparency of symbols is greatest when the symbols are real objects representing themselves. With very young children or children with cognitive delays, AAC is typically introduced using real objects. One primary goal of AAC intervention is to design a system of communicative techniques that provides an immediate method of communication (Mizuko, 1987). Thus, symbols that are learned easily are usually selected for implementation.

The finding that objects are transparent to children is supported by research on child development. Developmentally, discrimination studies have found that children 27 months of age can see differences between two different objects (i.e., a ball and a bucket); however, if given two of the same object that have differences be-

tween them (e.g., two balls with different sizes, patterns, or colors), a child of this age may view them as two different objects and not conceptualize them as belonging together (Daehler, Perlmutter, & Myers, 1976). This means that individuals with severe cognitive impairments may not have the ability to generalize from one example of an object to another. For example, they may not realize that the empty green bowl in front of them is a symbol to request the red bowl that they typically eat from. Daehler et al. (1976) reported that by the age of 2 to 3 years, color saliency surpasses form saliency in discrimination tasks. This may contribute to the increased transparency of color photographs over black and white photographs.

With regard to objects being used as symbols, there are differences between normal-sized objects versus miniature objects. Miniature objects are less transparent than normal-sized objects, color photographs, or black and white photographs (see Figure 4–4). It is suggested this is due to the diminutive scale of these objects, making it more difficult to see their representativeness (Mirenda & Locke, 1989).

The studies previously noted described a hierarchy, with objects as least difficult, followed by color photos, black and white photos, and miniature objects. However, this hierarchy should not imply that AAC communicators must move through the hierarchy as they use AAC techniques. Multiple symbol types are frequently employed in AAC systems. The selection of specific symbols is an individual decision, based on the characteristics of the communicator and the various communicative environments encountered. Finally, other types of object symbols have recently emerged with physical characteristics that do not fit into the existing symbol hierarchy. Two examples of these object-based symbols are tangible symbols and tactile symbols.

Tangible Symbols

Tangible symbols are permanent three-dimensional symbols that can be tactually discriminated and physically manipulated by the AAC communicator (Rowland & Schweigert, 1989). For those individuals who have extreme difficulty associating symbols with objects, identical objects should be used as symbols. These will provide the highest level of concreteness and representativeness (Mathy-Laikko, Iacono, Ratcliff, Villarruel, Yoder, & Vanderheiden, 1989). For example, as a symbol for *drink*, an identical cup can be used. If the establishment of symbolic communication is the goal, it is important to use an identical cup only as a symbol (i.e., the cup represents *drink* but is not actually used for drinking, the drink is poured into a different cup). From identical symbols, the progression of symbols is to partial objects or associated objects. For example, a few chainlinks can be used to indicate *swing* or the wand from a bubbles bottle can be used to represent *bubbles*. At times, it may be necessary to make an artificial association between a symbol and its referent. For ex-

ample, a carpet piece might indicate laying on the floor. In the presentation and use of tangible symbols, the AAC communicator might pick up a symbol to give to the listener or simply point to the symbol for communication. Tangible symbols may place less demands on cognition, memory, and vision than other symbol types due to their direct relationships to their referents (Rowland & Schweigert, 1989).

Tactile Symbols

Tactile symbols can also be used to develop AAC systems. Tactile symbols are particularly suited for individuals who have visual impairments or dual sensory impairments (e.g., who have both deafness and blindness) but adequate tactile exploration skills (Mathy-Laikko et al., 1989). For example, a terry cloth texture can serve as the symbol for bathroom or personal grooming whereas a piece of blanket is associated with resting. Associations are established between certain textures and specific referents. Tactile symbols can also be tangible symbols as in the use of a blanket to represent resting. Tactile symbol systems can incorporate multiple symbol types and should not be restricted to one specific set of items. In certain environments, or with certain listeners, one type of symbol may be more effective or more efficient than another. The Maryland School for the Blind has developed a tactile symbol system for communication that incorporates both tangible and tactile symbols (Cole, Sommer, Cole, Smith, Mondloch & Eidelman, 1993). For example, the symbol for *shoe* is a small, laced bow similar to a shoelace tied in a bow. On the other hand, *drink* is a smooth curved plastic surface similar to a plastic cup. The symbols are initially mounted on separate cards and taught during functional activities. Eventually, symbols are mounted together to create communication displays capable of meeting multiple communicative needs.

AAC intervention can also incorporate symbols that help the AAC communicator transition from three-dimensional objects to two-dimensional symbols. For example, an identical plastic cup may be the original symbol for *drink*. Once established as a symbol, the cup is cut in half and mounted on a flat surface. The symbol would then consist of both three-dimensional and two-dimensional features. Eventually, the cup would be whittled down to until it was a two-dimensional piece of plastic against a flat, two-dimensional background. This progression can be used with boxes of food, where the boxes are eventually reduced to two-dimensional cut-outs of box logos or pictures. As an added example, one child was not able to make the transition from the three-dimensional puffy microwave popcorn bag to a two-dimensional cut-out of the front of the bag. To assist in the transition, cotton was placed under the bag cut-out to make it puffy. This puffy symbol was then mounted on a two-dimensional surface.

Finally, Dixon (1981) found another technique that can assist in transitioning an AAC communicator from objects to two-dimensional symbols. In a study using photographs, the results suggested that a figure cut from a photograph led to its being classified as a three-dimensional object. Therefore, Dixon proposed the initial use of cut-out photos, followed by the gradual addition of background to the photo. Techniques such as these, and those noted in the previous paragraph, aid in the individual's progression to two-dimensional symbols; symbols that are more convenient and easier to organize, store, and carry from one environment to another (Dixon, 1981).

Two-Dimensional Symbols: Photos to Line Drawings

The most commonly used symbols for communication are two-dimensional symbols such as photographs or line drawings. Picture representation skills emerge early in a child's development. By 15 months of age, a normal infant is able to label not only objects but also pictures (Dixon, 1981). In addition, research has found that photos and objects are equivalent for children as young as 24 months of age (Dixon, 1981). Therefore, photographs are definitely a viable option when designing symbol systems for young AAC communicators. With regard to their relative transparency, color photographs are more transparent than black and white photographs, photographs are more transparent than line drawings, and line drawings are more transparent than traditional orthography. Frequently, an AAC system will include photographs, color magazine or catalog pictures, pictures from food ads, coupon pictures, real object/food labels, and line drawings (Mirenda, 1985).

Pictures and photographs are particularly suited for representing nouns and objects (Lloyd & Karlan, 1984). Pictures and photographs clearly depict many object features that lead to their recognition and identification, particularly when high-quality photos are used (Bloomberg et al., 1990; Dixon, 1981; Mirenda, 1985). Photographs require minimal symbolic ability due to this representativeness. This makes them appropriate for individuals with low levels of symbolic development (Mirenda, 1985). Pictures range from those that are exact matches to more symbolic, abstract pictures. Pictures that are exact matches may be difficult to obtain and can be costly if high-quality equipment and film are used. It is important to encourage continued symbolic growth and generalization by introducing more abstract pictures when the individual is developmentally ready for this transition. Finally, individuals who are able to use nonidentical pictures are most likely ready for black and white line drawings (Mirenda, 1985).

Photographs can be very transparent as symbols for objects and other nouns.

However, they are not as effective when attempting to represent actions and modifiers (Lloyd & Karlan, 1984). Line drawings are sometimes more effective than photos for these word classes. Unlike photos that are fixed and static, graphic drawings often use multiple cues to illustrate motion two-dimensionally. These cues include postural cues suggesting movement and cartoon movement cues (e.g., arrows, dots, and lines to indicate moving or shaking; Bloomberg et al., 1990). Modifiers are typically presented by associating the description with a known referent. Bloomberg et al. (1990) reported that the most translucent modifiers were those that referred to attributes of a noun. For example, the descriptor *hot*, referring to temperature, may be depicted by fire, a hand near a stove, or an individual sweating with a sun in the background. The selection of the specific symbol is based on the background of the communicator and reflects the graphic that is most meaningful to the communicator.

Line drawings can be purchased commercially in symbol sets or hand drawn. Commercial sets offer several advantages: they are readily available and are relatively inexpensive, and although the quality may vary from set to set, picture quality is generally good. Some symbol sets are now available in both color and black and white versions, along with a wide variety of symbol sizes (see Appendix A). The most significant drawback to commercial symbol sets is the potential for limiting the design and selection of vocabulary to symbols contained in a specific symbol set (Miranda, 1985). It is critical that AAC vocabulary be determined by the communicative needs and abilities of the individual, and not the constraints of the symbol set.

Types of Picture Languages

AAC communication boards and electronic communication systems are often based on using two-dimensional symbols to communicate messages. Two-dimensional symbols can range from photographs to line drawings to commercial symbol sets (Hurlbut, Iwata, & Green, 1982; McDonald & Schultz, 1973). A low tech picture communication display consists of carefully organized picture communication symbols, including traditional orthography (i.e., printed words). Many commercially available symbol sets frequently used by AAC communicators are high in iconicity which reduces the amount of training needed to learn to use them (Hurlbut et al., 1982). Therefore, these sets are commonly used when designing and constructing picture communication displays. Appendix A in this book lists product information for commercially available symbol sets.

Picture communication displays provide a means for sharing internal states, feelings, ideas, and experiences (McNaughton, 1993). Most of these systems have a logographic function where one symbol expresses one word or semantic concept (Clark, 1981; Poock & Blackstone, 1992). A logographic system of communication transcribes spoken communication into a graphic form of written communication, with a visual symbol representing each word or morpheme (e.g., Chinese scripts; Bishop, Rankin, & Mirenda, 1994). Early Chinese scripts contained thousands of pictographs and ideographs (Bishop et al., 1994; Bliss, 1965). Pictographs are simple pictures representing actual things such as symbols for *drink, tree,* or *bus* and ideographs are pictures representing ideas and concepts, such as symbols for *first, under,* or *lonely* (Bishop et al., 1994; Bliss, 1965). AAC symbol systems include both pictographs and ideographs, frequently accompanied by traditional orthography (Bishop et al., 1994; Burroughs, Albritton, Eaton, & Montague, 1990). Picture communication displays frequently convey communication in whole thought units. Expression is sometimes telegraphic, with main words or concepts presented in or out of sequence. For example, an individual communicating that he would like to go to a restaurant might point to *I + eat + restaurant;* or *restaurant + hungry.*

The effectiveness of a communicative attempt is determined by the partner's ability to interpret the meaning of the symbol selections made (Poock & Blackstone, 1992). Blissymbols is a symbol system that is generative in nature, allowing for new meanings and ideas to be created by combining the components of the basic symbol set. The various potential combinations of symbols and indicators will generate expressions of different meanings (Bliss, 1965). Figure 4–6 illustrates how combining the symbol for *feeling* (i.e., heart) with positive orthographic symbols (i.e., + and !) indicates *like* whereas combining the same heart symbol with symbols representing *food* means *hungry.* As an added example, the symbol for *mother* is a combination of the symbols for *woman* and *shelter.* Although this system has not been found to be transparent to unfamiliar partners and requires a longer training period to learn, its generative nature may make it preferable for some individuals (Mizuko, 1987).

Graphic symbol systems also provide the means to access messages programmed in electronic voice output AAC devices. Frequently messages are retrieved by activating symbols or symbol sequences from overlays. At times, these symbols are identical to those used on nonelectronic picture communication displays. On the other hand, a device may use a symbol system unique to that product (e.g., DynaSyms with the Dynavox, or Unity symbols with a Prentke Romich device).

A picture symbol-based technique offers several advantages as well as some potential disadvantages. One of the greatest advantages of symbol systems is their ease of use, requiring relatively low cognitive demands from the user or the listening partner. There is no need to depend on recall for symbol selection. This places less strain on the user's memory (Clark, 1981; Iacono et al., 1993). In studies of line drawn symbol systems, iconic line drawings were learned relatively quickly and maintained over time (Bloomberg et al., 1990; Romski et al., 1988). In addition, they were more easily generalized and used communicatively.

The effects of pictographic symbol systems on literacy have recently been questioned (McNaughton, 1993; Rankin, Harwood, & Mirenda, 1994). Specifically, McNaughton questioned whether certain symbol systems may be developmentally more appropriate than others, depending on the stage of development of the child. In addition, she posed several questions regarding the potential impact of graphic representational systems on literacy. For example, do certain symbol systems contribute more to the literacy process and therefore better support future literacy skills? Bishop et al. suggested that the rules that apply to the use of picture communication symbols differ from those that apply to orthography. Although symbol systems may increase certain aspects of an individual's print and word awareness, there are also several processes required in reading that are only minimally affected through the use of graphic symbol systems, if at all. Future research is needed in this area of AAC intervention and may some day offer answers to these questions and issues.

Ferguson (1975) studied pictographs and prereading skills with children. A symbol test was constructed that presented a picture language, with symbols expressing simple phrases and sentences. Children were asked to read, memorize, and comprehend the symbolic expressions. Ferguson described comparisons between this type of symbol interaction and reading. These included the translation of symbols into words and sentences as well as scanning symbols from left to right across a page. He found this type of activity to be

BLISSYMBOLS

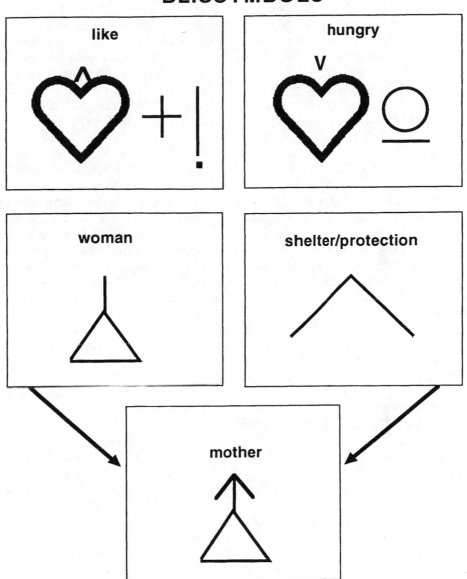

Figure 4–6. Using Blissymbols generatively to create new symbols.

more closely related to reading than some of the tasks presented in existing readiness tests. He also recommended the use of pictographs and ideographs to teach prereading skills to preschool children. As noted previously, this area of symbol sys-

tem research has recently seen a resurgence of interest. The reader is referred to Chapter 8 in this book for more information on literacy and AAC.

Graphic representational systems are picture languages. Individuals who are familiar with this type of communication and have access to large numbers of picture symbols are able to construct expressions and share their internal perceptions with the external world. The next section of this chapter provides descriptions of several pictographic symbol systems used in AAC intervention. Figures depicting nouns, verbs, modifiers, and questions for each symbol set are depicted when available.

Rebus

Rebuses were designed in the late 1960s to teach reading to children (Woodcock & Davies, 1969). The term *rebus* means thing. In this unique program, the rebus is a picture symbol that represents an entire word or part of a word. Most rebuses represent morphemes (Clark, 1981). The rebus may be pictorial, geometric, or abstract, although most rebuses are pictographic and iconic (Clark, 1981; Lloyd & Karlan, 1984). In the original Rebus reading program, all words were initially represented by rebuses, with a gradual replacement of rebuses with traditional orthography as the child's reading skills improved. The Standard Rebus Glossary contains 818 individual rebuses, symbols that are used for communication purposes as well as for reading instruction (see Figure 4–7). As a communication symbol system, Rebus offers several benefits. As noted earlier in the hierarchy section, Rebus is one of the most transparent symbol systems of the five systems studied. It is an open-ended system that permits a direct transcription from English (Clark, 1981).

Picture Communication Symbols

One of the most widely used symbol sets is Picture Communication Symbols (PCS) (Johnson, 1981). As noted before, PCS was one of the most transparent symbol systems in studies comparing five symbol sets, regardless of word class. Currently, three books of symbols are available, con-

taining more than 3,000 one-inch or two-inch symbols in the following categories: Social, People, Verbs, Descriptive, Foods, Leisure, Nouns, and Miscellaneous. Symbols represent single words, commonly used phrases, sentences, and social exchanges. Certain symbols are partially designed (e.g., containers, people shapes, buildings) to allow for customization of the symbol. Many symbols have alternatives that are more or less abstract, depending on the needs of the AAC communicator (see Figure 4–8). A limited number of symbols depicting sign language movements are also included as alternatives for some words. PCS is available in a paper notebook format, as stamps that one can peel and stick, or as color graphics in communication software programs (i.e., Boardmaker). In the computer software programs, symbols can be produced for customized picture communication displays, with accurate sizing of the symbols for many electronic AAC devices.

Pictogram Ideogram Communication (PIC) Symbols

Pictogram Ideogram Communication (PIC) symbols were developed in 1980 by Maharaj (Maharaj, 1980 as noted in Beukelman & Mirenda, 1992). Because of similar names, PIC symbols are frequently confused with the next symbol system, Picsyms. PIC symbols follow Rebus and PCS with regard to their perceived transparency. The symbols are unique from other symbol systems because of their reverse contrast (i.e., white on black instead of black on white).

Picsyms

Picsyms is a hand-drawn symbol system developed by Faith Carlson (1986). Like Rebus and PCS, Picsyms are composed of black lines on a white background (see Figure 4–9). The results of transparency stud-

Rebus Symbols

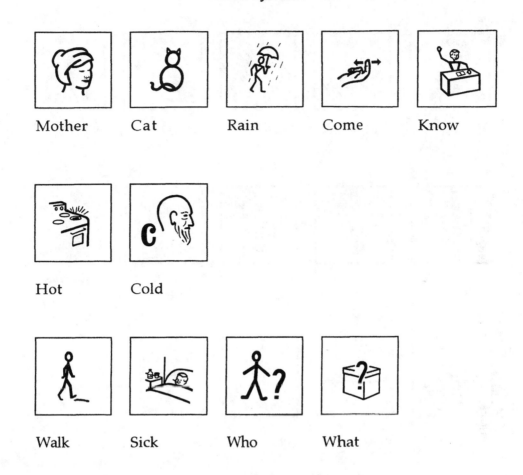

Figure 4–7. Rebus symbols.

ies with this symbol set were not as clear as other symbol sets (see Figure 4–5). One study found no significant differences between PCS and Picsyms for nouns, whereas another study found this symbol system less transparent. However, in studies of individual symbols, specific Picsym symbols were sometimes found to be the most transparent.

The Picsyms Categorical Dictionary contains approximately 850 symbols in regular, small-grid and large-grid sizes, grouped by categories. Blank grids and in-structions are provided for creating new symbols, modifying existing symbols, and combining symbols to create new meanings. Within the symbol set, actions are indicated by arrows, illustrating movement or the direction of movement. The target item in a symbol is in boldface, with other defining elements drawn with dotted lines. All spatial position symbols, such as *in* or *out*, use a box and a dot to indicate relative positions. Markers for plurality, tenses, and punctuation are included. Tags for morphological prefixes and suffixes are suggested.

Picture Communication Symbols (PCS)

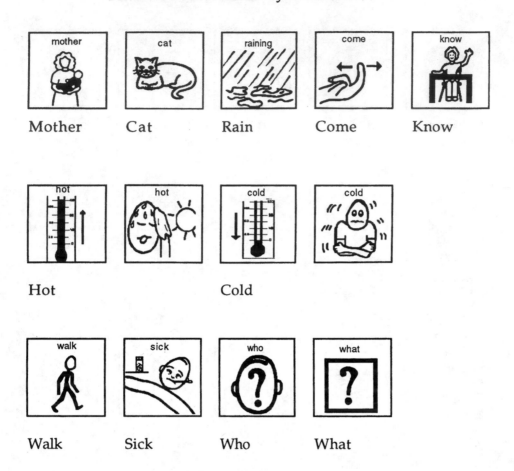

Figure 4–8. Picture Communication Symbols (PCS).

Blissymbols

Blissymbols were created by Charles Bliss in 1949 and later revised in 1965 (Bliss, 1965). His inspiration stemmed from his fascination with Chinese writing when he was stationed in China during World War II. Bliss was particularly impressed with the way the pictographs and ideographs of Chinese writing made it possible for him to interpret the writings. His goal was to devise a simple picture language that could be used to cross language barriers. Blissymbols is a generative symbol system, with specific rules regarding the placement and combination of symbols (Bliss, 1965; Burroughs et al., 1990). Many Blissymbols are pictographs, some are ideographs, and others are arbitrary or abstract (see Figure 4–10). Blissymbols contain 100 basic elements which are combined together using semantic rules to form many different meanings. For example, in Figure 4–11, a combination of the symbols, *person, give,* and *knowledge* yields the concept of *teacher.* Meaning is constructed by combining symbols. In addition, there are a variety of indicators such

Picsyms

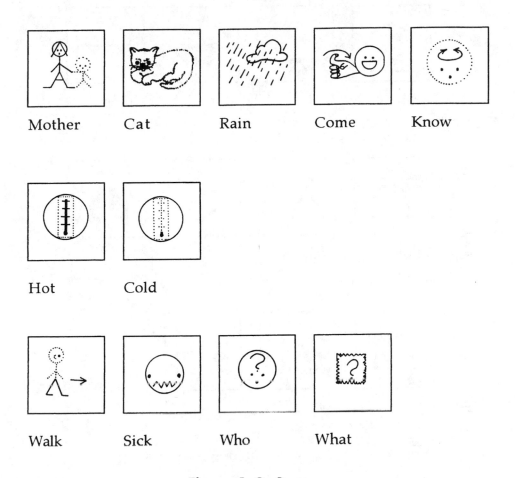

Figure 4–9. Picsyms.

as action indicators, plural indicators, description indicators (indicating adjectives or adverbs), and thing indicators that combine with other symbols to create specific meanings. The type of indicator placed above or near a symbol will guide its interpretation.

In hierarchical studies, Blissymbols were less translucent than Rebus, PCS, PIC, and Picsyms but were more translucent than traditional orthography. In studies with children, Blissymbols required approximately four times as many trials to

mastery (Hurlbut et al., 1982); in addition, they were significantly more difficult to recall than Rebus (Ecklund & Reichle, 1987).

Oakland Schools

The Oakland Schools symbols were developed by Ina Kirstein, a communication consultant, and illustrated by Carol Bernstein (Kirstein & Bernstein, 1981). Local school districts within Oakland County, Michigan, contributed to the conceptual development of this symbol set. The Oakland

Blissymbols

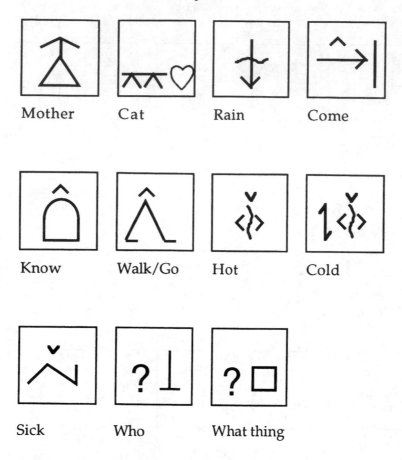

Figure 4–10. Blissymbols.

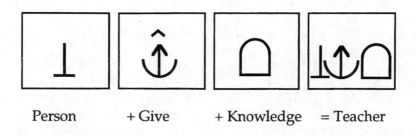

Figure 4–11. Construction of meaning with Blissymbols.

Schools Picture Dictionary consists of approximately 600 symbols in ½, 1, and 2 inch formats. Approximately 75% of the symbols are nouns (see Figure 4–12). The following categories are included: body parts; life cycle; calendar items; classroom items; clothing and accessories; emotions; food; high frequency requests; household; leisure time; nature; opposites; people; physical ailments and emergency situations; physical education, physical and occupational therapy; places; self-care; spatial relationships; transportation; verbs; and vocational training.

DynaSyms

DynaSyms is a relatively new symbol set, originally designed exclusively for the DynaVox augmentative communication device and more recently distributed in a paper format (Carlson, 1994). The new paper format provides over 1,000 symbols and is described as a starter set. DynaSyms was adapted from PicSyms, with specific structures for the types of symbols and specific rules for their creation and combination. A comparison of Figure 4–9 with Figure 4–13 illustrates similarities

Oakland Schools Symbols

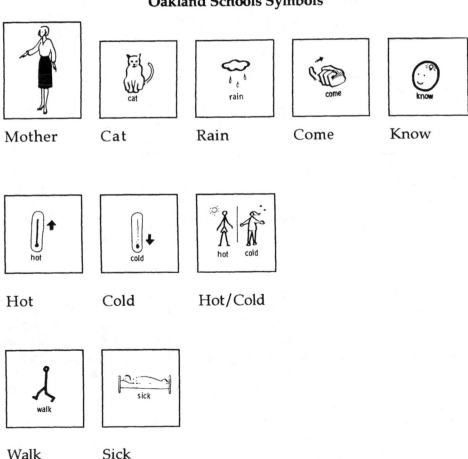

Figure 4–12. Oakland Schools symbols.

Dynasyms

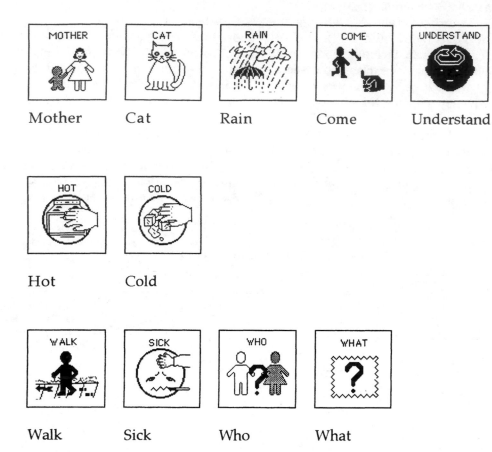

Figure 4–13. DynaSyms.

and differences between the two symbol sets. DynaSym objects are line drawings which are sometimes accompanied by background drawings of associated items to aid recognition (e.g., the *blanket* symbol has a small bed in the background). Actions are drawn with silhouette figures and arrows showing the type or direction of movement. Attribute symbols are circular, with several cues for identification. On the perimeter of the attribute's circle is a symbol drawn to identify the type of attribute (e.g., an eye if it is a visual attribute, a hand if it is a touch attribute, or a crayon if it is a color attribute); inside the circle is a drawing representing the attribute (e.g., a crooked line for *crooked*, a finger over closed lips for *quiet*, or an object with an identifiable color association, such as a leaf, a pumpkin, or an apple).

Minspeak

Minspeak refers to "minimum effort speech," a term and concept created by Bruce Baker (1986). Minspeak is different from other symbol sets presented in this section in that there is not a one-to-one correspondence between a symbol and its meaning. Minspeak symbols are typically created so that they incorporate a variety of details, allowing for multiple meanings to be assigned to a symbol. For example, one symbol pictured in Figure 4–14 shows a dog holding a newspaper. This symbol could be used in combination sequences with other symbols to represent the concepts of *dog, pet, news, newspaper, bring/get, furry, mouth,* and *taste* among others. Minspeak provides a means for coding language where combinations of multimeaning symbols yield specific messages (Bruno & Goehl, 1991; Musselwhite, 1985; Van Tatenhove, 1993). The AAC communicator assigns picture symbol sequences to specific words or messages, basing these assignments on associations between the symbols and the intended messages.

In theory, Minspeak can be used with any set of picture symbols to represent all types of vocabulary. Minspeak concepts can be followed to develop customized language systems using unique individual sequences of symbols as the encoding strategy. In reality, most individuals do not have the time or knowledge to develop and program customized picture sequences representing hundreds of words and phrases into an AAC device. There are software programs available for Prentke Romich AAC devices that consist of predetermined picture symbol sets and picture sequences which encode many functional words and phrases using Minspeak concepts. These preprogrammed vocabulary sets are called MAPs (Minspeak Application Programs). The AAC communicator is provided with symbol sequences for stored words and phrases as well as rationales for semantic associations for each vocabulary item. MAPs are designed to serve as starter vocabulary sets with the understanding that further customization and individualization will be required for each AAC user.

Messages or symbol combinations can be changed by the user, as long as care is taken to maintain the internal consistency of the program's language sequencing rules.

The examples provided in Figure 4–14 are from the Unity MAP symbol grid level 3 (Badman, Baker, Banajee, Cross, Lehr, Maro, & Zucco, 1995). Unity was designed to teach beginning language concepts through single symbol messages to young preschool children using a core set of picture symbols. As children learn initial concepts, symbol sequences are gradually added using the same picture symbol set with new additions. Unity grows across three different levels with the final stage appropriate for older children and adults. Many of the symbol sequences use categorization and association strategies to encode words. For example the word *Cat* requires sequencing 3 symbols together (Zebra + Dog + Bed). The first symbol Zebra, is used to start all animal words (i.e., *Cat, Horse, Monkey,* and *Dog*, all start with Zebra). The second symbol Dog, is used to indicate the subcategory of pets (i.e., *Cat* and *Dog* use Dog as the second symbol). The final symbol Bed, is an associative symbol for Cat because cats sleep on beds. Many of Unity's sequences rely on Part of Speech Markers to encode words. For example the word *Hot* is encoded using the Kitchen symbol (a boiling pot of water), followed by the Adjective symbol.

Sigsymbols

Sigsymbols were originally created in England by Cregan to provide a symbol system that served as a "bridge between iconic symbols such as pictographs and arbitrary symbols such as traditional orthography" (Cregan & Lloyd, 1990, p. iv). Sigsymbols are intended for individuals who know sign language or are learning sign language. The symbols consist of pictographs, ideographs, and sign-linked symbols. The sign-linked symbols represent the hand pos-

Words are derived by sequencing symbols together using underlying semantic or grammatical rule strategies. Examples of symbol sequences for words are provided below along with the underlying rationale.

Word	Symbols (Location) and Rationales		
Cat =	Zebra (D7) Animal Category	+ Dog (E6) Pet Subcategory	+ Bed (O7) Cats sleep on beds
Cold =	Kitchen (J6) Cooking Category	+ Mountain (H4) Mountain tops are cold	+ ADJ (I2) Part of Speech Marker
Come =	Dog (E6) Dogs come at your command	+ Verb (C2) Part of Speech Marker	
Coming =	Dog (E6) Dogs come at your command	+ Ing (E2) Part of Speech Marker	
Hot =	Kitchen (J6) Cooking Category The pot is boiling hot	+ ADJ (I2) Part of Speech Marker	
Hotter =	Kitchen (J6) Cooking Category The pot is boiling hot	+ ER (J2) Part of Speech Marker	
Know =	Know (F4) Person with idea	+ Verb (C2) Part of Speech Marker	
Mother =	Family (F6) Family Category	+ Family (F6) Near family Subcategory	+ Love (K6) Hug your mother
Rain =	Umbrella (I5) Weather Category	+ Umbrella (I5) You use umbrellas when its raining	+ Verb (C2) Part of Speech Marker
Sick =	Medical (M4) Health Category	+ ADJ (J2) Part of Speech Marker	
Walk =	Shoe (J3) You wear shoes to walk	+ Verb (C2) Part of Speech Marker	
What =	Question Word (J1) Question Category	+ Television (M7) Question Mark is located on symbol	
Who =	Question Word (J1) Question Category	+ Wanted (D5) Who is wanted in the picture?	

Figure 4–14. Symbol grid 3 for the Minspeak Unity/128 Level 3 MAP (From Badman, Baker, Banajee, Cross, Lehr, Maro, & Zucco, 1995. Reprinted with permission.)

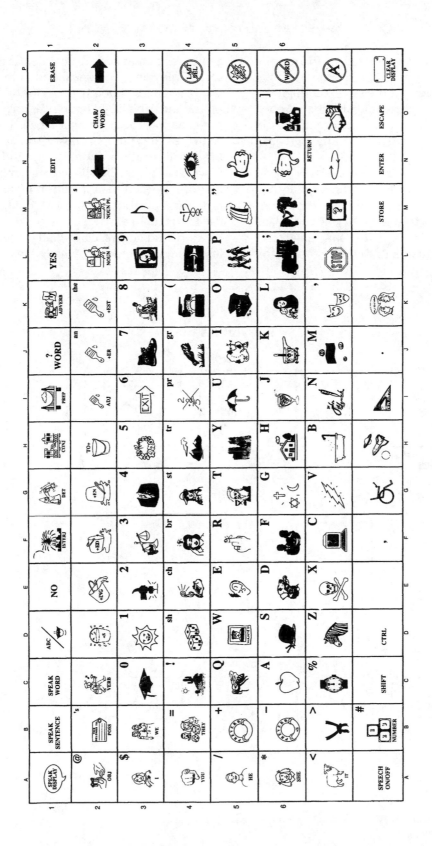

125

tures of signs in Signed English and may indicate the location of the sign on the body or the movement of the sign. Although the symbols can represent abstract concepts, they are based on the concrete motor responses for the corresponding sign (see Figure 4–15).

Symbol clarity is the primary criterion for Sigsymbols which requires using pictographs for many symbols. Color-coded arrows are added to some symbols, with black arrows indicating direction and red arrows indicating movement. Arrows refer to the symbol's referent and are not used as indicators of movement of signs. Red coloring is used on some symbols to provide added emphasis and to highlight targeted information. For example, the nose on a face is colored red when the symbol is *nose*. Triangles are used to illustrate locational terms and other adverbs of place. Sign-linked Sigsymbols illustrate the final hand position of a sign in red. Hand positions are drawn using standard formats to ease recognition (e.g., a flat hand, spread fingers, claw handshape are illustrated the same way). Finally, Sigsymbols

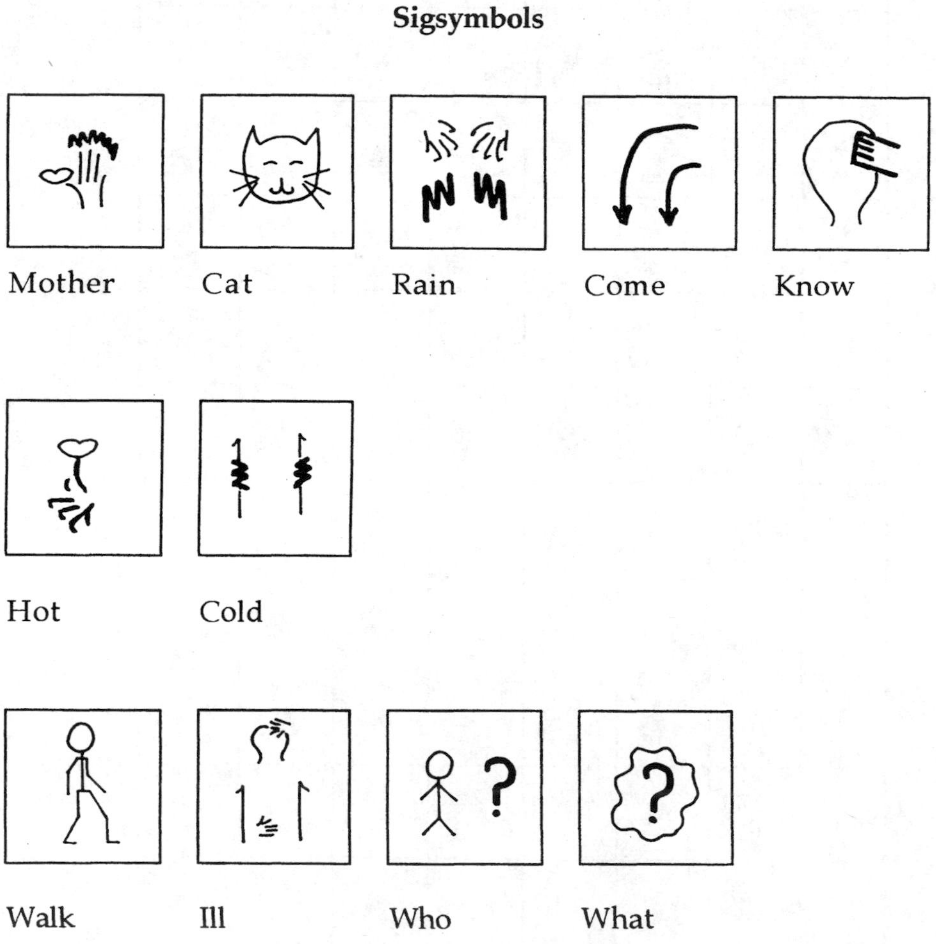

Sigsymbols

Mother   Cat   Rain   Come   Know

Hot   Cold

Walk   Ill   Who   What

Figure 4–15. Sigsymbols.

represent a mirror image of signs performed with the right hand.

Orthographic Symbol Systems

Pictographic systems can serve as a bridge to traditional orthography (Grove & Walker, 1990). Orthographic symbol systems directly correspond to spoken English or other spoken languages (Lloyd & Karlan, 1984). Traditional orthography (TO) consists of written letters that are combined together to form words, sentences, and other forms of written language. Other orthographic symbol systems include Morse Code, Braille, and phonemic symbols. In studies of the transparency of symbol systems, traditional orthography was the most difficult system to learn (Clark, 1981; Thorley, Ward, Binepal, & Dolan, 1991). Orthographic symbols are the most arbitrary of the symbol systems, with spelled words bearing no resemblance to the objects or concepts that they represent. However, orthographic systems are flexible and open symbol systems, with the capability of generating unique expressions with a small number of symbols. Orthography is frequently a system of choice for those capable of using this type of symbol system (Thorley et al., 1991). Many AAC communicators employ multiple language techniques that combine orthographic symbols with other pictographic symbol systems. For example, many adults who use AAC devices with Minspeak language systems rely on Minspeak picture sequences to quickly convey most of their vocabulary, and orthographic spelling to communicate words that are not preprogrammed into the system.

Traditional Orthography

Traditional orthography, or standard written print, was the least transparent symbol system for nonliterate individuals according to a study that compared Rebus, PCS, PIC, and Picsym symbol systems (Mirenda & Locke, 1989). Traditional orthography (TO) consists of the 26 letters of the alphabet, numbers, and other punctuation markers. Traditional orthography is a generative symbol system that enables an individual to construct unique and novel messages. The drawback is that spelling messages letter by letter can be slow and laborious and may not meet the temporal demands of a social conversation. Rate enhancement techniques such as word prediction can be used to reduce keystrokes and increase communication speed (Venkatagiri, 1993). The reader is referred to Chapter 3 in this text for more information on rate enhancement methods.

Morse Code

Standard International Morse Code, designed by Samuel Morse, is an orthographic symbol system that provides auditory or visual representation for letters of the alphabet and numbers, as well as the various punctuation markers of the spoken language. This representation is achieved through combinations of dits (.) and dahs (-), previously termed dots and dashes. Figure 4–16 shows the standard Morse Code symbol set. Adapted computers and dedicated AAC devices are able to interpret the dits and dahs of Morse Code, entered via a single switch or two switches. The information can then be spoken via speech synthesis. With practice, Morse Code is relatively easy to learn and provides an efficient AAC interface for clients who are limited to switch access methods of communication, or have slow direct selection abilities.

Braille

Braille is an orthographic symbol system that represents letters, numbers, punctuation marks, and music through combina-

MORSE CODE

.-	-...	-.-.	-..	.	..-.	--.	....	..
A	**B**	**C**	**D**	**E**	**F**	**G**	**H**	**I**
.---	-.-	.-..	--	-.	---	.--.	--.-	.-.
J	**K**	**L**	**M**	**N**	**O**	**P**	**Q**	**R**
...	-	..-	...-	.--	-..-	-.--	--..	
S	**T**	**U**	**V**	**W**	**X**	**Y**	**Z**	
.----	..---	...--	....-	.....				
1	**2**	**3**	**4**	**5**				
-....	--...	---..	----.	-----				
6	**7**	**8**	**9**	**0**				

Figure 4–16. Morse Code.

tions of small raised dots on paper. Individuals who are blind read Braille by running their fingers along the raised dots. Braille can be written electronically or via nonelectronic Braille aids. Braille can be used to access computers with specialized hardware and software. If the computer is adapted with a speech synthesizer and printer, Braille can be used to produce both written and spoken language. Braille symbols can also be used with dedicated AAC devices. Each Braille cell is three dots high and two dots wide, providing 63 possible combinations of dots. As shown in Figure 4–17, the first 10 letters of the alphabet use combinations of the top four dots. If preceded by a special number sign, these same 10 combinations represent the numbers 0 to 9. The addition of a lower left-hand dot to the initial 10 combinations makes the next 10 letters of the alphabet. The addition of a lower right-hand dot makes the last five letters of the alphabet and five commonly used words (and, for, of, the, with). Finally, the omission of the lower left-hand dot creates nine digraphs and the letter W.

Phonemic

Phonemic symbol systems represent spoken languages at the phonemic or sound level. One of the most well-known phonemic systems is the International Phonetic Alphabet (Faircloth & Faircloth, 1973; see Figure 4–18). Each speech sound is repre-

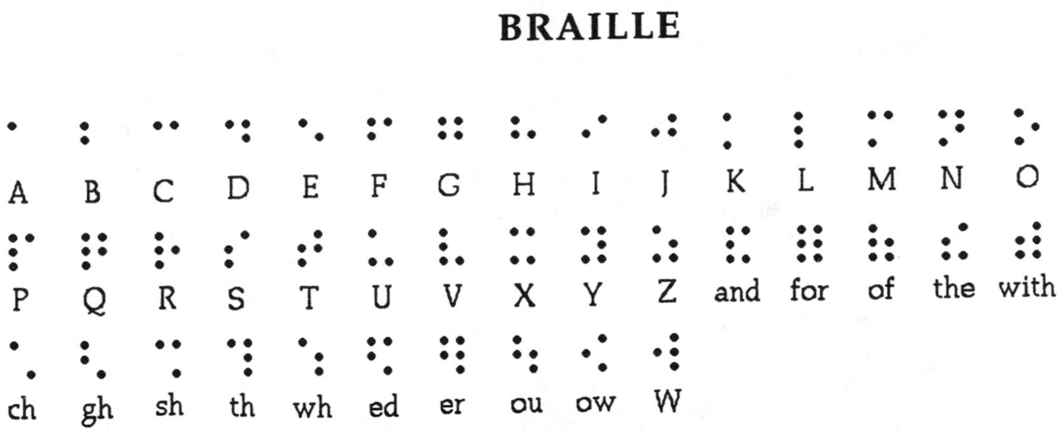

BRAILLE

Figure 4–17. Braille.

sented by a distinctive symbol and the phoneme set is not restricted to the English language. Many AAC devices use a form of phonemic orthography to repair pronunciations of programmed words and messages or to provide the text to speech translation vehicle through which messages are constructed. Finally, phonemic symbol systems are the most precise orthographic symbol systems for representing spoken language, due to the fact that their basic unit is the speech sound itself (Faircloth & Faircloth, 1973).

VOCABULARY AND SYMBOL SELECTION STRATEGIES

The next section of this chapter will provide an overview of methods used to (a) develop vocabulary and (b) select and organize symbols for AAC systems. Both steps are critical to the overall effectiveness of an AAC system. The first step is to match the vocabulary requirements of the user's communicative environment to the vocabulary capabilities of an AAC system (Doss et al., 1991). A needs assessment is conducted in order to determine required vocabulary across various communicative

environments. This vocabulary is then organized to maximize accessibility and functional use of the AAC system. The development and design of vocabulary requires careful consideration of the unique needs of each communicator (Grove & Walker, 1990; Mirenda, 1985). AAC communicators who are not able to spell messages have to depend upon the vocabulary decisions of others to create a working functional vocabulary (Carlson, 1981; Fried-Oken & More, 1992). All vocabulary decisions made for AAC communicators must include consideration of communicative needs, goals, listening partners, personal experiences, and environments (Mirenda, 1985; Romski & Sevcik, 1988).

Vocabulary Needs Assessment

Designing vocabulary for an individual's AAC system can be a difficult and time-consuming task. It requires the full participation of the AAC communicator as well as a team of people significant to that individual, including professionals, family, and friends (Berry, 1987; Beukelman, McGinnis, & Morrow, 1991). There are several

PHONEMIC UNITS

Vowels:

I   ə   æ   aI   i   ɛ   oU   ʌ   eI   ə   ɔ   ɑ   aU   u   U   ʒ˞   ɪ˞

Consonants:

Plosives: p   b   t   d   k   g   ʔ

Fricatives: f   v   θ   ð   s   z   ʃ   ʒ   h   hw

Glides: w   l   r   j

Nasals: m   n   ŋ

Affricates: tʃ   dʒ

Figure 4–18. Phonemic units.

techniques that can be employed that make this task less difficult. These techniques involve strategies for assessing vocabulary needs of individuals within daily environments. Helpful techniques for conducting a vocabulary needs assessment include ecological inventories, scripts, communication diaries, and standard vocabulary lists (Yorkston, Honsinger, Dowden, & Marriner, 1989). The use of these techniques can improve lexical diversity and functionality, enabling the AAC communicator to interact more effectively in a variety of places and with a variety of listening partners.

Different Vocabulary for Different Environments

We all interact across multiple environments in our daily lives. Vocabulary necessary for successful interaction in one environment may differ significantly from that needed in another environment. Different vocabulary is needed for communicating at home, school, the workplace, the grocery store, a hair salon, or a favorite restaurant. We choose different words and different expressions for each environment. In addition to the effects of the setting itself, the characteristics of the communication partners also contribute to the types of expressions we make as well as the vocabulary we choose to use. This is true of all communicators, including AAC communicators. There are several different strategies for determining the communicative needs of the AAC user across multiple environments. A progression of techniques to develop a lexicon might involve (a) interviews with significant persons in the AAC communicator's life, (b) ecological inventories of the primary daily environments, and (c) scripting.

Interview Methods. Structured interviews with significant persons in the AAC user's environment provide the following information: (a) the number and types of environments encountered on a daily basis as well as those faced occasionally; (b) the amount of time spent in each setting; (c) the names, numbers, and characteristics of communicative partners in those settings; (d) the types of activities occurring in those environments and communicative demands required to participate successfully; and (e) the types of objects present in those settings (Yorkston et al., 1989). An interview will provide a broad base of information, with general overviews as well as specific details.

Ecological Inventories. Information from direct observation of the AAC user is critical when designing and selecting vocabulary. Observations provide detailed information about communicative needs in specific settings. This information contributes directly to selecting vocabulary to meet individual expressive communication needs. An organized process for determining vocabulary needs of an AAC communicator that includes direct observation is the ecological inventory (Mirenda, 1985). There are six primary steps to an ecological inventory. These are listed as follows:

- determine the current home, school, community, and work environments;
- conduct detailed, on-site analyses of the communicative requirements of each setting (Fried-Oken & More, 1992; Mirenda, 1985);
- conduct detailed, on-site inventories of the AAC communicator's participation in each of these settings;
- conduct discrepancy analyses to determine any communicative deficits or needs of the AAC communicator;
- interview significant individuals concerning communicative needs that they have observed;

- create and design modifications or additions to the AAC system to alleviate these needs.

Analyses such as these, conducted in the primary environments encountered by the AAC communicator, can contribute tremendously to the effectiveness of the AAC system, ensuring vocabulary is relevant and functional in a variety of settings (Mirenda, 1985).

Ecological inventories serve two purposes, providing a process for assessing communicative needs in specific environments for individuals whose communication systems are initially being developed, providing a means to evaluate the effectiveness of an AAC system in various settings once it is developed and in use. For example, observation of the AAC communicator in a particular environment attempting to use an AAC system may reveal vocabulary to be inadequate or ineffective; conversely, observation may indicate that AAC vocabulary is adequate but further training with the user is needed. Finally, observations can sometimes highlight the need to provide training to the communication partners. This training might focus on increasing their understanding of the AAC techniques being used or teaching them to let the AAC user initiate communication in specific situations.

Several studies have used ecological approaches to determine the vocabulary needs of individuals across multiple communication settings. A study of preschool children at home and in school found similarities and differences in the content of their discussions, based on the setting (Marvin, Beukelman, Brockhaus, & Kast, 1994). At home, children were free to initiate and engage in conversation with adults, siblings, and other children. Discussions typically revolved around shared experiences; however, adults in the home frequently asked questions and made comments about events occurring outside of the home. At school, events and activities were structured, with topics frequently determined by the teacher. When children did engage in free conversation at school, their talk was primarily limited to topics dealing with the "here and now" although there were also occurrences when the children engaged in fantasy discussions and play. In both settings, the greatest percentage of talk centered around objects, followed by events, and then ideas about people. As expected, toys and food were the most common objects discussed. Actions that were referred to in both settings included jumping, getting, giving, sitting, walking, talking, and lying down. This study provided information that suggests that preschool children require vocabulary that is geared toward the here and now (e.g., common routines and activities) but also enables references to be made to distant events and occurrences. In addition, it was important to the interaction of these preschool children at school to be able to participate and engage in fantasy. These results highlight the importance of gaining direct information regarding the vocabulary needs of individuals across more than one setting.

Not only will social interactions change with advances in age but school-related vocabulary also changes as a child grows older. The increased emphasis on academic material and literacy instruction places greater demands on individuals to demonstrate knowledge of curricular material and comprehension of basic concepts and instruction (McGinnis & Beukelman, 1989). Therefore, as children increase in age, their vocabulary needs in school include a greater degree of specific curricular information in order to participate effectively in class discussions (McGinnis & Beukelman, 1989). This places additional demands on professionals and family members to update vocabulary frequently as curricular units change across the school year.

Scripting. After observing a particular environment or setting and conducting an ecological inventory of that setting, it is helpful to write a script, or scripts, of communicative expressions that are needed in the setting. Care should be taken to ensure that a variety of communicative functions are served by these expressions. These include requests for action, information, and objects; negation; regulation; evaluation; and commenting, to name a few (Spragale & Micucci, 1990). If the vocabulary is being developed for a picture communication display, key words in the scripts can then be underlined to assist in the collection of needed symbols for communication (see Figure 4–19).

It is also important to analyze the variety of word classes that are represented as well as the various communicative functions served by each message. Key words can be entered on a chart like the one in Figure 4–20 organized by various word classes (e.g., people, actions, objects, places, feelings, adjectives, questions, temporal words). This analysis will ensure that there is no imbalance of word classes. For example, many communication boards include an overrepresentation of a particular word class such as nouns. When AAC devices limit the number of words or messages that are available to the user, a word class analysis ensures that words that are selected for programming are based on a structured thoughtful process.

If an AAC device is the communication technique primarily used in a specific setting, the scripting activity will serve as a helpful tool for accessing relevant vocabulary in the device. For example, if a DynaVox2C is used, the script can assist in developing specific overlays, or pages, of vocabulary for a particular activity. If the device is a Liberator, the script can be transcribed, with appropriate symbol sequences noted beside the various words in the script. Finally, if the AAC communicator has specific limitations (e.g., cogni-

AAC THANKSGIVING SCRIPT

The script below provides a partial sample of expressions planned for an AAC

communicator participating in a classroom Thanksgiving activity. In this example,

several classes are making portions of a Thanksgiving dinner and the culminating

activity is a group dinner with all classes present. This script could be used to select

symbols for a picture communication display or to determine words and phrases that

need to be programmed into a high tech AAC device. Symbol words are capitalized.

WHAT did YOU MAKE for THANKSGIVING?
WE made TURKEY, DRESSING, MASHED POTATOES, SWEET POTATOES, BEANS,
      CORN, PUMPKIN PIE, BREAD, APPLE CIDER.
Was it FUN?
WHAt did YOU DO?
CAN I HELP MAKE the...
IT'S ABOUT TIME!
CAN I TASTE...
It TASTES DELICIOUS
It TASTES BAD
Do YOU CELEBRATE THANKSGIVING at YOUR HOUSE (home)?
If YOU EAT too much TURKEY DINNER, YOU might get FAT.
INDIANS and PILGRIMS ATE the FIRST THANKSGIVING
MY FAVORITE is...
I am THANKFUL for...

Figure 4–19. Writing a script for a class-based Thanksgiving dinner activity.

tive, motor, or visual) that restrict the number of symbols or expressions that can be used for communication, the scripted expressions can be prioritized, from most to least critical. For children and adults with limited vocabulary choices, it is helpful to develop more than one script for each activity. For example, the focus for one script might be hands-on participation in an activity. The prioritized words, statements, and questions would be those that involve the activity itself (e.g., supplies, requests, action words). On the other hand, if the focus of the same event shifted to the individual's perceptions and feelings about the activities, then personal statements and other evalu-

ative symbols might have priority (e.g., fun, boring). Therefore, ecological inventories and scripting activities can yield a wealth of information regarding the vocabulary needs and interactive potential of certain activities.

Vocabulary Lists. Research has focused on vocabulary needs of various individuals in specific environments in order to create master vocabulary lists of needed words and expressions. This research has yielded vocabulary lists that provide good resources for starter sets of words. Although vocabulary needs to be individualized for each AAC user, master vocabulary lists serve as templates that can be scanned to

SCRIPTED WORDS ANALYZED BY WORD CLASS

The partial vocabulary of symbol words scripted for the Thanksgiving Dinner Activity are analyzed by word class.

PEOPLE	ACTIONS	OBJECTS	DESCRIPTORS	QUESTIONS	MISCELLANEOUS
I (my)	make	Thanksgiving	fun	what	It's about time
you	help	turkey	delicious	can	
we	taste	dressing	bad		
Indians	celebrate	mashed potatoes	fat		
Pilgrims	eat	sweet potatoes	favorite		
		beans	first		
		corn	thankful		
		pumpkin pie			
		bread			
		apple cider			
		house			
		dinner			

Figure 4–20. Scripted words analyzed by word class.

fill in missing words from vocabulary developed from ecological inventories. Reviewing lists such as these can assist in reducing omissions of important vocabulary. These standard vocabulary lists have been developed for various ages, based on detailed analyses of specific environments (Francis, 1990; Fried-Oken & More, 1992; Yorkston et al., 1989). Of course, a word list will not serve all the communicative needs of an individual; however, these lists do provide an immediate lexicon for easy use.

Core Versus Fringe Vocabulary

There are two levels of vocabulary development for AAC systems, core vocabulary and fringe vocabulary. Core vocabulary consists of highly functional words and phrases, typically beginning with items related to basic functional needs, brief social exchanges, and other information necessary across most communication environments (Grove & Walker, 1990; McEwen & Lloyd, 1990; Spragale & Micucci, 1990). For example, core vocabulary for a child in elementary school would most likely include symbols for the following: *bathroom, go, eat, drink, mother, father, teacher, yes, no, stop, more, bus,* and *home.* An adult's core vocabulary might only include *go, eat, yes, no, stop* and *home.* In addition, there would be high frequency words relating to work. An adult's core vocabulary also reflects age-appropriate word differences (e.g., the use of the word *restroom* instead of *potty*). Regardless of age, core vocabulary for an AAC communicator must be highly reinforcing and responsive to the communicative and basic needs of the individual (Fried-Oken & More, 1992). It is also recommended that the core vocabulary reflect a wide variety of communicative functions. For example, a core vocabulary consisting entirely of requests (i.e., *I want . . .*) should be avoided, otherwise the AAC communicator might inter-

pret AAC techniques as request-only techniques (Romski & Sevcik, 1988). Although the request function can serve as a successful entry point for introducing AAC techniques, vocabulary needs to be expanded to avoid limiting the communicative potential of the individual. AAC users who have limited cognitive potential can still use their AAC systems in socially validated ways to communicate beyond the request level. For example, an adult AAC user who enjoyed social attention had a wolf whistle message recorded into his device. Although the message was certainly politically incorrect, it got him immediate attention from staff and peers every time he pressed the symbol!

Unlike core vocabulary, fringe vocabulary includes words and expressions that are particularly content-rich, topic-related, and specific to particular individuals, activities, or environments (McGinnis & Beukelman, 1989). For example, the fringe vocabulary for an AAC communication board specifically designed for the beach might include references to *suntan lotion, waves, bucket, pail, seagulls,* and possibly the verb *fry!* Fringe vocabulary contains expressions that customize the AAC system for the individual as well as for the specific interactions and situations in which the individual is involved. It is important that the AAC system's fringe vocabulary include diversity and language richness to enhance participation and interaction in various activities of daily living. Ecological inventories and standardized vocabulary lists provide two rich sources for the vocabulary development of AAC systems.

Fringe vocabulary needs to be accessible to the AAC user across activities. Some AAC users will be able to access fringe vocabulary independently, other AAC users will need to have adults or professionals set up fringe vocabulary when appropriate. Fringe vocabulary is essential to allow individuals to expand on communication topics. For example, one adult user had a *bowling* symbol on his primary communication board. But after he pointed to the symbol, he had nothing else he could tell the listener about his recent bowling outing. Fringe vocabulary specific to bowling was then added to his AAC system. Through fringe vocabulary he was able to comment on his bowling skills, the snacks he ate, how other bowlers performed, and who won the game.

Regardless of the various sources used, vocabulary development for an AAC system is an ongoing process. The system must remain dynamic and ever-changing as the communicative needs of the AAC communicator continue to change over time (Beukelman et al., 1991; Yorkston et al., 1989). New vocabulary will need to be added and other words and expressions will become stale and unused, thus prompting their eventual removal from the system. Once the vocabulary for an AAC system is developed, the next step is determining which symbols to use to represent the vocabulary, and how to organize the symbols for easy retrieval of the vocabulary. The next section of this chapter will review this process.

Selecting Symbols for Vocabulary

As described earlier in this chapter, there are a variety of symbol sets and symbols systems available for communication. Selecting appropriate symbols for an individual involves the consideration of a variety of factors. Some of these considerations are based on the environments in which communication takes place; others involve the characteristics of the communicative partners. Most importantly, it is critical to consider the preferences and abilities of the AAC user.

The communicative environment needs to be considered when selecting symbol systems. Information obtained through observations and interviews includes determining the physical characteristics of the environment. For example, will materials need to be waterproof, visible in the dark, or extremely durable? The need for portability of the symbol system also needs to be determined. Will the user need to carry the symbols from place to place independently? The characteristics of the listeners in the environment should also be evaluated. For example, if interaction partners cannot read, they won't be able to understand an AAC system based on traditional orthography. Similarly, sign languages are only useful with communication partners who are familiar with sign. The temporal demands of the interaction environment should be reviewed. A preschool setting where answers are immediately called out is very different from a preschool setting that requires raising a hand to participate. The first situation requires a symbol system designed for quick attention getting, the second situation would allow more time for the AAC communicator to access a device. The dynamics of group communication settings versus one-to-one settings should also be considered when developing the symbol set. These are some of the considerations that must be made when selecting symbol systems for an individual's AAC system.

In addition to the physical environment and listener characteristics, it is also important to consider the AAC communicator (Lloyd & Karlan, 1984). The AAC communicator's cognitive ability will influence the type of symbols selected (e.g., the degree of representativeness required) as well as the number of symbols displayed at one time (Lloyd & Karlan, 1984). For example, if the AAC communicator is a young child whose cause-effect or means-ends abilities are emerging, AAC intervention will most likely involve real objects and include activities to encourage the establishment of these skills. Display options might be limited to two to four items, with a gradual increase in the number of items as skills emerge. On the other hand, if the individual has picture representation skills, photographs, magazine pictures, and coupons would also be options. In addition, line drawings might be introduced. Finally, if the individual's cognitive skills are intact and reading and spelling skills are present, there are few limitations regarding the various symbol systems. Individual preferences and environmental conditions will guide the selection. If there are communicative partners who are non-readers, the AAC system must also include techniques or symbol systems that enable interactions to take place with those individuals (Musselwhite & Ruscello, 1984). The reader is referred to Chapter 5 in this text for more information on the evaluation process as it relates to symbol selection.

One consideration that should not be overlooked when symbol systems are selected for children is the effect of the symbol system on literacy and other language-related skills. There have not been a large number of studies that have investigated these relationships, particularly the relationship between literacy and symbol selection. Clark (1981) suggested that a logographic system (e.g., Rebus) may be the system of choice if a parallel to English is desired; on the other hand, if the individual requires a permanent system and has the capability to learn the complex rule system of a generative system, Blissymbols may be appropriate (Clark, 1981; Mizuko, 1987).

The motor skills and abilities of the AAC communicator are another factor that needs to be considered when selecting a symbol system. Individuals with severe physical disabilities will have difficulty using sign languages as a primary communication method. However, many AAC communicators with severe physical disabilities can learn to incorporate a few basic signs and natural gestures into their AAC lexicons to supplement their primary communication methods. After selecting the primary symbol set, further evaluation of motor abilities is needed to determine the number of available symbols that can be reliably accessed, the size and spacing of symbols, the overall size of any picture communication displays, even the actual design of the system itself (e.g., whether the design will include pages for turning). Chapter 7 in this text provides more information on the evaluation of motor abilities for AAC.

The AAC communicator's sensory skills will also have an impact on the symbol selection process. Visual acuity can affect the size of the symbols (Mirenda & Mathy-Laikko, 1989). In addition, if the AAC communicator has difficulty with figure-ground contrasts, several trials may be needed to find the appropriate contrast for the symbol system and background displays (Mirenda, 1985; Mirenda & Mathy-Laikko, 1989). It may be critical to use symbols that minimize the number and complexity of details (McNaughton, 1993). The individual may need a constant visual display that does not change. This impacts the type of symbols selected and also the types of AAC techniques that can be employed (Lloyd & Karlan, 1984). Finally, the spacing and placement of symbols may be determined largely by the individual's visual skills. For example, if the individual is unable to visually scan both horizontally and vertically, a row-column arrangement of symbols would be inappropriate and ineffective for that individual. Symbols may need to be placed one-per-page to avoid scanning problems (Mirenda, 1985), or organized with auditory feedback cues. Again, the reader is referred to Chapter 7 for more information regarding the assessment of visual abilities as they relate to AAC.

Finally, one of the most critical characteristics of a symbol system that may affect its adoption is its acceptability to the AAC communicator, to peers, and to other potential communicative partners (Lloyd & Karlan, 1984). If a symbol system is not considered acceptable by the AAC communicator, his family, peers, colleagues, or other communicative partners, it will probably not be used, regardless of its vocabulary potential. For example, many nonspeaking teenagers reject picture communication systems because they don't look sophisticated. If the teen does not have sufficient literacy skills to use traditional orthography, the AAC system will fail unless alternatives are developed. Therefore, the participation of the AAC communicator and other significant individuals in the development of the AAC system is useful and often essential (Beukelman et al., 1991).

Organizing a Vocabulary System

After a symbol system has been selected for the AAC communicator, the AAC system must then be physically and linguistically organized. Although there are organizational tasks that must be performed with electronic augmentative communication devices, this section will focus exclusively on nonelectronic, picture communication displays. However, many of the principles discussed in this section can be adapted for use in electronic AAC devices.

Physical Organization

Picture communication displays can take many different shapes. Selections can be made by pointing with an index finger or via eye gaze. The method of accessibility will have a direct impact on the physical organization of the display. A variety of organizational techniques are possible. Individual photographs can be covered in acrylic plastic and placed on rings organized by topic. The AAC communicator can use a small wallet, a small 5" × 8" book, and, at other times, a larger display.

If the individual has difficulty turning pages of a language book, foam spacers can be added to the pages to make page turning easier. The type of display will be determined by a variety of factors. For example, if an individual requires a highly portable display, a small wallet or a small book stored in a hip-pack can be used. If the individual will use the display when seated in a wheelchair with a tray, the display can be larger.

The purpose of the display can also affect its size and organization. A picture communication display for a holiday (e.g., a holiday topic board) can take the shape of a holiday symbol. The Jack-O-Lantern in Figure 4–21 is an example. Displays such as these can be quite colorful, aesthetic, and attract the interest of other children, thus serving as a "conversational piece." This attention then encourages the initiation of interactions and relationships with others.

Individuals who have problems with control over their motor movements and require a particularly durable language board may appreciate having a system made of plastic. Kydex plastic has been used to create language boards, offering many different thicknesses. If an individual requires a system that will not tear and is not affected by weather and moisture, a thin Kydex plastic board may be a possible solution, covered in shelf contact paper to add waterproofing. Thin types of this plastic can be cut with heavy duty scissors and holes can be added with an extra-strength hole-puncher. Tabs can be cut for the pages to aid page turning (see Figure 4–22). For individuals who require stiffness in order to turn pages as well as durability, a thicker Kydex board can be used. Thicker materials will require the use of a saber saw or scroll saw in order to cut the individual pages, and a drill to make holes.

Individuals who cannot use their hands or fingers for pointing can access picture communication displays using eye

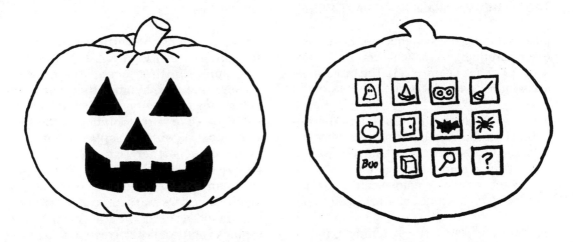

Figure 4-21. A Halloween topic board with both sides displayed.

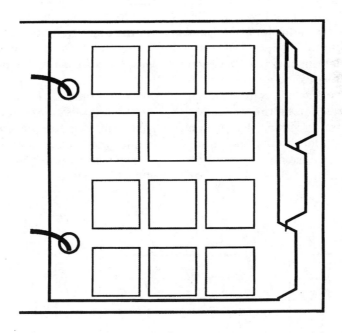

Figure 4-22. Plastic "pages" of a picture display system, with tabs cut and staggered to aid page turning.

gaze. All eye gaze systems use three-point eye referencing to make selections (Goossens, 1989; see Figure 4–23). The three steps are sequenced as follows:

- the AAC communicator scans the options on the communication display;
- he or she decides on the targeted symbol;
- the AAC communicator establishes eye contact with the communicative partner to indicate that a selection has been made.

Eye contact with the listening partner must be established immediately after the AAC communicator's eye gaze points toward the desired symbol in order for clear communication to occur.

Eye gaze picture communication displays offer a unique organizational challenge. A few of the most familiar formats for eye gaze systems include coded picture communication displays, coded books, picture frame displays, and cloth vests. The simplest design for an eye gaze display is one where the individual eye gazes at the desired symbol to communicate a message. A 1:1 relationship exists between the symbol and the desired message, with no coding or layering of symbols. With coded eye gaze responses, the communicator and the listener communicate via a coding system. Coded books and other displays are typically arranged in row-column matrices, with numbers, shapes, or

colors providing the vertical and horizontal markers (see Figure 4–24). The AAC communicator first locates the targeted symbol (e.g., the symbol that communicates *Love ya!*). He or she then communicates the code corresponding to the symbol's location on the display to the communication partner (e.g., red-moon). A picture frame eye gaze display can be used to communicate the code elements or symbols can be marked on a wheelchair tray. In either case, the AAC communicator looks at the color corresponding to the row (e.g., red), followed by eye gazing toward the shape corresponding to the appropriate column (e.g., moon).

Individuals who are literate and need a dynamic system that can keep up with fast moving discussions can use a dry-erase board as a simple communication system. Eye gaze coding symbols are permanently affixed to the corners of the dry-erase board. As the discussion ensues, relevant words, phrases, or expressions necessary for the conversation can be written on the board for the AAC communicator to select. As expressions are no longer needed, they are simply erased.

Two common formats for displaying symbols for eye gaze access include eye gaze vests and the picture frame eye gaze display (see Figure 4–25; Goossens, 1989). The eye gaze vest is particularly beneficial when the communication partner needs to

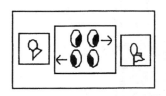

1) Eyes scan choices.

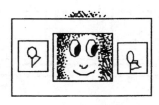

2) Eyes lock on choice.

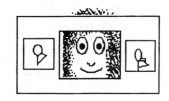

3) Eye contact with the listener.

Figure 4–23. Three-point referencing for eye gaze selections.

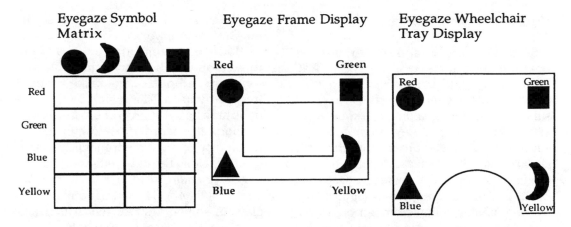

Figure 4–24. Coding methods for eye gaze communication.

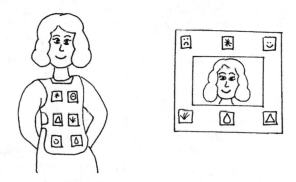

Figure 4–25. Eye gaze vest and picture frame eye gaze displays.

have his hands free. Velcro strips are sewn onto a cloth vest which is worn by the communication partner. Objects, pictures, or symbols are affixed to the velcro as needed. A vest can also be used to present a permanent display, with pictures or symbols permanently affixed, or there can be several displays on one vest. An eye gaze display with a picture frame format can be created using a clear, plastic display, with a center section cut out for face-to-face contact between the AAC communicator and his or her communicative partner. If the center is not cut out, it presents a visual and auditory barrier between the AAC

communicator and communicative partner. Objects, photographs, or picture symbols are placed along the periphery of the eye gaze display.

In summary, the physical organization of a picture communication display can vary greatly and is determined by a number of different factors. These include the individual's motor abilities, cognitive and linguistic constraints, the purpose of the AAC display, and the environment where the communication system will be used. Ecological inventories provide important information that contributes to decisions regarding the physical format of an AAC system.

Linguistic Organization

The linguistic organization of AAC displays does not affect the overall form of the AAC system as greatly as its physical organization. Most displays are organized in a format similar to the Fitzgerald Key (Bishop et al., 1994). The Fitzgerald Key format follows a left to right linguistic order in which words are arranged in classes according to their typical position in a sentence. Question words and people are typically found on the left of a display, followed by action words, then descriptors, and finally object nouns. Color coding the symbols by word class assists the AAC communicator in locating specific symbols. A common color coding system presents people symbols in yellow, verbs in green, descriptors in blue, nouns in orange or goldenrod, and social expressions in pink (Johnson, 1981). This system increases the efficiency of the system by providing an additional visual cue for the user. For example, if the AAC communicator is looking for the symbol for *big*, he or she will only need to visually scan the blue symbols.

The AAC display often includes some symbols that carry complete messages, usually social messages or frequently needed requests (e.g., *Hello, my name is . . . , Leave me alone,* or *Please reposition me*). In addition, there is typically a symbol such as *no symbol*, that indicates to the communicative partner that the AAC communicator would like to express a word or phrase that is not on the communication display. AAC systems that have complex coding schemes, such as eye gaze displays, need symbols that indicate *Mistake—Start the message over,* and *End of message.* All communication systems need to include a card or statement that describes how the communicator uses his or her AAC techniques. For users of simple communication boards, this explanation can be recorded on a loop tape or Big Mack switch to provide a verbal explanation to unfamiliar listeners. Users of electronic voice output systems can have a message key that describes how the system works.

If the communication aid is designed to include vocabulary for multiple environments, a book or book-like format is frequently used. The inside pages of the book may be cut narrower or shorter than the book size in order to allow for the continual display of some frequently needed symbols along the outer edges of the book (e.g., *I, you, hurt, sick, go, bathroom, What? Where? When?*). These sections of a display are sometimes referred to as the "always" section because they hold symbols that the AAC communicator wishes to have displayed at all times. The amount of space set aside for "always" symbols will be determined by the individual needs of the AAC communicator. Designing an always section serves several purposes: it saves time and space because symbols are not continually duplicated from page to page, and it allows the individual pages of the book to be topic specific.

Typically, the pages are narrower so that there are two lengths inside the book where symbols can be placed (see Figure 4–26). This arrangement is largely compatible with a left-right orientation. Some AAC communicators may prefer to have the always section at the top of the book. If more space is needed, the top and sides could be dedicated to this section. If there are quite a few symbols that require continual exposure, the always section can be designed to wrap around the pages, surrounding the topic-related vocabulary.

Within the book's pages it is important to organize vocabulary so that the AAC communicator can efficiently access needed words and phrases. Typically, communication books are organized so that each open area holds vocabulary for one topic or activity (i.e., when opened, the left and right pages of the display include vocabulary for the same topic or activity). Finally, a book can be organized further by attaching tabs or topic symbols to the sides of

Communication Boards with Continuous Displays

a. "Always" section on sides.

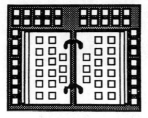

b. "Always" section on top.

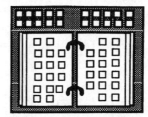

c. "Always" section on top and sides.

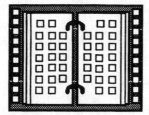

d. "Always" section surrounds pages.

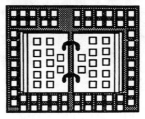

Figure 4–26. Examples of communication books, with areas for continuous display of specific symbols.

the relevant pages. Using tabs with picture symbols provides an additional cue to assist the user in locating the desired vocabulary (see Figure 4–27).

The concept of an always section can also be applied to electronic AAC devices. Dynamic display systems such as the Dynavox 2C, or Speaking Dynamically, can be programmed with templates of consistent always vocabulary appearing on every display page. AAC devices that use paper displays with multiple pages can also have always vocabulary that appear as a template on each overlay page. Some users combine their electronic AAC systems with a simple communication board that contains always vocabulary. For example, one young child who could not independently change the pages of his electronic AAC device had an always template designed on a U-shaped cut-out that wrapped around his AAC system. This always dis-

play had topic symbols that allowed him to select the communication page he wanted to use on his electronic device.

Eye gaze displays require additional creativity to linguistically organize the vocabulary. Because it is easy to misinterpret an eye gaze response, symbols with opposite meanings should be placed on opposite sides of the display (Goossens, 1989). The user might combine more than one eye gaze communication display to increase communication power. For example, the wheelchair tray might have permanent always symbols, and the clear display mounted in front of the user might contain changing symbols. Although eye gaze is quite effective for limited selections, the AAC communicator is typically limited to four to eight symbol areas at one time. Therefore, one common technique to expand the available vocabulary for the user involves branching overlays.

To branch eye gaze overlays, a master overlay is made that contains topic-related symbols. Once the AAC communicator selects the topic, another overlay is presented with secondary selections relating to that topic alone (see Figure 4–28). The number and type of branching are only limited by the organizational complexity of the displays. As long as the user understands how to access the various symbols, there is no upper limit to the number of overlays. Chapter 3 in this textbook describes other methods of configuring eye gaze systems to increase vocabulary options.

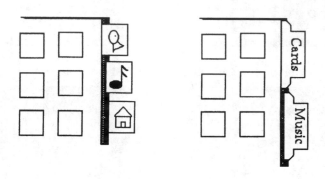

Figure 4–27. Organizational tabs by topic for communication books.

Branching Eyegaze Overlays

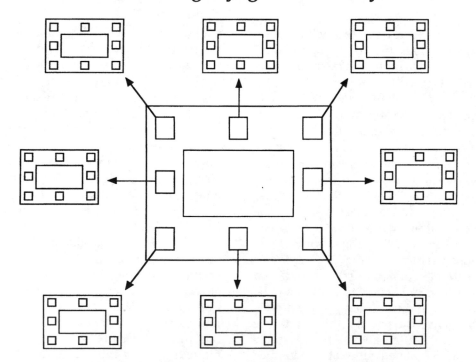

Figure 4–28. Branching eye gaze overlays.

SUMMARY

Selecting symbol systems and designing an AAC system for an individual are complex tasks requiring the input of a team of people, including the AAC communicator. The vocabulary of each AAC system should be open-ended and "sensitive to developmental, environmental and cultural changes" (Carlson, 1981, p. 244). As a matter of fact, it is recommended that when AAC systems have been rejected and are not being used, evaluate the effectiveness and efficiency of the vocabulary first (Yorkston et al., 1989). The available words and expressions may be limiting, boring, or not considered important to the AAC communicator. There may be more efficient means for expressing those same messages, thus making the AAC system inefficient and redundant. For example, one child was motorically limited to accessing six symbols at a time on his AAC device, including the messages yes, no, stop that, and mom. He initially was excited about his new talking system, but after several weeks gradually stopped using his AAC device. When reviewing the vocabulary, it was determined that he was able to produce most of the messages more efficiently using unaided communication strategies. Once the six messages were changed to motivating information that could not be conveyed using unaided methods, he immediately began to use his AAC system again.

The most meaningful way to evaluate the AAC symbol system is in action. The AAC communicator should be engaged in real situations where the use of a specific symbol results in real world responses (Poock & Blackston, 1992). Yorkston et al. (1989) recommended using a communication diary to keep a record of communication use and breakdowns with the AAC system. This will help to pinpoint new vocabulary that should be added to the AAC system or to indicate better methods of organizing or accessing vocabulary. It is also helpful if the communication diary documents anecdotal reports of particularly successful interactions with the system. An occasional review of the diary, along with an ecological inventory, serves as a periodic recheck on the effectiveness and efficiency of the AAC system. Just as the design of an AAC symbol system is an ongoing process, the evaluation of the system must also be ongoing.

REFERENCES

Badman, A., Baker, B., Banajee, M., Cross, R., Lehr, J., Maro, J., & Zucco, M. (1995). *Unity 128 Minspeak Application Program*. Wooster, OH: Prentke Romich Company.

Baker, B. (1986). Using images to generate speech. *Byte, 3*, 160–168.

Berry, J. O. (1987). Strategies for involving parents in programs for young children using augmentative and alternative communication. *Augmentative and Alternative Communication, 3*, 90–93.

Beukelman, D. R., McGinnis, J., & Morrow, D. (1991). Vocabulary selection in augmentative and alternative communication. *Augmentative and Alternative Communication, 7*, 171–185.

Beukelman, D. R., & Mirenda, P. (1992). *Augmentative and alternative communication: Management of severe communication disorders in children and adults*. Baltimore, MD: Paul H. Brookes Publishing Co.

Bishop, K., Rankin, J., & Mirenda, P. (1994). Impact of graphic symbol use on reading acquisition. *Augmentative and Alternative Communication, 10*, 113–125.

Bliss, C. K. (1965). *Blissymbolics*. Sydney, Australia: Semantography Publications.

Bloomberg, K., Karlan, G. R., & Lloyd, L. L. (1990). The comparative translucency of initial lexical items represented in five graphic symbol systems and sets. *Journal of Speech and Hearing Research, 33*, 717–725.

Bruno, J., & Goehl, H. (1991). Comparison of picture and word association performance in adults and preliterate children. *Augmentative and Alternative Communication, 7*, 70–79.

Burroughs, J. A., Albritton, E. G., Eaton, B. B., & Montague, J. C., Jr. (1990). A comparative study of language delayed preschool children's ability to recall symbols from two symbol systems. *Augmentative and Alternative Communication, 6,* 202–206.

Carlson, F. (1981). A format for selecting vocabulary for the nonspeaking child. *Language, Speech, and Hearing Services in Schools, 12,* 240–245.

Carlson, F. (1986). *Picsyms categorical dictionary.* Unity, ME: Baggeboda Press.

Carlson, F. (1994). *Poppin's cut and paste with 1000+ DynaSyms.* Arlington, VA: Poppin & Company.

Clark, C. R. (1981). Learning words using traditional orthography and the symbols of Rebus, Bliss, and Carrier. *Journal of Speech and Hearing Disorders, 46,* 191–196.

Cole, C., Sommer, R., Cole, M., Smith, L., Mondloch, B., & Eidelman, J. (1993). *Maryland School for the Blind Texture Communication List.* Unpublished paper, Maryland School for the Blind, Baltimore, MD.

Cregan, A. (1993). Sigsymbol system in a multimodal approach to speech elicitation: Classroom project involving an adolescent with severe mental retardation. *Augmentative and Alternative Communication, 9,* 146–160.

Cregan, A., & Lloyd, L. L. (1990). *Sigsymbols: American edition.* Wauconda, IL: Don Johnston Developmental Equipment, Inc.

Daehler, M. W., Perlmutter, M., & Myers, N. A. (1976). Equivalence of pictures and objects for very young children. *Child Development, 47,* 96–102.

DePaul, R., & Yoder, D. E. (1986). Iconicity in manual sign systems for the augmentative communication user: Is that all there is? *Augmentative and Alternative Communication, 2,* 1–10.

Dixon, L. S. (1981). A functional analysis of photo-object matching skills of severely retarded adolescents. *Journal of Applied Behavior Analysis, 14,* 465–478.

Doss, L. S., Locke, P. A., Johnston, S. S., Reichle, J., Sigafoos, J., Charpentier, P. J., & Foster, D. J. (1991). Initial comparison of the efficiency of a variety of AAC systems for ordering meals in fast food restaurants. *Augmentative and Alternative Communication, 7,* 256–265.

Duncan, J. L., & Silverman, F. H. (1977). Impacts of learning American Indian sign language on mentally retarded children: A preliminary report. *Perceptual and Motor Skills, 44,* 11–38.

Dunham, J. K. (1989). The transparency of manual signs in a linguistic and an environmental nonlinguistic context. *Augmentative and Alternative Communication, 5,* 214–225.

Ecklund, S., & Reichle, J. (1987). A comparison of normal children's ability to recall symbols from two logographic systems. *Language, Speech, and Hearing Services in the Schools, 18,* 34–40.

Faircloth, S. R., & Faircloth, M. A. (1973). *Phonetic science.* Englewood Cliffs, NJ: Prentice-Hall, Inc.

Ferguson, C. (1975). Pictographs and prereading skills. *Child Development, 46,* 786–789.

Francis, W. C. (1990). Letters to the Editor: Clinical and research issues of vocabulary lists: Comments on Yorkston, Dowden, Honsinger, Marriner and Smith. *Augmentative and Alternative Communication, 6,* 275–276.

Fried–Oken, M., & More, L. (1992). An initial vocabulary for nonspeaking preschool children based on developmental and environmental language sources. *Augmentative and Alternative Communication, 8,* 41–56.

Fuller, D. R., & Lloyd, L. L. (1991). Forum: Toward a common usage of iconicity terminology. *Augmentative and Alternative Communication, 7,* 215–220.

Goodman, J., & Remington, B. (1993). Acquisition of expressive signing: Comparison of reinforcement strategies. *Augmentative and Alternative Communication, 9,* 26–35.

Goossens, C. (1989). Aided communication intervention before assessment: A case study of a child with cerebral palsy. *Augmentative and Alternative Communication, 5,* 14–26.

Granlund, M., Strom, E., & Olsson, C. (1989). Iconicity and productive recall of a selected sample of signs from signed Swedish. *Augmentative and Alternative Communication, 5,* 173–182.

Grove, N., & Walker, M. (1990). The Makaton vocabulary: Using manual signs and graphic symbols to develop interpersonal communication. *Augmentative and Alternative Communication, 6,* 15–28.

Hurlbut, B. I., Iwata, B. A., & Green, J. D. (1982). Nonvocal language acquisition in adolescents with severe physical disabilities: Blissymbol versus iconic stimulus formats. *Journal of Applied Behavior Analysis, 15,* 241–258.

Iacono, T., Mirenda, P., & Beukelman, D. (1993). Comparison of unimodal and multimodal AAC techniques for children with intellectual disabilities. *Augmentative and Alternative Communication, 9,* 83–93.

Johnson, R. (1981). *The picture communication symbols.* Solana Beach, CA: Mayer-Johnson.

Kirstein, I. J., & Bernstein, C. (1981). *Oakland Schools Communication Enhancement Center Picture Dictionary.* Pontiac, MI: Oakland Schools.

Lloyd, L. L., & Karlan, G. R. (1984). Non-speech communication symbols and systems: Where have we been and where are we going? *Journal of Mental Deficiency Research, 28,* 3–20.

Loeding, B. L., Zangari, C., & Lloyd, L. L. (1990). A "working party" approach to planning inservice training in manual signs for an entire public school staff. *Augmentative and Alternative Communication, 6,* 38–49.

Lowenbraun, S., & Thompson, M. D. (1982). Hearing impairments. In N. G. Haring (Ed.), *Exceptional children and youth.* Columbus, OH: Charles E. Merrill Publishing Company.

Maharaj, S. (1980). *Pictogram ideogram communication.* Saskatchewan, Canada: The Pictogram Centre.

Marvin, C. A., Beukelman, D. R., Brockhaus, J., & Kast, L. (1994). "What are you talking about?": Semantic analysis of preschool children's conversational topics in home and preschool settings. *Augmentative and Alternative Communication, 10,* 75–86.

Mathy-Laikko, P., Iacono, T., Ratcliff, A., Villarruel, F., Yoder, D., & Vanderheiden, G. (1989). Teaching a child with multiple disabilities to use a tactile augmentative communication device. *Augmentative and Alternative Communication, 5,* 249–256.

McDonald, E. T., & Schultz, A. R. (1973). Communication boards for cerebral-palsied children. *Journal of Speech and Hearing Disorders, 38,* 73–88.

McEwen, I. R., & Lloyd, L. L. (1990). Some considerations about the motor requirements of manual signs. *Augmentative and Alternative Communication, 6,* 207–216.

McGinnis, J. S., & Beukelman, D. R. (1989). Vocabulary requirements for writing activities for the academically mainstreamed student with disabilities. *Augmentative and Alternative Communication, 5,* 183–191.

McNaughton, S. (1993). Graphic representational systems and literacy learning. *Topics in Language Disorders, 13,* 58–75.

Mirenda, P. (1985). Designing pictorial communication systems for physically able–bodied students with severe handicaps. *Augmentative and Alternative Communication, 1,* 58–64.

Mirenda, P., & Locke, P. A. (1989). A comparison of symbol transparency in nonspeaking persons with intellectual disabilities. *Journal of Speech and Hearing Disorders, 54,* 131–140.

Mirenda, P., & Mathy–Laikko, P. (1989). Augmentative and alternative communication applications for persons with severe congenital communication disorders: An introduction. *Augmentative and Alternative Communication, 5,* 3–13.

Mizuko, M. (1987). Transparency and ease of learning of symbols represented by Blissymbols, PCS, and Picsyms. *Augmentative and Alternative Communication, 3,* 129–136.

Musselwhite, C. R. (1985). What is minspeak? In *Touch Talker Training Manual.* Wooster, OH: Prentke Romich Company.

Musselwhite, C. R., & Ruscello, D. M. (1984). Transparency of three communication symbol systems. *Journal of Speech and Hearing Research, 27,* 436–443.

Musselwhite, C. R., & St. Louis, K. W. (1988). *Communication programming for persons with severe handicaps: Vocal and augmentative strategies.* Boston, MA: Little, Brown & Co.

Orlansky, M. D., & Bonvillian, J. D. (1984). The role of iconicity in early sign language acquisition. *Journal of Speech and Hearing Disorders, 49,* 287–292.

Poock, G. K., & Blackstone, S. W. (1992). Using information theory to measure effectiveness of an augmentative and alternative communication display. *Augmentative and Alternative Communication, 8,* 287–296.

Rankin, J. L., Harwood, K., & Mirenda, P. (1994). Influence of graphic symbol use on reading comprehension. *Augmentative and Alternative Communication, 10,* 269–281.

Reichle, J., Mirenda, P., Locke, P., Piche, L., & Johnston, S. (1992). Beginning augmentative communication systems. In S. F. Warren & J. Reichle (Eds.), *Causes and effects in communication and language intervention* (pp. 131–156). Baltimore, MD: Paul H. Brookes Publishing Co.

Romski, M. A., & Sevcik, R. A. (1988). Augmentative and alternative communication systems: Considerations for individuals with severe intellectual disabilities. *Augmentative and Alternative Communication, 4,* 83–93.

Romski, M. A., Sevcik, R. A., & Pate, J. L. (1988). Establishment of symbolic communication in persons with severe retardation. *Journal of Speech and Hearing Disorders, 53,* 94–107.

Romski, M. A., Sevcik, R. A., Pate, J. L., & Rumbaugh, D. M. (1985). Discrimination of lexigrams and traditional orthography by nonspeaking severely mentally retarded persons. *American Journal of Mental Deficiency, 90*(2), 185–189.

Rowland, C., & Schweigert, P. (1989). Tangible symbols: Symbolic communication for individuals with multisensory impairments. *Augmentative and Alternative Communication, 5,* 226–234.

Schuler, A. L., & Baldwin, M. (1981). Nonspeech communication and childhood autism. *Language, Speech, and Hearing Services in the Schools, 12,* 246–257.

Sevcik, R. A., Romski, M. A., & Wilkinson, K. M. (1991). Roles of graphic symbols in the language acquisition process for persons with severe cognitive disabilities. *Augmentative and Alternative Communication, 7,* 161–170.

Skelly, M., & Schinsky, L. (1979). *Amer-Ind gestural code based on universal American Indian Hand Talk.* New York: Elsevier North Holland.

Smith-Lewis, M. R. (1994). Discontinuity in the development of aided augmentative and alternative communication systems. *Augmentative and Alternative Communication, 10,* 14–26.

Spragale, D. M., & Micucci, D. (1990). Signs of the week: A functional approach to manual sign training. *Augmentative and Alternative Communication, 6,* 29–37.

Stillman, R. D., & Battle, C. W. (1984). Developing prelanguage communication in the severely handicapped: An interpretation of the Van Dijk method. *Seminars in Speech and Language, 5*(3), 159–170.

Thorley, B., Ward, J., Binepal, T., & Dolan, K. (1991). Communicating with printed words to augment signing: Case study of a severely disabled deaf-blind child. *Augmentative and Alternative Communication, 7,* 80–87.

VanTatenhove, G. (1993). *What is Minspeak?* Wooster, OH: Prentke Romich Company.

Vanderheiden, D. H., Brown, W. P., Reinen, S., MacKenzie, P., & Scheibel, C. (1975). Symbol communication for the mentally handicapped. *Mental Retardation, 13*(1), 34–36.

Vanderheiden, G. C., & Lloyd, L. L. (1986). Communication systems and their components. In S. W. Blackstone (Ed.), *Augmentative communication: An introduction* (pp. 49–161). Rockville, MD: American Speech-Language-Hearing Association.

Vanderheiden, G. C., & Yoder, D. E. (1986). Overview. In S. W. Blackstone (Ed.), *Augmentative communication: An introduction* (pp. 1–28). Rockville, MD: American Speech-Language-Hearing Association.

Venkatagiri, H. S. (1993). Efficiency of lexical prediction as a communication acceleration technique. *Augmentative and Alternative Communication, 9,* 161–167.

Watkins, L. T., Sprafkin, J. N., & Krolikowski, D. M. (1993). Using videotaped lessons to facilitate the development of manual sign skills in students with mental retardation. *Augmentative and Alternative Communication, 9,* 177–183.

Wetherby, A. M., & Prizant, B. M. (1992). Profiling young children's communicative competence. In S. F. Warren & J. Reichle (Eds.), *Causes and effects in communication and language intervention* (pp. 217–253). Baltimore, MD: Paul H. Brookes Publishing Company.

Wetherby, A. M., & Prizant, B. M. (1993). Profiling communication and symbolic abilities in young children. *Journal of Childhood Communication Disorders, 15*(1), 23–32.

Woodcock, R. W., & Davies, C. O. (1969). *The Peabody Rebus Reading Program.* Circle Pines, MN: American Guidance Service, Inc.

Yorkston, K. M., Honsinger, M. J., Dowden, P. A., & Marriner, N. (1989). Vocabulary selection: A case report. *Augmentative and Alternative Communication, 5,* 101–108.

Yovetich, W. S., & Young, T. A. (1988). The effects of representativeness and concreteness on the "guessability" of Blissymbols. *Augmentative and Alternative Communication, 4,* 35–39.

Chapter 5

AUGMENTATIVE AND ALTERNATIVE COMMUNICATION ASSESSMENT STRATEGIES

Sharon L. Glennen

Many professional disciplines have developed established assessment procedures based upon a long history of experience within the field. In contrast, the field of augmentative and alternative communication (AAC) has yet to develop a consensus concerning best practices for conducting AAC assessments. AAC evaluation procedures vary widely from facility to facility, which produces variations in assessment outcomes. Some professionals evaluate by simply trying a wide variety of devices with various nonspeaking individuals. Other professional teams exhaustively evaluate all aspects of an individual's skills before trying any AAC systems. Evaluation procedures range from naturalistic observations of the individual (Beukelman & Mirenda, 1992), to the use of formal and informal tests (Elder, 1987), to the use of computerized assessment systems (Garrett, Andrews, Olsson, & Seeger, 1990).

The lack of systematic AAC evaluation procedures has caused difficulty for nonspeaking individuals who require AAC systems. Recommendations for AAC devices range widely, making it difficult for families and consumers to decide which communication options to implement. Third party payers are reluctant to fund AAC devices when the assessment process does not provide sufficient justification or evidence to support the recommendations. AAC devices are sometimes abandoned by users due to mismatches between skills, expectations, and the device's capabilities (Culp, Ambriosi, Berniger, & Mitchell, 1986; Jinks & Sinteff, 1994). The American Speech-Language-Hearing Association developed a consensus paper that outlines professional skills necessary for working with persons with severe communication impairments (ASHA, 1989). However, this document limits itself to professional training and experiences, and does not provide a blueprint of best practices for the assessment process itself.

AAC evaluations are a complex interaction of assessment procedures across multiple domains. This chapter is the first of three chapters that will provide the reader with AAC evaluation guidelines. In an attempt to simplify the assessment process, procedures have been categorized into the following areas: evaluation of the communicative environment, evaluation of cognitive and linguistic abilities, assessment of seating and positioning, evaluating motor access abilities, and examination of visual skills. Although the book reviews these evaluation procedures neatly in sequence, in reality AAC evaluations are an intricate process that crosses multiple assessment areas and plays out differently each time. Because of the many assessment domains that need to be addressed, AAC evaluations are frequently ongoing and require multiple sessions.

The guidelines presented across these three chapters will provide the reader with a road map to follow through the AAC evaluation process. Like any road map, detours and alternate routes may be necessary for different situations and environments. Professionals who are learning the AAC evaluation process for the first time will need to stick closely to the procedures outlined in these chapters. More experienced professionals will have the skills necessary for knowing when to bypass certain evaluation procedures and when to delve deeper into other assessment areas. This chapter will review assessment procedures designed to evaluate the environment where AAC will be implemented and to evaluate an individual's cognitive, linguistic, and symbolic skills necessary for the AAC decision-making process. Chapters 6 and 7 provide more information for assessing seating and positioning concerns, visual abilities, and motor access skills for nonspeaking individuals with physical disabilities.

AAC ASSESSMENT AS THEORY

Historical Perspectives

During the early 1980s, some of the pioneering facilities providing AAC services began to disseminate their evaluation procedures to others (Goosens & Crain, 1985; Montgomery, 1980; Shane, 1980). An example of these assessment procedures comes from the Plavan School in Fountain Valley, California, which published extensive assessment guidelines (Montgomery, 1980). Plavan School's model included evaluating motor abilities, perceptual skills, cognitive and academic skills, psycholinguistic abilities, communication needs of the individual, seating and positioning, device accessing, and switch use. Although these assessment models were a good beginning for a relatively new field, they were sometimes vague when it came to the specifics of the assessment process.

Many of the early assessment models focused on evaluating prerequisite cognitive skills necessary for operating AAC systems. Shane and Bashir (1980) developed a 10-step AAC decision matrix for clinicians. The first step of the decision matrix asked whether the individual had reached Stage V of Piaget's sensorimotor intelligence (i.e., cause-effect, or means-end skills). If the answer was negative, the clinician was directed to delay implementing AAC. Similarly, Alpert (1980) developed a model for assessing AAC with autistic children. The first phase of the model consisted of training attending skills, motor imitation, and imitative matching. Once these skills were mastered, then an AAC system could be considered.

Later in the 1980s, professionals in the field began to challenge the need to learn prerequisite cognitive skills before implementing an AAC system (Kangas & Lloyd, 1988; Reichle & Karlan, 1985; Romski, Sevcik, & Pate, 1988). The processes of teaching attending, visual tracking, matching, and imitation skills were seen as incidental to the ultimate goal of teaching communication. Rather than wasting years trying to train these prerequisite skills, it was proposed that individuals with severe communication and cognitive impairments should be exposed to learning activities that would teach the process of communication through the use of AAC strategies. This change in views eliminated the use of detailed cognitive candidacy criteria guidelines which were prevalent during the early years of AAC.

In addition to cognitive candidacy criteria, many of the early assessment models also focused on evaluating the individual's potential ability to acquire speech. The prevailing view was that AAC was a "last resort" to be tried when all attempts to improve speech intelligibility had failed (Silverman, 1980). Many professionals feared that the introduction of an AAC system would delay or inhibit the production of speech. Shane and Bashir's (1980) AAC Decision Matrix contained questions that reviewed an individual's speech motor abilities, age level, and history of previous speech therapy as part of the decision-making process. Children and adults who had the potential to improve their speech were not considered for AAC systems. As recently as 1982 this author worked at a facility that was reluctant to allow the use of AAC systems with children with multiple disabilities in the belief that it would inhibit speech development. Children who were candidates for AAC interventions had to be reviewed and approved by a professional supervisor at the facility before any unaided or aided communication techniques could be implemented. Many children with severe expressive communication disorders spent years in traditional speech therapy before AAC devices were finally implemented.

Today's perspective is quite different. The use of AAC systems is encouraged with all individuals with severe communication impairments, regardless of the potential to acquire speech. Case study and research evidence suggest that the use of AAC does not inhibit the development of spoken language, and in some cases it may even enhance the acquisition of speech (Goosens, 1989; Light, Beesley, & Collier,

1988; Silverman, 1980; Weller & Mahoney, 1983). Current assessment theory has moved from focusing on detailed candidacy criteria to simply focusing on an individual's need for improved communication. This perspective was first proposed by Beukelman, Yorkston, and Dowden (1985) as the Communication Needs Model. This model examines an individual's communicative demands within the natural environment, and recommends implementation of AAC interventions when unmet communicative needs are present.

AAC Team Assessment

The AAC evaluation process has always been practiced as a team effort. Early assessment models stressed the team concept as being necessary because of the need to consider cognitive, language, physical, perceptual, emotional, and technical issues in the evaluation process (Goosens & Crain, 1985; Montgomery, 1980; Shane, 1980). Professional team members might include speech-language pathologists, special educators, rehabilitation specialists, psychologists, occupational therapists, physical therapists, and rehabilitation engineers. In addition, nonspeaking individuals and their families should also be included as members of the team. In practice, the exact composition of the professional portion of the team varies from one program to another depending on the age and mix of individuals seen for service.

The process of providing team evaluations can also vary across programs. Some programs conduct arena assessments, in which all team members are present throughout the entire evaluation, each making contributions as needed. In an arena assessment, discipline boundaries are often eliminated, with each team member providing expertise across a wide range of skills. The benefit of the arena assessment model is the constant interaction among team members during the evaluation. This interaction makes it possible to make decisions quickly regarding various AAC options. The drawback of this model is its high cost due to large personnel and labor expenses.

To reduce costs, some programs conduct separate evaluations by professionals, who come together near the end of the process as a team. The nonspeaking individual might first be evaluated by the speech-language pathologist, followed by the special educator, the physical therapist, and the occupational therapist. At the end of the evaluation, the team comes together with recommendations. The drawback of this model is the lack of information sharing throughout the decision-making process. This sometimes causes duplication in evaluation procedures, and prevents the development of cohesive integrated recommendations for the nonspeaking client.

Some programs have developed team evaluations that are based on arena assessment models, but implement the model in a more cost-effective manner. One method is to discuss all upcoming assessments ahead of time in order to determine which team members are necessary. A nonspeaking individual with cerebral palsy who wishes to have an AAC system integrated with a laptop computer, power wheelchair, and environmental controls will probably require the services of a complete team. In contrast, a young preschooler who has a severe apraxia of speech with no other physical impairments might only require the services of the speech-language pathologist and the occupational therapist. Chapter 2 in this book provides more extensive information on teaming and service delivery methods.

AAC Assessment Models

Many of the early assessment models focused on candidacy issues. Once candidacy for an AAC device was established, there was little information to guide the practitioner into making a decision about which communication system to implement. Over time, other assessment models have been devel-

oped which focus instead on evaluating the skills and capabilities necessary for operating an AAC system. Yorkston and Karlan (1986) reviewed the evaluation process from this capability assessment viewpoint. Capability assessment consists of evaluating an individual's skills or capabilities across a wide variety of areas necessary for implementation of an AAC system. The end result of the capability assessment is a profile of skills which is used to determine which AAC strategies to evaluate further.

There is currently a lack of consensus about what constitutes a necessary AAC skill. Different capability assessment models have developed different methods of implementing the evaluation process. Beukelman and Mirenda (1992) further categorized various capability assessment models into the groupings of Maximal Assessment, Criteria-Based Assessment, and Predictive Assessment.

Maximal Assessment Models

The maximal assessment process consists of exhaustively evaluating an individual's abilities across cognitive, academic, perceptual, linguistic, and motor areas. Information is gathered across all domains in order to determine which AAC system to implement. The Nonspeech Test (Huer, 1983) is an example of an assessment procedure that uses the maximal assessment model. Several early AAC evaluation guidelines also used this approach (Montgomery, 1980). Maximal assessment is a thorough process that can lead to appropriate AAC recommendations. The difficulty with the procedure is that it is extremely time consuming. Lots of information critical to the AAC decision-making process is gathered, along with information that is probably unnecessary. Inexperienced professionals often rely on the maximal assessment model because they are unable to determine which AAC skills are important for the decision-making process.

Criteria-Based Assessment

Criteria-based assessment is another capability assessment model. Criteria-based assessment formalizes the decision-making process into a series of branching yes/no questions. Information about the client is obtained through observation, records review, and evaluation. This information is then discussed by the team using the decision-making branching process. By concentrating on the information necessary for answering the questions, unnecessary assessment information is weeded out of the process. The Non-Oral Communication Assessment (Fell, Linn, & Morrison, 1984) is an example of criteria-based assessment procedures.

Criteria-based assessment is a useful model for evaluating AAC users whose skills divide nicely into neat yes/no categories. The branching process saves time in the evaluation by guiding the team toward appropriate AAC strategies. However, many individuals do not fit neatly into dichotomous groupings. For example, one of the first questions asked by many criteria-based models is whether the individual can access an AAC system using direct selection. If the answer is no, then scanning methods of access are reviewed. If the answer is yes, then scanning options are presumably ignored.

Many children with physical handicaps do not have access skills that can be cleanly divided into direct selection versus scanning options. There are many young children who initially do not have good range of motion, target accuracy, or muscle pressure to use a direct selection system with enough symbol choices to meet their communicative needs. However, with motor maturation and training, many of these children can learn to access devices using direct selection. These children often require systems that will initially allow them to access their devices using both direct selection and scanning methods. Over a long period of time the preferred method of access can then be determined.

Predictive Assessment: Feature Matching

Predictive AAC assessment is the process of obtaining information that will predict which AAC system or systems should be considered for actual use (Yorkston & Karlan, 1986). The evaluation process is goal-oriented toward determining which AAC system will best meet an individual's needs. Only those skills necessary for developing an AAC prescription are evaluated. Because the evaluation is focused on specific skills, the assessment process is often streamlined.

This assessment model is sometimes referred to as a feature-matching process (Swengel & Varga, 1993). The skills of the nonspeaking individual are matched to the features of a given AAC system. This model requires expert knowledge of various AAC options and strategies. Team members must be able to determine what linguistic, cognitive, perceptual, and motor skills are needed to operate an AAC device, and then systematically evaluate those skills. In addition, the individual's environment, motivation, and need for using AAC are evaluated. The AAC skills of the individual and information about the individual's communication environment are then matched to a system that has the desired features. Figure 5–1 provides a visual model for the feature-matching process used in the predictive assessment model.

Although the predictive model provides the field with a practical theory of assessment, implementation of the model is still in its early stages. There are broad-based guidelines describing what skills need to be assessed in the evaluation process (Yorkston & Karlan, 1986; Swengel & Varga, 1993). However, there is little specific information regarding how to evaluate these skills.

AAC ASSESSMENT: FROM THEORY TO PRACTICE

The predictive model provides a frame-

AAC Predictive Assessment Model

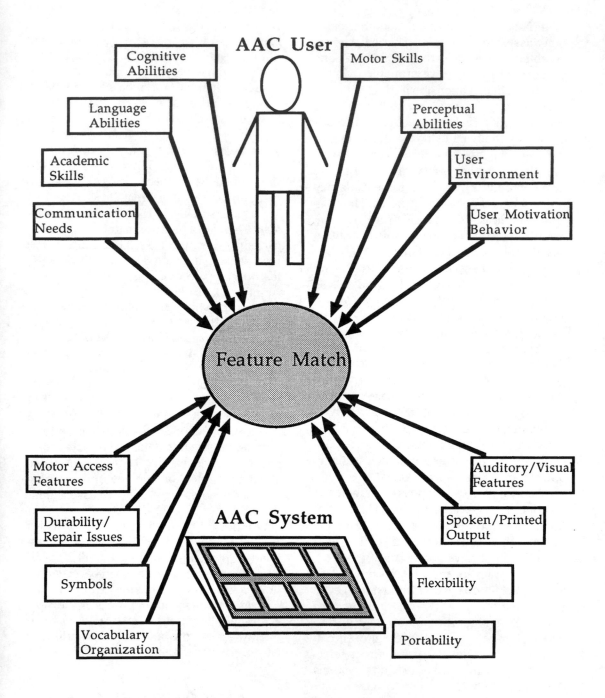

Figure 5–1. AAC Predictive Assessment Model.

work that can be used to develop actual AAC assessment practice patterns. The predictive model helps to guide the thinking process necessary for developing evaluation procedures. The goal of the assessment is to determine which skills are necessary for operating an AAC device, and to break those skills down into specific criteria that can be measured. In order for the predictive evaluation process to work well, it must be systematic, it must be replicable, and it must provide accountability for the decisions that are ultimately made. The remainder of this chapter will provide a road map for implementing the predictive feature match assessment process with specific guidelines for evaluating skills necessary for AAC device operation.

THE AAC PREDICTIVE ASSESSMENT PROCESS

The AAC assessment procedures described in this chapter combine many different forms of evaluation into a single process. Family and client interviews, formal and informal assessment tasks, and field observations are all part of the process. Table 5–1 provides an overview of the AAC assessment process. The evaluation begins by assessing the communication needs and existing communication environment of the nonspeaking individual. This is followed by an assessment of the individual's current methods of expressive communication. In order to complete the evaluation, a method of direct selection for testing is then determined. Using direct selection methods, the individual's language and symbolic skills necessary for the AAC decision-making process are systematically evaluated. All of this information is then used to develop a list of AAC systems to consider. If needed, seating and positioning are evaluated and adjustments are made to improve postural stability. A method of motorically accessing the recommended AAC system is then determined. Finally, the nonspeaking individual is given an opportunity to field test any recommended equipment before making final decisions. These procedures will be outlined further in this chapter and in Chapters 6 and 7.

AAC Needs Assessment

The AAC assessment process begins with an evaluation of the nonspeaking individual's need for an AAC system. The needs assessment helps the evaluation team to determine factors that will impact the implementation of AAC interventions. Establishing the communicative need for AAC

Table 5–1. Overview of the AAC predictive feature match assessment process.

- Evaluate the individual's communication needs and communication environment.
- Evaluate the individual's ability to use existing expressive communication modes.
- Determine a direct selection method that the individual can use to respond during the assessment process.
- Systematically evaluate language and symbolic skills necessary for the AAC decision-making process.
- Use assessment information to develop a list of AAC devices to consider for further evaluation.
- Evaluate seating and positioning. Adjust existing positioning equipment or fabricate new seating systems when necessary.
- Determine a motor response for accessing an AAC system.
- Field test recommended AAC systems.

also helps the evaluation team to focus on specific areas of communicative concern. For example, a child who can speak intelligibly to those who know her well but requires an AAC system when interacting with strangers requires a different type of AAC system than a child who has no intelligible speech. Interviews with consumers, families, and professionals are combined with direct observations of the consumer to obtain this information. Methods of evaluating AAC needs will be reviewed in this section of the chapter.

The evaluation process typically begins by interviewing all parties, including the nonspeaking individual, family, and professionals who interact with the nonspeaking person on a regular basis. Components of the interview consist of determining the individual's current methods of communication and the relative success of those methods. In addition, the interview asks for information about the environments where AAC is needed and the interaction partners within those environments. Information regarding the client's physical skills, mobility, wheelchair seating systems, and ambulation is obtained. The individual's visual and auditory skills are also reviewed in order to determine if any sensory deficits would affect use of an AAC device. Use of other technologies that may impact on AAC use is also addressed. Finally, the expectations of the family, professionals, and most importantly, the nonspeaking individual are discussed. Figure 5–2 presents an AAC Needs Assessment Form which can be used to collect this information.

In addition to interviews, the needs assessment process also involves observing the nonspeaking individual interacting in natural environments. Beukelman and Mirenda (1992) developed a method of documenting communication needs by comparing the nonspeaking individual's ability to communicate and participate in a given environment with peer models. Nonspeaking individuals are observed participating in naturally occurring situations throughout the day. Participation levels of the nonspeaking individual and peers within the environment are rated according to the performance standards listed in Table 5–2. Participation levels for the nonspeaking individual and typical peers can range from fully independent to unable to participate. Areas that have discrepancies between the nonspeaking individual and his or her peers are areas to target for AAC or other types of environmental intervention.

For example, Tommy is a preschooler with physical disabilities who attends a neighborhood private preschool program. He was observed interacting with his friends while playing with clay. In contrast to his school-mates, Tommy was unable to get the clay by himself. He needed the teacher or peer to place the clay on the table in front of him. The other children were able to use rolling pins, spoons, dull knives, and cookie cutters to play with the clay. Tommy was unable to use any of these items unless the teacher provided hand-over-hand assistance. Tommy had a communication board with pictures available to request clay, and to indicate when he was finished. Once he requested the clay, the communication board was removed from the table so it wouldn't get messy. Tommy was not able to request specific colors of clay, to request tools to play with the clay, or to request assistance from his friends or teachers when playing with the clay. He also was unable to comment, ask questions, or make statements to friends when playing with the clay. According to Beukelman and Mirenda's Participation Patterns, Tommy's peers would be fully independent when playing with clay. Tommy would be rated as requiring physical assistance. Due to the discrepancy between Tommy's ability when compared to his peers, AAC intervention is needed in this situation. Although Tommy may never be able to physically play with clay independently, AAC intervention will

Augmentative and Alternative Communication
Information and Needs Assessment

Client Name: _____   Date: _____

Clinician: _____   DOB/Age: _____

         Name   Relationship

Informants: _____   _____

                  _____   _____

                  _____   _____

                  _____   _____

I. CURRENT METHODS OF COMMUNICATION:

Modality Checklist	Description	Vocabulary Size	Intelligibility
_____ Speech			
_____ Vocalizations			
_____ Sign language			
_____ Gestures/Points			
_____ Head Nods			
_____ Eye Gaze			
_____ Facial Expressions			
_____ AAC Device			
_____ Other			

(continued)

Figure 5–2. AAC information and needs assessment interview forms.

Figure 5–2. *(continued)*

II. PAST AAC EXPERIENCE:

2a) Has this individual ever used a picture or letter based AAC device in the past? If yes, describe the system.

Name of Device: Length of Time Used:

Number of Symbols: Size of Symbols:

Symbol System Used: Organization of Symbols:

Access Method:

2b) What were the strengths and limitations of the AAC system described above?

III. COMMUNICATION ENVIRONMENTS: Where will AAC be used?

Environment Checklist   Description   Interaction Partners

_____ Home

_____ School

_____ Work

_____ Community

_____ Other

3a) What barriers to AAC implementation exist in any of the environments listed above?

IV. MOBILITY AND ACCESS: How will the client transport an AAC device?

Mobility Checklist   Description   Environment Used

_____ Fully Ambulatory

_____ Ambulatory with assistance

_____ Manual Wheelchair

_____ Power Wheelchair

_____ Other

4a) Are there any mobility, seating or positioning concerns that will effect the implementation of an AAC system? (If yes, describe).

Functional Access Checklist: What extremities are functional for AAC access?

	Description	Access Limitations
_____ Left Arm/Hand		
_____ Right Arm/Hand		
_____ Head		
_____ Left Leg/Foot		
_____ Right Leg/Foot		
_____ Eye Gaze		
_____Other		

V. OTHER TECHNOLOGIES: What other technologies will need to integrate with an AAC system?

Technology Checklist	Description	Environment Used
_____ Wheelchair		
_____ Computer		
_____ Environmental Controls		
_____ Switch Toys		
_____ Other		

VI. AAC EXPECTATIONS: What goals could be achieved if the client had access to an AAC system?

allow him to independently direct others and communicate during the play experience.

Assessment of Environmental Barriers

Beukelman and Mirenda (1992) also developed a systematic method to identify environmental barriers that affect the implementation of an AAC system. Proceeding with the AAC assessment process without consideration of these barriers is a formula for failed AAC outcomes. These barriers need to be discussed ahead of time as part of the needs assessment process. There are two groups of barriers that need to be considered: opportunity and access barriers. Opportunity barriers are those that are imposed by other persons or obstacles in the consumer's environment. They include official and unofficial policies that affect use of AAC devices in the classroom, attitudes and opinions of persons who interact with nonspeaking individuals, and lack of knowledge regarding AAC practices. For example, a regular education teacher who has limited experience with computers and is reluctant to have special needs children in her classroom has knowledge and attitude barriers toward AAC that need to be addressed. Failure to address the teacher's concerns will result in an AAC system that is rarely used in the classroom. Opportunity barriers are outlined further in Table 5–3.

Communicative barriers are a special category of opportunity barriers which need to be addressed. Glennen and Delsandro (1994) defined communicative barriers as those that prevent the nonspeaking individual from communicating optimally within an environment. Communicative barriers are often the result of knowledge and attitude barriers on the part of professionals and peers within the individual's environment. Communicative barriers include a lack of opportunities to communicate with others, participation in activities that are not conducive to communication, lack of recognition of existing communication

Table 5–2. Participation pattern levels.

Independent: An individual who is fully independent within an activity is able to get all materials for the activity, independently complete the activity, and communicate all needs at any time.

Independent with Setup: Minor intervention is required to prepare for an activity. For example, a teacher might need to put a communication board designed for a specific activity on an individual's wheelchair tray before beginning the activity.

Verbal Assistance: Repeated directions and verbal guidance are given throughout the activity. This might include modeling the vocabulary necessary for the activity, or breaking down the steps for the activity into short, simple command sequences.

Physical Assistance: Some individuals require physical help from others to participate in an activity. For example, a child with physical disabilities may not be able to cut paper, draw, or shape clay independently without adult or peer assistance.

Unable to Participate: There are times when nonspeaking individuals are excluded from participation in an activity. The classroom might be playing kickball while the nonspeaking child sits and watches on the sidelines.

Source: Adapted from Beukelman and Mirenda (1992).

Table 5–3. Opportunity barriers.

Policy Barriers: On the broad level, policy barriers occur when governmental or legal decisions are made that affect the implementation of AAC. School policies that segregate nonspeaking persons into separate classrooms or schools are examples of policy barriers.

Practice Barriers: Many barriers are discussed as if they are official policies, when instead they are simply procedures or conventions that have become commonly used. For example, a school district may state that it is their policy not to send home AAC devices that were purchased by the school. Further examination often finds that there is no such written policy, or that the practice is in violation of federal or state mandates.

Attitude Barriers: Attitude barriers occur when individual beliefs and opinions affect the implementation of AAC. Some regular education teachers are resentful when nonspeaking children are integrated into their classrooms. They may refuse to alter curriculum or testing procedures to accommodate the child's needs.

Knowledge Barriers: A lack of knowledge or information on the part of teachers, peers, or families can often limit a nonspeaking individual's progress. This lack of knowledge can range from professionals who are technophobic to those who wish to learn more but do not know how to find necessary resources.

Communicative Barriers: These barriers occur when the existing environment is not conducive to facilitating optimal communication for a nonspeaking individual. For example, a consumer may be seated at a work station that is situated away from peers, or not provided with opportunities to respond during classroom lessons.

Source: Adapted from Beukelman and Mirenda (1992).

modalities, and an inability to interpret attempts to communicate. The best AAC system in the world will not be successful if the communicative environment does not give the consumer an opportunity to communicate meaningfully with others.

Communicative environments that are not designed for interaction will need to be

AAC Activity Analysis

Name:_____   Date: _____

Environment: _____   Activity:_____

I. Communication Partners

Does the activity involve more than one peer?   Yes   No

Are the participants able to take turns communicating?   Yes   No

Does the consumer interact with peers during the
    activity?   Yes   No

Does the activity involve communication with
    an adult or supervisor?   Yes   No

List the communication partners. Indicate whether the partners are peers, or adult supervisors. Indicate whether the consumer is able to communicate with each partner. If communication does not occur, explain why.

Partner   Role   Able to Communicate Together?

Improving Partner Interactions:

A. How can the activity be changed to facilitate interactions between the consumer and peers?

B. How can the activity be changed to facilitate turn taking within the activity?

(continued)

Figure 5–3. AAC Activity Analysis (Glennen & Delsandro, 1994).

Figure 5–3. *(continued)*

II. Purpose of the Activity

Does the activity involve manipulation of materials by the consumer?	Yes	No
Does the consumer need to request assistance to manipulate the materials or complete the activity?	Yes	No
Is there a tangible goal or end product for the activity?	Yes	No
Does the activity involve manipulation of materials by more than one peer at a time?	Yes	No
Is the activity age appropriate for the consumer?	Yes	No

Improving the Purpose of the Activity

A. How can the activity be changed to increase the consumer's need to communicate to complete the activity?

B. How can the consumer play a more active role in manipulating materials in the activity?

C. How can peers be involved in manipulating materials with the consumer?

III. **Style of Communication During the Activity**

Are multiple modalities of communication encouraged? Yes   No

Is the consumer able to make requests during the activity? Yes   No

Is the consumer able to make statements?   Yes   No

Is the consumer able to ask questions?   Yes   No

Does the leader of the activity provide opportunities
      for the consumer to initiate communication?   Yes   No

Does the leader of the activity model appropriate
      communication for the consumer?   Yes   No

Improving Communication Style

A. How can the consumer be encouraged to initiate communication during this activity?

B. What changes to the consumer's AAC system are needed to change the ability to make requests, statements, or ask questions?

C. What other modalities of communication are available to the consumer during the activity?

changed prior to implementing AAC. It is difficult for AAC professionals to enact these changes without the full cooperation and understanding of those individuals who control the communicative situation. Figure 5–3 presents an AAC Activity Analysis that can be used to evaluate a specific communication activity (Glennen & Delsandro, 1994). Videotapes of the activity are viewed by a team consisting of professionals with AAC experience and individuals who directly control the communicative environment (i.e., teachers, parents, aides). The Activity Analysis form is completed by all team members through group discussion. This process is designed to help those in control of the situation realize that the communicative environment needs to change, and to provide them with structured guidance to make the necessary changes. Once changes are implemented, the revised activity can be videotaped and analyzed for improvement using the same procedures.

Access barriers are the other category of barriers outlined by Beukelman and Mirenda (1992). Access barriers refer to the capabilities and needs of the nonspeaking person. Access barriers might include cognitive skills, physical abilities, perceptual skills, previous experience with AAC or other technologies, and personal opinions of the AAC user. For example, teenagers are painfully aware of differences between them- selves and others. Because of this, nonspeaking teenagers are sometimes reluctant to use AAC systems with picture symbol strategies. They frequently insist on using devices that resemble laptop computers, even though their literacy skills aren't sufficient to take full advantage of a laptop system. This access barrier would need to be addressed as part of the needs assessment process.

Evaluation of Expressive Communication Modalities

Once the need for AAC and the barriers that will impact use of AAC are identified, the actual client assessment process begins. Because one goal of the assessment is to determine if an AAC system would improve an individual's communication ability, careful documentation of existing expressive communication skills needs to be part of the process. This is especially important when trying to justify funding of AAC equipment with third party payers, educational programs, or vocational programs. Documentation of current expressive communication abilities helps to explain why an AAC system is necessary for the nonspeaking individual.

The expressive communication evaluation process begins by observing the individual communicating in a natural situation or activity. This process is similar to collecting a spontaneous expressive language sample for a speaking child. For young children, spontaneous interactions during play activities can be observed to evaluate communication abilities. It is more difficult to obtain a good expressive language sample for older children and adults. Teenagers and adults are often in natural situations where communication opportunities are severely limited (Elder & Goosens, 1994). For example, an adult may work in a setting where every individual is seated at a separate table, making peer interactions difficult to observe.

If the natural environment does not lend itself to observing an individual's best communication abilities, structured situations designed to encourage maximum communication may need to be implemented. One method of structuring communication interactions with older individuals is to use barrier games. During a barrier game, the nonspeaking individual conveys information about a topic or activity to a listener who has been kept blind to the information. For example, a nonspeaking individual might describe a picture or retell a narrative story to a listener who has not seen the picture or heard the story.

The communication that occurs during these interactions can be analyzed in many different ways. Detailed procedures have been developed for research purposes that survey all aspects of an individual's communication (Buzolich & Wiemann, 1988; Glennen, 1989; Light, Collier, & Parnes, 1985). Although these procedures are exhaustive, they are more detailed than necessary for the purposes of evaluation. Realistically, the evaluator should be able to record interaction skills on-line during direct observations. Several checklist procedures have been developed for this assessment process (Bolton & Dashiell, 1984; Calculator & Luchko, 1983). Most checklists evaluate the communication modes used by the nonspeaking individual, the communicative acts that can be conveyed, and the occurrence of communication breakdowns. Figure 5–4 presents an Augmentative Communication Interaction Checklist that can be used for evaluation purposes (Glennen, 1992).

The Augmentative Communication Interaction Checklist begins by listing the expressive communication modes of interest across the top of the grid. Information obtained from the Needs Assessment can be used to determine which communication modalities should be analyzed. Communication modalities might include speech, other vocalizations, sign language, head nods, eye gaze, and pointing, among oth-

Augmentative Communication Interaction Checklist

Instructions: List the communication modes to be analyzed in the blank spaces across the top of the grid. Observe the individual interacting with other persons while participating in a fun activity for 30 minutes. Check the communication act categories that occur spontaneously by marking an "S" in the appropriate grid. Check communication act categories that can be elicited with specific cues by marking an "E" in the appropriate grid. Communication act categories not observed should be left blank.

Communication Act Categories	Communication Mode Categories				
Examples in Parentheses					
Request Objects (Want ball)					
Request Actions (Throw ball)					
Request Other (Where's ball?)					
Statement (Big ball)					
Yes/No Response (Want the ball? Yes)					
Wh Question Response (Where's the ball? There)					
Acknowledgment (It's round. Uh-Huh.)					
Other Response (Do you want this? This.)					
No Response					

Figure 5-4. AAC Communication Interaction Checklist. *Note:* from *The Handbook of Assistive Technology.* G. Church & S. Glennen, (Eds.), 1992. San Diego: Singular Publishing Group. Reprinted by permission.

ers. The individual is observed interacting during naturally occurring activities. Communication skills observed within the activity are then categorized by modality and by communication act categories. Communication act categories are used to analyze the functions of language that a nonspeaking individual is able to convey either spontaneously or with elicitation from others. Communication act categories modified from the work of Dore (1978) are further described in Table 5–4. This procedure is often completed in conjunction with the AAC Activity Analysis presented in Figure 5–3.

Once the interaction checklist has been given, the data should be analyzed to determine if the individual is able to communicate a wide range of communication acts using the available modalities of expressive communication. A pattern that often emerges with nonspeaking individuals is heavy reliance on the communication act categories that are respondent in nature (Calculator & Dollaghan, 1982; Glennen, 1989; Light, Collier, & Parnes, 1985). That is, the individual is responding to the requests, questions, and statements of others, usually with a simple yes/no response or acknowledgment. Communication act categories that involve initiating or maintaining interactions are observed less frequently, if at all. These include making requests and statements. Individuals who are unable to convey a wide range of communicative acts are in need of AAC intervention to enhance their existing communication abilities.

Evaluation of Speech Intelligibility

Individuals who have some intelligible speech need to have a thorough evaluation of their speech and oral motor abilities. This evaluation is important to document intelligibility, and to determine if additional speech therapy might improve articulation and phonological abilities. Even though an AAC system might still be recommended, additional recommendations to continue traditional speech and language therapy might also be warranted. The AAC system then becomes a transitional device, to be used as a method of enhancing existing speech abilities, or as a bridge to learning new expressive verbal skills.

It is also important to determine the individual's level of speech intelligibility across different listeners and environments. Those who are only unintelligible to strangers often require different AAC interventions when compared to those who are unintelligible most of the time. Documentation of articulation and phonological skills, oral motor skills, intelligibility in single word, phrase, and sentence contexts, and intelligibility across familiar and unfamiliar listeners need to be part of the assessment process.

Intelligibility is a broad functional measure of communication ability, but there is little consensus regarding how it should be assessed. Kent, Miolo, and Bloedel (1994) provided a comprehensive tutorial over-view of methods that can be used to evaluate intelligibility. Informally, family members and others can be asked to describe the percentage of the nonspeaking individual's speech that can be understood, or can complete an informal rating scale. This is typically done as part of the Needs Assessment interview.

A systematic method of obtaining intelligibility information from the family is the Meaningful Use of Speech Scale (MUSS; Osberger, 1992). This scale consists of 10 levels of intelligibility that are determined through parent interview questions (see Table 5–5). The focus of MUSS is to determine the individual's ability to effectively use speech for functional communication.

There are several standardized methods to assess intelligibility at single word and sentence levels. These include the CID Word Spine (Monsen, 1981) and CID Picture Spine (Monsen, Moog, & Geers, 1988).

These two measures require the individual to name consonant-vowel-consonant (CVC) words that differ by a single phonemic feature (e.g., *bat, back, bag, bad*). The individual being evaluated is randomly asked to name one of the words. A listener records which of the four word choices was produced. The percentage of words correctly perceived by the listener is used to estimate intelligibility. Intelligibility can also

Table 5-4. Communication act categories.

Request Objects: The individual can ask for an object or thing.

Verbal Example: "I want the dolly."
AAC Example: Points to the doll, or looks at the doll.
                      Points to a "doll" symbol on a communication board.

Request Actions: The individual can ask for an action to occur.

Verbal Example: "Give dolly a bath."
AAC Example: Signs "wash" then points to the doll.
                      Points to a "wash" symbol on the communication board.

Request Information: The individual can ask for information from others.

Verbal Example: "Where's the dolly's brush?"
AAC Example: Points to dolly's hair, then vocalizes with a question inflection.
                      Points to a "question" symbol on the communication board
                      followed by pointing to the doll's hair.

Statement: The individual can describe objects, actions, thoughts, feelings, or events.

Verbal Example: "I feel sad."
AAC Example: Begins to cry and whine.
                      Points to a "sad" symbol on the communication board.

Yes/No Response: The individual can answer yes/no questions.

Verbal Example: "No."
AAC Example: Head nod "no."
                      Eyes look down and a frown for "no."

Wh Question Response: The individual can answer Wh questions.

Verbal Example: Adult: "Where's the doll?" Child: "On the table."
AAC Example: Child responds by pointing to the doll.
                      Points to a symbol for "table" on the communication board.

Acknowledgment: The individual can noncommitally respond to statements or communications of others.

Verbal Example: Adult: "It's a pretty dolly." Child: "Uh-huh."
AAC Example: Child vocalizes after adult statement.
                      Child nods and smiles after adult statement.

Other Response: Communicative acts such as echolalia, perseveration, or other categories that do not belong to any of the proceeding categories.

Verbal Example: Adult: "Do you want the doll?" Child: "Doll."
AAC Example: Child points to "doll" after the adult's request.

No Response: The individual does not make a response when requested.

Verbal Example: Adult: "Where is the doll?" Child: no response
AAC Example: Child ignores the adult.

Table 5–5. Ten probes on the meaningful use of speech scale (MUSS).

1. Vocalizes during communicative interactions.
2. Uses speech to attract other's attention.
3. Vocalizations vary with content and intent of messages.
4. Is willing to use speech primarily to communicate with familiar persons on known topics.
5. Is willing to use speech primarily to communicate with unfamiliar persons on known topics.
6. Is willing to use speech primarily to communicate with familiar persons on novel topics or with reduced contextual information.
7. Is willing to use speech primarily to communicate with unfamiliar persons on novel topics or with reduced contextual information.
8. Messages are understood by persons familiar with the individual's speech.
9. Messages are understood by persons unfamiliar with the individual's speech.
10. Uses appropriate repair and clarification strategies when not understood.

Source: Osberger (1992).

be measured by systematically analyzing an individual's phonological patterns and deriving a severity index from the results (Hodson & Paden, 1983; Webb & Duckett, 1990). Other procedures involve having a naive listener transcribe single words and continuous speech. Intelligibility scores are then calculated from these measures (Weiss, 1982; Wilcox, Schooling, & Morris, 1991; Yorkston & Beukelman, 1981).

One difficulty encountered when using these procedures with young children and adults with developmental delays is a lack of familiarity with the test vocabulary. For example, the *Preschool Speech Intelligibility Measure* (Wilcox et al., 1991) was designed for young children, yet uses words such as *occur, defers, reserve, converge, absurd,* and *obscure* within a single word set (Kent et al., 1994). One method of assessing intelligibility using words within the child's developmental level is to have the child name pictures from age-appropriate expressive vocabulary tests such as the Expressive *One Word Picture Vocabulary Test—Revised* (Gardiner, 1990). The child's productions are written down by a listener who is unable to see the test pictures. The percentage of words transcribed correctly

can then be used to estimate single word intelligibility. Although vocabulary tests are not phonologically designed to evaluate intelligibility across all phonemic contexts, the simplified vocabulary results in more spontaneous word productions.

A factor that needs to be considered when assessing intelligibility is defining the listener. Standardized procedures are traditionally interpreted and scored by the examiner, or a naive judge. Although intelligibility levels with unfamiliar listeners need to be assessed, it is also important to determine the individual's intelligibility with familiar listeners. Many individuals can be extremely unintelligible, yet their families, teachers, and other familiar listeners are able to understand a significant portion of their speech.

Once measures of speech and phonological abilities are completed, the team needs to determine if AAC intervention is needed. This decision-making process is a difficult one with many gray areas. Discrepancies between the child's receptive language and expressive speech abilities and discrepancies between expressive language and phonological abilities need to be reviewed. Young preschool children who are making good developmental progress toward acquiring spoken language may not require AAC intervention. When in doubt, it is always better to err on the side of overprescribing AAC interventions. Several studies have anecdotally found that use of AAC results in increased attempts to use speech, or that overall expressive communication abilities were enhanced (Goosens, 1989; Light et al., 1988; Romski & Ruder, 1984; Silverman, 1980). In addition, AAC can be used as a method to train spoken language development using aided language stimulation procedures.

Determining a Motor Response for Assessment

The next portion of the evaluation involves assessing the individual's linguistic and cognitive abilities. Before these skills can be assessed, the best method for evaluating these abilities needs to be determined. The team must decide if test procedures need to be adapted for the individual being assessed. Receptive language and other cognitive skills should always be evaluated using direct selection modalities that the nonspeaking person is able to motorically access easily. Individuals might point with fingers, hands, head sticks, light pointers, or use eye gaze as their direct selection mode.

It is important that linguistic and cognitive assessments be conducted through direct selection modes because scanning adds another dimension of cognitive and motoric difficulty to the process. A child who is not responding appropriately to test items presented using scanning methods may not understand how the scanning process works, may not be able to access a switch in time to select the correct answer during the scanning process, or may have forgotten the test question while waiting for the system to scan to the correct response. Ratcliff (1994) evaluated the ability of normal children to use a Light Talker to respond to standardized test items. Two different access methods with the Light Talker were compared: direct selection via an optical light pointer, and single switch row column scanning. Ratcliff found that, regardless of age, error rates for responding were always higher when scanning methods were used. The only time scanning methods of assessment should be used to evaluate existing cognitive or language skills is when the nonspeaking person comes into the assessment with previous experience successfully and accurately using a scanning method of communication.

For individuals who may not be able to follow verbal directions, motor skills necessary for direct selection responding can be determined through play activities. The person's hand, arm, head, and eye gaze functions should be observed by the AAC assessment team during play. Tempting toys can be held out for the child to reach for, visual tracking of colorful toys can be observed, and toys can be moved around to determine if the individual can cross midline and the range of motion available for direct selection tasks. Small toys can be placed in arrays, and the child's ability to reach and touch or eye gaze toward individual items can be determined. The number of items in the toy array can be enlarged or reduced depending on the child's abilities. In addition, the spacing and arrangement of the toy items can be adjusted. At the end of this process the team should have a good sense of which modality appears easiest for the child, and the arrangement of test materials and items within that modality. Readers are referred to Chapter 7 in this text for more information about evaluating motor abilities.

Older children and adults who are able to follow simple commands can be assessed more quickly. The nonspeaking person is asked to point to specific locations and items using either hands, eye gaze, head sticks, or some other form of direct selection. The individual can be asked to point to pictures on standardized test pages, or to point to other materials. During this part of the assessment, the non-speaking person is not asked to respond to any test items. Instead, the individual is simply asked to "touch this picture," or "look at this one." Again, the goal is to determine whether standardized test procedures need adaptation, and the range and accuracy of responding with the direct selection method of choice.

Sometimes it is difficult to establish a direct selection method of accessing test materials. If this is the case, nonspeaking individuals with highly reliable yes/no responses can be evaluated to determine if their yes/no system can be used for assessment. Developmentally appropriate yet simple yes/no questions with obvious answers can be asked (e.g., "Is your name Big Bird?," "Is mommy here?" or "Is this a doggy?"). The individual's ability to respond correctly to these simple questions will indicate if yes/no responding can be used as a method of assessment. Yes/no responding should only be used for assessment when other direct selection modalities are inefficient or unreliable and the yes/no response is clear and accurate. Specific procedures for yes/no verbal scanning methods of assessment are outlined later in this chapter.

Before proceeding further in the assessment process, the individual must have a direct selection or yes/no method of responding which has been documented to be reliable. In addition, the efficiency of responding should also be considered. For example, child may be able to make choices between two items using his or her hands when the arms and body are fully extended. However, the motoric effort necessary may result in the child fatiguing quickly. Eye gaze might be a faster, more efficient method of responding that would allow the child to complete the assessment pro-cess quickly.

For individuals who can use direct selection to respond, but cannot always reliably select items in a manner that can be interpreted by the team, additional components to the response mode can be incorporated. For example, a young child using a head stick might slide the pointer across several pictures until the correct item is reached. Because of a slow response time, the evaluator may have difficulty knowing when the child has reached the final choice. Test procedures might be adapted by having the child lift up the pointer and look at the examiner after choosing an item or by having the child tap the picture twice once the correct item is reached. It cannot be emphasized enough that all adaptations and test procedures need to be practiced repeatedly by the individual before the actual evaluation process begins.

Assessment of Receptive Language, Cognitive, and Academic Capabilities

Formal evaluation of receptive language abilities, cognitive functioning, and academic skills certainly assists in the AAC feature matching process, but is not always necessary. Knowledge of an individual's ability to comprehend language, to process information, and to learn educational material provides the assessment team with data that help with AAC decision making. However, an individual's score on a language, cognitive, or educational assessment does not directly correlate to prescribing a specific AAC system. The assessment of these skills will provide the AAC evaluation team with information about gaps between existing expressive communication abilities and the individual's receptive, cognitive, and educational potential. When a significant gap exists between these two areas AAC intervention is recommended to assist the individual in communicating at a level that is commensurate with other abilities. At this point in time, there is no set level to define what constitutes a significant gap. Blackstone (1986) stated that AAC intervention is required when "cognitive dissonance" between receptive and expressive language exists.

It has also been proposed that prerequisite skills are not required prior to implementation of an AAC program (Kangas & Lloyd, 1988; Reichle & Karlan, 1985; Romski et al., 1988). The purpose of evaluating receptive language, cognitive, and acade-

mic skills is not to determine who would benefit from AAC intervention. Instead, this information should be used to determine how best to implement AAC interventions with a particular individual. The final decision to provide AAC intervention should be based on an individual's communication needs in the natural environment (Beukelman et al., 1985).

The receptive language, cognitive, and academic abilities of nonspeaking individuals can be evaluated using any standardized or nonstandardized assessment proce-

Table 5–6. Standardized assessment procedures using multiple-choice pointing testing formats.

Test Name	Format	Skills Assessed
CELF Preschool (selected subtests) (Wiig, Secord, & Semel, 1992)	Multiple Choice Pointing to Visual Stimuli	• Receptive vocabulary • Comprehension of syntax • Comprehension of directions
Clinical Evaluations of Language Functions–3 (selected subtests) (Wiig & Semel, 1995)	Multiple Choice Pointing to Visual Stimuli	• Comprehension of directions • Comprehension of syntax
Peabody Picture Vocabulary Test–Revised (Dunn & Dunn, 1981)	Multiple Choice Pointing to Visual Stimuli	• Receptive vocabulary
Preschool Language Scale III. Auditory Comprension Scale (Zimmerman, Steiner, & Evatt-Pond, 1991)	Multiple Choice Pointing to Visual Stimuli	• Receptive vocabulary • Comprehension of syntax • Sequencing events
Receptive One Word Picture Vocabulary Test (Gardner, 1985)	Multiple Choice Pointing to Visual Stimuli	• Receptive vocabulary
Test of Auditory Comprehension of Language–Revised (Carrow-Woolfolk, 1985)	Multiple Choice Pointing to Visual Stimuli	• Receptive vocabulary • Comprehension of syntax
Test of Early Reading Ability–2 (selected items) (Reid, Hresko, & Hammill, 1989)	Multiple Choice Pointing to Visual Stimuli	• Letter Identification • Sign/Symbol Identification • Sight Word Reading • Reading sentences
Test of Nonverbal Intelligence–2 (Brown, Sherbenou, & Johnsen, 1982)	Multiple Choice Pointing to Visual Stimuli	• Visual Spatial Skills • Visual Spatial Sequencing
Motor Free Visual Perception Test (Colarusso & Hammill, 1972)	Multiple Choice Pointing to Visual Stimuli	• Visual Perception
Peabody Individual Acheivement Test–Revised (most subtests) (Markwardt, 1989)	Multiple Choice Pointing to Visual Stimuli	• Reading Comprehension • Reading Recognition • Spelling • Mathematics
Woodcock Johnson Tests of Cognitive Ability–Revised (selected subtests) (Woodcock & Bonner-Johnson, 1989)	Multiple Choice Pointing to Visual Stimuli	• Visual Processing Speed • Visual Matching • Spatial Relations

dure that relies on responding to multiple choice items or answering yes/no questions. Table 5–6 lists some standardized assessment tools that can be given using these formats. The direct selection method of access that was identified in the previous part of the assessment is used to respond to test items. Before giving any items, the individual's ability to respond by pointing or answering yes/no questions should be assessed using the standard test formats. For example, a child might be asked to touch all of the picture choices on a test page to determine if adequate responses to the test items can be obtained. Sample and practice questions provided for most standardized assessments can be used to assist in this process.

Methods of Adapting Testing Procedures

When standard testing formats are not feasible, adaptations to test materials are needed. Test pages can be cut apart into separate items. The separate items can then be arranged in a different pattern, spread further apart, or moved closer together. It is helpful to have cut-up versions of tests available in an AAC evaluation center so that the assessment team can immediately adapt testing procedures. Cut-up pictures can be stored in file boxes, with each picture set separated by index dividers; stored in photo albums with plastic pockets for the item groups; or stored in file drawers with envelopes or file folders used to divide the test items.

Sometimes nonspeaking individuals are unable to respond to test items using the traditional number of choices. For example, a child might not be able to reliably point between four picture choices, but can make reliable choices between two pictures at a time. The number of test stimuli will need to be reduced, which can compromise test results. During normal test administration, a four choice picture format provides the individual with a 25%

chance of guessing the correct answer. These chance levels are taken into consideration when normative data for the assessment are developed. Reducing the choices down to two pictures increases this chance level of responding to 50%, thus invalidating the use of standard test norms. One method to compensate for this problem is to reduce the number of test stimuli but repeatedly test each target (correct) item against every foil (incorrect) item. For example, in the standardized format, the child might be asked to choose the picture bus from a group of four pictures (*bus, car, ball, horse*). In a two choice format, the child would first be asked to point to *bus* when it is paired with *car*. The child would then have *bus* paired with *ball* for another selection, and finally would have *bus* paired with *horse*. The child would need to get all three attempts correct to have the test item scored as correct.

There is one significant factor that will invalidate assessment results if the adaptation procedures previously described are followed. Many individuals will be able to recognize which picture is being shown repeatedly across the three trials. The first attempt to respond to the test item might have been a guess, but when the individual sees the very same picture on the next item, he is cued into making the correct response. In order to eliminate these cues, test items should be given in a rotating order. Table 5–7 provides an outline of how to test using a rotating item order. Children ages 2 or 3 can rotate test items with only a few trials between tasks. Older children and adults may need 15 to 20 items or more between trial rotations to prevent memorization or recognition of correct answers.

Another method of assessment that works well for older children and adults is to use yes/no verbal scanning. This assessment method can only be used with individuals who have a reliable yes/no response. Following the presentation of a

Table 5–7. Rotation of standardized test items used during adapted testing.

Trial	Test Item	Correct Picture	Foil Picture
1	1	Car	Spoon
2	2	Plant	Bottle
3	3	Bee	Chair
4	1	Car	Baby
5	2	Plant	Cup
6	3	Bee	Fly
7	1	Car	Bus
8	2	Plant	House
9	3	Bee	Horse

test item, the evaluator asks the nonspeaking individual yes/no questions to determine the desired answer. For example, the individual can be asked to indicate with yes/no answers which picture from a group of four represents the target vocabulary word. The evaluator systematically points to all possible choices and asks "Is this a _____?" after each item. The nonspeaking individual then responds yes or no to the questions. It is important that the evaluator not provide any cues during the assessment process. Cueing can take the form of varying the question order across test items, changing the intonation patterns of the questions, or only looking directly at the nonspeaking individual when a yes response is required.

Assessment of Symbolic Language Abilities for Aided AAC Systems

Communicating with an aided AAC system at a symbolic level requires the nonspeaking individual to understand and use object, tactile, or picture symbols or written language. Different commercially available AAC systems vary in the way symbols are organized and manipulated, or in the methods that written language is processed. In order to best match a nonspeaking individual to an appropriate AAC system these skills need to be systematically assessed.

When reviewing commercially available aided AAC devices that use picture symbols as a communication mode, there are several symbolic skills that are necessary in order to successfully use the systems. At a base level, an individual needs to understand that the act of pointing to a picture or object is communicative. In order to progress further, discrimination between multiple symbol choices must be learned. To increase communication potential, the individual needs to learn to sequence symbols together to communicate messages. At higher levels, the individual needs to learn how to categorize and associate words or phrases into logical semantic and syntactic groupings. Finally, the individual needs to be able to remember picture codes or other symbolic cues. Table 5–8 lists the picture-based symbolic skills commonly used in commercially available AAC devices.

When written language is used as a communication modality, different skills are necessary. At the earliest level, the individual needs to be able to recognize let-

Table 5–8. AAC picture-based symbolic skills.

- **Expressive use of picture symbols:** Does the individual understand that touching or looking at a symbol is communicative?

- **Receptive understanding of picture symbols:** Is the individual able to discriminate between picture symbols?

- **Picture symbol sequencing:** Can the individual combine two or three pictures to communicate a message?

- **Categorization and associations with picture symbols:** Does the individual understand semantic, syntactic, and functional vocabulary categories as they relate to picture symbols?

- **Complex picture symbol sequencing:** Can the individual use categorization and association concepts to encode language using a picture-based system?

ters and sight read basic words. The ability to spell words by rote and to phonetically spell novel words is also needed. In order to speed up the written language process, the individual may need to understand word prediction strategies or abbreviation-expansion strategies. Table 5–9 lists skills necessary for using AAC devices that require written communication abilities. These skills also need to be evaluated as part of the AAC assessment process.

The next section of this chapter outlines symbolic AAC assessment procedures developed at the Kennedy Krieger Institute (Glennen, 1992). These procedures are developmentally ordered for both picture-based and writing-based aided AAC device features. These assessment procedures were developed to be completed without the use of high tech AAC devices. There are two reasons for developing assessment procedures in this manner. First, many professionals do not have access to a wide array of AAC systems and would not be able to perform assessments that relied heavily on using a specific AAC device. Second, many young children with developmental delays get extremely excited when using voice output AAC technology for the first time. It can become difficult to maintain attention on assessment tasks if the individual is more interested in randomly pushing buttons to hear the device speak.

The AAC skills presented in this section were designed to be evaluated devel-

opmentally. For example, individuals who come into the assessment process demonstrating good use of an existing simple picture communication board will have already shown competence for early developing AAC symbolic skills. The evaluator would move up the AAC hierarchy to begin the assessment by examining higher level picture symbol or written language skills. In some cases, formal assessment of receptive language and academic abilities or informal observation of the individual's existing expressive communication abilities will have already provided the professional team with some of the information needed for the AAC evaluation process. When this occurs, some of the procedures outlined here will not be necessary. The next section outlines specific assessment procedures. The process of using evaluation data to make predictive AAC feature matching decisions will follow each assessment section.

Picture Symbol Assessment Strategies

Early Expressive Use and Receptive Understanding of Symbols. At early stages of implementing aided AAC interventions, there are several skills that need to be evaluated in order to make a feature match between the individual and an AAC system. Beginning at a level of using objects as symbols, the individual's ability to understand the functional use of an object should be assessed. That is, does the individual know what to

Table 5–9. Written language AAC assessment skills.

- **Letter identification:** Can the individual identify letters by name?

- **Sight word reading:** Can the individual read sight words at a third-grade reading level?

- **Single word spelling:** Can the individual spell words and create simple sentences intelligibly at a third-grade writing level?

- **Word prediction:** Can the individual write grammatically ordered sentences? Can the individual correctly spell the first two to three letters of a predicted word? Can the individual select a desired word from a list of highly similar words?

- **Abbreviation expansion:** Can the individual select alphabet-based codes to represent language, and then remember those codes?

do with common objects or toys (e.g., brush hair with a brush, eat with a spoon, brush teeth with a toothbrush)? Functional use of objects can be informally observed with able-bodied individuals during play or other naturally occurring activities. Individuals with severe physical impairments may know what objects are used for, but may be unable to physically demonstrate their knowledge. Methods of informally evaluating this knowledge might involve interviewing the family or classroom teacher. Are there certain toys or objects that consistently excite or upset the individual when they are shown? For example, a child might consistently vocalize excitedly when shown keys in anticipation of a car ride. Does the child laugh if items are used inappropriately (e.g., the evaluator attempts to feed a baby with a brush, or attempts to comb the baby's hair with a spoon)?

In addition to knowing the functions of objects, the individual also needs to understand that touching or looking at objects or pictures can be communicative to others. At the level of using objects, an array of favorite items can be placed so that the individual can access them. Observe whether the individual spontaneously reaches for the objects, or whether physical or verbal prompts need to be given. If the individual can touch objects communicatively, the objects should be moved out of reach but within sight and replaced

with a single corresponding concrete picture symbol (e.g., photographs or realistic drawings) for the object that the person preferred. The individual's ability to touch the picture symbol to request the preferred object is then evaluated. If the individual continues to reach toward the object, rather than toward the picture, physical and verbal prompts should be given to try to teach the skill within the evaluation setting. The goal is to determine if the individual can learn the cause-effect link between touching a picture and receiving a desired object.

Once the concept of touching a single picture to obtain an object is established, two to three additional pictures can be added to the task to see if the individual is able to discriminate between them to request preferred objects. It is important that the pictures be concrete and visually salient from one another. If the individual does not immediately make the discrimination, cueing and prompting should be used to train the skill within the evaluation. If the individual is able to discriminate to request a preferred object from a group of pictures, the evaluator can then randomly move the pictures around to determine whether the picture symbol itself was the discriminating factor, or whether the individual was responding to the location of the symbol.

Finally, the individual's ability to associate objects or picture symbols with spoken words is evaluated. An array of pictures representing early developing vocabulary words is arranged so that the individual can access them. The individual is asked to touch or look at each item by name. If possible, standardized tests such as the *Peabody Picture Vocabulary Test—Revised* (Dunn & Dunn, 1981) can be used for this portion of the assessment. If the individual cannot recognize black and white line drawings, vocabulary comprehension can be evaluated with objects or visually salient photographs.

AAC Feature Matching. At the end of this portion of the evaluation, the examiner will know if the individual can: recognize simple objects and their functions; understand the communicative cause-effect relationship of touching an object or picture, and subsequently receiving the item; make discriminations between symbols to request objects; and understand vocabulary words in order to make associations between spoken words and their corresponding objects, actions, and/or pictures.

Individuals who cannot do any of these skills are still candidates for AAC intervention. Intervention might consist of teaching a simple cause-effect request for a highly motivating reward. For example, a child who responds excitedly to music might be taught to touch a tape recorder to request turning on the music. This cause-effect skill teaches the concept of reach-pointing, and the association between an object (tape recorder) and its function (music).

Individuals who have object preferences and understand object functions but are unable to understand that pointing to a picture is communicative are candidates for simple picture-based AAC choice making. At early levels, the individual would be provided with physical and verbal guidance to touch pictures to receive a motivating reinforcer. Discrimination between picture choices is not important. Instead, the individual needs to understand the cause-effect relationship that touching the pictures will obtain a desired reward. Simple high tech AAC strategies can be used at this level to provide voice output, music, or visual cues when the child touches the picture. For example, the picture can be placed on a Big Mack switch that activates a recorded message when touched. Once the individual is spontaneously attempting to touch picture symbols, discrimination between picture choices can be taught.

Individuals who are able to discriminate between picture symbols and/or identify objects or pictures by name are ready for simple AAC communication boards or high tech devices with several picture or object symbol choices. Some individuals are able to discriminate between picture symbols without being able to identify the pictures by name (i.e., they know what they want without knowing what the object is called). These individuals are also ready for simple choice-making activities using AAC communication systems. Chapters 12 and 17 in this book provide more information on AAC programming for individuals functioning at these early symbolic communicative levels.

Picture Symbol Sequencing. This portion of the evaluation is designed to assess the individual's ability to combine picture symbols to communicate messages. One method of obtaining this information is to interact with the nonspeaking individual during naturally occurring activities such as playing with toys or listening to music. The individual is given a simple communication board to use during the activity with vocabulary designed to promote concrete picture symbol sequencing. Individuals who already have AAC systems can use them if the vocabulary lends itself to sequencing. Otherwise, the individual will need to be provided with a simple picture communication board to complete this portion of the assessment. In order to keep the assessment task cognitively and physically easy, the number of picture symbols on newly created communication boards is limited to four or six items. Table 5–10 provides ex-amples of picture communication board vocabulary for this part of the assessment.

During the play activity, the individual has constant access to the communica-tion board. The examiner begins by modeling picture sequences on the communication board during the play activity. Modeling involves pointing to the pictures while simultaneously verbalizing the picture sequences. The individual is encouraged to imitate the models. If necessary, physical and verbal prompting is given. The examiner should also set up situa-

Table 5–10. Methods used for evaluating picture symbol sequencing.

Topic of Communication	Picture Symbols	Objects Needed
Play with Baby Doll	I/Mommy Baby Bottle Diaper	Baby Doll Bottle Doll's Diaper
Play with Cars	I/Me Car Crash Go	Two or More Cars Toy Garage
Listen to Music	I/Me Tape Go/Play Stop	Cassette Player Two or More Tapes

Table 5–11. Picture symbol sequencing assessment script.

Evaluator Verbalizations	Modeled Use of Communication Board	Child's Use of Communication Board
Baby is hungry.	(Baby + Bottle)	
Do you think baby is hungry?	(Baby + Bottle)	Baby (I = imitated)
Yes. This baby needs her bottle.	(Baby + Bottle)	Bottle (I)
What should we do?		Bottle (S = spontaneous)
Oh. The bottle.	(Bottle)	
Let's give baby a bottle.	(Baby + Bottle)	Baby + Bottle (P = physical) (hand over hand)
Yes. The baby wants a bottle.		Bottle (S)
Tell me all of it.	(points to board)	Baby + Bottle (V)
Who should feed the baby this bottle?		points to self
Oh. Do you want to feed the baby?	(I/Me + Baby)	I/Me + Baby (I)
Good job. You can feed the baby.	(I/Me + Bottle + Baby)	Baby (I)

tions or ask questions designed to elicit use of the communication board during play. Table 5–11 gives a sample script for this portion of the evaluation.

The individual's attempts to use the communication board should be recorded for analysis. Each attempt to use the pictures communicatively is recorded, along with codes indicating the level of prompting necessary to elicit the utterances. Spontaneous (S) use occurs when the child uses the board without immediate models. If the evaluator physically models a symbol sequence which is then imitated by the individual, the sequence is marked as being imitated (I). Verbal prompts (V) can range from direct commands that tell the individual what pictures to touch (e.g., "You need to show me the baby") to indirect questions or commands which will elicit more from the individual (e.g., "Tell me more"). Physical prompts (P) occur when the examiner physically assists the individual in touching the pictures.

AAC Feature Matching. By the end of this phase of the assessment, the evaluator will know if the individual is able to sequence picture symbols, what level of cueing is necessary to prompt symbol sequences, and the individual's frequency of attempting to use the communication boards. Some individuals, despite frequent modeling, are unable to point to more than a single symbol unless physical prompts are used. These individuals are candidates for using AAC systems with vocabulary designed for single symbol messages. Individuals who are able to sequence pictures together with imitative or verbal prompts are candidates for AAC devices that have sequencing capabilities. However, single symbol messages would need to predominate on the AAC system until sequencing skills develop further. Individuals who can sequence symbols together spontaneously need to be matched to AAC systems that will allow them to use this feature to expand their ability to communicate.

In addition to examining picture symbol sequencing, the evaluator will also have collected data on the child's frequency of attempting to use the communication boards. Some children may ignore the board in favor of unaided methods of communication during the play activity. Other children may initially use unaided methods of communication, then turn to the board to clarify information. Infrequent use of the board may mean that AAC systems designed to enhance existing unaided methods of communication should be considered, or that training will need to focus on pragmatically teaching the child which method of communication is most effective in different environments.

Picture Symbol Categorization and Association. Individuals who are able to sequence picture symbols are candidates for using AAC systems with complex picture-based vocabulary organization strategies that allow them access to hundreds of words or more. These include AAC systems that use Minspeak software (Baker, 1986), and those that organize vocabulary into separate category pages such as the Dynavox, or the computer-based picture symbol software programs Speaking Dynamically, or Talking Symbols. Chapter 3 provides an overview of how these picture symbol-based AAC devices operate.

In order to use these AAC systems effectively, the individual needs to have an understanding of how vocabulary words can be associated and categorized using picture symbols. The following categories are commonly used as methods to organize picture-based vocabulary systems: object names, object functions, category names, part/whole concepts, descriptive concepts, similar item associations, location concepts, size/shape concepts, color concepts, rhyming words, phonetic associations, and semantic-grammatical concepts. Table 5–12 provides examples of these categories.

There are standardized language tests that assess a child's understanding of some of these concepts. For example, the *Pre-*

Table 5–12. Semantic categorization strategies used to encode vocabulary in picture-based AAC systems.

Semantic Categorization Strategy		Assessment Example
Symbol Name	Identification of a picture by name.	Where's the dog? Points to dog.
Object Function	Associating an object with its functions.	What do we ride on? Points to bus.
Category Name	Associates an object with its category referent.	Where's the animal? Points to dog.
Part/Whole Concepts	Can identify a named part of a whole object.	Where's the pillow? Points to bed.
Similar Item Associations	Associates items that belong together in groups.	What goes together with cat? Points to dog.
Location Concepts	Can associate an object with its typical location.	What belongs in the bedroom? Points to bed.
Size/Shape Concepts	Associates size and shape terms with objects.	Find a circle. Points to sun.
Color Concepts	Can identify colors.	Find something yellow. Points to sun.
Other Descriptive Concepts	Associates other descriptive terms with a picture.	Find something soft. Points to bed.
Rhyming and Phonetic Concepts	Associates words that rhyme or sound alike.	Which word sounds like frog? Points to dog.
Grammatical Concepts	Can understand grammatical terms such as action, verb, object.	Show me an action. Points to dog running.

school *Language Scale—3* (Zimmerman, Steiner, & Evatt-Pond, 1991) assesses understanding of colors, categories, size, and a limited number of grammatical concepts. These tests can be used to partially evaluate these AAC skills.

A method of assessing comprehension of concepts specifically for AAC purposes was first developed by Elder (1987). Elder's assessment protocol evaluated an individual's ability to make vocabulary associations with a variety of picture symbols. Her assessment methods were further refined by Glennen (1992). A limited set of four picture symbols is used to evaluate comprehension of vocabulary concepts necessary for encoding language in picture-based AAC devices. The nonspeaking individual is asked to make increasingly

abstract vocabulary associations with the same picture symbol set. Multiple sets of four pictures are used for the assessment process. Table 5–12 lists specific assessment questions used for a set of four picture symbols (*dog, bus, bed, sun*).

AAC Feature Matching. The assessment team should realize that this portion of the evaluation is by no means standardized. Instead, it is simply an information gathering process. Assessing these skills will provide the team with information about which picture-based vocabulary encoding strategies will be conceptually easy for a nonspeaking individual to use, versus those encoding strategies that will need to be trained. For example, if a nonspeaking child understands concepts related to object names, object functions, and category names, the AAC system should be developed to rely heavily on those vocabulary encoding strategies. Vocabulary concepts that have not been mastered can be trained, but the time to learn new vocabulary will be increased since the picture symbol encoding strategies will not be transparent or intuitively obvious to the child. In order for an AAC system to be immediately functional for communication purposes, it will need to be customized so that the individual can access needed vocabulary using encoding strategies that are already understood.

Complex Picture Symbol Sequencing and Memory.

The previous assessment procedure evaluated an individual's ability to understand increasingly abstract vocabulary concepts as they related to picture symbols. In addition, nonspeaking individuals also need to be able to logically sequence encoded picture symbols together when using AAC systems based on Minspeak software (Baker, 1986). Minspeak is currently available in Prentke Romich equipment. Other devices that have the capability to link keys in sequence rely upon these Minspeak concepts as well. This task is relatively easy when the pictures being sequenced relate directly to the underlying vocabulary (e.g., *"I want a drink"* = *I/Me* + *Drink*). However, the task becomes more difficult when the sequence order can be easily reversed, or the sequence is relatively abstract (e.g., *"Bus"* = *Car* + *Banana*).

Many individuals with language learning disabilities have difficulty with short- and long-term memory related to remembering sequences of items. This skill needs to be evaluated before considering use of AAC systems that require memorization of symbol sequences.

These evaluation procedures were modified from assessment methods originally developed by Elder (1987). For this portion of the evaluation, the individual is asked to select two pictures from a set of four to represent the following: a sentence that is concretely associated with the picture symbol set; a single word associated with the symbol set; and a sentence that is abstractly associated with the symbol set. Table 5–13 gives examples for this portion of the assessment.

Several trials are given across each of the three skill levels using different picture symbol sets. The first portion of the assessment analyzes whether the individual is able to make picture symbol associations at these more complex levels. Picture symbol associations at the concrete and single word level are usually straightforward when a limited set of four pictures is used. Picture symbol associations for abstract sentences usually involve more than one potentially correct answer. For example, the sentence stimuli used in Table 5–13 for the abstract level is "My breakfast is too hot." In the table, the picture sequence *Bed* + *Sun* is listed as the correct sequence. However, the individual could just as easily associate the picture of *Bus* with breakfast, because breakfast is

Table 5–13. Complex picture symbol sequencing.

Picture Symbol Set	Dog	Bus	Bed	Sun

Sentence/Word Stimulus		Picture Symbol Sequence
Concrete Sentence:	The dog rides the bus.	Dog + Bus
Single Word:	Teddy Bear	Dog + Bed
Abstract Sentence:	My breakfast is too hot.	Bed + Sun

eaten before the bus arrives every morning. In addition, the picture *Dog* could also be associated if the person feeds their dog breakfast every morning.

What is more important at the abstract and single word level is the second portion of this assessment procedure, which involves a memory test. The individual is told that he or she will need to remember the symbols selected and recall them at a later time. Ten to 15 minutes after the initial items are assessed the items are given again. The individual's ability to remember what symbols were chosen and the correct order of the symbols is then evaluated. Individuals who choose symbol sequences that logical for them usually are able to remember the chosen sequence during the memory retest. Those who choose symbols arbitrarily often have difficulty with this portion of the assessment.

AAC Feature Matching. The ability to sequence abstract picture symbols together is a necessary skill for using high level picture-based AAC strategies relying on Minspeak concepts such as Unity, Interaction Education and Play +, and Words Strategy. Individuals who are able to sequence concrete symbols, but cannot sequence when using more abstract concepts, will need to have their picture-based AAC systems customized to emphasize concrete sequencing strategies in which the picture symbols directly represent the underlying vocabulary. Individuals who are able to sequence abstract concepts are candidates for picture-based encoding systems that rely upon abstract sequencing.

The ability to remember sequences in order is also an important consideration. AAC systems that use symbol sequencing require the individual to recall the sequence in the correct order. Reversing the sequence will often result in an incorrect word or no vocabulary output. Individuals who are unable to remember symbol sequences in the correct order will require

additional cueing strategies in order to use AAC systems that are sequence dependent. Cueing strategies might involve using light prediction cues such as those available in Prentke Romich's Liberator, Delta Talker, and AlphaTalker. AAC system features that eliminate activation of incorrect symbols can also be used. Other cueing strategies might involve color coding symbols that are the initial pictures in a symbol sequence, or organizing all symbols that initiate sequences into a certain location on the device.

Summary of Picture Symbol Assessment Procedures. This portion of the assessment process was designed to provide predictive information for implementing picture-based AAC systems. Using this information, the evaluator should be able to predict which devices will be easy or difficult for an individual to use. Evaluators are cautioned that predictive information does not always directly translate into actual performance capabilities. For example, during the evaluation an individual may be able to sequence symbols together using complex vocabulary concepts with a limited set of four pictures. The ability to sequence symbols together with a set of 128 pictures on an AAC device is a much more difficult process. Many individuals can demonstrate competence using picture symbols in predictive testing, yet have difficulty translating that competence into actual device use. Following the predictive portion of the assessment, nonspeaking individuals should then be evaluated using the actual AAC devices being considered. More information about that portion of the assessment is given later in this chapter.

Written Language Assessment Strategies

Some nonspeaking individuals come into the assessment process with well-documented information pertaining to their ability to read and write. Written language scores from standardized tests, information from teachers, and demonstration of writing competence using computers or AAC systems can all be used to analyze a person's ability to communicate using written language modalities. However, many individuals come into the assessment process with limited information about their written language abilities. The following procedures were developed at Kennedy Krieger Institute to quickly screen early written language skills with nonspeaking individuals when other information is not available (Glennen, 1992). Additional written language skills necessary for using word acceleration and prediction strategies are then assessed to obtain predictive information necessary for the AAC feature matching process. Similar to the predictive evaluation of picture-based symbolic skills, the evaluator should not duplicate the assessment process by re-evaluating skills already demonstrated by the nonspeaking individual through other means of evaluation.

Literacy Screening. The screening of literacy skills is done to determine if a nonspeaking individual has sufficient literacy abilities to consider using written language as a communication modality. At the earliest level, an individual's ability to identify alphabet letters is screened. Children with good physical abilities can quickly point to named letters from an alphabet arrayed on a communication board or on a computer keyboard. Children with more limited physical abilities can point to named letters from a limited number of choices arranged on test cards which can be spread apart or arranged to promote access to the choices. If a limited number of choices is used, there probably is not sufficient time for evaluating the individual's ability to identify all 26 letters. Instead, a limited number of letters are screened by the evaluator. At Kennedy Krieger Institute, the AAC team typically screens for recognition of the letters *A, D, E, I, P, R, S, T.* These letters are used

because they can be combined to form a number of words when screening spelling abilities later in the assessment process. When a limited set of letters is screened, the evaluator should be aware of situations in which the majority of letters screened occur in the individual's first or last name. Many youngsters learn to identify the letters in their name, yet cannot identify the entire alphabet. Additional letters that are not contained in the individual's name will need to be screened.

Sight word reading skills also need to be screened. Subtests from standardized tests such as the *Peabody Individual Achievement Test—Revised* (Markwardt, 1989) can be used for this purpose. The Kennedy Krieger Institute uses word lists adapted from *The Handbook of Diagnostic Teaching* (Mann & Suiter, 1974) to screen sight word reading. The individual is presented with up to four word choices on cards and is asked to identify the named word. Individuals who are able to identify single words should also have their ability to comprehend text in phrases, sentences, or paragraphs evaluated. Again, standardized tests of written language can be used to evaluate these skills with minor adaptations. Table 5–6, which was presented previously in this chapter, outlines reading tests which can be adapted to yes/no questions or are designed for multiple choice methods of responding. Many individuals have good reading comprehension skills, yet have difficulty expressing themselves using written language. Learning disabilities, or a lack of practice in writing, often contribute to these difficulties. Readers are referred to Chapter 8 for more information about literacy abilities and their impact on nonspeaking individuals. As part of the predictive assessment process, the ability to spell words, phrases, and sentences needs to be evaluated. Again, there are many standardized assessments that can be used to evaluate these skills. The majority require the individual to write using paper and pencil or a computer. It is very difficult to adapt these procedures for individuals with severe physical disabilities.

At Kennedy Krieger Institute, the AAC team screens for the ability to spell single words that can be derived from a small set of letters. This speeds up the screening process for individuals with limited physical abilities. The same eight letters used in the letter identification portion of the screening are used (*A, D, E, I, P, R, S, T*). Individuals are asked to point or eye gaze to letter cards to spell increasingly more complex words (see Table 5–14). The words were adapted from Mann and Suiter (1974). At the easiest level, the words are simple CVC combinations. At the next level, spelling conventions such as silent E and consonant blends are added to single syllable words. At the highest level, these skills are combined into one and two syllable words.

AAC Feature Matching. The screening of literacy skills is necessary to determine which nonspeaking individuals require access to written language in their AAC systems. Individuals who are unable to identify letters, sight read words, or spell can use AAC devices that rely solely on picture symbol methods of communication. Individuals who have beginning literacy abilities (e.g., letter identification and some sight word reading) will still need to rely on picture-based communication systems, but should be considered for devices that provide printed output of picture symbol choices, and the capability of communicating using writing if those skills can be developed. This is also true for young nonspeaking children who do not demonstrate reading or writing abilities, but are expected to develop those skills in the near future. Individuals who are able to spell single words, even if the spellings are only phonetically close approximations (e.g., *Periat* for *Pirate*), definitely require access to written language in their AAC systems. AAC devices that combine picture-based communication with written language capabilities should be considered.

Finally, nonspeaking individuals who are able to spell intelligibly, but not necessarily correctly, at a phrase or sentence level are candidates for considering AAC systems that rely completely on written language as a method of communication. This is not to say that communication using picture-based symbol systems should be ignored. There are many nonspeaking adults who are capable of communicating through written language, but prefer using picture-based AAC systems because of past experience, communication speed, or other factors. The feature matching process for nonspeaking individuals who are capable written communicators should not rule out the use of picture-based AAC devices.

Table 5–14. Screening spelling abilities using a limited letter set.

Letters	A, D, E, I, P, R, S, T		
Primer Words	Sad	Red	Sit
	See	It	Is
Level One	Said	Drip	Ride
	Tear	Read	Tape
Level Two	Trade	Stripe	Pirate
	Parade	Dressed	Easter

Word Prediction and Abbreviation Expansion. Nonspeaking individuals who are capable users of written language and are considering using AAC devices based upon written language as a communication method may need to use advanced features designed to accelerate the communication process. These two features are word prediction and abbreviation-expansion for letter codes. Chapter 3 has further information about these two AAC system features. Methods of informally evaluating skills in these two areas that were developed at Kennedy Krieger Institute will be reviewed (Glennen, 1992).

Word Prediction. Users of AAC systems with word prediction capabilities need the ability to read text and to select the word that comes next from a list of choices. Many individuals are able to find a specific word from a list of words when the words differ by the initial consonant-vowel combination (e.g., *grape, ball, juice, car*). However, most word prediction programs present word lists that have highly similar spelling sequences (e.g., *the, this, that, then, there*). In order to select the correct word, the individual needs to be able to discriminate among them. To evaluate the ability to make these discriminations, written sentences are shown to the nonspeaking individual with the final word left blank. The individual is given a word prediction list of four choices to complete the sentence. Table 5–15 lists several examples of word prediction assessment stimuli. Some items evaluate the ability to find the correct word from lists of similarly spelled words. Other items evaluate the ability to comprehend grammatical word ordering. The word prediction lists can be arranged on cards which are then pointed to by the individual to complete the sentence.

Abbreviation-Expansion. AAC devices that have abbreviation-expansion capabilities use letter codes as abbreviations for retrieving prestored words, phrases, or sentences. For example, the sentence *Hello, how are you?* might be stored under the sequence of *H + Y.* The sentence might just as easily be stored under the sequence of *H + H,* or *H + E.* Using abbreviation expansion as a communication strategy requires the individual to select appropriate abbreviation codes and remember the codes in the correct sequence. At Kennedy Krieger Institute this skill is informally evaluated by presenting short phrases, single words, and lengthy sentences and asking

Table 5–15. Word prediction assessment.

Test Item	Word Choices
Similar Spelling Pattern Completions	
1. Let's go for a drive in my new _____.	Car, Can, Carpet, Cap
2. I want to pet the _____.	Dog, Door, Done, Dot
3. Close the _____.	Dog, Door, Done, Dot
4. I want to put it _____.	That, There, This, The
Grammatical Phrase Completions	
1. The dog _____.	Is, Are, Can, Were
2. The cat is _____.	Eating, Are, Give, Sit
3. Do you _____.	Like, What, New, My
4. I want _____.	The, Is, There, Get

the individual to select two letters to represent the stimulus from a limited set. The same eight letters used previously to evaluate letter identification and letter spelling are used (e.g., *A, D, E, I, P, R, S, T*). Table 5–16 lists some of the test items that are used for the assessment process.

In addition to being able to select appropriate letter sequences, the nonspeaking individual's ability to remember the letter sequences is evaluated on a memory retest. The individual is informed that the sequences that are selected will be reviewed later in the evaluation session. After 10 minutes of completing other activities, the individual is re-administered the test items and asked to recall the originally selected letter codes.

AAC Feature Matching. Individuals who are capable spellers, and are able to choose appropriate words from prediction lists and create and remember abbreviation-expansion codes should certainly be considered for AAC devices that provide these features. The use of word prediction and abbreviation-expansion significantly speeds up the communication process for individuals who have slow AAC access

methods. The grammatical and spelling support provided by both features also allows some individuals to improve the quality and complexity of their writing.

Summary of Written Language Assessment. Once this portion of the evaluation is completed, information pertaining to using written language as a potential communication mode can be used to determine which AAC systems to assess further. Consideration should be given to an individual's current written language abilities, and the potential to develop those abilities in the future. Young children with beginning literacy abilities should certainly be considered for AAC systems that will allow them to develop these skills in the future. Older adults with developmental delays may not require written language as an AAC device feature if they are functioning at early literacy levels.

Individuals with the ability to write sentences should be considered for AAC systems that rely heavily on written language as a communication tool. Features that enhance use of written language such as abbreviation-expansion and word pre-

Table 5–16. Abbreviation expansion assessment.

Letters	A, D, E, I, P, R, S, T
Single Choice Phrases	*Abbreviations*
Please stop	P + S
Don't play	D + P
I'm tired	I + T
Single Words	
Stop	S + T, or S + P
Please	P + S, or P + E
Apple	A + P, or A + E
Multiple Choice Phrases	
Time to eat doughnuts.	T + E, or E + D, or T + D. . .
Don't pet that dog.	D + P, or P + D, or T + D. . .
Eat a red apple today.	E + R, or E + A, or R + A. . .

diction should be assessed further. As stated previously, the predictive assessment process can be used to guide the evaluator toward choosing AAC systems that will best meet an individual's needs and abilities. However, predictive assessment does not always translate into actual performance. For example, a child may not be able to discriminate between word prediction choices that are spelled similarly. However, several word prediction software programs allow the use of customized word prediction dictionaries. A custom dictionary composed only of words the child can easily read might allow the child to take advantage of learning word prediction features. Further assessment and a trial period of using an AAC system is needed before final decisions are made.

FEATURE MATCHING: THE DECISION PROCESS

Predictive AAC assessment is the process of obtaining information that is necessary for predicting which AAC system or systems should be considered for actual use. Like any complex decision-making process, the information obtained in the evaluation does not always lead to easy answers.

At this point in the assessment, the team should have information to guide them in predicting which AAC devices should be considered further for a given individual. The ability to use predictive assessment information to make these decisions is heavily dependent on having expert knowledge of various AAC options. Professionals who have limited experience or knowledge of the wide array of AAC systems available need to refer the final decision-making process to professionals who specialize in AAC. Many times, the decision-making process is a collaborative effort between field professionals who have daily contact with the nonspeak-

ing individual and an AAC team with expert knowledge of AAC options. Field professionals can often gather needs assessment information, evaluate existing expressive language and speech abilities, and screen predictive skills necessary for using AAC systems. The expert AAC team then reviews the information and selects several AAC options to evaluate further.

Many factors need to be considered in the decision making process. Figure 5–1, which was discussed earlier in this chapter, indicated some of these decision-making factors. The evaluation procedures outlined in this chapter provide guidance for collecting information on some of these factors. Collecting information is relatively easy. The process of deciding which factors are important and which are secondary is more difficult and is different for every nonspeaking individual. For example, some ambulatory individuals may feel that portability is more important than any other AAC system feature. Even though they are capable of using an AAC system with more advanced features, if the system weighs too much or is overly large it will not be used. AAC systems with fewer features that are smaller in size may be preferred. Other nonspeaking individuals may have ease of operation and programming high on their priority lists. For example, adults who live in assisted living arrangements often require easy to operate systems because of problems with high staff turnover. An AAC system that is more difficult to operate or program has a higher likelihood of being misused by new staff who have not been adequately trained. Some information about priorities is gathered during the initial needs assessment portion of the evaluation. However, at this point in the evaluation, additional questions may arise that need to be answered before determining which AAC systems to consider. The nonspeaking individual, family members, and professionals who have regular contact with the individual should be consulted for additional information if needed.

Once all of the information is gathered and reviewed, the AAC team should come to a consensus about which AAC strategies to consider for further assessment. The next step in the evaluation process is to determine how the nonspeaking person will motorically access the AAC devices being considered. Individuals with good physical and visual abilities will probably not require extensive access evaluations and can move right into trying various AAC options. Individuals with physical disabilities may need to have adjustments in seating and positioning before proceeding further with the evaluation. Extensive evaluation of physical access skills may be necessary before finding a method of accessing that is quick, efficient, accurate, and not fatiguing. Individuals with visual disabilities will need further assessment of their ability to visually identify symbols of different sizes, colors, and backgrounds, to scan visually across large numbers of symbols, and to take advantage of auditory cues when using AAC systems. Chapter 6 presents information about improving seating and positioning. Chapter 7 reviews evaluation procedures used to assess motor access and visual abilities necessary for using AAC devices.

EVALUATING AAC PERFORMANCE: FIELD TESTING

Once the AAC evaluation team has determined which AAC devices to consider, and has found accurate methods to access each device, the individual's performance with the actual system needs to be assessed. During the evaluation an individual can be presented with several devices as options to consider. The physical ability to access each device, the ability to understand how to use the device, and the

ability to communicate using the device can be explored during the evaluation session. Sometimes during this portion of the assessment the team can rule out AAC devices that are not successful options for the individual. However, typically there are several AAC systems that appear to work well, or work well enough to be worth considering further, with different pros and cons related to each option. At this point in the evaluation process, a field test with recommended AAC systems is often warranted.

Some nonspeaking individuals reach this stage of the assessment process with borderline skills for using AAC devices with more advanced options and features. For example, a child who can easily use single picture symbol messages, but requires frequent structured prompting to sequence symbols together, may require more experience and training with a device before a final decision is made. Devices that have sequencing features are typically more expensive than devices without these features. Before spending hundreds or thousands of unnecessary dollars, field testing with an AAC system is warranted.

Finally, some nonspeaking individuals complete the initial assessment process and may not appear to be good candidates for using aided systems. Despite these findings, a field test with an AAC system may still be warranted. This author often counsels beginning professionals to "never say never," or never use results from an initial evaluation to completely rule out an AAC strategy. A young 4-year-old with autism once came in for an AAC assessment with a history of not using picture communication boards or sign gestures functionally. Across two evaluation sessions he did not respond appropriately to any picture stimuli, sign gestures, simple communication choice boards, or voice output devices. However, his mother insisted that if he had the opportunity to use a voice output AAC system over a longer period of time he could learn to use the device. The family was reluctantly loaned an IntroTalker for a 6-week trial period. When the family returned, the device had been programmed with 10 single symbol messages, with corresponding photographs on the overlay. As soon as the IntroTalker was pulled out of the bag, the child walked over to the device, pressed *I want gum please* and then walked over to his mother while holding out his hand for gum. He continued to use the device appropriately to make other simple requests. Needless to say, the final AAC recommendations changed following the field test.

Field testing is a process whereby an individual gets to "test drive" an AAC system before any final decisions are made. AAC devices are obtained through short-term loan or rented for 1 week to 1 month trials in the natural environment. It is important that the field test be implemented in a manner that allows the nonspeaking individual the opportunity to use the AAC system across all neccesary environments. It is only through field testing that actual barriers to using AAC in the natural setting can be identified (Sloand-Armstrong & Jones, 1994).

The field test will help to resolve logistical barriers such as who will charge the system, how the system can be accessed in unusual situations, weight and portability of the device, transporting the device from one environment to another, and whether the device batteries will last throughout an entire day. AAC device barriers such as learning a new symbol system, learning to sequence symbols, or use of written communication within the system can be further evaluated during the field test. Family and professional barriers such as teaching a family or teacher to program the system, integrating the device into existing communication activities, and negative opinions toward using AAC can be delineated. Finally, for those individuals who have existing unaided or aided methods of communication, a field test often determines whether use of a new AAC system actually enhances existing communication abilities, or whether it is rarely used.

At the end of the field test period, the nonspeaking individual is evaluated again by the AAC team. Whenever possible, this final evaluation should take place within the natural setting. The individual's ability to use the field tested AAC equipment is evaluated by observing interactions in the natural environment. The nonspeaking individual, professionals involved in the field test process, and family are further interviewed to determine pros and cons that were identified during the field test process.

Sometimes the field test outcome is so successful that an immediate decision can be made to implement the tested AAC system. At other times, additional questions are raised that can only be answered by extending the field test for a longer period of time with a few modifications to the system. Another outcome is for the field test to be unsuccessful. The AAC system is rejected by the nonspeaking individual or others in the environment during the field test period. Nonspeaking individuals who reject an AAC system are then given the option to try other AAC devices. At times, following field testing an individual will reject the system and decide that implementation of any aided AAC system is not feasible.

Obtaining equipment for field testing can be a difficult process for many nonspeaking individuals. In an effort to improve this situation, some states or regions have established free device libraries that allow state residents to "check out" equipment for trial. The loan period for these libraries ranges from 1 week to 1 month and often there are waiting lists for loaning popular AAC devices. Many progressive school districts have small libraries of AAC equipment available for short-term trials. AAC equipment manufacturers have also recognized the need for field testing devices before making a final decision. Loan equipment is available for short-term rental, with a portion of the rental fee applied to the purchase price. However, equipment rentals are often expensive and many families and individuals cannot afford the fees. Insurance companies and third party payers will sometimes pay for equipment rentals, however, the process of obtaining funding for renting equipment is often lengthy and paperwork intensive.

THE AAC PRESCRIPTION AND FUNDING

Once the field test process is completed, the AAC assessment team will need to develop a prescription for the AAC equipment and develop recommendations for implementing and training use of the equipment in the natural environment. The AAC prescription is a listing of all items that are necessary for implementing an aided AAC system. These will include the device itself along with symbol sets, mounting equipment, keyguards, battery chargers, equipment to integrate the device with a computer, software, and carrying cases, among others. It is important that the prescription be complete, detailed, and thorough. Information obtained during the field test process often determines equipment items necessary for the final prescription. For example, many children use a power chair at school and a manual chair at home. Equipment necessary for mounting an AAC system on both chairs will need to be part of the prescription.

Once the prescription is completed, the AAC team is ready to approach sources to obtain funding for the recommended equipment. It is important that the team not let funding restrictions guide the prescription process. It is common to hear professionals lament that "we'll never get funding for this device, so we shouldn't bother recommending it." Every non-speaking individual needs to have access to an appropriate AAC system, regardless of cost. Funding can be obtained for expensive equipment. It requires perseverance, tenacity, and knowledge of how to work the funding system. It also requires careful documentation of the assessment process, with clear presentation of data regarding why AAC is essential to the individual, and why other AAC options will not suffice. Chapter 9 further outlines strategies for the funding process.

In addition to a listing of prescribed equipment, the AAC assessment team also needs to develop specific recommendations necessary for implementing AAC strategies. Recommendations should review how to integrate existing methods of communication with newly recommended AAC strategies, sequential training strategies to teach use of an aided communication system, methods of eliminating barriers to AAC implementation, and recommendations for using unaided or low tech strategies in situations where an aided system is not feasible.

SUMMARY

This chapter outlined predictive assessment procedures used to evaluate nonspeaking individuals. The procedures began with an assessment of an individual's communicative needs, progressed to an evaluation of existing expressive communication modes, and moved on to evaluating symbolic and linguistic skills necessary for using aided AAC systems. Once motor access and visual issues were addressed, the nonspeaking individual then had the opportunity to field test any recommended equipment before making a final decision.

It should be noted that AAC evaluations are usually lengthy, and often require more than a single assessment session. Nonspeaking individuals who are able-bodied with good attention to task can sometimes be evaluated in a single session, with a field test to follow. Nonspeaking individuals who have physical disabilities may need multiple sessions to address seating and positioning concerns along with motor access strategies before a field test can begin. Individuals with cognitive and attentional difficulties may not respond well to new situations or settings. Again, multiple sessions may be required as part of the AAC assessment process. Finally, young children who are nonspeaking can be difficult to assess because of constantly changing developmental skills and abilities. For example, a young child's ability to physically access a system often improves or changes over time. In addition, the underlying symbolic language skills of the child often mature at a rapid rate. Again, a long-term evaluation process may be necessary, with short-term AAC training strategies implemented throughout the assessment period.

REFERENCES

Alpert, C. (1980). Procedures for determining the optimal nonspeech mode with the autistic child. In R. L. Schiefulbusch (Ed.), *Nonspeech language and communication: Analysis and intervention* (pp. 389–420). Baltimore: University Park Press.

American Speech-Language-Hearing Association. (1989). Competencies for speech language pathologists providing services in augmenative communication. *ASHA, 31*, 107–110.

Baker, B. (1986). Using images to generate speech. *Byte*, 160–168.

Beukelman, D. R., & Mirenda, P. (1992). *Augmentative and alternative communication: Management of severe communication disorders in children and adults*. Baltimore: Paul H. Brookes.

Beukelman, D. R., Yorkston, K., & Dowden, P. (1985). *Communication augmentation: A casebook of clinical management*. San Diego, CA: College-Hill Press.

Blackstone, S. (Ed.). (1986). *Augmentative communication: an introduction*. Rockville, MD: American Speech-Language-Hearing Association.

Bolton, S., & Dashiell, S. (1984). *INCH: Interaction checklist for augmentative communication*. Wauconda, IL: Don Johnston Developmental Equipment Inc.

Brown, L., Sherbenou, R., & Johnsen, S. (1982). *Test of Nonverbal Intelligence—2*. Circle Pines, MN: AGS.

Buzolich, M., & Wiemann, J. (1988). Turntaking in atypical conversations: The case of the speaker/augmentated communicator dyad. *Journal of Speech and Hearing Research, 31*, 3–18.

Calculator, S., & Dollaghan, C. (1982). The use of communication boards in a residential setting: An evaluation. *Journal of Speech and Hearing Disorders, 47*, 281–287.

Calculator, S., & Luchko, C. (1983). Evaluating the effectiveness of a communication board training program. *Journal of Speech and Hearing Disorders, 48*, 185–199.

Carrow-Woolfolk, E. (1985). *Test of Auditory Comprehension of Language–Revised*. Chicago, IL: Riverside Publishing.

Colarusso, R., & Hammil, D. (1972). *Motor free visual perception test*. Novato, CA: Academic Therapy Publications.

Culp, D., Ambriosi, D., Berninger, T., & Mitchell, J. (1986). Augmentative communication aid use–A follow-up study. *Augmentative and Alternative Communication, 2*, 19–24.

Dore, J. (1978). Requestive systems in nursery school conversations: Analysis of talk in its social context. In R. Campbell & P. Smith (Eds.), *Recent advances in the psychology of language: Language development and mother-child interaction* (pp. 271–292). New York, NY: Plenum Press.

Dunn, L., & Dunn, L. (1981). *Peabody Picture Vocabulary Test—Revised*. Circle Pines MN: American Guidance Service.

Elder, P. (1987). Assessment for semantic compaction competency. *Proceedings of the third annual Minspeak conference*. Wooster, OH: Prentke Romich Company.

Elder, P., & Goossens, C. (1994). *Engineering training environments for interactive augmentative communication*. Birmingham: Southeast Augmentative Communication Conference Publications Clinician Series.

Fell, A., Lynn, E., & Morrison, K. (1984). *Non-oral communication assessment*. Ann Arbor, MI: Alternatives to Speech.

Gardner, M. (1990). *Expressive one word picture vocabulary test-revised.* Novato, CA: Academic Therapy Publications.

Gardner, M. (1985). *Receptive One Word Picture Vocabulary Test–Revised.* Novato, CA: Academic Therapy Publications.

Garrett, R., Andrews, P., Olsson, C., & Seeger, B. (1990). Development of a computer-based expert system for the selection of assistive communication devices. *Proceedings of the RESNA 13th Annual Conference.* Washington DC: RESNA Press.

Glennen, S. (1989). *The effect of communication aid characteristics on the interaction skills of nonspeaking persons and their adult speaking partners.* Unpublished doctoral dissertation, Pennsylvania State University, State College.

Glennen, S. (1992). Augmentative and alternative communication. In G. Church & S. Glennen, *The handbook of assistive technology* (pp. 93–122). San Diego, CA: Singular Publishing Group.

Glennen, S., & Delsandro, E. (1994). *AAC activity analysis.* Unpublished manuscript, The Kennedy Krieger Institute, Baltimore, MD.

Goosens, C. (1989). Aided communication before assessment: A case study of a child with cerebral palsy. *Augmentative and Alternative Communication, 5,* 14–26.

Goosens, C., & Crain, S. (1985). *Augmentative communication assessment resource.* Wauconda, IL: Don Johnston Developmental Equipment Inc.

Hodson, B. W., & Paden, E. (1983) *Targeting intelligible speech* (2nd ed.). San Diego: College-Hill Press.

Huer, M. (1983). *The nonspeech test.* Wauconda, IL: Don Johnston Developmental Equipment Inc.

Jinks, A., & Sinteff, B. (1994). Consumer response to AAC devices: Acquisition, training, use and satisfaction. *Augmentative and Alternative Communication, 10,* 184–189.

Kangas, K., & Lloyd, L. (1988). Early cognitive skills as prerequisites to AAC use: What are we waiting for? *Augmentative and Alternative Communication, 3,* 211–221.

Kent, R. D., Miolo, G., & Bloedel, S. (1994). The intelligibility of children's speech: A review of evaluation procedures. *American Journal of Speech Language Pathology, 3,* 81–95.

Light, J., Beesley, M., & Collier, B. (1988). Transition through multiple augmentative and alternative communication systems: A three year case study of a head injured adolescent. *Augmentative and Alternative Communication, 4,* 2–14.

Light, J., Collier, B., & Parnes, P. (1985). Communicative interactions between young nonspeaking physically disabled children and their primary caregivers: Part I, discourse patterns. *Augmentative and Alternative Communication, 1,* 74–83.

Mann, P., & Suiter, P. (1974). *Handbook in diagnostic teaching.* Boston, MA: Allyn & Bacon.

Markwardt, F. C. (1989). *Peabody Individual Achievement Test–Revised.* Circle Pines, MN: AGS.

Monsen, R. B. (1981). A usable test for the speech intelligibility of deaf talkers. *American Annals of the Deaf, 126,* 845–852.

Monsen, R. B., Moog, J. S., & Geers, A. E. (1988). *CID Picture SPINE.* St Louis: Central Institute for the Deaf.

Montgomery, J. (1980). *Non oral communication.* Fountain Valley, CA: California State Department of Education.

Osberger, M. J. (1992). Speech intelligibility in the hearing impaired: Research and clinical implications. In R. D. Kent (Ed.), *Speech intelligibility in speech disorders: Theory, measurement, and management* (pp. 233–264). Amsterdam: John Benjamins.

Ratcliff, A. (1994). Comparison of relative demands implicated in direct selection and scanning: Considerations from normal children. *Augmentative and Alternative Communication, 10,* 67–74.

Reichle, J., & Karlan, G. (1985). Decision rules for the adoption of augmentative techniques. In R. L. Schiefulbusch & L. Lloyd (Eds), *Language perspectives II* (pp. 321–339). Austin TX: Pro-Ed.

Reid, D. K., Hresko, W. P., & Hammill, D. D. (1981). *Test of Early Reading Ability—2.* Austin TX: Pro-Ed.

Romski, M. A., & Ruder, K. (1984). Effects of speech and speech + sign instruction in oral language learning and generalization of action + object combinations by Down's syndrome children. *Journal of Speech and Hearing Disorders, 49,* 293–302.

Romski, M. A., Sevcik, R., & Pate, J. (1988). The establishment of symbolic communication in persons with severe mental retardation. *Journal of Speech and Hearing Disorders, 53,* 97–107.

Shane, H. (1980). Approaches to assessing the communication of nonspeaking persons. In R. L. Schiefulbusch (Ed.), *Nonspeech language and communication: Analysis and intervention* (pp. 197–224). Baltimore, MD: University Park Press.

Shane, H., & Bashir, A. (1980). Election criteria for the adoption of an augmentative communication system: Preliminary considerations. *Journal of Speech and Hearing Disorders, 45*, 408–414.

Silverman, F. (1980). *Communication for the speechless.* Engelwood Cliffs, NJ: Prentice-Hall.

Sloand-Armstrong, J., & Jones, K. (1994). Assistive technology and young children: Getting off to a great start. *Closing the Gap, 13,* 31–32.

Swengel, K., & Varga, T. (1993). *Assistive technology assessment: The feature match process.* Paper presented at Closing the Gap Conference, Minneapolis, MN.

Webb, J. C., & Duckett, B. (1990). *The RULES phonological evaluation.* Vero Beach, FL: The Speech Bin.

Weiss, C. E. (1982). *Weiss Intelligibility Test.* Tigard, OR: CC Publications.

Weller, E., & Mahoney, G. (1983). A comparison of oral and total communication modalities on the language training of young mentally handicapped children. *Mental Retardation, 21*, 123–132.

Wiig, E., Secord, W., & Semel, E. (1992). Clinical evaluation of language functions —preschool. San Antonio, TX: The Psychological Corporation.

Wiig, E., & Semel, E. (1995). *Clinical Evaluations of Language Function—3.* San Antonio, TX: The Psychological Corporation.

Wilcox, K. A., Schooling, T. L., & Morris, S. R. (1991). *The Preschool Speech Intelligibility Measure (P-SIM).* Paper presented at the Annual Convention of the American Speech-Language-Hearing Association, Atlanta, GA.

Woodcock, R., & Bonner-Johnson, M. (1989). *Woodcock Johnson Tests of Cognitive Ability.* Allen, TX: DLM Teaching Resources.

Yorkston, K., & Beukelman, D. R. (1981). Communication efficiency of dysarthric speakers as measured by sentence intelligibility and speaking rate. *Journal of Speech and Hearing Disorders, 46*, 296–301.

Yorkston, K., & Karlan, G., (1986). Assessment procedures. In S. Blackstone (Ed.), *Augmentative communication: An introduction* (pp. 163–196). Rockville, MD: ASHA.

Zimmerman, I., Steiner, V., & Evatt-Pond, R. (1991). *The Preschool Language Scale III.* San Antonio, TX: The Psychological Corporation.

Chapter 6

AUGMENTATIVE AND ALTERNATIVE COMMUNICATION ASSESSMENT STRATEGIES: SEATING AND POSITIONING

Ulrika Radell

Augmentative and alternative communication (AAC) assessment is a complex process that involves communicative, cognitive, linguistic, sensory, and motor components. The preceding chapter provided a framework to evaluate the communicative, cognitive, and linguistic components of the AAC evaluation process. For many individuals the evaluation of those components is only one part of AAC assessment. Children and adults with physical disabilities require further assessment of their motor skills by physical and occupational therapists who have experience evaluating individuals with neuromotor disabilities. These team members are an integral part of the AAC assessment process. Their role in evaluating motor abilities will be the focus of this chapter and Chapter 7.

Individuals with physical disabilities often use their AAC devices while seated. Those who are able to walk, either independently or with assistance, often cannot coordinate using an aided communication device while simultaneously maintaining their balance. They typically need to sit down in a chair or on the floor in order to access their systems. Individuals with more severe physical difficulties may use a wheelchair or other seating and positioning system for all or part of their day. Seating and positioning directly affects the ability to successfully use an AAC device. A poorly designed seating system can negatively affect the ability to motorically access an AAC system, the ability to use the AAC system without fatigue, the ability to see symbols and text on the AAC device, or a combination of motor and sensory difficulties. It is important that seating and positioning be addressed before proceeding with the motor accessing component of an AAC evaluation. This chapter will provide the reader with basics for improved seating and positioning in wheelchairs or other seating systems. Chapter 7 reviews methods of evaluating AAC motor access strategies and visual skills.

SEATING:
THE PHYSICAL BASE

With our bodies we experience and learn, we communicate and act. Body language is often a reflection of a person's state of mind. For people dependent on wheelchairs, the wheelchair can be thought of as a body orthosis, or brace, that creates the physical base for an ever-changing, ever-growing person. The wheelchair is a very important base. Seating position not only impacts upon physical well-being but also makes optimal motor function possible and thus affords greater opportunities for success in daily activities, including communicating with others.

One of the most challenging tasks for professionals has been to find a functional sitting position that enhances function and postural control while simultaneously decreasing spasticity or involuntary movements (Steen, Radell, Lanshammar, & Fristedt, 1991). The goal is to develop safe and aesthetically acceptable solutions that maximize function and keep costs at a reasonable level. Due to financial constraints, many individuals can get only one chair, which needs to function in a variety of situations: during transport, while watching television, when working at a desk, when driving a power chair, while playing games, and during other activities. Considering these many and varied uses, it is clear that there is a need for chairs that allow for changes in positioning.

The need to change position throughout the day needs to be planned into any seating system. For example, you will probably change positions a number of times while reading this chapter. It is normal and a necessity, as it is hard work to sit absolutely still! After sitting for a period of time, certain muscle groups increase their static muscle activity, which in turn causes fatigue. Subconsciously, a person either stands up or tries to increase body stability. According to Engstrom (1993), the three most commonly used methods to try to stabilize the upper body are crossing the legs, crossing the arms across the chest, and sliding down on the seat. It is important to remember that these stabilizing compensations are natural.

Wheelchair users also need to have some freedom of movement in their chairs to make similar compensations in positioning. It is quite common that this natural need is forgotten when it comes to children or adults with physical disabilities. They are often restrained; their only choice of movement is to press against the back or neck support, or "stand up" by extending in their chairs. Therapists often look at the tendency to push back as an abnormal pattern and attach additional restraints, which further restricts movement in the chair. This practice is well meaning but is founded on the assumption that the extension pattern is a primary problem, not a compensation for a need to change position. This does not mean that the extension pattern is something to encourage, but it is important to have knowledge of what is normal and how spasticity and other problems are affected by the sitting position itself. With this knowledge, changes in position can be made that are appropriate for the individual's situation.

NEUROMOTOR SYMPTOMS

Many individuals who use AAC systems or other assistive technologies will have a variety of neurological and physical disabilities. Many display neurological and motor symptoms such as changes in muscle tone, balance, or coordination that are common in disorders of the brain. These symptoms will be reviewed in this section.

Muscle Tone Changes

Muscle tone changes involve increased tone, which is commonly seen in the extremities, and low muscle tone in the trunk. Too much muscle tone makes voluntary movements of the extremities difficult to produce. Hands may be fisted, thus making it difficult to hit a key on a keyboard. There are different kinds of high muscle tone, one example being spasticity, which is an increase of muscle tone in certain movement patterns such as flexion of the arms and hands and extension of the legs (see Figure 6–1). Another example of high muscle tone is rigidity, where muscle groups

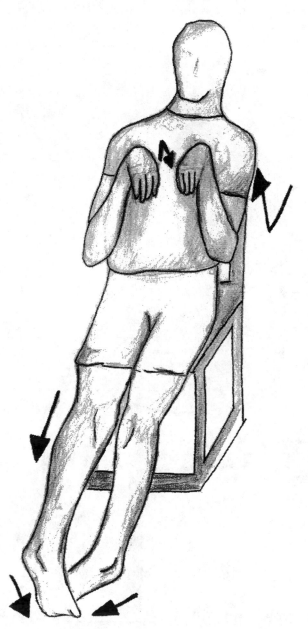

Figure. 6–1. Spasticity is a form of high muscle tone that leads to a tendency for flexion of the arms and extension and scissoring of the legs.

on both sides of a joint are activated simultaneously, creating a stiff, extended limb. Problems related to low muscle tone are inadequate postural control, inadequate static balance, and difficulty applying force (see Figure 6–2). Many persons with neurological impairments display a mixture of low and high muscle tone, with low tone in the trunk and high tone in the extremities.

Impaired Balance

Learning to balance is a complex process. A simplified description of the development of balance includes developing the ability to right the body, maintaining equilibrium, and using protective saving reactions. These concepts can be illustrated by thinking of a baby who is learning to sit. In order for the baby to learn how to sit he

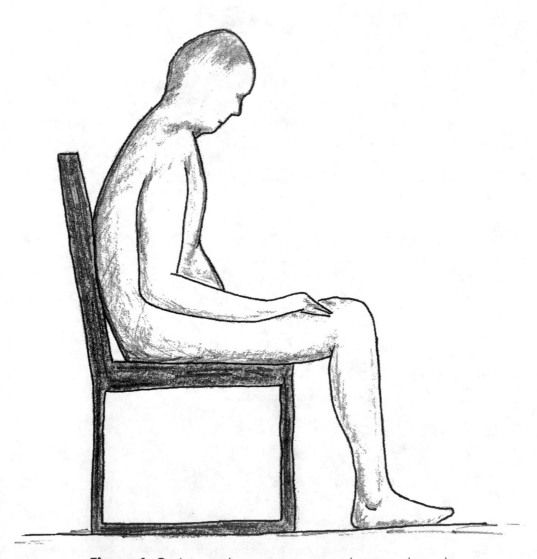

Figure 6–2. Low muscle tone is most commonly seen in the trunk.

or she needs to be able to lift the upper body against gravity into a vertical position. This ability to raise the trunk against gravity is accomplished by using the righting reaction. However, the fact that a baby can bring the trunk up to a seated position is not by itself sufficient for independent sitting. When reaching for a toy, the center of gravity will move to the side of the reaching arm (see Figure 6–3). In order not to fall, the baby needs to counteract the lifting up and extension of the arm by activating muscles on the opposite side of the body. This is an equilibrium reaction.

The equilibrium reaction can be elicited by an internal force, such as reaching with the arm, and in this case, the reaction naturally precedes the reaching action. The equilibrium reaction can also be elicited by an external force such as somebody gently pushing the baby to one side. In this instance, the equilibrium reaction occurs after the external force is applied. The equilibrium reaction counteracts the push and the child will remain upright. Most children develop equilibrium reactions in a specific order. First they learn to counteract falling forward, then they learn to counteract falling to the side, and finally they can counteract falling backward.

Protective saving reactions are similar to equilibrium reactions, but they function on a higher level where one needs to maintain balance during acceleration or quick changes in position. An example of this is the ability to remain seated when pulled on a bouncing sled. Vision and vestibular organs are other components of the balance system.

Primitive Reflexes

Newborn, full-term babies all display many different neonatal reflexes. Examples of these are the sucking reflex, grasping reflex, automatic stepping reaction, and asymmetric tonic neck reflex. These reflexes normally disappear at different times during infancy. Reflexes that are persistent and easily produced after specific developmental ages are a sign of neurological disability. One can commonly see these

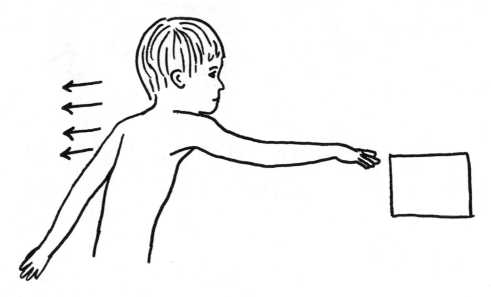

Figure 6–3. A change in the location of the body's center of gravity, such as when reaching, is counteracted by an equilibrium reaction.

reflexes in persons with neurological disorders of the brain. Children with spastic cerebral palsy (CP) often display the asymmetric tonic neck reflex (ATNR). It is a response to passive or active turning of the head. When the head turns to the side, the arm and leg on the side to which the face is turned increase in extensor tone while the opposite side increases in flexor tone (see Figure 6–4). This response is normal in babies between 2 and 5 months of age. The ATNR reflex pattern is pathologic when it is persistent and is easily elicited in children over 6 months of age. The symmetric tonic neck reflex (STNR) is a response to flexion (i.e., bending) or extension of the neck. Extension of the neck results in the arms extending outward and in flexion of

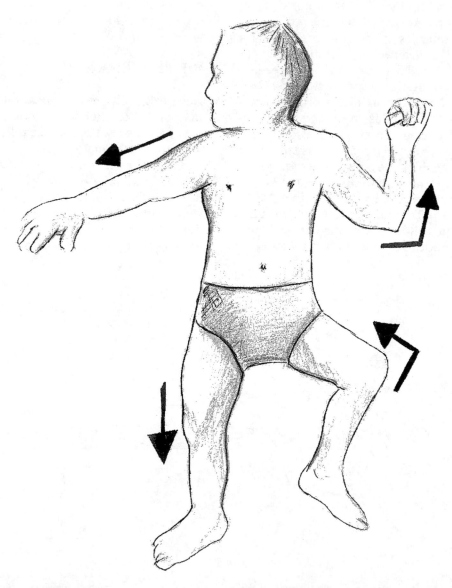

Figure 6–4. The asymmetric tonic neck reflex (ATNR), with head turning to the right, the right arm and leg increase extensor tone and the left extremities increase flexor tone.

the hips. Flexion of the neck results in flexion of the arms and extension of the hips.

Deformities

Deformities can have many causes, among them the tendency to adopt habitual postures of one part of the body. They result in an inability to move a joint through its full range of motion. Different joints have different structures and therefore allow different movements. For example, the elbow joint can only move in flexion and extension, whereas the shoulder joint also can rotate and move in and out to the side. A deformity may partially or totally limit movement in a specific direction. Asymmetry results in deformities and unequal distribution of muscle tone. Deformities of all sorts need to be prevented as the body often tries to compensate for deformity by changing its alignment in adjacent parts of the body, thus creating a risk of further deformities.

A commonly observed example of physical deformity is the Windblown Hip Syndrome (Letts, Shapiro, Mulder, & Klassen, 1984). This deformity includes the triad of hip dislocation, pelvic obliquity, and scoliosis (see Figure 6–5). With spasticity of the legs there is a risk of shortening the muscles on the anterior side of the hip, which results in the hip coming out of its joint (i.e.,

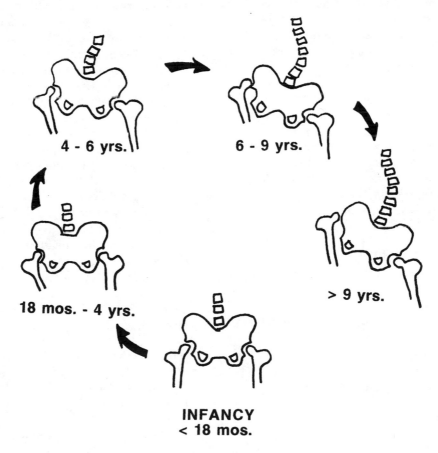

Figure 6–5. The genesis of the windblown hip syndrome starting with dislocation of the hip, followed by pelvic obliquity and finally scoliosis. *Note:* From "The Windblown Hip Syndrome in Total Body Cerebral Palsy," by K. Letts, L. Shapiro, D. Mulder, & O. Klassen, 1984, *Journal of Pediatrics Orthopedica, 4*, p. 57. Copyright 1984 by Lippincott-Raven Publishers. Reprinted with permission.

a dislocation). The hip has a higher position on the side of the dislocation which in turn leads to the pelvis tilting (i.e., obliquity) with a high pelvic position on the same side as the hip dislocation. The body naturally strives to maintain the eyes in the horizontal position and it compensates for the obliquity at the hip by bending the spine in the opposite direction in order to reach an upright position of the head. This leads to scoliosis of the spine, which means that the spine is curved in the frontal plane.

Dyscoordination

Lesions in the basal ganglia of the brain can cause movement disorders such as Athetosis and Dystonia. Movement disorders are characterized by an impairment of postural fixation of the trunk and by the presence of involuntary movements during muscle activation. These involuntary movements occur mostly in the face and limbs. They are usually not present at rest, but become exaggerated when trying to perform a task. Despite the sometimes unusual distorted postures produced when trying to attend to a task, people with movement disorders can often become proficient in using their head or arms for accessing assistive technology.

OPTIMAL SEATING AND POSITIONING: RESEARCH REVIEW

In a functional sitting position, we strive for:

• Stability
• Mobility
• Head, trunk, and foot control
• Arm and hand function
• Comfort.

A greater understanding of these issues can be drawn from basic sciences such as anatomy, neurophysiology, orthopedics, biomechanics, ergonomics, and kinesiolo-

gy. Because motivation is a crucial element in the ability to function, important information can also be gained from psychology and from the study of motor control and motor learning. This section of the chapter will review information from these disciplines as they relate to the development of a functional sitting position.

Balance: Vision and Head Control

The body always strives to maintain the eyes in a horizontal position. The eyes are an important part of the control mechanism for maintaining balance because they provide information about body position in space. If we move or lose balance, the eyes automatically send signals that initiate a response from muscle groups in order to maintain or regain balance. The head and neck influence the distribution of muscle tone (i.e., muscle activity) through- out the body, and therefore have a strong influence on posture and movement. An abnormal position of the head in space or lack of head control adversely influences posture and movement of the rest of body. In order to use vision effectively, an individual must learn to hold his or her head steady in space in the midposition in relation to the shoulders. When seated, head and neck control are necessary to initiate normal, purposeful movement (Galley & Forster, 1982).

Preferred Working Sitting Positions

While investigating a working position for nonimpaired clients, Mandal (1984) gave school children the opportunity to choose their preferred sitting positions. The preferred seat was capable of sloping forward 10 to 15 degrees with the forward-sliding tendency counteracted by a small fixed cushion at the front edge of the seat. The preferred table top sloped 10 to 15 degrees and the child's visual focus distance was best at about 30 centimeters (12 inches). Mandal also concluded that chair seat height should be at least one-third the person's height, and table height at least one-half the person's height. In contrast, Mandal showed that a backward sloping seat increased flexion (forward bending) of the lumbar region (lower back; see Figure 6–6a), and that a chair low to the ground did the same (see Figure 6–6b).

Flexion of the lumbar region often causes problems such as compression, fatigue of muscles, and stretching of ligaments of the spine, all resulting in pain. Raising the table decreased flexion of the lumbar region (see Figure 6–6c). When individuals are seated with their thighs horizontal, the hip joint flexes about 60 degrees and the lumbar back about 30 to 35 degrees. This "correct" position in reality creates about 35 degrees of lumbar flexion with strain on the joints, tendons, and muscles of the lumbar back. Mandal showed that with 60 degrees of hip flexion but on a seat elevated about 20 centimeters (7.8 inches), one can sit upright with a vertical pelvis (i.e., neither forward nor backward tilted) without bending the lumbar back. Traditionally, it was recommended that all individuals, both nonimpaired and those with disabilities, use a sitting position with 90 degrees of hip and knee flexion, with a straight back and erect head (see Figure 6–7). Subsequent research has found that it is impossible to maintain this posture while working, and this position is considered unrealistic for long periods of sustained sitting (Mandal, 1984; Pope, Bowes, & Booth, 1994).

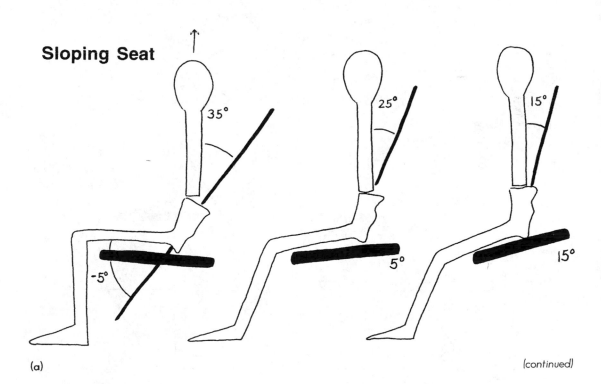

(a)

(continued)

Figure 6–6. (a) Flexion of the lumbar spine can be decreased by changing the seat inclination from a backward sloping seat to a forward sloping seat and also by **(b)** increasing the height of the seat or **(c)** the height of the table. *Note:* From "The Correct Height of School Furniture," by A. C. Mandal, 1984, *Physiotherapy, 70,* p. 50-51. Copyright 1984 by the Physiotherapy Journal. Reprinted with permission.

Figure 6–6. *(continued)*

Low Chair

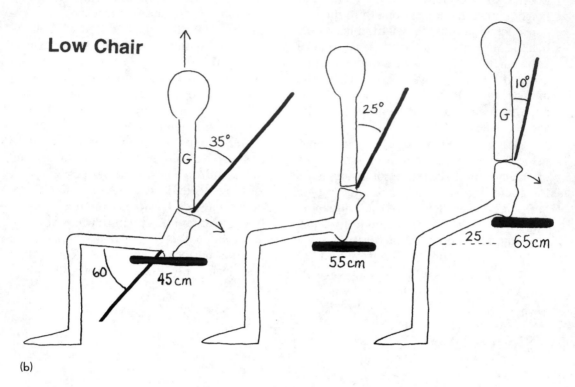

(b)

Low Table

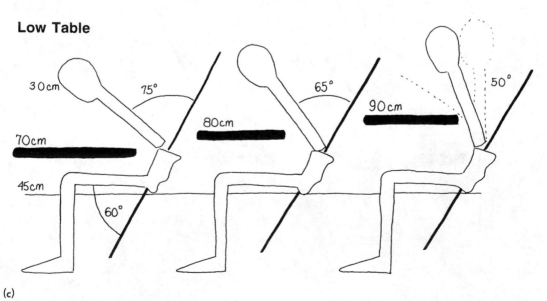

(c)

202

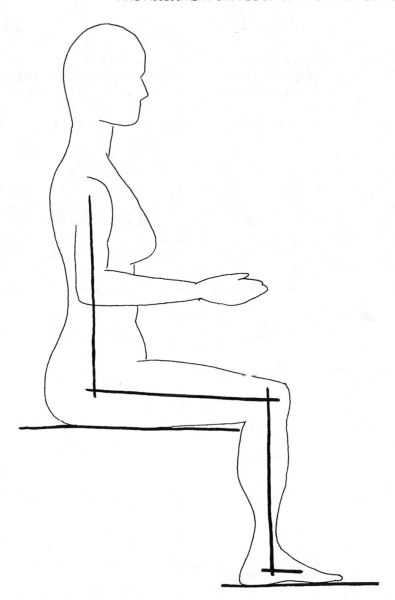

Figure 6–7. Traditional schematic model representing "correct posture" in reality creates about 35 degrees of lumbar flexion with strain on the joints, tendons, and muscles of the lumbar back.

Factors That Decrease Spasticity and Improve Postural Control

In recent years, studies have focused on the body position in relation to gravity. Nwaobi, Brubacker, Cosich, and Sussman (1983) and Nwaobi (1986) showed that with the same joint positions (e.g., 90 degrees of hip and knee flexion), but with a different postural tilt in space (either tilted forward, seated upright, or tilted backward), muscle activity in the spastic muscles changed in response to body orientation in space. These studies found that muscle activity was least when children with cerebral palsy sat in an upright position when compared with the reclined position. Reid, Sochaniwskyu, and Milner (1991) investigated the effects of flat and forward inclined seats on postural sway at the level of the seventh cervical vertebrae in children with CP, groups of children without impairments, and children with head injuries. In comparing the effects of seat base positions on sway, no difference was evident for any group. However, qualitative analysis indicated that in 50% of the children with CP, a seat inclined slightly forward, from planar (flat) up to 10 degrees, reduced postural sway. This group of children was able to obtain a more upright position. Of interest was that these children were those clinically identified to have tight hamstring muscles, generalized low tone, and trunk hypotonia. The other children with CP in the study displayed an increased sway but improvement in spinal posture on the inclined seat.

In a series of articles, Myhr and von Wendt (1990, 1991, 1993) and Myhr, von Wendt, Norrlin, and Radell (1995) identified factors that decreased spasticity and enhanced postural control during sitting in children with CP. They studied sitting function by placing children in several sitting positions, with variable seat and backrest inclinations. They found that spasticity lessened and postural control improved when children were placed into a forward leaning position (see Figure 6–8a). A forward leaning position could be reached both from a horizontal and a forward inclined seat and it should be emphasized that it was not the seat incination itself that

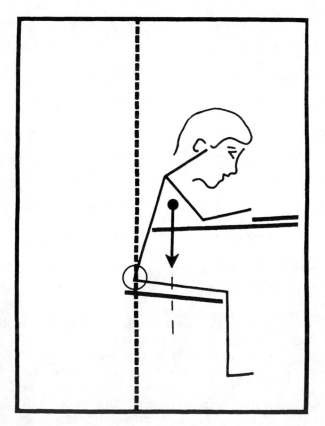

(a)

Figure 6-8 (a), (b), and (c). Spasticity was least and postural control best in a forward-leaning position. Spasticity increased and postural control decreased as the center of gravity moved behind the hip joint. *Note:* From "Reducing Spasticity and Enhancing Postural Control for the Creation of a Functional Sitting Position in Children with Cerebral Palsy: A Pilot Study," by U. Myhr and L. vonWendt, 1990, *Physiotherapy Theory and Practice,* 6, pp. 70–71. Copyright 1990 by Erlbaum Taylor & Francis. Reprinted with permission.

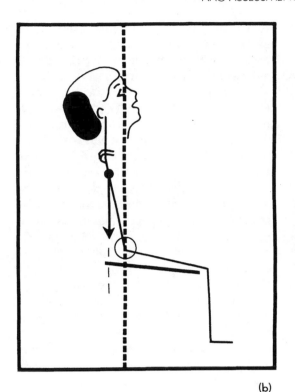

(b)

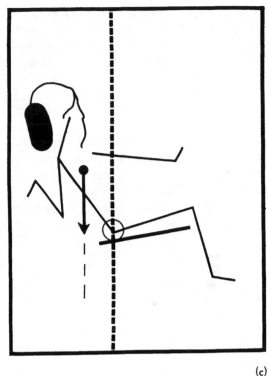

(c)

was of most importance, but the upper body's anterior location in relation to the hip joint. Spasticity increased and postural control decreased when the center of gravity moved behind the hip joint (see Figures 6–8b and 6–8c). Based upon this information, Myhr and von Wendt designed a so-called functional sitting position, which was described as a position with the pelvis stabilized in a neutral or forward-leaning symmetric position, with abducted legs (i.e., moved apart), and with the line of gravity for the upper body anterior to the fulcrum at the ischial tuberosities (i.e., sitting bones at the base of the pelvis). This required using foot plates on the chair that were parallel to the floor without hindering straps at the back, fixating the pelvis in place with a hip belt, providing a stable base (the chair seat), and using an abduction orthosis (i.e., dynamic leg divider).

Myhr and von Wendt's evaluation methods included using the Sitting Assess-

ment Scale for analysis of head, trunk, and foot control and arm/hand function; photographs to analyze the position of different body segments in relation to movement axes; and surface electromyography (EMG) to measure leg muscle activity. Their results showed that the total median score according to the Sitting Assessment Scale improved significantly in the functional sitting position previously described, when compared to the child's original sitting position. Muscle activity in the legs, measured by EMG was significantly lower in the functional sitting position. Muscle tone was noted to be highest in reclined positions and in flat positions with a vertical back rest, without the abduction orthosis. When EMG responses and reactionsto various seating positions were compared to individuals without disabilities, they found that the patterns were essentially similar.

The conclusion that the reclined position caused increased activity in muscles that create the spastic pattern, in both the group with impairments and the group without impairments, led to the question of whether it was the sitting position itself and not the impairment that triggered the spastic movement pattern of the legs. Among 10 children with cerebral palsy who were followed up 5 years after first being introduced to the functional sitting position, 8 children who still sat according to the principles of the functional sitting position had slight but significant improvement of their motor control, whereas the other 2 who were seated differently had deteriorated (Myhr et al., 1995).

Hirschfeld (1992) showed that the ability to make postural adjustments during sitting seems to develop prior to the development of sitting stability. Motor commands are calibrated on the basis of experience and lead to improvement over time (Ghez, 1991). Skilled motor performance is therefore highly dependent on learning. This leads to the understanding that, even if an individual cannot sit independently, professionals need to create regular opportunities for practicing postural control in sitting. Children with neurological impairments often lack the ability to achieve a normal balanced seated position. This results in the lack of a reference point for what is normal, which in turn makes it difficult to know what position to strive for when making postural adjustments. Providing children with opportunities to experience more normal sitting positions can result in improved head control and arm and hand function (Steen, Radell, Lanshammar, & Fristedt, 1991).

Hirschfeld (1992) found that the somatosensory signals derived from the rotation of the pelvis play a main role in triggering postural adjustments. Responses were more easily triggered when falling backward than forward since loss of stability is more immediate when moving backward. Reese, Msall, diAmato, Pictor, and Gillespie (1990) studied the correlation be-

tween the presence of a persistent ATNR and dislocated hips. They concluded that a neurological examination and primitive reflex profile correctly predicted the side of dislocation in 78 percent of the cases studied. Myhr and von Wendt (1990) saw that the presence of ATNR in the reclined position could be eliminated when seated in a position with the center of gravity above the sitting bones (see Figures 6–9a and 6–9b). As the presence of ATNR is common in individuals with CP, it is crucial to realize the importance of trying to eliminate its occurrence. Eliminating the ATNR reflex greatly reduces the risk for hip subluxation (i.e., dislocation) and thus reduces the need for expensive and painful hip surgeries.

All of these studies indicate that many of the problems individuals with physical disabilities encounter can often be attributed to the sitting position itself. Placing an individual in a chair where he or she has to work against the effects of gravity makes it difficult for to gain a balanced work position. Problems such as spasticity and primitive reflexes are also exacerbated. The rationale behind existing seating recommendations has often been lacking (Myhr 1994), and neurophysiological approaches to treatment are often founded on assumptions that recently have been questioned and modified (Bower & McLellan, 1992). It is important to incorporate new concepts of motor control when developing seating assessment instruments (Fife et al., 1991) and to always observe the uniqueness of the individual when trying to find the best possible solution to seating problems.

THE FUNCTIONAL SITTING POSITION

Throughout this chapter it will be evident that what is strived for is a sitting position that to a great degree resembles the way individuals without disabilities sit when they perform different tasks. Able-bodied

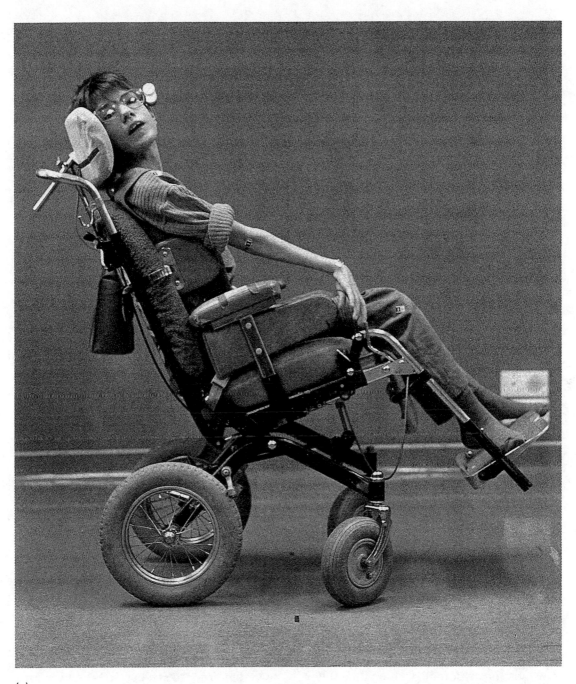

(a)

Figure 6–9. (a) Sitting in a reclined chair this girl elicits the asymmetric tonic neck reflex (ATNR) every time she turns her head. (b) The same girl in a functional sitting position with her center of gravity above her base of support. She is able to turn her head without eliciting the ATNR. *Note:* From "Improvement of Functional Sitting Position for Children with Cerebral Palsy," by U. Myhr and L. vonWendt, 1991, *Developmental Medicine and Child Neurology, 33,* p. 249. Copyright 1991 by Mac Keith Press.

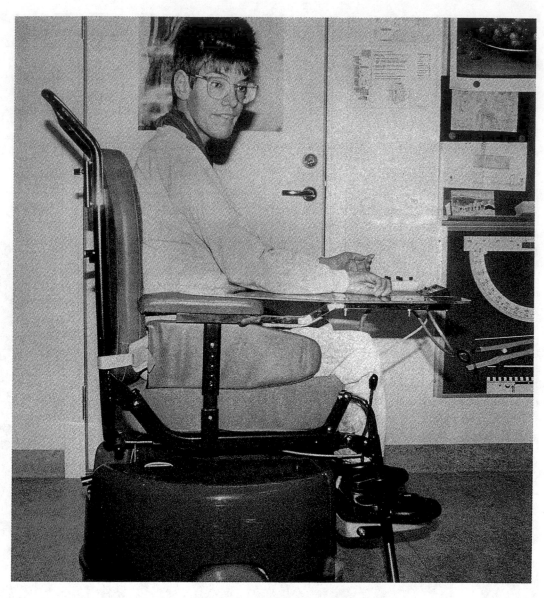

(b)

persons use different positions for different tasks. When relaxing in front of the television, a recliner is used for a reclined or curled up position. When driving a car and simultaneously using feet, arms, and eyes, drivers sit erect with a slightly reclined back support. If there is a big rainstorm drivers slow down and also lean forward in order to see better. When working at a table surface, most people lean forward with their trunk, as it improves eye-hand coordination. Feet are commonly placed under the chair. Most augmentative communication (AAC) device users need to be in an active, upright position to best access their devices. There will be times when they need to recline in order to relax, or be placed in therapeutic positions. In those positions they may need other methods of accessing their AAC systems.

The focus in this chapter is a functional sitting position, which is defined as a sitting position in which postural control is such that the child can obtain the maximum possible degree of independent function when performing arm and hand or other movements for purposeful tasks (Myhr & von Wendt, 1990, 1991). Individuals who use assistive technology may strive for the use of an AAC device or the ability to drive a power wheelchair. In some instances the individual may use the head or foot instead of arms and hands to access the technology. The reason for focusing on a functional sitting position rather than a resting position is that it is more natural to sit upright when using assistive technology. There is a great need for knowledge about functional sitting. Current research has provided insight on how to create a dynamic relaxed functional sitting position for people with severe physical handicaps. Use of a functional sitting position can enable children with severe physical disabilities to increase motor control and function over time. This contradicts earlier beliefs that after reaching a plateau in motor control, deterioration in an individual's physical status was to be expected over time.

Basic Functional Sitting Position Concepts

There are three concepts that need to be understood before positioning an individual: (1) equilibrium—how it is affected by gravity and by changes in location of the center of gravity; (2) balance—how forces affect one another to create stability; and (3) postural control—the difference between postural muscles versus voluntary muscle actions and the location of postural muscle groups.

Equilibrium and Balance

Gravity affects all physical bodies. All physical bodies have a center of mass which is pulled by gravity. The center of mass is also called the center of gravity and it is the place in the body where weight is located if drawn to one central point. In standing, the center of gravity falls anterior to the second lumbar vertebra. In sitting, the center of gravity varies depending on body size but normally falls in front of the ninth thoracic vertebra (see Figure 6–10).

The body is more stable when the center of gravity is low and the base of support for the body is wide. The base of support refers to the supporting area beneath the body. It includes the points of contact with the supporting surface and the area between them (Galley & Forster, 1982). Think, for example, of a beginner downhill skier. With knees bent, poles spread far apart and skis apart, the skier is creating a wide base of support with the center of gravity at a low point. After becoming more proficient, the skier stands up straighter, placing the skis together with the poles only slightly touching the snow close to the body. The base of support is smaller and the center of gravity is located higher up. Equilibrium is achieved when the forces that act upon the body balance one another so that the center of gravity falls within the base of support. If the skier's center of gravity falls outside the base of support, the forces pulling down on one side will cause him or her to lose equilibrium and fall. With proficiency, the skier has better control of the forces acting on the body and, therefore, can maintain equilibrium with a higher center of gravity and smaller base of support.

When building a tower of blocks, the center of gravity lies above the base of support in different ways (see Figure 6–11). Again, loss of equilibrium occurs when the center of gravity falls outside of the base of support. If the center of gravity falls outside of its supporting base, a force needs to counteract the tendency to fall in order to create balance. In the human, the force that creates balance is applied by muscle force or, in some cases, by an outside support such as a wall to lean against.

Postural Control

A baby learns to lift its head, crawl, sit, and stand by using postural muscles to extend the body against gravity. Postural muscles are also called antigravity muscles. They are located on the posterior side of the body, and include muscles in the back of the neck, a multitude of small muscles in the back, and some leg muscles. Postural muscles work in groups and different groups of muscles are activated depending on the position of the body. A baby evolves from flexion in the fetal position to extension in standing. Development is cranio-caudal, which means that it begins with the head and continues in a downward direction. Postural muscle tone has been described as "the state of continuous

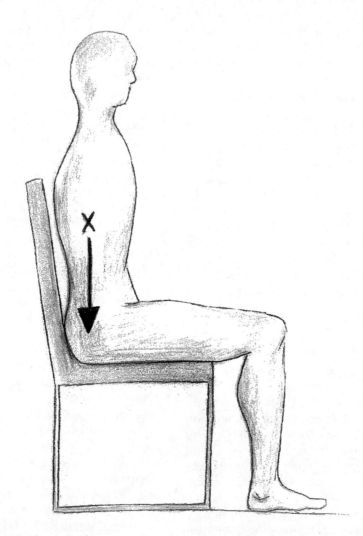

Figure 6–10. A person's center of gravity in the seated position falls in front of the ninth thoracic vertebra.

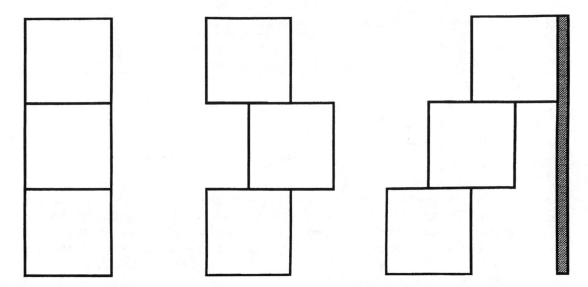

Figure 6–11. Three different ways of maintaining equilibrium in a tower of blocks.

muscles that is needed to overcome gravity and maintain posture" (Foley, 1977, p. 277). In other words, postural muscles are continuously active but their activity is regulated automatically and we do not have to think about it. Postural muscles differ from muscles used in voluntary movements of the extremities. Postural muscle tone creates the subconscious background to voluntary movement and tends to be unnoticed by the individual.

Included in the development of postural control are several skills. These include the ability to raise the body up against gravity, for example, a baby lifting his or her head. It also involves the ability to maintain equilibrium (e.g., maintaining a stable trunk while shifting weight to one side such as when reaching out with one arm). Finally, it requires development of the ability to counteract an altered balance (e.g., maintaining head and trunk control while someone pulls a rug out from under a person when they are sitting on it).

Recent studies indicate that postural responses from muscles are not innate, but instead emerge gradually with experience (Wollacott, 1993). For children who lack equilibrium reactions, such as some children with CP, external supports are used to create a stable trunk in sitting. By experiencing the seated position with the center of gravity in the correct location, the child gets a chance to develop a reference point to strive for when practicing unsupported sitting.

FINDING THE OPTIMAL FUNCTIONAL SITTING POSITION

An ideal functional sitting position includes a forward tilted secured pelvis, symmetric weight bearing, the upper body center of gravity above or in front of the ischial tuberosities, legs allowed to move backward, head control, arm and hand function, and trunk control (see Table 6–1 and Figure 6–12). The uniqueness of the individual must always be taken into account, and it may not be possible for all individuals to achieve this position. However, the principles for gaining postural

Table 6–1. Features of the functional sitting position.

- Symmetric weight bearing
- The upper body center of gravity is above or in front of the ischial tuberosities
- Stable trunk control
- Legs allowed freedom to move backwards
- Good head control
- Promotes arm and hand function

control and motor function must always be addressed. Therefore, the long-term seating goal for function needs to focus on the upright or forward leaning position.

The process of developing a functional sitting position can be divided into both stable and dynamic components. Stable seating components include the pelvis and thighs, which provide the base of support for functional activities. Dynamic seating components need to move and change depending on the activity. Dynamic components include the trunk, feet, head, arms, and hands. It must be emphasized that generalized guidelines cannot overshadow each individual's need to be assessed for his or her unique qualities. For example, depending on the type and severity of the disability, the trunk can sometimes be a stable component in sitting. This occurs more frequently in persons with severe movement disorders and less often in persons with neuromotor disabilities that are characterized by spasticity. The development of a functional sitting position across these seating components will be reviewed in the next section of the chapter.

The Stable Base of Support in Sitting

Pelvis

The upper and lower body rotate around the base created by the pelvis, together with the thighs. A change in pelvic position creates a change in the rest of the body. It is therefore of great importance to secure the pelvis in a good position and to start with the pelvis when creating a functional sitting position. An ideal seating position has the following components:

- Equal weight bearing on the ischial tuberosities (i.e., the sitting bones);
- Pelvis forward tilted or neutral;
- Stability by securing the pelvis to the chair with the pull of a hip belt in a posterior, inferior direction.

Equal weight bearing on the ischial tuberosities is sought to avoid the development of pelvic obliquity and scoliosis. If there already is a fixed pelvic obliquity, the seat needs to allow for it and maximize proper alignment to prevent further deterioration. The pelvic position creates the starting point for good alignment and control of the legs and feet, and also the upper body and head (see Figure 6–13). A forward tilted pelvis facilitates a straight back (see Figure 6–14). It also locks joints in the lumbar back that allow lateral (sideways) movements. Sitting stability is increased when sideways movement of the trunk is limited, but anterior and posterior movement is allowed. Some individuals with severe scoliosis and pelvic obliquity cannot get their pelvis aligned into a neutral position while simultaneously maintaining acceptable trunk and head alignment. In these cases it is better to focus on gaining a vertical head position and allowing the trunk and pelvis to be tilted and rotated (Carlson & Ramsey,

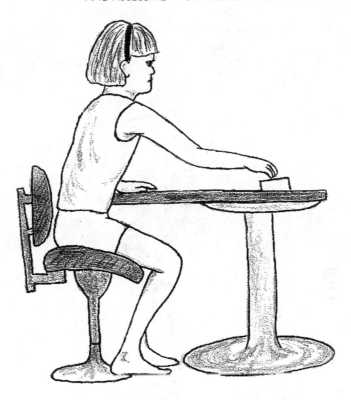

Figure 6–12. A functional sitting position.

1994). There are different options for securing the pelvis to the chair, for example, a belt can be placed in the pelvic-femoral angle and secured under the seat (see Figure 6–15). Pelvic straps are secured at midline at the posterior edge of the seat (see Figure 6–16). The straps are positioned under the crotch and loop around the thighs in the pelvic femoral angle. They fasten laterally onto the posterior edge of the seat. A sub-ASIS bar is another option for stabilization and is used to position individuals who have severe difficulty staying secured on the seat (see Figure 6–17).

The Optimal Seat

An optimal seat has the following features:

- A seat depth 1–2 inches shorter than the length of the individual's thigh.

- Horizontal or slightly forward tilted (up to 10 degrees) seat inclination.
- Comfort and avoidance of pressure sores and sliding on the seat.

If the seat depth is longer than the thighs, the individual compensates by sliding down on the sacrum with the pelvis tilted posteriorly in order to bend the knees. This shifts the location of the upper body so that it falls behind the preferred base of support. Instead of using postural muscle groups to hold the trunk up, stomach muscles must then work against gravity to move the body forward (see Figure 6–18). In contrast, a seat depth that is too short creates no changes in alignment but moves the location of the center of gravity forward. A seat depth that is too short decreases the base of support and therefore decreases the stable base for sitting. It can also create problems for persons sensitive to pressure areas. For them, it is important to have a large base of support in order to spread weightbearing on a large surface, thus creating less pressure per square inch.

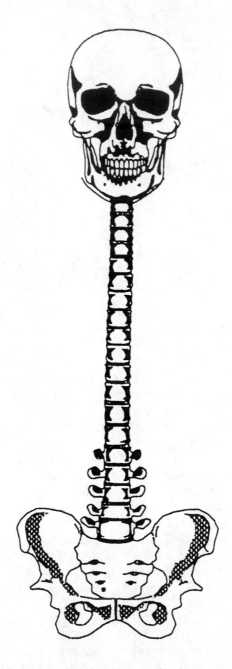

Figure 6–13. The spine balances the head, and the pelvis bears weight on the ischial tuberosities (i.e., sitting bones). *Note:* From *Ergonomics Wheelchairs and Positioning* (Figure 10), by B. Engstrom, 1993. Stockholm, Sweden: Bromma Tryck AB. Copyright 1993 by Bengt Engstrom. Reprinted with permission.

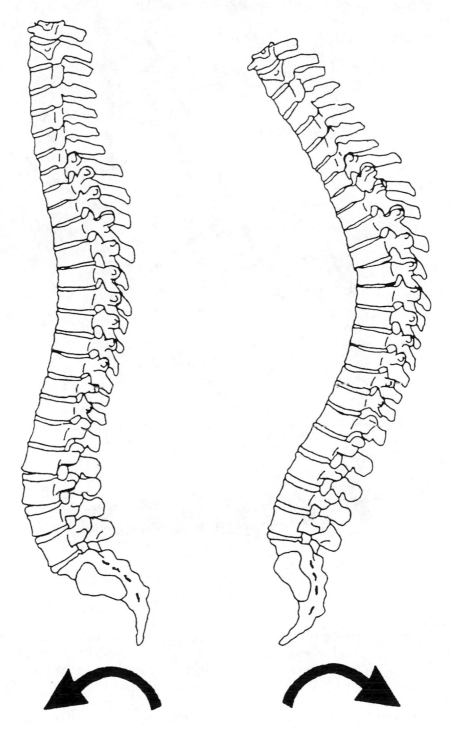

Figure 6–14. Tilting the pelvis results in changes of the shape of the spine. A forward tilted pelvis creates an erect spine whereas a backward tilted pelvis leads to rounding of the lumbar spine. *Note:* From *Ergonomics Wheelchairs and Positioning* (Figure 11), by B. Engstrom, 1993, Stockholm, Sweden: Bromma Tryck AB. Copyright 1993 by Bengt Engstrom. Reprinted with permission.

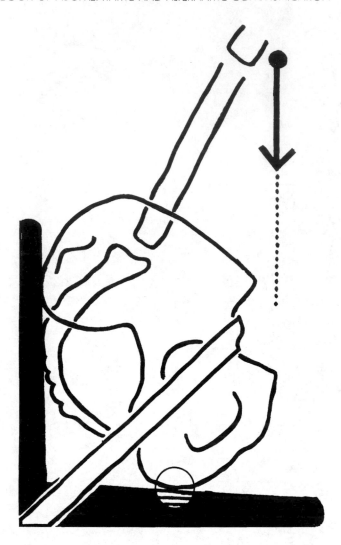

Figure 6–15. A forward tilted pelvis with weight bearing on the sitting bones and a hip belt with a posterior, inferior pull, secured in the pelvic femoral angle. *Note:* unpublished figure, by Ulla Myhr (1995). Reprinted with permission.

A forward leaning seat (up to 10 degrees) creates a greater forward pelvic tilt and makes it easier for the upper body to come forward (see Figure 6–19). However, it is important not to tilt the seat inclination too far forward. A seat inclination of 15 degrees or more can have adverse effects on balance. Increased muscle activity in the antigravity muscles was seen in children seated on a 15 degree tilted surface, when compared to a seat with a forward in-

cline of only 10 degrees. This suggests that, when the seat is inclined too far forward, the individual needs to exert conscious effort to maintain the upright posture.

On a flat planar seat, the weight of the thighs can also create a slightly forward tilted pelvis (see Figure 6–20). Hipguides can be used to prevent a sideways shift of the pelvis (see Figure 6–16). Custom molded seats are made from a mold of the client's body. They increase stability and decrease the tendency

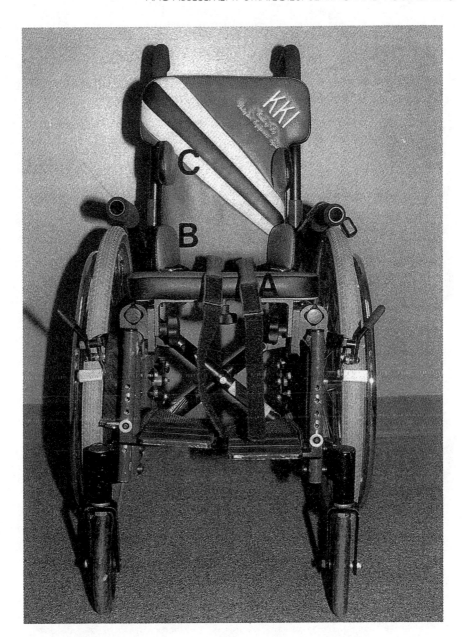

Figure 6–16. Seating insert components. **(A)** Pelvic straps for securing the pelvis; **(B)** hip guides for centering the pelvis; and **(C)** lateral trunk supports for maintaining the trunk at midline.

to slide forward if the seat is tilted forward (see Figure 6–21). In a custom molded seat, areas sensitive to pressure can be cut out and filled with gels or other materials which lessens the risk for pressure sores. A back-

ward tilted seat may be appropriate for a resting position but should be avoided in a functional sitting position. It increases the tendency to sit on the sacrum with decreased stability from side to side. The back

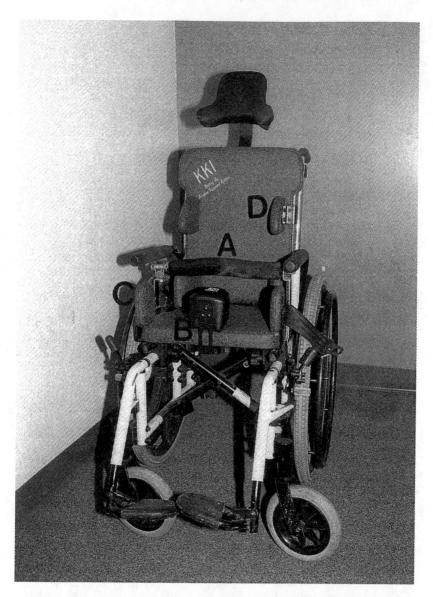

Figure 6–17. Seating insert components. **(A)** Sub-ASIS bar for securing the pelvis; **(B)** flip away solid abductor; **(C)** adductor supports; and **(D)** lateral trunk supports.

becomes kyphotic (rounded) and stomach muscles have to work to move the body forward (see Figure 6–22). When reclined, it becomes more difficult to maintain the center of gravity above the ischial tuberosities. The process of trying to come forward can be likened to doing a situp. It is fatiguing and

too much energy is spent trying to come forward instead of attending to tasks with the hands. One exception to this principle is the client with severe muscular dystrophy who, because of extreme muscular weakness, cannot maintain an upright sitting posture. Some individuals with extreme movement disorders are also exceptions because of their need to maximize postural support in order to use their hands.

Thighs on the Seat

The thighs, together with the sitting bones, create the base of support in sitting, over which the upper body's center of gravity balances. The preferred seating position includes having the thighs relaxed and spread apart. The base becomes broader and therefore increases stability if the legs are separated. For people with physical disabilities, spasticity of the legs is common and often manifests itself by a ten-

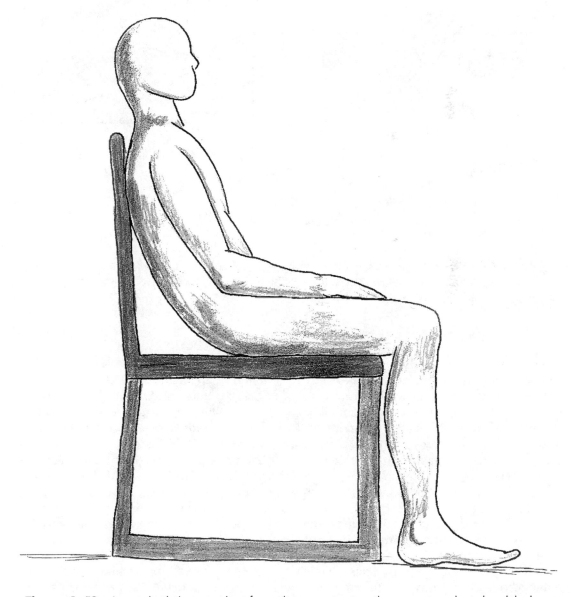

Figure 6–18. A seat depth that is too long forces the person to sit on the sacrum in order to bend the knees.

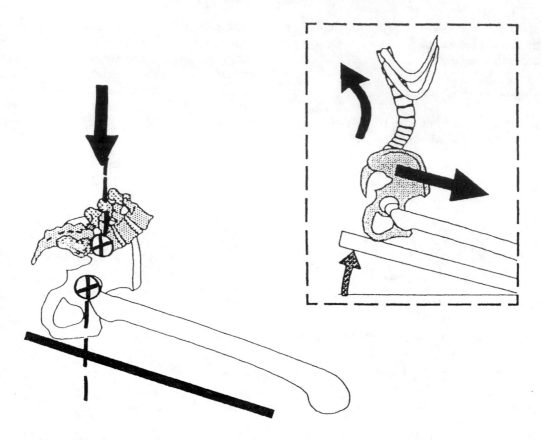

Figure 6–19. Anterior slope results in an anterior pelvis and spinal extension. *Note:* From *Ergonomics Wheelchairs and Positioning* (Figure 58), by B. Engstrom, 1993, Stockholm, Sweden: Bromma Tryck AB. Copyright 1993 by Bengt Engstrom. Reprinted with permission.

dency for scissoring of the legs. Scissoring occurs when the thighs adduct (move together) at the same time as they rotate internally. This movement pattern makes the base of support smaller and more unstable. The tendency toward scissoring has been called a spastic pattern. However, understanding of what spasticity actually is remains vague and a universal definition is lacking.

The tendency toward scissoring commonly occurs when showing excitement or emotion. It is also present when struggling to use arms and hands. Scissoring is a dangerous behavior if it occurs frequently. It can lead to subluxation of the hip,

which in turn can lead to luxation, pelvic obliquity, and scoliosis (Letts et al., 1984).

Myhr and von Wendt (1993) showed that individuals without disabilities activated the adductors and internal rotators of the thigh while seated in a restrained reclined position using their hands. The fact that these individuals had the same tendency for scissoring in the reclined position leads us to question if the reclined sitting position in itself evokes spasticity for those with neurological handicaps. The tendency for scissoring decreased for both persons with physical disabilities and those without disabilities when sitting upright or leaning forward.

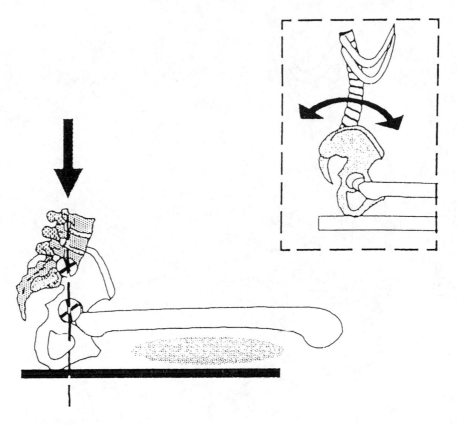

Figure 6–20. Horizontal seat results in a neutral pelvis. *Note:* From *Ergonomics Wheelchairs and Positioning* (Figure 59), by B. Engstrom, 1993, Stockholm, Sweden: Bromma Tryck AB. Copyright 1993 by Bengt Engstrom. Reprinted with permission.

In order to decrease scissoring, it is desirable to create an upright sitting position with the upper body's center of gravity above or in front of the ischial tuberosities, and to use abductors to separate the legs. Abductors can be either solid or dynamic. The most commonly used ones are well padded, solid wedge pieces that are located between the knees, up about one-third of the thigh. They are wider at the base by the knees. They can be placed on a swing-away mount to facilitate easy transfers in and out of the chair (see Figure 6–17). An abduction orthosis is a dynamic device that slightly rotates the thighs externally at the same time as it separates the legs. The coiled spring allows for moving the legs together and aids in separating the legs when relaxing (see Figure 6–23). One advantage of this is that it creates rotation and long-term stretch to adductor muscles, which is key to decreasing spasticity (Odeen 1981). Another advantage is that it helps greatly to create a symmetrical base in sitting. The Miller Swing Away Dynamic Abductor is an oval-shaped leg divider that also consists of a dynamic material that allows the unwanted pressing of legs together, yet assists in returning the legs to the desired position (see Figure 6–24).

Dynamic abduction devices allow movement of the legs but return the legs to a desired position. When using a static device

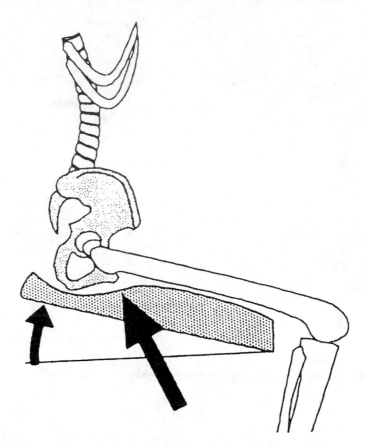

Figure 6–21. Contours prevent sliding on an anteriorly sloped seat. *Note:* From *Ergonomics Wheelchairs and Positioning* (Figure 60), by B. Engstrom, 1993, Stockholm, Sweden: Bromma Tryck AB. Copyright 1993 by Bengt Engstrom. Reprinted with permission.

one runs the risk of not allowing movement to take place such that the forces created at the knee will be transferred, for example, to the hip joint area and thus promote hip subluxation. Without the dynamic component, the leg divider can sometimes stimulate leg muscles to press the legs together and therefore increase spasticity. It is crucial to observe each individual's reaction to the leg divider chosen. A static device may be sufficient or preferred to no device at all. A dynamic device is best but may not be needed if spasticity decreases in the upright or forward leaning position.

The Dynamic Part of Sitting

Individuals create a base of support with their sitting bones and thighs. As mentioned earlier, the body's center of gravity should fall within the limits of the base of support. The base is the stable unit around which the person is able to move feet, trunk, head, and arms. Moveable body parts constitute the dynamic component of sitting. In order to prepare a natural alignment of the upper body above the base, the pelvis is positioned in a slightly forward tilted position. This position naturally aligns the spine in an erect position in contrast to a backward tilted pelvis,

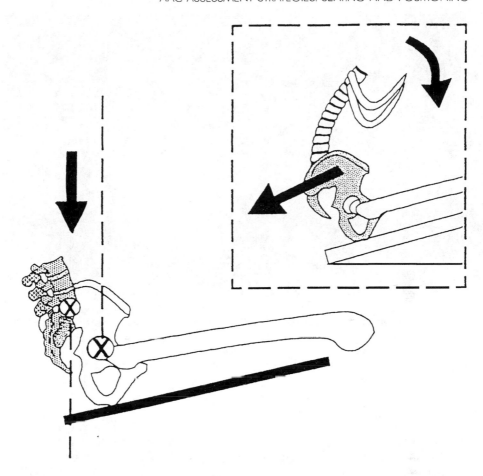

Figure 6–22. Posterior slope results in a posterior pelvis and spinal flexion (i.e., collapse). *Note:* From *Ergonomics Wheelchairs and Positioning* (Figure 61), by B. Engstrom, 1993, Stockholm, Sweden: Bromma Tryck AB. Copyright 1993 by Bengt Engstrom. Reprinted with permission.

which creates a kyphosis, or rounding of the back, and makes it more difficult to align the upper body on top of its base.

Trunk

An ideal seating position consists of the following components:

- An upright or forward leaning trunk
- Support for the trunk when needed.

In the upright and forward leaning position, the head and eyes are able to function properly for upper body activities. The upper body's center of gravity falls above or in front of the sitting bones. This allows postural muscles located posteriorly to the head and trunk to hold the body balanced and erect.

Certain observations need to be made to determine when to let a person sit in a forward leaning position versus straight up. A prerequisite for using a forward leaning position is that the client has the physical ability to re-erect the body to an upright position. Some clients have the capability to re-erect themselves but have a

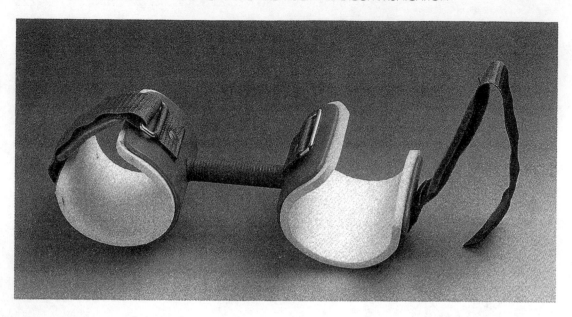

Figure 6–23. Dynamic abduction orthosis, consisting of two C-shaped braces, each fitting around the femur just proximal to distal condyles and connected by a progressive spring. *Note:* From "Influence of Different Sitting Positions and Abduction Orthosis on Leg Muscle Activity in Children with Cerebral Palsy," by U. Myhr and L. vonWendt, 1993, *Developmental Medicine and Child Neurology, 35,* p. 872. Copyright 1993 by Mac Keith Press. Reprinted with permission.

tendency to nose dive into whatever is in front of them on the table. If this occurs, the forward leaning position can still be used as a therapeutic intervention for limited periods of time to practice postural control. Additionally, trunk supports that allow leaning forward only within certain stability limits can be used. These limits can be gradually increased as postural control improves. It is not possible to practice postural control in a reclined position as the whole body creates the base of support. There are no forces balancing over the base.

The Seat Back. The seat back is an important part of a seating system. There are many details to consider and different options to choose from. The spine is naturally curved, and if the individual needs a large contact area for comfort or to avoid pressure points, then the seat back needs to be contoured to follow this curvature of the back. For increased comfort, the low-

est part of the seat back can be cut out in order to allow room for the buttocks. Back support is provided at the level of the thoracic vertebrae.

When allowing room for spinal curvature without using a contoured seat, the inclination of the back rest will change depending on the height of the back support (see Figure 6–25). Seat backs commonly end at the level of the scapula. They may be higher if needed to attach trunk supports. If a planar (i.e., flat) back is designed only to support the pelvis and lumbar area of the back, it can be angled slightly forward. When increasing seat back height to midthoracic level, the back needs to be vertical to accommodate the natural spinal curve. When increasing the back height even more, it needs to be reclined in order to allow room for the natural kyphosis (e.g., curvature) of the thorax. In other words, the seat back is slightly reclined but the individual's trunk is actually upright without

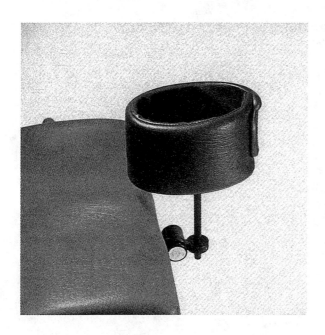

Figure 6–24. Miller's swing away dynamic abductor. Photo courtesy of Miller's Adaptive Technologies.

support at the lower parts of the back. A contoured seat back can more easily create support for the different parts of the back and is preferred, especially if the client is sensitive to pressure over small areas. The higher the back support, the more reclined it needs to be to accommodate the natural curvature of the spine.

Trunk Supports And Restraints. Supports and restraints for the upper body can be placed behind or in front of the body. Forward supports include a tray or table in front of the body. These enable the person to support body weight on the forearms or hands. Lateral trunk supports are used in order to keep the trunk in midline and avoid excessive leaning to one side (see Figure 6–26). Lateral trunk supports need to fit snugly. There should be ½ inch of space between the client's body and the trunk supports for an optimal fit. All-season brackets can be used to provide room for a heavy coat during the winter season. They allow easy sideways adjustment of the lateral supports. Lateral supports should extend past the individual's midline when viewed from the side (Harryman & War-

ren, 1992). Vests and shoulder retractors are anterior trunk supports that hold the client upright and stable in the sagittal plane in which the upper body moves forward and backward (see Figures 6–26 and 6–27). When using these supports, it is important that the head of the humerus is free for movement of the arm.

Vests and shoulder retractors are functional when the individual needs to be seated in an erect position. When a client needs to lean forward, these supports do not allow for forward movement. Individuals will sometimes compensate for this lack of movement by bending the neck at a sharp angle to come forward. There is currently a lack of trunk support options that will allow for forward movement of the trunk within a controlled range without fully restraining the shoulders and head.

Feet

The position of the feet is influenced by the position of the pelvis and the upper body. An ideal seating position has the following components:

- The ability to move the feet backward behind the knee joint when the upper body moves forward
- Chair foot plates or resting surface in a horizontal position
- The absence of heel cups, straps, or other restrictive devices unless needed.

It is normal to counteract changes in the center of gravity of the upper body by moving the feet in the opposite direction. If the upper body goes forward when seated, the feet go backward. If the body moves posteriorly when seated, then the feet move anteriorly. Heel cups and foot straps hinder these compensatory movements of the feet as do angled foot plates. If footrests cannot be placed in a horizontal position, it may be preferred that they be removed when working at a desk. The individual can then support the feet flat on the floor. If the feet do not touch the floor, small step stools or step boxes can be placed under the feet to create a flat surface.

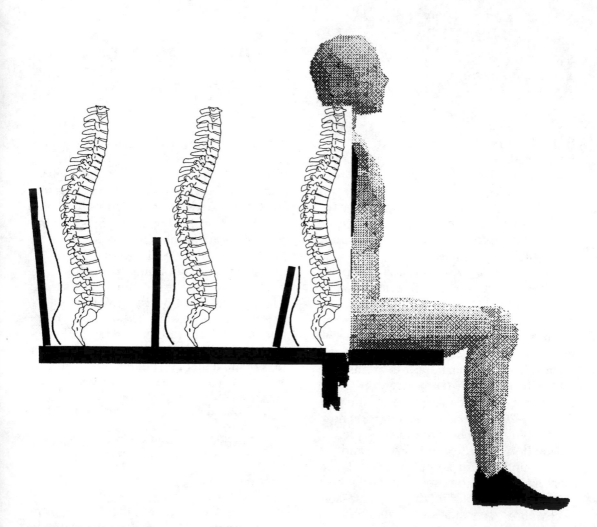

Figure 6–25. Back height and angles. *Note: From Ergonomics Wheelchairs and Positioning* (Figure 67), by B. Engstrom, 1993, Stockholm, Sweden: Bromma Tryck AB. Copyright 1993 by Bengt Engstrom. Reprinted with permission.

Arms

A good sitting position creates an opportunity for optimal arm and hand function with an absence of reflex movement patterns of the arms. The quality and amount of arm/hand function that a client has will vary with different types of physical disabilities. The sitting position itself cannot change certain aspects of fine motor arm and hand function. However, positioning can greatly influence an individual's capacity to use the hands by creating optimal postural control when sitting. By creating a relaxed and balanced sitting position one can avoid using the arms to counteract improper balance.

A sign of improper balance is the so-called alarm or hands up position where the elbows are flexed and hands are held fisted at the shoulders (see Figure 6–28a). It is often caused by the upper body's center of gravity being placed too far posteriorly, which creates a sensation of falling backward. It is difficult to bring the arms forward from this position unless the whole sitting position is changed to one where the body is balanced over the seat surface. A table or tray for forearm support will usually add stability and increase control and improve hand function (see Figure 6–28b). Some children like to hold onto a vertical dowel placed on the tray in order to stabilize one arm while using the other (see Figure 6–29).

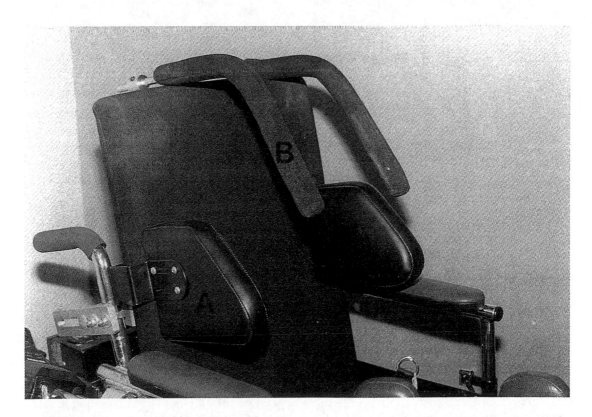

Figure 6–26. Seating insert components. **(A)** lateral supports for trunk stability; and **(B)** shoulder retractors for anterior trunk stability.

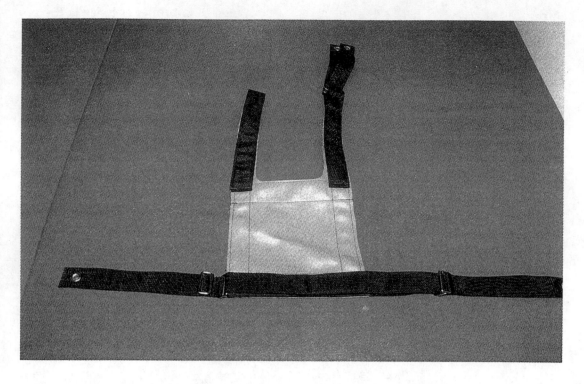

Figure 6–27. Vest for trunk support.

Head

An ideal seating position has the following components:

- Optimal head control
- Optimal visual field
- Optimal eye-hand coordination.

Head control in a seated position is something that most children, even with severe disabilities, can learn to achieve if given the opportunity to practice head control in the upright position. There is a common misconception that lack of head control is due to lack of muscle strength and fatigue. In fact, if the head is balanced correctly on the spine, minimal muscle activity is needed to keep it upright. Instead, lack of head control is often due to lack of postural control or balance. Since keeping the head

postured downward is detrimental for visual regard when learning, children who have not yet developed head control and who are weak due to decreased postural muscle tone are commonly placed in chairs that are reclined. This initially may be necessary when concentrating on learning tasks, including using an AAC system. However, from the long-term perspective, it is important to provide opportunities to sit upright and practice head control on a daily basis. Through practice, a child can learn to improve head control and develop a better working position. A seating orthosis, which is discussed later in this chapter, can be used for practicing head control. There are exceptions to trying to gain an upright or slightly forward flexed head position. For example, people in late stages of muscular dystrophy lack muscle strength almost entirely and need a good

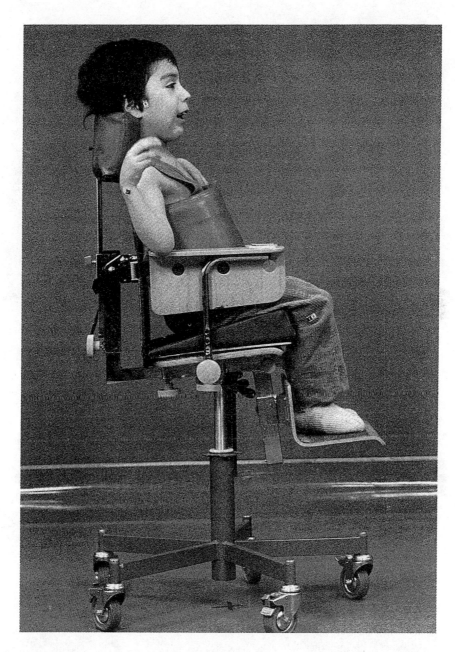

(a)   (continued)

Figure 6–28. (a) Arms held back in unbalanced position. (b) Arms free for function in balanced position. *Note:* From "Reducing Spasticity and Enhancing Postural Control for the Creation of a Functional Sitting Position in Children with Cerebral Palsy: A Pilot Study," by U. Myhr and L. vonWendt, 1990, *Physiotherapy Theory and Practice, 6,* p. 68. Copyright 1990 by Erlbaum Taylor & Francis. Reprinted with permission.

Figure 6–28. (continued)

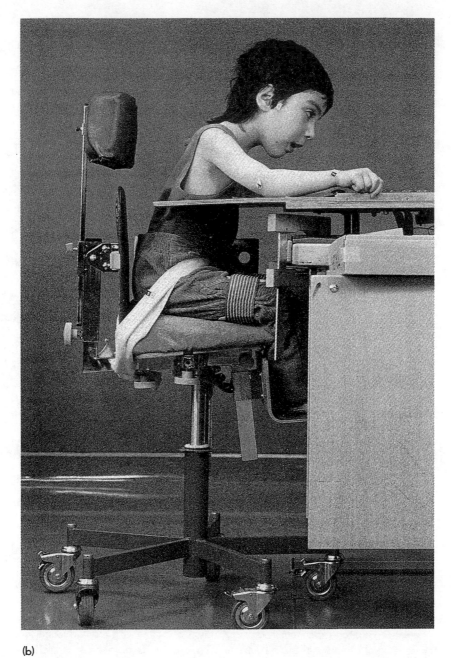

(b)

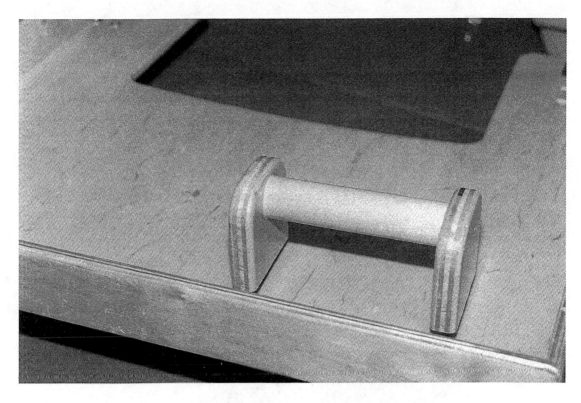

Figure 6–29. Vertical dowel. The individual holds onto the dowel which increases trunk stability.

head support and a neck rest for safety reasons. If they lose head control and the head falls forward, they lack the ability to bring the head back up, thus creating a dangerous situation with risks of suffocation.

It is important to have a motivating task to attend to when evaluating and practicing head control. Parents are the best sources of information when trying to map a child's performance span. Therapists and parents need to evaluate whether the child's downward head position is a behavioral condition. A child may be able to hold the head up for long periods of time when watching television or when absorbed by watching something that catches his or her interest, yet when sitting at a desk in a learning situation the head remains in a down position. Many children who are physically disabled cannot independently move their wheel-

chairs and often look down to escape boring or difficult situations.

Professionals also need to consider head position when determining where to visually place learning materials, including AAC devices. Because many individuals with physical disabilities have visual impairments, individual visual needs may differ. In general, direct selection AAC systems should be placed about 12 inches from the eyes for optimal focal distance, with the device or table surface reclined 10 to 15 degrees. This placement will vary depending on the size of the symbols, the individual's need to visually attend to the AAC system, and the individual's upper extremity motor accessing skills. Additional information regarding vision as it relates to augmentative communication is presented in Chapter 7.

In the optimal functional sitting position, head supports are not always needed as the individual will be able to balance the head over the seating surface. However, head supports may be needed until the person is able to independently maintain the functional sitting position for extended periods of time (see Figure 6–30). Each person must be assessed individually when determining the need for neck and head supports. Some individuals, such as those with different types of muscular dystrophy, may need them for continuous support across all activities. Other individuals will only need them when resting and during transportation. In the latter example, the head support should be placed at a distance behind the head. By placing the support at a distance it will still fulfill its function of supporting the head when leaning back to rest or serving as a safety device during an abrupt stop. With children with cerebral palsy, a head support placed too close to the head may have negative consequences. The head support can stimulate the tonic labyrinthine reflex, causing the child to constantly press the head back into the head support. A safety issue to consider is that some children move their heads to the side before extending back. The child can then end up with his or her head caught behind the head support. A sideways extension of the head support may be needed to stop this movement.

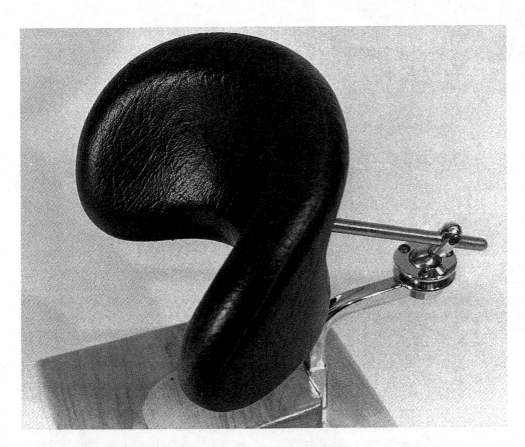

Figure 6–30. Ottobock Head support. Photo courtesy of Ottobock.

THE SEATING ORTHOSIS

Small children naturally sit and play on the floor, or perhaps in a sandbox or the bath tub. There are floor sitters that can create a stable base for sitting while following the same guidelines as those for creating a functional sitting position in a chair, namely, to have the pelvis neutral or anteriorly tipped with upper body alignment above or in front of the sitting bones. Negative aspects of traditional floor sitters are that they are heavy and use restraints that limit arm and hand function. An alternative to the traditional floor sitter is the seating orthosis (see Figures 6–31 and 6–32). It is a lightweight orthosis consisting of a back and trunk piece with removable back supports. Easily removable head and chin supports can be added if needed. The seating orthosis can be used in a variety of chairs and situations, in water, on the floor, on a sled, or in a regular chair. The seating orthosis has been shown in a controlled study to increase head control and arm and hand function in children with neurological handicaps (Steen et al., 1991). Instead of putting the unstable child in a very stable chair or insert, the seating orthosis enables the child to sit in different places and also learn postural control through the use of the orthosis.

SEATING FOR CHILDREN WITH MILD NEUROLOGICAL DISABILITIES

It may not be obvious that ambulatory children with Attention Deficit Hyperactivity Disorder or mental retardation also benefit from seating interventions. These children may seem clumsy but can still function quite well motorically. The fact that they are so motorically active makes many believe that there is nothing wrong with their

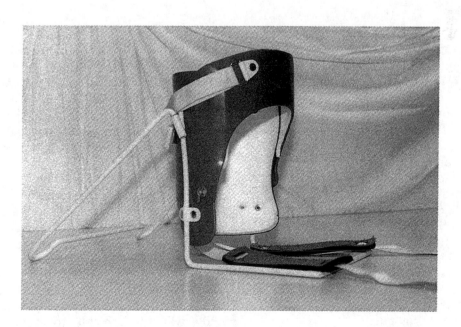

Figure 6–31. The seating orthosis, a lightweight, versatile seating device which en-hances function and postural control.

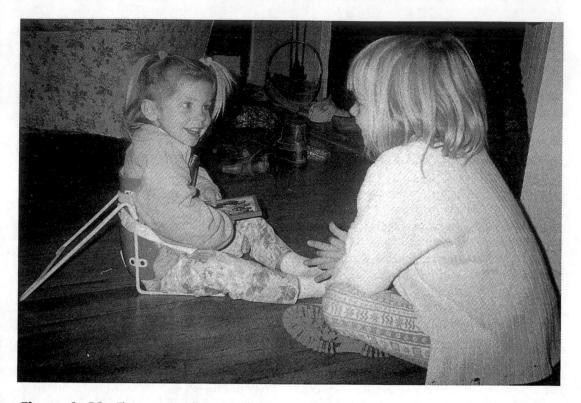

Figure 6–32. The seating orthosis used by a young child for interactive play when sitting on the floor.

gross motor function. However it is very common that these children have moderately low to very low postural muscle tone. This lack of postural muscle tone makes it difficult for them to hold a specific body position for some time (see Figure 6–33). They are great runners and jumpers but have difficulty standing still on one leg, or performing any activities that require static balance. Sitting at a desk is difficult for many of these children as it requires postural muscle activation and shoulder stability for fine motor activities. A working position where the child sits on a posteriorly tilted chair may make it difficult for the child to concentrate on school work as much energy goes to trying to change position when muscle groups fatigue.

Letting those children sit in a forward leaning position with about 45 degrees of hip flexion provides a balance between muscles at the front and back of the pelvis and naturally aligns the spine in an erect position (Mandal, 1984). This position can be likened to sitting slightly crouched on a horse or a motorcycle. When balance is reached there is less need for postural muscle activity and the child will subsequently increase endurance for sitting at a desk. Most children naturally strive to reach this position by tilting the chair forward when reading or writing at a table and also by leaning backward when resting. A chair that accommodates the need to move from sitting forward to resting in a backward leaning position is preferred. A regular chair with a slightly forward sloping front edge will allow the child to come forward on the seat when working. When listening to the teacher for a longer time the child

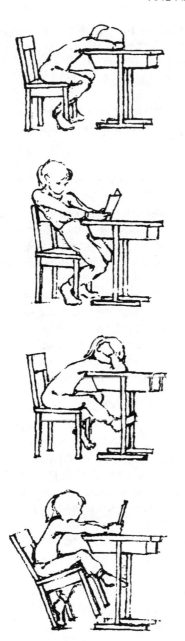

Figure 6–33. Low postural muscle tone in children with ADHD or mental retardation leads to difficulty in maintaining a static sitting posture. *Note:* From *MBD Barn* (Figure 33) by B. Bille and K. Brieditis 1984, technical illustrations by M. Nordquist. Copyright 1984 by M. Nord-quist. Reprinted with permission.

can move back to a resting position by placing the foot on a horizontal bar between the front legs of the desk, giving an opportunity to lean back against the back support.

THE SEATING EVALUATION

The most commonly used approach when trying to find the optimal position for an augmentative communication device is to have a team of experts evaluate the individual's physical abilities. Optimally, this allows for a greater understanding of the complex problems involved and also potential solutions. It is sometimes overwhelming for a young child to be surrounded by a team of adults who are observing and intervening at the same time. In order to make the situation fun, professionals should gather as much information as possible before the actual appointment. Information should be obtained regarding existing seating and positioning and also regarding what tasks or toys are highly motivating for the child. A motivating task can help improve motor performance. It is crucial to realize the importance of motivating the individual both cognitively and motorically within the assessment pro-cess. When evaluating seating and positioning, the props used should create opportunities to observe the following motor skills:

- Reaching forward and touching or grasping and re-erecting
- Looking from side to side
- Transferring from one hand to another
- Two-handed activities.

Objective Evaluation Measures

One way of improving the seating assessment process is by using objective outcome measures. Videotaping seating assessments and using standardized evaluation methods to measure improvements in the person's ability to function when seated are recommended. Using videotapes of the evaluation is a relatively inexpensive and practical way to assess seating options objectively. Another advantage of using video is that it allows for evaluation after the actual session with the client. Instead of performing the trials and evaluation at the same time, professionals can concentrate on the different seating trials in the session, then analyze their effects in a thorough detailed manner after the evaluation.

When using video filming during an assessment it is important to film the whole person throughout the entire evaluation. For example, when the feet are fastened to footplates it may increase spasticity of the arms and hands. A videotape that focuses only on the upper body will miss the influence of the foot and leg position. One benefit of videotaping seating assessments is that the film serves as a document and reference point when dealing with a client across many years. Another advantage of the video camera is that it can be taken to the individual's home or school environment. This increases the validity and functionality of the assessment process.

Sitting Assessment Scale

Currently there is a lack of valid, reliable, and easy-to-use seating evaluation methods. Some exist and can be administered quite easily, such as the Sitting Assessment Scale (Myhr & von Wendt 1991, 1993; Myhr et al., 1995) and The Seated Postural Control Measure (Fife et al., 1991). The Sitting Assessment Scale was designed to be used when evaluating video films. It is used to assess head, trunk, and foot control and also arm and hand function (see Figure 6–34). It consists of a scale from 1 to 4 where 1 represents no control or no function and 4 equals good control or good

function. Each item on the scale has a descriptive objective corresponding to the number. Observations are done during 5 minutes of video filming in different positions. The Sitting Assessment Scale has shown high interrater and intrarater reliability (Myhr & von Wendt, 1993; Myhr et al., 1995).

Counting Pathologic Movements

Another objective seating evaluation method is to count pathological movements during a specific time period and to compare the number of pathological movements across different positions (Myhr & von Wendt, 1990). Instead of counting all possible pathological movements, another option is to count the pathological movement that occurs most often for a given individual. Examples of such patterns are extensor spasticity of the legs, the asymmetric tonic neck reflex, or the hands up movement of the arms with flexed elbows and hands at the shoulders. After choosing the most common pathological pattern, one must establish exactly how strong the response must be in order to qualify as a pathological movement. For example, if the chosen pattern is the hands up reaction, one must determine how far up the hands have to come in order to be counted as a pathological movement (for example, to the level of the head of the humerus). These movements are then counted in a systematic manner across seating and positioning trials.

Biomechanical Analysis

An individual's movement patterns can be analyzed using biomechanical analysis. When photographing the client in different positions, one strives to take the picture in a situation that is representative of the typical behavior in that specific position.

SITTING ASSESSMENT SCALE

HEAD CONTROL

1. None: unable to hold head erect or needs neck support.
2. Poor: holds the head erect for ≤ 2 minutes* easily loses control.
3. Fair: holds head erect but displaces with acceleration/rotation.
4. Good: holds head upright and able to rotate.

TRUNK CONTROL

1. None: lacks control of trunk or needs back support.
2. Poor: holds trunk erect only when supported by forearms or hand
3. Fair: holds trunk erect supported by one forearm or hand, some degree of lateral flexion can occur.
4. Good: holds trunk erect with and without forearm or hand support, with pelvis supported or unsupported.

FOOT CONTROL

1. None: unable to hold feet against underlying surface without fixation.
2. Poor: holds feet against underlying surface for ≤ 2 minutes*.
3. Fair: good control of one foot, less control of the other.
4. Good: holds feet against underlying surface for entire period.

ARM FUNCTION

1. None: unable to control arms at will.
2. Poor: uses arms for support, but easily loses control: stretches arms towards objects but in uncontrolled movements.
3. Fair: uses one arm for support and stretches other arm towards objects intentionally.
4. Good: uses one or both arms for support, stretches arms towards objects intentionally or uses arms for functional movements.

HAND FUNCTION

1. None: unable to grasp objects, knocks object with one hand.
2. Poor: grasps and holds objects using uncontrolled movements.
3. Fair: good function in one hand, less control of the other.
4. Good: good function in both hands, or able to consciously grasp, hold and release objects.

---

* Accumulation duration, maximum two minutes out of five.

Figure 6–34. Sitting Assessment Scale. *Note:* From "Improvement of Functional Sitting Position for Children with Cerebral Palsy" by U. Myhr and L. vonWendt, 1991, *Developmental Medicine and Child Neurology, 33,* p. 251. Copyright 1991 by Mac Keith Press. Reprinted with permission.

It is possible by drawing a vertical line on the photograph through the hip joint, to evaluate how the position of the upper and lower body influences the movement pattern in relation to the hip joint (Myhr & von Wendt, 1990, 1991). It is helpful to mark the movement axis of different joints, for example the shoulder, elbow, ankle, and knee, in order to analyze arm, knee, and foot positions relative to the pelvis. Photographs can also be used for evaluation with The Sitting Assessment Scale, although it has not been tested for reliability in this way.

Seating Evaluation Procedures

The variety of physical disabilities makes it difficult to have a cookie cutter approach to assessing seating and positioning. Differences in physical ability can vary greatly between two persons with the same neuromotor diagnosis. The evaluation needs to begin by assessing each client in a systematic, standardized way. First, the individual is observed in the existing chair, the way he or she is positioned when coming to the appointment. If the person needs to use an AAC system in other positions, those positions also need to be observed. Movement patterns, stability, and comfort are observed as well as body alignment and the location of the person's center of gravity. Seat depth and sideways stability also need to be assessed.

Second, the individual is taken out of the chair and the chair itself is examined and measured. Seat and back angles and their relationship to one another are observed. Other components of the chair are noted along with the type of seating system; for example, a contoured seat and back or a solid seat and back insert. The relationship between the chair and its components and the previously obtained observations of the individual positioned in the chair are then addressed.

Third, the person needs to be assessed out of the chair. Musculoskeletal deformities, pressure sores, and any other physical problems need to be evaluated. For example, individuals with hip contractures may be impossible to seat with 90 degrees of hip flexion. These physical problems need to be taken into account when developing recommendations for improved positioning. If physical problems are found, referrals to orthopedic specialists are needed before making any changes to the seating system.

When these three processes have been completed and the findings discussed, changes can be implemented that will improve positioning. Changes in positioning should always start at the pelvis. By securing the pelvis and creating a stable base, the alignment of the upper and lower body automatically follows. It is important to pay attention to the seat surface inclination and how it affects movement patterns and balance. Once the position of the pelvis is determined, changes to seating should follow the order presented in this chapter. The stable components of seating (i.e., pelvis, thighs, and hips) are positioned first. The dynamic components of seating are then evaluated beginning with the trunk, then working distally to the arms and hands, feet and legs, and finally the head and neck. The assessment conditions should simulate normal working situations for the individual whenever possible.

Orthopedic Versus Neurological Effects

Traditionally, seating has been evaluated from an orthopedic approach that assesses the effects of the seating system on stability and movement. When working with individuals with neurological impairments it is of great importance that we also evaluate the effects of positioning on postural control and spasticity. There are several differences in the evaluation process when comparing orthopedic effects versus neurological effects. The orthopedic evaluation can take place immediately after the person has been positioned. In contrast, the neurological evaluation should be delayed to allow time to learn and adjust to new positions before measures are taken. For example, when evaluating the effects of tilting the pelvis forward, the often spastic "hamstring" muscle is stretched, which can initially cause some discomfort. However, after about 5 minutes the prolonged stretch of this muscle often decreases spasticity and enhances postural control. Time is also a factor in giving the client an opportunity to practice head control when placed in a forward leaning position. Initially, the client may use a strong extension pattern to bring the head back up from the forward position, but with time and practice the movement becomes more controlled by voluntary muscle activation.

LOOKING AT THE HORIZON

In the last decade there has been tremendous improvement in the construction of both manual and power wheelchairs. Although testing of the technical aspects of the chairs has improved, little attention has been given to the sitting position itself. Despite efforts to improve seating, there have been studies showing that individuals with physical disabilities continue to sit in positions that do not address their unique deformities and may cause physical deterioration over time (Mulcahy, Pountney, Nelham, Green, & Billington, 1988). Current research offers knowledge that has great potential for improved seating. Despite these research findings, this current knowledge is not always implemented in everyday rehabilitation settings.

Although electronics and lightweight materials have improved the frame of wheelchairs, the seating systems themselves have not gone through the same revolution. Seating materials often remain rigid and heavy. In the future, chairs need to be developed that allow for easy changes in position; from forward leaning to reclined, from sitting with 90 degrees of hip and knee flexion to a seated position on an elevated seat for increased comfort when working at a desk. Chairs are needed that allow for freedom of movement without promoting spastic patterns. The chairs themselves need to allow for changes in seat and back support in order to avoid heavy seat inserts. By creating a flexible support system for the individual, and by thinking of the chair as a body orthosis that needs to have as many options for positioning as possible, it is possible to prevent problems of deformity and enable the individual to grow and learn according to his or her abilities.

A chair that functions optimally will improve the person's ability to function more independently, which in turn increases self-esteem and the desire to communicate. For the potential AAC user, an optimal seating position also provides the best condition for motorically accessing an AAC device. Poor positioning affects the ability to easily and accurately move body extremities, increases fatigue, and causes long-term behavioral and physical changes that significantly impact on the ability to use an AAC system. It is important that the AAC team address seating and positioning concerns at the beginning of the assessment process to ensure optimum communication outcomes.

REFERENCES

Bille, B., & Brieditis, K. (1984). *MBD barn. (translation: MBD children)*. Uppsala, Sweden: Esselte Herzogs.

Bower, E., & McLellan, D. L. (1992). Effect of increased exposure to physiotherapy on skill acquisition of children with cerebral palsy. *Developmental Medicine and Child Neurology, 34*, 25–39.

Carlson, S. J., & Ramsey, C. (1994). Assistive technology. In S. Campbell (Ed.), *Physical therapy for children,* Philadelphia, PA: W. B. Saunders.

Engstrom, B. (1993). *Ergonomics wheelchairs and positioning,* Stockholm: Bromma Tryck AB.

Fife, S. E., Roxborough, L. A., Armstrong, R. W., Harris, S. R., Gregson, J. L., & Field, D. (1991). Development of a clinical measure of postural control for assessment of adaptive seating in children with neuromotor disabilities. *Physical Therapy, 71*, 981–993.

Foley, J. (1977). Cerebral palsy: Physical aspects. In C. M. Drillien & M. B. Drumond (Eds.), *Neurodevelopmental problems in early childhood* (p. 277). Oxford: Blackwell Scientific Publications Limited.

Galley, P. M., & Forster, A. L. (1982). *Human movement.* Edinburgh: Churchill Livingstone.

Ghez, C. (1991). Motor systems of the brain: The control of movement. In E. R. Kandel, J. H. Schwartz, & R. Jessel (Eds.), *Principles of neural science* (pp. 143–172). New York: Elsevier.

Harryman, S., & Warren, L. (1992). Positioning and power mobility. In G. Church & S. Glennen (Eds.), *The handbook of assistive technology.* (pp. 55–92). San Diego: Singular Publishing Group.

Hirschfeld, H. (1992). *On the integration of posture, locomotion and voluntary movement in humans: Normal and impaired development.* Unpublished thesis, Karolinska Institute, Stockholm, Sweden.

Letts, K., Shapiro, L., Mulder, D., & Klassen, O. (1984). The Windblown Hip Syndrome in total body cerebral palsy. *Journal of Pediatrics Orthopedica, 4*, 55–60.

Mandal, A. C. (1984). The correct height of school furniture. *Physiotherapy, 70*, 48–53.

McClenaghan, B. A., Thombs, L. & Milner, M. (1992). Effects of seat-surface inclination on postural stability and function of the upper extremities of children with cerebral palsy. *Developmental Medicine and Child Neurology, 34*, 40–48.

Mulcahy, C. M, Pountney, T. E., Nelham, R. L., Green, E. M., & Billington, G. D. (1988). Adaptive seating for the motor handicapped, problems, a solution, assessment and prescription. *Physiotherapy, 74*, 531–536.

Myhr, U., & vonWendt, L. (1990). Reducing spasticity and enhancing postural control for the creation of a functional sitting position in children with cerebral palsy: A pilot study. *Physiotherapy Theory and Practice, 6*, 65–76.

Myhr, U., & vonWendt, L. (1991). Improvement of functional sitting position for children with cerebral palsy. *Developmental Medicine and Child Neurology, 33*, 246–256.

Myhr, U., & vonWendt, L. (1993). Influence of different sitting positions and abduction orthosis on leg muscle activity in children with cerebral palsy. *Developmental Medicine and Child Neurology, 35*, 870–880.

Myhr, U., vonWendt, L., Norrlin, S., & Radell, U. (1995). A 5-year follow-up of a functional sitting position in children with cerebral palsy. *Developmental Medicine and Child Neurology, 37*, 587–596.

Nwaobi, O. M. (1986). Effects of body orientation in space on tonic muscle activity of patients with cerebral palsy. *Developmental Medicine and Child Neurology, 28*, 41–44.

Nwaobi, O. M., Brubacker, C. E, Cosich B., & Sussman, M. D. (1983). Electromyographic investigation of extensor activity in cerebral palsied children in different seating positions. *Developmental Medicine and Child Neurology, 25*, 175–183.

Odeen, I. (1981). Reduction of muscular hypertonus by long-term muscle stretch. *Scandinavian Journal of Rehabilitation Medicine, 13*, 93–99.

Pope, P. M., Bowes, C. E., & Booth, E. (1994). Postural control in sitting with the Sam system: Evaluation of use over three years. *Developmental Medicine and Child Neurology, 36*, 241–245.

Reese, M., Msall, M. E., diAmato, C., Pictor, S., & Gillespie, R. (1990). *The influence of asymmetric primitive reflexes and tone on orthopedic deformity in children with cerebral palsy.* Paper presented at the American Academy of Cerebral Palsy and Developmental Medicine, Orlando, Fl.

Reid, D. T., Sochaniwskyu, A., & Milner, M. (1991). An investigation of postural sway in sitting of normal children and children with neurological disorders. *Physical and Occupational Therapy in Pediatrics, 11*, 19–34.

Steen, M., Radell, U., Lanshammar, H., & Fristedt, A. (1991). Sittskalet - ett hjalpmedel for gravt rorelse hindrade barn och ungdomar. *Sjukgym-nasten, Vetenskapligt supplement, 12,* 25–30.

Woolacott, M. H. (1993). Early postnatal development of posture control: Normal and ab-normal aspects. In A. Kalverboer, B. Hopkins, & R. Geuze (Eds.), *Motor development in early and later childhood: Longitudinal approaches* (pp. 43–67). Cambridge University Press.

Chapter 7

AUGMENTATIVE AND ALTERNATIVE COMMUNICATION ASSESSMENT STRATEGIES: MOTOR ACCESS AND VISUAL CONSIDERATIONS

Denise C. DeCoste

Augmentative and alternative communication (AAC) assessment requires the convergence of information across different aspects of an individual's development and communication environments. Critical paths of information must come together to accomplish the AAC feature match evaluation process (Swengel & Varga, 1993), as discussed in Chapter 5. As part of the AAC assessment process, information pertaining to cognitive, linguistic, and environmental factors is combined with information on motor and visual components. All together, this information strengthens the AAC feature match assessment, in which the skills of the individual are matched to the AAC system that has the desired features.

The evaluation of motor access is a critical component of AAC assessment. Motor access refers to the ways in which an individual will physically approach and use AAC systems. Access evaluation begins with the assessment of seating and positioning, followed by the assessment of motor skills. The goal is to delineate the best system for accessing picture- or word-based symbols for purposes of communication. In order to accomplish this, seating, positioning, motor, and visual-perceptual issues must be carefully examined. Identifying proper seating and positioning is a logical first step because this significantly affects the areas of assessment that follow (see Chapter 6). Central trunk stability with ample mobility must be established in order to evaluate reliable movements for pointing or using a switch with an AAC system. Visual and perceptual issues also have an impact on the positioning of AAC systems, the types of communication symbols used, the need for auditory feedback, and the size and layout of the symbols. Confidence in the recommended design of an AAC system is best achieved when the assessment is carried out in a logical and comprehensive manner. Systematic assessment will carefully factor out elements that will impede effective communication with an AAC system.

This chapter focuses on the motor and visual components of the AAC assessment process. It begins with a discussion of general issues related to motor access evaluation, and the impact of visual abilities on the AAC feature match process, focusing on the visual-motor and visual-perceptual elements of targeting symbols. Thereafter, a systematic assessment of motor access is described, the range of methods available for direct and indirect selection (i.e., scanning) are outlined, related research is discussed, and access training methods are addressed.

THE NATURE OF THE ACCESS EVALUATION PROCESS

The access portion of an AAC evaluation is a relatively discrete area of assessment, but it is only part of the total AAC evaluation process. Chapter 5 discusses the predictive feature match process relative to cognitive, linguistic, and environmental elements of the AAC assessment process. As discussed in Chapter 5, the AAC evaluation process often begins with a needs assessment and an evaluation of communication environment issues. Thereafter, speech-language pathologists will need to evaluate expressive and receptive communication abilities, as well as existing symbolic language abilities. Additional evaluations by psychologists and educators may be necessary to further evaluate cognitive and academic abilities. Together, this information delineates available skills and potential abilities which contributes to the predictive aspect of the AAC feature match process.

To conduct the seating, positioning, and motor access portion of the AAC evaluation, occupational therapists and physical therapists are considered key players. A vision specialist may be needed for a client with vision impairments. For more on team development and models of service delivery, the reader is directed to Chapter 2. For additional information on the overall assessment process specific to individuals with physical disabilities, see Chapter 10.

AAC assessment, including the access portion of the evaluation, is not a one-shot deal. Motor access assessments may take more than one session to complete. Seating and positioning evaluations are rarely resolved in one session. Generally, seating systems and seating modifications need time for construction and are then tried out at a later date. The individual with disabilities often needs additional time with a new or adapted seating system to be sure the seating modifications are optimal. Motor, visual, and symbol selection evaluations can also take time and may or may not be accomplished in one session. Multiple evaluations on one day can be overwhelming and fatiguing for an individual. With others, attention span and limited cooperation can be an issue.

Some parts of the AAC access evaluation may need to be repeated at regular intervals to monitor an individual's changing needs. Motor skills can improve or decline depending upon the individual's health or developmental status. It is important to add that there are some clients for whom a reliable, satisfactory motor access method is never found. This can be the case for clients with severely limited volitional motor control, characterized by wildly fluctuating movements or severe abnormal reflexes. Although this is rare, professionals will need to choose whatever is best (usually, eye gaze, as described in Chapter 3) and push it to the maximum potential of the client. For these clients, repeated motor access evaluations at regular intervals will still be needed, as there is no justification for "giving up" on a client. This is especially true for children. For example, in the case of a young girl with spastic athetoid quadriplegia, no method of motor access, including eye gaze, was found over repeated evaluations during the first 12 years of her life. It was not until her teenage years, when she learned to exert some cognitive control over her volitional movement and muscle tone, that a more reliable method of motor access was finally identified.

Assessment Across Multiple Environments

AAC access evaluations must also look at skills across multiple communication systems. Different environments demand different communication methods. Communication in the community setting may require a small, lightweight, nonelectrical system, whereas communication in the school setting may require a combination of high-tech and low-tech systems. Each of these systems may require different motor skills to operate, different mounting systems, and different communication symbol layouts. Different environments may also require AAC systems for different positions; for example, access may be needed for a side-lying position or for a prone standing position.

Short-Term Versus Long-Term Evaluation Issues

AAC evaluation is often classified as a predictive evaluation (Yorkston & Karlan, 1986) because short-term abilities as well as long-term efficiency must be considered. It is important to take into consideration the immediate AAC needs of a child, as well as future needs based on reasonable predictions. For example, a young toddler may have sufficient fine motor coordi-

nation to access a communication overlay of eight picture symbols. However, based on his or her current rate of language development, he or she may require access to many more symbols in the near future. Motor access evaluation will need to consider features of AAC systems that will keep pace with the child's developing language needs. Likewise, a young child with traumatic brain injury may be able to use scanning to communicate for the time being, but may be expected over time to gain improvement in upper extremity skills and progress to direct selection access methods. A young toddler may currently use low-tech AAC strategies when positioned in an adapted chair or seat insert in a stroller, but may need to advance to a wheelchair within the year. Hence, an AAC access evaluation must look objectively at existing skills, while simultaneously considering long-term issues.

THE IMPACT OF VISUAL ABILITIES ON AAC

Visual abilities can have an impact on the selection of AAC systems. For example, visual problems can affect the types of symbols used, the layout of symbols, and the positioning of AAC systems. Prior to the discussion of motor access assessment, it is important to consider the role of vision.

Vision has three optical elements: sight, transmission, and interpretation (Beukelman, Mirenda, Franklin, & Newman, 1992). Sight involves the sensory reception of the eye itself, transmission involves the optic nerve, and interpretation involves the processing of the image in the visual cortex of the brain. In addition to optical concerns, when evaluating the effects of vision on the use of AAC ocular motor issues also must be considered. For example, poor control of eye movements can affect the individual's ability to visually scan and localize target symbols on a communication overlay. On top of this, environmental factors that may affect vision must be addressed. The following subsections will discuss the impact of these issues on AAC.

Optical Considerations in AAC

Visual acuity is a critical factor when evaluating the use of visually based AAC systems. Vision testing to establish acuity levels may be necessary prior to any access evaluation. Existing information on visual acuity should be obtained as part of the background information at the time of referral. Acuity affects the size of symbols, the type of symbols, and the spacing of symbols. It also affects the positioning of the AAC system relative to the user. Light and color are also factors affected by acuity (Beukelman, Mirenda, Franklin & Newman, 1992). Nearsighted individuals often prefer a display that is well lit. Individuals with decreased visual acuity may benefit from symbols that are color-cued to locate symbols on their display more easily.

Visual field is another optical consideration. "Visual field refers to the area in which objects are visible to the eye without a shift in gaze, normally extending in arcs of 150 degrees from right to left and 120 degrees up and down" (Jose, 1983). Visual field losses may require modifications to the arrangement of visual symbols on an AAC display and also to the position of the AAC system relative to the user.

The visual processing of information is another factor that can have serious ramifications on the effective use of AAC. In situations involving milder impairments, the individual may have visual discrimination difficulties that are remedied by the use of background or foreground color cues or by highlighting a critical part of the symbol. When visual figure–ground problems arise, accommodations include fewer symbols on a page, separating symbols, or grouping symbols in a logical way

(e.g., by parts of speech or by activity). The type of symbols selected will also be important. Some symbols will have to be simplified in order to eliminate extraneous details. Enlarging symbols can also be effective to counteract visual perceptual problems.

In some cases, severe visual processing problems will negatively impact or even preclude the use of a visually based AAC system. These individuals have difficulty interpreting what they see. The root of the problem is not acuity, because these individuals can often identify people from far away and also small items near them, and cognition is not the critical issue. Individuals with severe visual processing often cannot visually discriminate among objects and pictures that are similar in size and contour, but they can answer higher level associative questions about these items. For example, one young boy could not discriminate a horse from a cow in photo, picture, or toy formats, and yet when asked about these animals, he was able to verbally provide information about the sounds the animals make, and that cows give milk and live on a farm. Individuals with severe visual processing problems may do better with AAC systems designed to provide auditory cues to locate messages.

In some situations, vision may not be stable. Fluctuating vision on a daily basis may be due to environmental conditions (e.g., light or glare) or due to the physical nature of the individual's condition. A gradual decline in vision can also be caused by progressive disease and aging.

Oculomotor Considerations in AAC

Eye muscles are normally coordinated to move together smoothly in all directions. When this does not occur, as in nystagmus (involuntary rhythmical movement of the eyes) or strabismus (focusing problems due to muscular imbalance), it can affect the individual's ability to visually scan, track, and localize. It can also compromise the AAC user's ability to visually survey and fixate on symbol arrays. For individuals using visual scanning, it may affect their speed and accuracy. Symbol layout and spacing, as well as the positioning of the AAC system, are all accommodations to be considered in individuals demonstrating oculomotor difficulties.

Environmental Effects on Vision

Insufficient lighting and poor natural lighting are common environmental problems that can compromise the use of AAC. Glare is a byproduct of poor lighting conditions and can be caused by harsh natural light or by overhead lighting reflected off the AAC user's communication display. Glare shields or changing the position of the device or the user can sometimes mitigate the effects of glare. AAC devices with dynamic displays and laptop computers with passive matrix screens are often difficult to see clearly from different angles. Individuals with physical disabilities with extraneous head or trunk movement may have difficulty viewing these systems if they move out of the midline area of the device.

Assessing Visual Abilities for AAC

Some aspects of visual ability, such as acuity and visual field loss, should be formally evaluated by opthalmologists, optometrists, or vision specialists prior to the AAC evaluation. During the access portion of the AAC assessment, it is useful to examine functional visual and perceptual abilities. Screening can be done utilizing traditional clinical methods to examine skills in isolation, or can be incorporated into the course of the evaluation using more of a criterion referenced approach.

Oculomotor skills can be screened by evaluating the individual's ability to do the following tasks:

- Look at a moving target to assess tracking skills and the ability of the eyes to work together.
- Maintain gaze on a fixed target to assess visual fixation skills (this should be evaluated relative to head movement and visual range).
- Quickly find a picture symbol or word on a page to assess localizing skills (gradually increase the number of items on the page).
- Scan rows or columns of symbols to assess visual scanning skills. (gradually increase the number of items within the rows and columns).

It is important to note that even though an individual demonstrates difficulty with oculomotor control, it does not necessarily follow that he or she will be unable to use a visually based communication system. Individuals are quite capable of adaptation, and oculomotor problems do not always prevent successful use of AAC systems.

When examining oculomotor skills, it is equally important to look at these skills in direct use with appropriate AAC systems. It is difficult to examine visual skills in isolation when assessing the use of AAC devices. Visual abilities interact with motor, cognitive, and language abilities. However, observations during repeated practice trials with an AAC system will provide needed information on oculomotor functioning relative to AAC use. Modifications may include changing the layout of symbols, enlarging symbols, and highlighting symbols with color. Adding tactile cues through the use of tactual symbols or grid markers may also be beneficial. For AAC consumers who use scanning, slowing the scan speed or adding auditory cues may improve success.

The visual processing of symbols can be sequentially assessed by asking the individual to identify different types of individual pictures or symbols (e.g., photographs, colored drawings, black and white drawings, picture communication symbols, or text). Using cognitively appropriate types of pictures or symbols, assess the ability to identify the smallest viable size, ranging from largest (3 to 4 inch) to smallest (½ inch) pictures or symbols.

Using standard grid sizes from AAC devices, the evaluator can then assess the individual's ability to visually discriminate pictures or symbols from different types of overlays (e.g., 8 location, 20 location, 32 location, and up to 128 location grids). If direct selection motor skills are problematic or if visual scanning is a consideration, then the types of overlays presented should be in keeping with available pointing or scanning skills. Once the evaluator has an estimate of the type of overlay, refinements to the arrangement of pictures or symbols on the overlay can be examined. Also, the type of color enhancements that are beneficial (background color, highlighting the background of individuals symbols, coloring the symbols) can be assessed. This evaluation is generally not completed in a single session and usually represents an ongoing aspect of evaluation as vocabulary is developed and overlays are modified in design. For additional information on visual accents to enhance communication symbols, the reader is referred to Bailey and Downing (1994).

During this assessment of visual skills related to AAC, it is beneficial once again to look at positioning with respect to visual considerations. If the individual can point, should the overlay be positioned flat on a table, at an angle, or at eye level? Is there less glare in certain environments with the overlay or device in a different position? For individuals using visual scanning, should the device be angled, positioned low or high, or mounted to the left, center, or to the right? Whenever possible, the system should not block the user's line of vision.

Due to the fact that many AAC systems are visually based systems, the impact of visual abilities described in the preceding paragraphs must be carefully considered when conducting AAC evaluations. In the next section, which focuses on motor access evaluation, visual considerations will continue to play a role. It is important to emphasize that AAC evaluation is a dynamic process and that one area of assessment can have an effect on another area; visual abilities and motor abilities along with cognitive and linguistic abilities are usually intertwined.

EVALUATING MOTOR ACCESS

Literature on Motor Access

More and more is being written on the subject of AAC in professional journals, books, parent magazines, and trade newsletters. There is a growing number of articles on subjects related to assistive technology, including motor input and its effect on AAC. Angelo and Smith (1993) conducted a review of technology-related articles in occupational therapy (O.T.) periodicals and other O.T. sources over an 11-year period from 1978 through 1988 and found 174 articles pertaining to assistive technology. The types of articles reviewed included research, client training, informational, and training articles. Research-oriented articles employed case study, survey, and single subject design methodologies, but constituted a small percentage of articles found. Overall, there is a lack of research-oriented articles that address motor access issues. The field of AAC is still quite young and this is expected to change in the years to come.

Articles on motor access and AAC appear to fall into three main categories: descriptions or comparisons of input methods and AAC systems, normative studies using able-bodied individuals to examine input methods and strategies, and descriptive case studies or single subject designs. According to Szeto, Allen, and Littrell (1993), objective comparisons of AAC devices and input methods are complicated by the ever-changing number and types of devices available, and the difficulty of finding individuals with similar disabilities using similar devices to take part in controlled studies. Although the number of empirical studies is increasing, there is still a paucity of research on the many variables that affect decisions on motor access and AAC. Research data are needed on how different AAC configurations affect the speed, accuracy, and ease of communication (Mathy-Laikko & Yoder, 1986; Smith, Thurston, Light, Parnes, & O'Keefe, 1989).

Most professionals agree and existing studies show that direct selection is faster than scanning. For example, Szeto et al. (1993) conducted a study with 16 able-bodied college students, using four electronic devices paired with three input devices to copy text and to communicate. Direct selection using a light pointer was fastest, followed by joystick control. Single switch scanning was slowest. In a study by Levine, Gauger, and Bowers (1986), mouthstick use was compared to Morse code using a sip-and-puff switch with able-bodied subjects. Again, the direct selection method (mouthstick) resulted in a higher number of words per minute. This study also included one C2 quadriplegic subject who used Morse code at a faster rate than the able-bodied subjects, which raises the issue of the generalizability of research conducted with able-bodied subjects. Speed is not the only factor for consideration, however. Other issues must also be taken into consideration, such as ease of use and degree of fatigue, when deciding between direct selection and indirect scanning methods.

Ratcliff (1994) conducted a study with 100 able-bodied children in grades 1 to 5 to evaluate the use of an optical pointer versus row column scanning. She determined that row column scanning produced more errors than direct selection using an optical head pointer. Ratcliff's assertions are consistent with conventional beliefs that scanning is slower, more physically difficult, and more cognitively complex. Passive waiting (Harris, 1982) and memory load (Beukelman & Mirenda, 1992) are two issues that may contribute to the greater degree of difficulty associated with row column scanning. Ratcliff also postulated that the difficult demands of row column scanning may be related to the type of electronic device being used; scanning features may be better on some devices than on others. Fried-Oken (1989) looked specifically at visual scanning, auditory scanning, and combined visual-auditory scanning. In a study of 90 able-bodied adults, response accuracy and reaction times were best for visual scanning and poorest for auditory scanning. Combined visual-auditory scanning scored between the two.

Szeto et al. (1993) found that the type of switch had more of an effect on speed than accuracy. The most common errors across all methods were the insertion or omission of characters or spaces, totaling over 60 percent of all errors. The best row column scanning rate for copying tasks after four trial sessions was three words per minute, suggesting the need for acceleration or rate enhancement techniques, such as word prediction, when using scanning. By comparison, the keyboarding rates of able-bodied experienced and inexperienced typists for written expression (not transcription) fell around 27 and 16 words per minutes, respectively, in a study conducted by Weeks, Kelly, and Chapanis, (1974). Thus, in the absence of acceleration techniques, scanning is significantly slower than typing for purposes of written expression.

In Blackstone's issue of *Augmentative Communication News* (1989), which focused on visual scanning, she asserted that there was no set hierarchy for teaching different scanning skills. She further stated that there was no research that demonstrated the age at which scanning could be taught, though some experts report children as young as 4 (developmentally) achieving success with row column scanning. In Blackstone's synthesis of expert opinion, the following emerged as prerequisites to the introduction of visual scanning: seating and positioning must facilitate function; movement, control site, and switch options must be delineated; the switch and device must be well positioned; and scanning instruction may require conceptual task analysis. In a discussion on scanning considerations with respect to children with severe physical disabilities, Treviranus and Tannock (1987) suggested that scanning systems must have built-in flexibility, provide a range of scanning methods, allow for changes in speed, and allow for numerous displays that can be customized for layout design, quantity, and size of symbols.

Seating and positioning can have an effect on direct selection as well as scanning. Bay (1991) used a single subject design with an adult with spastic quadriplegia and choreoathetosis who used a Light Talker with an optical pointer. The study demonstrated that changes in positioning caused improvements in typing rate of speed and in typing rate of accuracy.

Everson and Goodwyn (1987) conducted a comparison of the use of switches by adolescents with cerebral palsy. In their discussion on the use of switches, they reported that reliable motor responses appeared to depend on optimal seating and positioning, the position and mounting of the switches, the quality and control of the individual's movement, and the motivation and cooperation of the student.

Evaluating Motor Skills

The evaluation of motor skills is a process that becomes more comfortable for professionals over time. Initially, it is best to observe professionals who are experienced in motor access evaluations. Based on this author's experience, mentoring is useful because it takes experience with approximately 25 to 50 AAC access evaluations before one becomes comfortable with this type of assessment and begins to see patterns emerge (e.g., seating issues as they relate to motor skills, motor skills as they relate to symbol selection, or visual skills as they relate to symbol selection).

There are no comprehensive, standardized, norm-referenced motor access evaluations available. Norm-referenced standardized tests are based on the performance of typical age peers. AAC users generally require adapted test methods using nonstandardized presentations due to time limits, limited speaking skills, or lack of fine motor skills. Consequently, norm-referenced tests do not apply. Motor access evaluations are more often criterion-referenced and have a direct tie to specific AAC system features. Criterion-referenced evaluations involve yes/no decisions which help to narrow down the AAC options. For example, can the individual point? This must be assessed for all body parts, including eye and head movements. If the individual cannot point effectively, then AAC systems utilizing scanning should be considered. Can the individual manage linear step scanning? If the answer is yes, can the individual move to circular automatic scanning or group-item scanning? Recommendations regarding AAC rely on a decision-making branching process across many variables. More often, motor access recommendations are tied directly to the specific features of available AAC systems.

According to Beukelman and Mirenda, "the goal of the motor access assessment in AAC is to discover motor capabilities, not to describe motor deficits" (1992, p. 122). In light of this goal, some attempts have been made to formalize the assessment of motor access. Formal assessments follow a specific set of guidelines. Lee and Thomas (1990) devised a comprehensive clinical access assessment manual which provided step by step procedures for a nine stage Control Assessment Protocol. The manual also included 14 sample assessment forms. Other formal assessments are software-based such as the *Switch Assessment Program* and the *Text Entry Assessment Program*. These software programs, available through the Assistive Device Center at California State University (School of Engineering and Computer Science, California State University, Sacramento, CA 95819), provide hard data on the hold and release time of switch use or a client's ability to use switches to enter text.

Informal assessments provide general guidelines and follow a less structured protocol (Beukelman & Mirenda, 1992; Goossens & Crain, 1986, 1992; Wright & Nomura, 1985). Informal protocols also allow for flexibility in how the assessment is presented. Anson (1994) devised a decision matrix called the Roadmap to Computer Access Technology as a tool to help therapists make decisions regarding access methods. Goossens and Crain (1986) described an informal MSIP assessment devised by staff at the Hugh MacMillan Medical Center which includes four basic areas of motor access assessment: M = movement pattern, S = control site, I = input method (originally referred to as switch "interface"), and P = position. The MSIP assessment was originally designed for evaluating single switch use. As a set of guidelines, it can also be applied to the evaluation of direct selection (e.g., finger pointing, head pointing, and light pointing). It has served this author well, with some adaptations, over the years because it offers a systematic outline for technology-based motor assessments. To the original four components of MSIP this author has also added a new component, T= Targeting.

Using the adapted MSIPT format, each of the components is examined as part of the access evaluation. There is a sequential and cumulative aspect to the MSIPT components. For example, once a movement pattern is delineated, then the control site is identified. Thereafter, information on movement and site is applied to decisions regarding input method. Positioning decisions hinge on movement-site-input decisions. Targeting decisions depend on information gleaned from the previous areas of assessment. The consequence of this sequential yet cumulative effect is that the variables must be examined in relation to other variables and only one MSIPT variable can be changed at a time in order to assess the impact. As professionals advance their skill and experience with MSIPT components and their application to a wide variety of clients, then multiple MSIPT variables can be manipulated simultaneously during the course of an evaluation. For the purposes of this chapter, MSIPT components will be described as a sequential process.

The MSIPT approach, adapted from the Hugh MacMillan Medical Center MSIP assessment (Goossens & Crain, 1986), provides an outline of critical areas of motor access evaluation. It can be used to steer the assessment process without holding the evaluator to a rigid protocol. For the purposes of this chapter, MSIPT provides a schema for motor access assessment.

MSIPT Assessment

MSIPT assessment involves the systematic examination of five major components: movement, control site, input method, position, and targeting. Prior to the beginning of the actual MSIPT assessment, it is important to describe the position of the individual and any adaptations made to positioning. Changes to the individual's positioning will often affect the performance of different motor skills; therefore, it is critical to describe carefully the seating and positioning used during each MSIPT combination. For example, if a client is positioned poorly in his wheelchair with his body curved to one side, body alignment is affected. This will result in poor head positioning, which will compromise any assessment of the individual's ability to access a switch with his head. Using another example, if a client has slid forward and down in her wheelchair (creating a posteriorly tilted pelvis), it will be more difficult for the individual to bring her upper body forward to reach, thereby compromising the assessment of direct selection. Documenting the positions used during assessment is also important for practice trials at a later date.

With young children and individuals with cognitive impairments, it is important to incorporate motivating and meaningful activities into the assessment process, and it is important to document the activities that were used as motivators or reinforcers during the MSIPT assessment. These activities, however, should not be cognitively loaded. The activity demands should be simple and well within the individual's cognitive, language, and visual abilities. For example, when evaluating motor access with Maria, we used a simple overlay in conjunction with a nail polish activity. Using picture communication symbols, Maria could choose to file her nails, choose a nail polish color, use some lotion, comment on how her nails looked, and so forth. When evaluating pointing accuracy, you may want to use colorful stickers to assess the range of motion of a child's pointing skills. Beukelman and Mirenda (1992) suggested using coins that the child can keep when evaluating pointing skills. When evaluating switch access, you may want to use a simple switch toy, a tape recorder with some popular tapes, or favorite songs programmed into a voice output device. Information regarding motivating or reinforcing activities is

also useful later when outlining MSIPT training strategies.

When the individual is first referred, it is important to obtain general information on the individual's motor skills. Can the child point and to what size target? Does the individual have good head control? Table 7–1 lists these and other questions that can provide useful up-front information. For example, a parent or teacher may be asked in advance whether the child can point. If the answer reflects that the child can point using gross shoulder movement and a whole hand approach, then questions regarding the size and number of targets should be asked. The first step in the actual MSIPT assessment would then begin with an objective assessment of upper extremity direct selection to determine the exact range of pointing accuracy. Prior observation or videotaping is often helpful in narrowing down the potential MSIPT combinations that will be evaluated as part of the motor assessment.

Generally, at the conclusion of the MSIPT assessment, one to three effective MSIPT combinations can be identified. Using repeated practice trials, the evaluator can delineate MSIPT combinations that are optimal for that individual. The evaluator can also identify emerging combinations that may require additional motor training for future consideration. Notes on issues such as overall speed, accuracy, reliability, and quality are recorded for each MSIPT combination upon completion of the evaluation. Field trials by way of short-term equipment loans using one or more of the identified MSIPT combinations are often helpful to further document the efficacy of each combination. When this is recommended, training and implementation plans should be outlined.

The next section details the sequential yet cumulative elements of MSIPT assessment. Figure 7–1 provides an example of a form for recording MSIPT observations and provides an example of actual client

Table 7–1. Interview questions prior to conducting a motor access assessment.

1. What types of seating and positioning are used throughout the individual's day?

2. Are there unsolved seating and positioning problems?

3. What assistive technology or augmentative communication systems have been used previously with success?

4. Are there any visual or perceptual problems?

5. Can the individual point? __ yes   __ no

    If yes, how does the individual point best?

        __ using fingers, __ left __ right

        __ using the whole hand, __ left __ right

        __ headpointer or chinstick

        __ other _____

    If no, does the individual have controlled voluntary movement   in some part of the body? Describe this.

        __ eyes _____

        __ head _____

        __ arms _____

        __ legs _____

        __ feet _____

6. What topics or activities are of high interest to the individual?

7. How long can the individual attend without undue fatigue?

data. A blank MSIPT form can be found in Appendix 7–A. The client, "Maria," is a 7-year-old girl with spastic quadriplegia and mild to moderate mental retardation. References to Maria throughout the next section will help to illustrate the MSIPT assessment process.

M: Evaluating Movement

General Guidelines. When evaluating movement, identify the individual's best possible movement patterns, taking into consideration the range of movement, the ease of movement, and the time it takes to contact and release the method of input. Look for overall movements that have good reliability and accuracy and can be performed with the least amount of effort without undue abnormal muscle tone or overflow movements (e.g., increased spasticity, abnormal reflex-

es; Goossens & Crain 1992). Speed of movement, unless very laborious, is generally less of a concern at the initial evaluation stage. The speed with which a person hits a switch or the surface of an AAC device is often less critical than the speed with which they can release the movement.

Informal activities that allow an occupational and a physical therapist to obtain an overall picture of an individual's voluntary and involuntary movement patterns are initially helpful. Reliable, voluntary movements can used as a means of motor access. Upper extremity movement (arms, hands, fingers) and head movements are more commonly used for motor access. Upper extremity and head movements are generally considered more natural methods of access and allow for greater dexterity of movement as compared to lower extremity movement. More often, the AAC

MSIPT ASSESSMENT

Client: Maria _____ Date: _____ Evaluator: _____

Date:	MSIPT # 1	MSIPT # 2	MSIPT # 3
Position of Client	Wheelchair Customized seat insert Tray, chest harness	Wheelchair Customized seat insert Tray, chest harness	Wheelchair Customized seat insert Tray, chest harness
Positioning Adaptations	harness loosened for forward trunk mobility		
Motivators	Nail polish activity	Nail polish activity	Nail polish activity
M: Movement	Forward, right shoulder flexion	Small range head movements	Wrist flexion/extension
Movement concerns	Increased spasticity with volitional movement, wrist flexion with ulnar deviation	Dificulty holding head steady to keep light on 3/8″ sensor	May need forearem stabilization
S: Control Site	Right distal thumb pad	(Optical pointer)	Base of the palm
Site adaptations		Optical pointer angled downward	
I: Input Method	8 location Macaw	Lightpointer on a 32 location AlphaTalker	Light touch plate switch 128 location DeltaTalker
Direct Selection Features: (Keyboard size and configuration, keyguards/grids, pressure sensitivity)	8 location grid Standard acceptance time	Acceptance time set at 1 second	
Scanning Features: Scan method, scan pattern, scan speed, reactivation time, switch hold down time, auditory scan, audiory feedback			Row-column automatic scanning mode Scan speed set at 2.5 sec. Auditory prompting Light pressure switch with click feedback
P: Position of Input Method (Device/switch)	To the right of midline on the wheelchair tray; device on a 45 degree slant	Mounted to the right of midline at eye level	Switch angled 40 degrees on the right side of the tray. Device mounted to the right of midline at eye level
T: Targeting method (Target size, number of keys/ cells, number of active keys/cells)	8 2-inch picture symbols with programmed messages	15 1 & 1/2-inch picture symbols with messages, spaced apart every other cell	25 1/2-inch symbols (5 x 5 layout) with columns separated
Speed of overall response	Too slow to be efficient for communication	Variable	Adequate speed; scan speed may be increased later
Accuracy of overall method	100% accuracy	50% accuracy with many accidental activations. Needs additional practice trials	70% accuracy (7 out of 10 trials) Distractibility affected accuracy
Reliability	Reliability affected by fatigue	Insufficient at this time	Good reliability over a 20 minute period
Overall quality	Severely limits vocabulary for communication	Erratic, distractibilty may be affecting accuracy	Best option at this time
Additional comments	Direct selection limits communication potential, but can be used for some communication activities	This method may have potential, low tech parrallel training is needed	Provides the most vocabulary with good accuracy, without undue effort

Training and Implementation Plan:
1) Four week field trial period and loan of a DeltaTalker.
2) Provide daily opportunities for use of the Liberator, using open-ended activities which allow her to gain proficiency with the motor and visual elements of operating the Liberator.
3) When accuracy reaches about 80%, then initiate activities which require Maria to access a sequence of two symbols using the prediction feature*. (This will help evaluate her potential with Minspeak symbol systems with icon predicion.)
4) Provide low tech parallel training opportunities in the use of a light pointer. Make a customized head mount using low temperature plastics.

Figure. 7–1. MSIPT assessment for Maria.

254

consumer can see what he or she is doing motorically when using arm or head movement. Lower extremity movement is usually evaluated when no effective upper extremity and head movement can be identified. Chin, mouth, and shoulder control are also possible movement areas. Figure 7–2 depicts major potential movement and control sites and serves as a way to help the evaluator envision where to begin. Additional movements and control sites are possible; the important element is to critically analyze the client's motor abilities in order to identify reliable movements which can be used for AAC access. Movement analysis relative to the upper extremities, the head, and lower extremities will be presented, followed by some discussion on abnormal reflexes. Thereafter, the assessment of movement will be discussed relative to direct selection and indirect selection.

Upper Extremity Movement Analysis. To begin, physical or occupational therapists should examine the ease of shoulder, arm, and hand movements for use with direct or indirect selection relative to the following specific movement patterns:

- Forward shoulder flexion and extension
- Horizontal abduction and adduction of the arm
- Internal and external rotation of the arm
- Forearm flexion and extension
- Forearm pronation and supination
- Wrist flexion and extension
- Finger and thumb extension and isolation of movement.

The most common form of direct selection using the upper extremities involves simple finger pointing. For this, forward and horizontal shoulder movement is combined with the ability to isolate an extended finger. Maria (Figure 7–1) used shoulder flexion to bring her right arm forward and activated the Macaw cells with her thumb. Although she was able to use this movement to point, the initiation of the movement was characterized by an increase in spasticity and an awkward angle (ulnar deviation) in her right wrist. Her speed of selecting items was slow and the target size was enlarged. This resulted in a slow method of communication, it caused fatigue, and her vocabulary was then limited to a small number of large symbols.

For individuals with adequate shoulder movement, who are not able to finger point, commercial manual pointing devices (Figure 7–3) and customized splints may assist with direct selection. For individuals with poorly controlled shoulder movement, but who have the ability to control distal finger movement, mobile arm supports (e.g., suspension arm slings or arm positioners that are hinged to promote arm movement) may allow for direct selection. Individuals with moderate to severely limited upper extremity range of movement, but who have some distal hand control, may be able to use a hand-held light pointer, switch-activated device or use a trackball, trackpad, or mouse emulator.

When direct selection upper extremity movements do not offer sufficient control relative to the communication needs of an individual (as in the case of Maria in Figure 7–1), and when other methods of direct selection have been ruled out (e.g., optical pointing or head pointing), then scanning is a consideration. Use of the upper extremities with switch scanning is an option when shoulder movement is limited in range, but is sufficient to access a switch with reasonable speed and efficiency. In Maria's case, her upper extremity movement was adequate to control the timed activation needed to operate the row column scanning of the DeltaTalker. An individual with adequate upper extremity speed may be able to use forward shoulder flexion to punch forward to activate a vertically positioned switch or access a switch with his or her elbow using

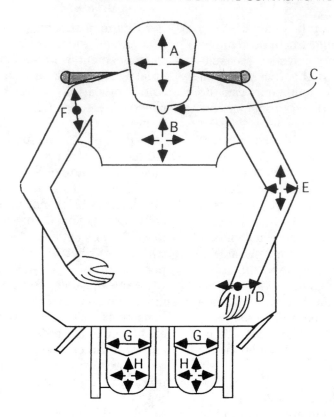

A.   Head Control - forward/backward and left/right movement of the head

B.   Chin Control - forward/backward and left/right movement of the chin, as with a chin controlled joystick

C.   Mouth/Tongue/Lip or Puff/Sip Control

D.   Hand Control - up/down and left/right hand movement

E.   Arm/Elbow Control - movement of the elbow outwards or sliding the arm forward and backward

F.   Shoulder Control - elevation/depression or protraction/retraction of the shoulder

G.   Leg/Knee Control - inward/outward movement of the knee

H.   Foot Control - left/right and up/down movement of the foot

Figure 7–2. Potential movement and control sites. *Note:* From D. M. Bayer, 1984, *DU-IT,* Control Systems Group, Inc., 8765 Township Rd., Shreve, OH. Adapted with permission.

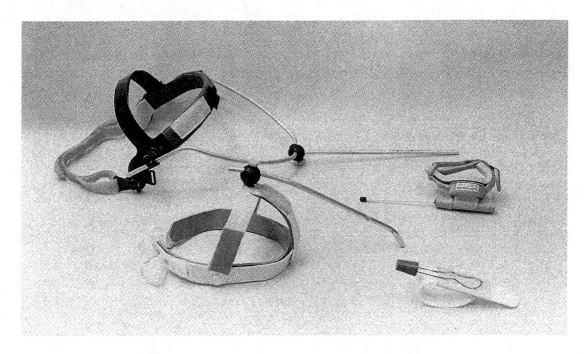

Figure 7–3. Manual pointers and head pointers.

shoulder extension (using a backward movement) or abduction (using a sideways movement). When distal finger or thumb movement is intact, but shoulder and arm movement is limited, as in the case of individuals with muscular dystrophy, then motor access via scanning using a small, light-touch switch is an option. However, when upper extremity movements are unreliable, difficult, too slow, or too fatiguing for an individual then head movements should be investigated.

Head Movement Analysis. In general, physical or occupational therapists will examine head movement for use with direct selection or scanning relative to the following movement patterns.

- Forward flexion and extension of the neck
- Lateral neck flexion
- Neck rotation.

Common methods of motor access using head movement for direct selection include the use of headpointers, chinsticks, and mouthsticks. These movements generally require good head control in a variety of movement planes. Light pointers and optical pointers require less range of movement, but require more sustained, steady control. In Maria's case (Figure 7–1), she was able to control small range head movements in order to move the light across the surface of the device. However, her light pointing lacked accuracy because she could not keep her head steady. This meant that she could not keep the light fixed on the AlphaTalker's tiny ⅜ inch light sensor long enough to activate the cell. Low tech, nonelectronic eye gaze boards (e.g., E-Trans) do not require a great deal of head control; however, high tech computerized pointing systems (e.g., Headmaster, Freewheel) require steady head movements and have a high cognitive load.

Common methods of accessing a switch using the head include moving the head back or to the side to hit a switch. Less common but no less effective movements involve forward head movement for chin or forehead activation.

Lower Extremity Movement Analysis. When head and upper extremity movements have been ruled out, then lower extremity movements such as hip/knee movements (adduction/abduction) or foot movements (plantar flexion/dorsiflexion) can be explored. Again, the best possible movement patterns should be evaluated relative to the range of movement, the ease of movement, and the time it takes to contact and release the method of input. Reliable and accurate movements that can be performed without undue fatigue are preferable. It is important to select lower extremity movements that do not exacerbate pelvic alignment issues (see Chapter 6).

Abnormal Reflex Patterns. It is best to avoid movements that are dominated by abnormal reflex patterns. For example, pointing that is dominated by an ATNR (asymmetric tonic neck reflex, as described in Chapter 6 and shown in Figure 6–4) is often inaccurate and is best avoided. For individuals using head rotation to activate a switch, the effect of the ATNR pulls the child's visual gaze away from the AAC device and interferes with visual scanning. The STNR (symmetric tonic neck reflex as described in Chapter 6) affects motor access because, as the individual extends his or her arms to point or activate a switch, the head and neck extend and the individual may lose visual contact with the AAC device or symbol overlay.

Movements that cause a significant increase in abnormal tone should also be avoided. For example, if the individual using neck extension (moving the head back) to activate a rear-mounted head switch must rely on high amounts of total body extension (straightening and stiffening of the body), then alternative movements should be identified to diminish this. Abnormal movement patterns, such as excessive internal rotation of the arm (i.e., the arm turned inward) and wrist deviation (i.e., angled laterally), should also be avoided or, again, adaptations should be explored to minimize these abnormal movement patterns.

At times it is difficult to avoid completely the influence of abnormal reflexes. When the only available reliable movement has a measure of abnormal movement associated with it, then use the abnormal movement with the objective to gradually phase away from the abnormal pattern. For example, when a child can only hit a switch positioned to the side, which activates the ATNR, then gradually over time move the position of the switch more toward the center or closer to the body to lessen this effect. For additional information on adaptations to mitigate the effects of abnormal reflexes, the reader is referred to Goossens and Crain's discussion of movement pattern selection (1992). For more information regarding normal and abnormal movement patterns, it is important to consult with experienced occupational and physical therapists.

Manipulating Critical Variables. During the evaluation of movement skills, it is critical to change only one variable at a time and in small increments. For example, if it is determined that an individual can use lateral head movement to hit a plate switch, then conduct trials with the switch at the side of the head. The individual should try to hit the switch 5 to 10 times at the side before it is moved to a new position such as closer to the cheek or closer to the back of the head. While trying to determine the optimal position, the evaluator should not change any other variable, such as introducing a different type of switch, or attaching the switch to a new device.

Movement Assessment Specific to Direct Selection. Direct selection is an "access method that allows the user to indicate choices directly by pointing with a body part or technology aid to make a selection" (Church & Glennen, 1992, p. 348). Movements that allow for direct selection are usually the first order of priority for motor access. Direct selection is generally faster than scanning. Goossens and Crain described optimal direct selection as the "response mode that will allow the individual the largest range of motion to accurately target the smallest cell size possible within the least amount of time" (1986, p. 91). The hierarchy of direct selection assessment according to Lee and Thomas (1990) is to focus first on the upper extremities, then the area of the head, face, and mouth, and the lower extremities.

Pointing with a finger, the most common and most acceptable form of direct selection, is usually fastest for communication. When upper extremity use is very limited, pointing with a headstick, a mouthstick, or a light or optical pointer is generally faster than switch scanning. At times, these methods require too much head control for some individuals and fatigue factors must be considered. Parents of young children often have difficulty with the look of headpointers and some light pointers and this must be sensitively addressed. These cosmetic effects should not be ignored, because they increase the likelihood of AAC system abandonment. Eye movement is another form of direct selection for use with eye gaze boards.

In the MSIPT case study of Maria (Figure 7–1), direct selection using her right upper extremity to point was evaluated first. When it became clear that her upper extremity movement was too slow and too limiting to meet her communication needs, then direct selection using an optical pointer was evaluated. Because this method proved to have a high degree of inaccuracy, scanning was then pursued.

Direction selection methods fall into three categories: contact with physical pressure or depression, contact with no physical pressure, or no contact pointing (Beukelman & Mirenda, 1992). Contact via physical pressure or depression requires the individual to push on a membrane surface, touch screen, or keyboard using a finger, pointer stick, etc. Adaptations to these methods can include changing the sensitivity or acceptance time (i.e., the amount of time you must maintain contact with the surface before initial activation) or increasing the repeat delay (the amount of time between key activations). The former is an option for individuals with erratic movement; the latter is for those with tremulous movement or who tend to push too long on a surface or key, causing unwanted repetitive activations.

Contact with no physical pressure occurs when an individual points to a non-electronic picture communication board with a finger, headpointer, mouthstick, or other adaptation for pointing (Figure 7–3). Adaptations for different types of pointing include custom-made splints, commercially available manual pointers, or even the eraser end of a pencil.

No contact pointing includes optical pointers, light pointers (Figure 7–4, or eye gaze. Optical pointers operate via sonar (Headmaster) or are infrared (FreeWheel, Liberator, AlphaTalker, DeltaTalker). A light pointer can be generated by a miniature high intensity flashlight with a focused beam and can be attached to a headband, glasses, or customized head gear. Light pointers are also commercially available (Ability Research, Crestwood, Innocomp and Prentke Romich). Nonelectronic eye gaze involves eye pointing to symbols or text on a transparent eye gaze board, often called an E-Tran. Symbols or text can also be attached by velcro to an eye gaze frame made of PVC pipe, or attached to a communication vest worn by the communication partner (Goossens,

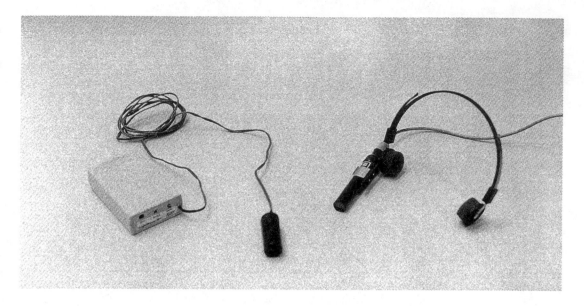

Figure 7—4. Light pointers and optical pointers.

Crain, & Elder, l992). For more information on specific devices and their characteristics, the reader is referred to Chapter 3.

Movement Assessment Specific to Scanning. Scanning is an access method that "involves intermediate selection steps between indicating the choice and actually sending a keystroke or command" (Church & Glennen, 1992, p. 348). Scanning should be evaluated when direct selection movements are limited, too fatiguing, or lack accuracy. For example, Maria (Figure 7–1) had limited arm movement and could only point using gross arm movements to eight large picture communication symbols, but her vocabulary needs were far greater than this. Scanning gave her access to more vocabulary via picture communication symbols.

According to Beukelman and Mirenda (1992), there are six components of switch control and three techniques for scanning. Each will be addressed in turn in the following discussion. Decisions regarding movement must be evaluated in the context of these variables.

The six components of electronic switch control, are waiting, activating, holding, releasing, waiting, and reactivating. The individual must first be able to wait for the appropriate moment to hit the switch, accurately activate the switch, be able to hold the switch for the requisite amount of time, appropriately release the switch, and, as needed, continue the process by waiting and then reactivating the switch. With each of these steps, problems can occur due to individual inabilities. For example, a child may not be able to sustain the visual attention necessary to wait, or may not be able to inhibit extraneous movement, resulting in accidental switch activations. Activation and release abilities may demonstrate inconsistent accuracy due to motor control problems. Some individuals have sufficient motor control to hit and activate a switch, but the movement required to release the switch is not as accurate.

During a motor access evaluation to examine scanning skills, it is important to look at all six components of switch control. In the case of Maria (Figure 7–1), switch activation and release using a light pressure plate switch was adequate. Accuracy errors appeared to be due to distractibility during the waiting period when the light was moving but had not yet reached the desired target.

Scanning techniques refer to the methods by which an individual uses his or her switch to select a communication symbol (e.g., picture or text). Scanning techniques include step scanning, directed scanning, and automatic scanning. Figures 7–5 through 7–7 illustrate scanning techniques employing a voice output device (using a linear scanning pattern which is discussed later in this chapter) to select an "ice cream" picture symbol. With step scanning (Figure 7–5), the indicator moves across one item at a time each time the switch is activated. Using directed scanning (Figure 7–6), the indicator moves as long as the switch is pressed or activated. When the switch is released or deactivated, the indicator then stops at the selected item. In automatic scanning (Figure 7–7), the indicator moves automatically and continuously once the switch is hit until the AAC user hits his or her switch again to interrupt the scanning at the selected communication item. During the motor access evaluation, it may be necessary to provide trials with each of these techniques.

Automatic scanning is often best for individuals who are better at activating a switch and can control wait-time, whereas directed scanning is best for individuals who are better at maintaining and releasing switch activation (Beukelman & Mirenda, 1992; Goossens & Crain, 1992). Both methods require the individual to scan in ways that require timing control. Automatic scanning is a common scanning technique, but directed scanning is considered to be potentially faster. However, directed scanning is also considered to be motorically and cognitively more difficult than step or automatic scanning, as well as potentially more fatiguing (Goossens & Crain, 1992).

Step scanning is generally considered the easiest method of scanning and is used with individuals who can initiate and release a switch repeatedly without undue fatigue, but cannot control a timing element. Step scanning is a slow scanning technique that can only be used with a limited number of symbols. For this reason, step scanning is often used as an initial scanning strategy while training is underway to teach automatic or directed scanning skills (Goossens & Crain, 1992).

S: Evaluating the Control Site

The control site refers to the point of contact with the input device. For direct selection using a touch screen (DynaVox, Touch Screen, SynergyMAC) this may be a body surface such as the index finger or middle finger, or it may be the end of a manual pointer or headpointer. Site is less applicable when evaluating eye gaze or the use of a light beam or optical pointer, as there is no direct contact with the surface of the input device.

When evaluating scanning, it is very important to clearly identify the site of contact. If the best possible movement is head movement, it is important to specify the contact site (e.g., back of the head, right temple, left cheek). Specifying the site of switch contact is particularly important for people who are attempting to replicate this method of access for purposes of reassessment or training. Any positioning adaptations that bring about improvement to the site should be noted. Positioning adaptations could include adjustment of the wheelchair head rest, the angle of a headpointer stick, or the design of a splint to help support the wrist and hand for direct selection.

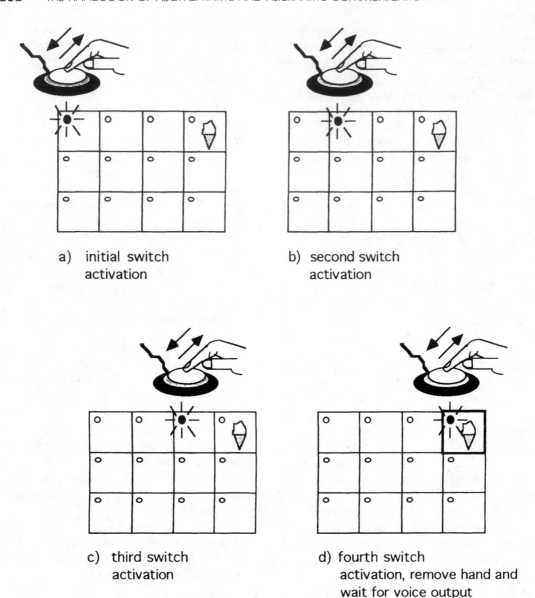

Figure 7–5. Step scanning technique (linear scanning pattern).

I: Evaluating Input Method

Input method refers to the equipment the individual will use to communicate. The input mode can be a standard keyboard, a TouchWindow, or an eye gaze board. It can be a single switch or a joystick, or it can be a combination of equipment, such as a headpointer with a standard keyboard, or a switch with a dynamic screen, voice output device.

Once reliable movements and their control sites have been identified, it is then time to pair these with various input

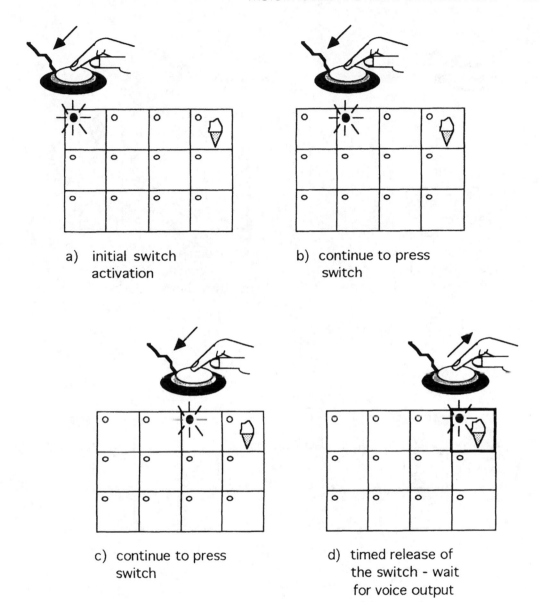

a) initial switch
    activation

b) continue to press
    switch

c) continue to press
    switch

d) timed release of
    the switch - wait
    for voice output

Figure 7–6. Directed scanning technique (linear scanning pattern).

methods. Again, it is important to recognize the sequential yet cumulative path of the MSIPT evaluation. Information regarding movement contributes to the input method phase of the evaluation. Factors that must be considered during this part of the evaluation include: (a) the appropriate type of input method relative to the individual's movement skills, and (b) the accuracy associated with the combined movement and input method. Choices of input methods will depend upon whether the individual is using direct selection or scanning.

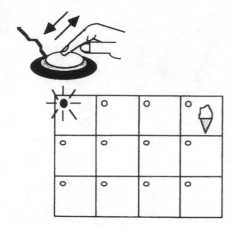

a) initial switch
    activation

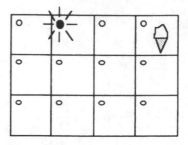

b) indicator light moves
    automatically in preset
    timed intervals

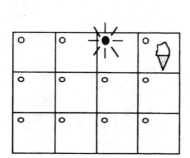

c) indicator light moves
    automatically in preset
    timed intervals

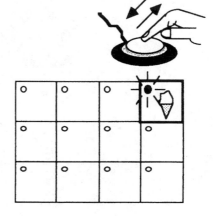

d) timed switch
    activation stops
    indicator light - wait
    for voice output

Figure 7–7. Automatic scanning technique (linear scanning pattern).

Input Methods for Direct Selection. When the individual is using direct selection, input methods are combined in logical ways. Hands, feet, and adapted pointers can be combined with different types of keyboards. Eye gaze is associated with transparent eye gaze boards or frames. Sometimes switches are a direct method of communication, such as AbleNet's BigMack or Enabling Devices's Talking Rocking Plate switch. Using this type of device, voice output is activated as soon as the switch is activated. Figure 7–8 illustrates the relationship between different methods of direct selection and types of input devices.

INPUT METHODS	INPUT DEVICES

Hand/digit(s)
Feet/Toe(s)
Manual pointer
Chinstick
Headpointer
Mouthstick
Adapted splints
	Standard keyboard
	Assisted keyboard
	Alternate keyboard
	    Membrane
	    Depressable
	Low tech communication boards

Eye gaze	Eye gaze board (ETRAN) Eye gaze frame
Light pointer Optical pointer	Eye gaze board Low tech communication boards Light activated keyboard Sonar or infrared sensor to on-screen keyboard
Mouse/mouse emulator Trackball, Trackpad Joystick, multiple directional switches	On-screen keyboard Communication displays
Switch	Direct switch activation, e.g., voice output talking switches

Figure 7–8 Feature match for direct selection. *Note: From Feature Match: PennTech's AAC Assessment Process,* by K. Swengel and T. Varga, 1993, October. Paper presented at the Closing the Gap Conference, Minneapolis, MN. Adapted with permission.

In the case of Maria (Figure 7-1), direct selection using an eight location Macaw was evaluated first to gauge the extent of her upper extremity control. Due to difficulties with that method, direct selection via an optical pointer with the AlphaTalker was attempted to assess the use of small range head control for direct selection. A headpointer was not tried because Maria did not appear to have the large range head control needed to control the use of a headpointer.

Computer-based AAC systems often use arrow keys, the mouse, trackballs, trackpads, and mouse emulators to control the cursor. The individual moves the cursor using one of these methods and clicks to activate the cell that has been programmed for voice output (e.g., Speaking Dynamically). A mouse requires more range of motion than the other methods of input. Although a significant amount of fine motor control is needed to operate these cursor control devices, they should not be ruled out without some clinical trial. Make no assumptions—children and older individuals with physical disabilities often do surprisingly well with these methods.

Figure 7–9 provides a cursor control evaluation form and outlines the major variables that should be addressed to evaluate an individual's ability to control cursor functions via a mouse, trackball, or trackpad. Variables include the type of device (e.g., mouse, trackball, trackpad) and its position, the type of button mechanism, adjustments for the speed at which the cursor moves (i.e., tracking speed), double click speed (i.e., how quickly the button needs to be repeatedly pressed), and the visual size of the on-screen cursor. Targeting accuracy will depend on these variables. Target size will depend on the software. For example, an on-screen keyboard generally has a small target size, whereas dynamic screen AAC devices have variable, customized target size options. The overall quality of an individual's

ability to use cursor control devices will in large part depend on the person's ability to maneuver the cursor in all directions and the degree to which they can master button functions. For additional information on these input methods, the reader is referred to Chapter 3, Figure 3–6.

Input Methods and Scanning. When an individual is using scanning, there are four principal features that must be evaluated relative to a scanning system. Figure 7–10 illustrates the different components: scanning techniques, scanning patterns, switch types, and switch action. Each component must be addressed in order to match features to the AAC system under consideration. Scanning techniques, described previously, include step scanning, automatic scanning, and directed or inverse scanning. Scanning patterns will be discussed in the section on targeting and are also described in Chapter 3 (Figure 3–5). The type of switch chosen during this part of the evaluation will depend on such factors as size, force or pressure, feedback, amount of travel, weight, moisture resistance, safety, and whether single, dual, or multiple switches are needed (Goossens & Crain, 1992).

Scanning speed is another critical variable. Scanning speed is the amount of time it takes for the cursor to move from one cell to the next. Most AAC devices have ways to change the scanning speed. Scanning speed should not be set so high that accuracy is compromised. For more information on switches and scanning methods, the reader should refer to Chapter 3 and Figures 3–7 and 3–8. Switch features and switch actions as described by Goossens and Crain (1992) will be summarized in the following section.

Switch size often depends on the body site or the degree of movement accuracy at the site. The amount of force or pressure required to activate the switch will vary depending on the type of touch

CURSOR CONTROL EVALUATION

Name: _____ Clinician: _____ Date: ___

Movement pattern and control site: _____

ACCESS COMPONENTS	Trial 1	Trial 2	Trial 3	Trial 4
Type of input device				
Position/angle of device				
Software				
Button mechanism (note any adaptations)				
Cursor tracking speed				
Double click speed				
Cursor size				
Target Size				
Directionality/ Targeting Accuracy				
Button Click Accuracy				
Button Down/Drag & Drop Accuracy				

NOTES:

Figure 7–9. Cursor control evaluation. *Note:* From S. Glennen, E. Delsandro, R. Radell, and S. Schiaffino, 1995. Unpublished paper, Kennedy Krieger Institute, Department of Assistive Technology, Baltimore, MD. Adapted with permission.

A SCANNING TECHNIQUES	B SCANNING PATTERNS	C SWITCH TYPES	D SWITCH ACTIONS
Step Automatic Directed or Inverse	Linear Circular Group-item 　　Row-column 　　Column-row 　　Block	Pressure Pneumatic (air sensitive) Motion (mercury, infrared) Photosensitive Physioelectric (muscle tension) Sound activated	Single Dual Multiple

Figure 7–10. Scanning system features. Features from each of the four columns are identified to determine a scanning system. *Note: From Feature Match: PennTech's AAC Assessment Process,* by K. Swengel and T. Varga, 1993, October. Paper presented at the Closing the Gap Conference, Minneapolis, MN. Adapted with permission.

switch. This information is usually available through the individual manufacturers. Feedback refers to information that a switch gives back to the individual to indicate whether the switch is on or off. Switch feedback can be auditory in the form of beeps or clicks, visual, tactile, proprioceptive, or vibrotactile (Goossens & Crain, 1992). The amount of travel refers to the distance from the point of rest to the point of activation. For some switch users, too little travel distance means an increase in accidental activations. For others, too much travel distance results in incomplete activations. Weight is more of an issue when the switch is mounted on the individual's body (e.g., a Du-IT Chin Switch Controller on a Kydex Collar) or held in some way. Individuals with muscular dystrophy who have significant muscle weakness may choose to hold a small switch in

their hand. In this case, a small, lightweight, light action switch such as the TASH Micro Light may be appropriate. Moisture resistance is a factor when the switch is positioned near the mouth and when drooling is an issue. Safety is not to be overlooked. For example, an individual who uses a switch positioned near his or her temple should not use a switch that could cause accidental damage to the eye.

In the case of Maria (Figure 7–1), a light touch plate switch that provided an audible click when activated was selected for use with scanning on the DeltaTalker. The 2 × 4 inch surface of the switch was an adequate size and the light pressure did not require increased force which might result in abnormal upper extremity movement patterns or overflow movements (e.g., oral-facial movements such as tongue protrusion or jaw protrusion).

In addition to single switches, multiple switches are available. Multiple switches give the individual more control when using directed scanning. The use of a joystick or four separate directional switches can control the up, down, left, and right movements of an on-screen cursor. Dual switches or pneumatic switches such as a sip and puff can be used with Morse code. Individuals using a dual switch, who may be Morse code candidates, must be evaluated on their ability to sequence activations across two switches. Individuals using Morse code must eventually memorize input codes requiring a sequence of one to five switch activations using a dual switch (a single switch using a long and short hold-down time can also be used). Joystick and multiple directional switches (e.g., wafer boards) require an evaluation of the individual's ability to manage the motoric and spatial-perceptual elements that link switch actions with the direction of the on-screen cursor. For more information on how to evaluate multiple switch use, the reader is directed to Lee and Thomas (1990).

Switch features are an important consideration when evaluating input methods with scanning or direct selection. Durability is another feature to consider when purchasing a switch. The large number of commercially available switches (Figure 7–11) from companies such as AbleNet, Creative Switch Industries, Don Johnston, DU-IT, Enabling Devices, Prentke Romich, TASH, and Zygo give the evaluator and the client a broad range of options.

Input Methods and Cognitive Considerations. Observations on the level of comfort and the cognitive understanding of

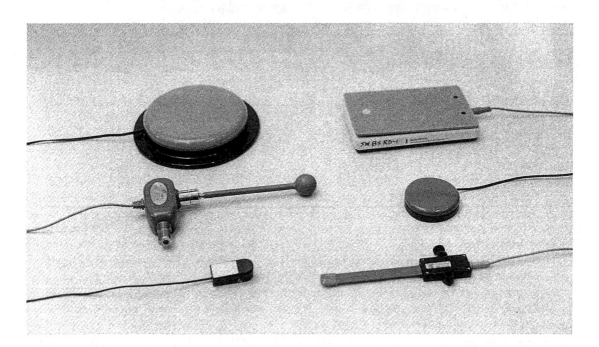

Figure 7–11. Different types of switches. Clockwise from the upper right corner. Don Johnston Bass Switch, TASH Buddy Switch, Zygo Leaf Switch, TASH Micro Light Switch, Toys for Special Children Ultimate Switch, and Able Net Big Red Switch.

the input method is also key. Dynamic touch screens can be confusing to some individuals who become disoriented when the symbol overlay frequently disappears and changes. Scanning is a complex skill and may not be readily understood by the user. However, it is advisable not to jump to hard conclusions about what an individual can or cannot comprehend. At this point in the AAC assessment, it is more important to examine MSIPT combinations with good potential. It will take additional trials and guided practice to determine which input modes are optimal.

P: Evaluating the Position of the Input Method

It is important to clearly delineate the placement of switches and AAC devices. Movement, control site, and input method data are consolidated and applied to decisions relative to the placement of the input method. Motor and visual skills will contribute significantly to decisions on this. The type of AAC device and/or switch will also drive these decisions. However, it is important to note that positioning issues are examined at a variety of points throughout the total MSIPT assessment. For example, the positioning of a head switch will need to be examined while the evaluator is determining movement relative to an input device. Likewise, the positioning of a keyboard will also need to be considered early in the MSIPT process. In Maria's situation (Figure 7–1), the input methods and the positioning of the input methods were evaluated simultaneously. The best position for her plate switch was toward the right side of her tray with the switch placed at a 40 degree angle. The best position for the DeltaTalker was at eye level to the right of midline. Additional positioning issues, such as the exact type of mounting bar for a device or the best switch mount, are evaluated later in the MSIPT process.

The optimal position for a switch or input device relative to the movement site is within the individual's range of motion, but not so close that accidental activations occur. A direct access AAC device may need to be positioned on the wheelchair tray more toward the side, rather than at the midline. The device may need to be on a slant and so the angle of position must be measured. For an individual using scanning, a head switch may need to be positioned next to the cheek, the temple, or the back of the head, and the AAC device may need to be attached to a mounting bar and positioned at midline near eye level. Positioning of the input device should not interfere with the AAC user's line of vision or with routine daily activities. It is often helpful to draw, describe in writing, videotape, or take a picture of the position of the equipment. These methods of documentation will also be helpful later for purposes of reassessment and training.

Using a sequential trial and error approach, try different positions to determine the best arrangement relative to motor skills, visual abilities and input methods. Mounts for devices are usually available through the device manufacturer or representative; switch mounts are also commercially available (Zygo, Tash, Don Johnston, Ablenet). When constructing or purchasing commercial mounts, attention must be paid to the type of clamp that will attach the mount to the wheelchair, table, sidelyer, etc.; to the type of frame (rigid or flexible); and to the method by which the switch or device will be attached to the mount (adjustability and locking mechanisms). The reader is directed to Goossens and Crain (1992) for more information on commercial mounts and how to construct customized mounting systems. Above all, mounts should provide flexibility for positioning switches or input devices, but ultimately must be stable and safe.

T: Evaluating Targeting Methods

Targeting refers to the ability of an individual to access a desired symbol using direct selection or scanning. It typically requires a combination of visual and motor skills, though for individuals relying on auditory scanning, it requires auditory plus motor skills. Targeting skills also involve cognition and memory, especially when scanning is the method of targeting. The design of the communication overlay is a critical element of targeting. Targeting accuracy is affected by the layout of symbols, symbol size, and spacing. When using scanning, scanning patterns are key factors.

In the MSIPT assessment, targeting is initially addressed during the evaluation of movement and during the selection of appropriate input methods. Toward the end of the MSIPT assessment, targeting is addressed in more detail so that overlays can be designed. Detailed targeting assessment may not take place during the initial MSIPT evaluation session, due to the complexity of the individual's access needs and abilities, as well as the fatigue of the individual. Additional appointments may be needed to complete this portion of the assessment.

Targeting assessment will need to take into consideration different access methods across multiple environments and short-term versus long-term communication needs. The design of the overlay might start out with a small number of symbols for trial use and training, with the understanding that symbols will be added over time. Targeting assessment will help to determine the maximum number of symbols, the minimum size of symbols, and the minimum spacing between symbols that can be accessed with accuracy and reliability.

Assessing Targeting with Direct Selection.

Targeting as it relates to pointing can be assessed using a grid paper that simulates the size and shape of the input devices being considered. Grid paper can be divided into ½ inch, 1 inch, 2 inch, or larger squares. The individual is requested to point to places on the grid paper until the pattern of targeting is clear, taking into consideration the individual's speed, accuracy, and range of movement. The individual may be able to reach ½ inch spaces in all quadrants of the surface, or due to motor difficulties, the evaluator may determine that 2 inch squares have the best accuracy and reliability at the midline or on the right side of the grid. It is also important to indicate the position of the grid, including angle, relative to the position of the individual at the time of the evaluation.

This approach can be used to evaluate pointing using fingers, manual pointer adaptations, headsticks, and keyguard adaptations, as well as the use of eye gaze or light pointers. It can be used to evaluate standard or alternate keyboards, as well as fixed or dynamic displays. For these devices, the practitioner can evaluate directly on the device using built-in display options or simulate the device layout on grid paper. Do not require the individual to aim for every square in the grid. Empty spaces adjacent to target spaces will help to illustrate "misses" as well as "hits." Target all four corners of the grid and then target various locations on the grid (see Figure 7–12). In the case of Maria (Figure 7–1), targeting was first evaluated directly on the device. When using the optical headpointer, only half of the cells were programmed to evaluate targeting. Empty spaces were left between cells to better assess accuracy.

Electronic methods of direct selection involving optical pointers and mouse emulators can be evaluated by placing laminated paper on the computer screen or through the use of appropriate on-screen keyboard software. Electronic methods of direct selection using AAC devices usually require added elements of control which must be assessed relative to targeting, such as the ability to hold the light pointer

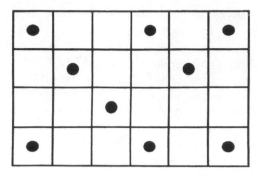

Figure 7–12. Example of a targeting grid.

on the targeted symbol for the required amount of time, and the ability to hold the cursor steady. With fixed, and especially with dynamic touch screens, it is important to look at targeting accuracy relative to accidental activations. Good accuracy is important because numerous accidental activations diminish communication effectiveness.

When evaluating the targeting skills of children, it is helpful to use a game approach (e.g., shine a light at different points on the grid and ask the child to catch the light) or use stickers or pennies as targets on the grid (Beukelman & Mirenda, 1992). Goossens and Crain (1986a) suggested using laminated grids with vinyl colorforms.

Assessing Targeting with Scanning. For individuals using electronic scanning, targeting must be evaluated relative to the type of switch employed as an input device and the type of scanning pattern. Types of switches relative to size and pressure, and so forth, were discussed previously in this chapter. Scanning patterns refer to the visual layout of the pictures, symbols, or text and the manner in which the indicator moves across patterns. (See Figure 3–5 in Chapter 3 for examples of scanning patterns.) The three scanning patterns are linear, circular, and group-item scanning (Beukelman & Mirenda,

1992). With linear scanning, the cursor highlights one item or set of items at a time in a line by line pattern. It is often combined with automatic or step scanning techniques. This pattern is generally easy to learn, but slow and inefficient beyond 10 items. When using auditory linear scanning, items are spoken one at a time.

With circular scanning, items are displayed in a circular layout and highlighted one at a time. Circular scanning can be combined with step, directed, or automatic scanning techniques. Several commercially available circular scanners resemble clocks that use one large dial to point to items (see the Product Directory in Appendix A) or a circular array of lights to highlight items (the VersaScan). Goossens and Crain (1992) provided a description of how to construct a clock scanner. Circular scanning is considered easy to learn, but limited in the number of items that can be presented.

Group item scanning patterns increase the efficiency of scanning when larger numbers of items are being scanned. Group item scanning is usually associated with automatic scanning techniques. Row column scanning is a frequently used method of group item scanning. With this type of scanning, the individual activates his or her switch for the first time and whole rows of items are sequentially highlighted. The individual activates his or her switch a second time to select the desired row of items. Then individual items are highlighted across the row and the user activates his or her switch a third time to select the item of choice. Group item scanning requires more switch activations than linear and circular patterns. Whereas, linear and circular scan patterns require one or two switch activations, group item scanning patterns require three or more activations. Consequently, the individual needs to be able to activate and release a switch repeatedly with good accuracy. It can take months or years to increase speed and accuracy with this approach.

When evaluating scanning, it is important for the evaluator to be familiar with scanning techniques and scanning patterns, and how they can be combined using various AAC systems. For an individual who has never experienced scanning, it is often useful to first assess circular scanning with auditory cueing. If circular scanning proves successful, then move to row column with auditory scanning or another type of group item scanning. The auditory prompts are an option that can be turned off once the scanning pattern is understood. If the device does not have auditory scanning built in, then the evaluator acts as the auditory scan prompt.

In Maria's case (Figure 7–1), she was able to demonstrate immediate success with single switch scanning with audible prompts when limited to the first horizontal row of picture symbols. As a result, row column scanning was introduced with good success for a beginning scanner. It is important to stress that determining what scanning method works best must be based upon the needs and abilities of the AAC consumer. It should not be based on what the evaluator is most familiar with or most comfortable teaching.

There are different types of group item scanning patterns depending upon the patterns that are built into various electronic AAC devices. There is horizontal group scanning, column row scanning, top half-bottom half group scanning patterns, and other forms of block scanning. To view these and other types of scanning, it is best to get to know available patterns associated with specific devices. Again, all of these group-item scanning patterns are designed to increase the efficiency of scanning when access is needed for larger numbers of pictures, symbols or letters, numbers, and function keys. The "pop-up" windows of the DynaVox 2 provide access to additional supplementary vocabulary while maintaining scanning efficiency.

It is not uncommon for individuals who use scanning to use more than one type of scanning pattern. For example, an individual may use group item scanning with his or her communication system, but also use a low tech circular scanning device which has fewer symbol choices during a reading lesson. It is also not uncommon for individuals to use different patterns combined with the various scanning techniques. A child with cerebral palsy may use a simple horizontal step scan for use with numbers 0 to 9, but also use row column scanning for communication. The choice of scanning techniques and scanning patterns relies not only on the abilities of the individual, but also on the nature of different daily activities.

Targeting and the Layout of Symbols. The placement of symbols on a device, whether high-tech or low-tech, should be approached logically from the perspective of the user. In initial trial practices, the evaluator can place vocabulary items in easy access areas. When appropriate, the evaluator may want to consider placing highly motivating symbols in areas that are more difficult to access in order to facilitate the individual's range of control. A strategy that is especially useful for individuals using scanning is to place the most frequently used symbols in areas most easily accessed (Goossens & Crain, 1992).

For example, if a person is using row column scanning, then frequently used symbols would be positioned in the upper left quadrant of the device as this area is accessed with the least amount of wait time. If a person is using direct selection with a finger or headpointer, then frequently used symbols might congregate in the center of the communication board, where the individual demonstrates his or her best pointing accuracy. Other symbol system arrangements and the rationale for their uses are discussed in Chapter 4.

MSIPT Options

At the conclusion of the motor evaluation, there may be one very clear option or two or three MSIPT combinations that look promising. Upon the completion of Maria's evaluation, there was one best option (single switch scanning), one option with possible future potential (optical pointing), and a direct selection option (thumb pointing) which could be used for limited activities.

Qualitative Observations. For each MSIPT option, it is important to record observations regarding speed of response, accuracy, and reliability. The overall quality of the MSIPT option should take into consideration relative ease of movement, short- and long-term fatigue, and communication effectiveness. In Maria's situation (Figure 7–1), the first MSIPT combination involving pointing was direct and accurate, but her performance was slower overall due to increased muscle tone, and she demonstrated a tendency to fatigue. Because of the need for larger symbols, this method also severely limited her access to vocabulary. The second MSIPT involving the use of an optical pointer was only accurate 50% of the time, and therefore, was not an effective method at this time. It may be a method that would improve if Maria were given sufficient training. The third MSIPT option involving

scanning was 70 percent accurate and offered the most in terms of access to vocabulary. Scanning proved to be reliable and she did not show signs of undue effort or fatigue. It was concluded that additional trials over a period of weeks were needed to gain more information on these MSIPT options.

It is also possible that more than one MSIPT option is appropriate. Motor access via pointing to a low tech, eight location communication board may be appropriate for Maria for certain activities such as snack time, which involves a limited predictable vocabulary, whereas single switch scanning is more appropriate for conversational activities. Many AAC devices on the market have direct selection as well as scanning methods built in, which gives the individual the option to change methods within a given day or over a period of time. When purchasing a device for an individual, consideration should be given to a device that will allow the individual to communicate with more than one motor access option. This is important for progressive diseases and traumatic injuries, as well as for static conditions. Above all, recommended access methods should reflect the needs and abilities of the individual and not the biased preferences of the team.

Issues to Consider When Making Recommendations. When the AAC evaluation team meets to discuss evaluation findings, it is important to view the results of the motor access evaluation in light of other considerations. Client preference is the key. If the best method of access is not one the client or his or her family likes, then the likelihood of it being used is lessened. For example, some clients dislike wearing headgear to which an optical pointer is mounted. Affordability is a major concern when there are limited funding options. Durability and repair arrangements should be considered, as well as size, weight, and battery power. Portability and mounting issues must also be addressed. The degree to which the device provides intersystem capability and optional types of input will be important for some consumers. For example, individuals who drive power wheelchairs and use AAC devices will need to transition from one to the other independently. Some individuals use direct selection for part of the day, and as fatigue sets in, need to switch to scanning. And most importantly, will the device have sufficient memory or space to display an increasing number of symbols in order to keep pace with the developing communication needs and capabilities of the individual? Goodness-of-fit depends on many elements. It is up to the AAC team to attend to all of them.

The MSIPT approach is a general outline for how to step through the motor access evaluation. It provides a logical and sequential, yet cumulative, approach to the evaluation of motor skills relative to AAC systems. Again, motor access evaluation takes time and experience to master. It involves problem solving skills and task analysis skills. Therapists who have training and experience in analyzing normal and abnormal movement, combined with AAC specialists who are familiar with the features of a wide range of AAC equipment, are needed to ensure a comprehensive assessment. Video taping the motor access assessment is not only helpful for documentation, but also useful for professionals who are just beginning to conduct these assessments. For beginners or advanced evaluators, video taping provides a way to check impressions and to take an objective second look at motor skills relative to communication abilities.

TRAINING ACCESS SKILLS

Identifying the best methods of access is not enough. Once consensus is reached and a recommendation is made, there is still work to be done relative to motor access. Even before a recommended AAC system is put in place, training needs should be addressed. Light, et al. (1988) as cited in Goossens and Crain (1992), described augmentative communication training as "the process of acquiring operational, linguistic, and social knowledge. Very generally, the child must be able to reliably and effortlessly access an augmentative communication system (operational knowledge) to effectively utilize that system for communicative exchange (social and linguistic knowledge)" (p. 157). To achieve operational knowledge, training is needed. In this final section of the chapter, training as a natural follow-up to access evaluation is discussed.

Regardless of whether this is an initial access assessment or part of the ongoing assessment process, it is likely that additional trials will be necessary to confirm the parameters of a newly identified MSIPT. To ensure the best use of the additional trials, it is imperative to clearly describe the parameters of the MSIPT and to outline training and implementation plans. Parallel training is another reason for providing training strategies. According to Goossens and Crain (1992), when conducting parallel training, "the skills required by the next-more-advanced selection technique are trained concurrent to the child's communicative use of a less taxing technique" (p. 158). Upgrading to new methods of symbol selection may be necessary because the individual needs access to a greater number of communication symbols, or because the individual may ultimately need a faster AAC technique. In the case of Maria (Figure 7–1), field training was recommended for a 4-week trial period using the DeltaTalker and single switch scanning. Longer term parallel training was also recommended using an optical pointer with simple communication boards in appropriate classroom activities. If her accuracy improves, optical pointing would ultimately be faster for Maria than scanning.

At times, motor access training needs isolated instruction prior to use in the natural environment. Clearly, the overarching goal is to integrate communication skills into functional and relevant everyday activities. However, because of the complexity of motor access skills, there are times when skill development may need a period of one-on-one attention. This is not to suggest that absolute skill mastery is a prerequisite to use of an AAC system in the natural environment, only that there are times when pull-out training sessions are necessary (e.g., to reduce distraction and to concentrate on the learning of a new or challenging skill).

Another training concept is that of "layering" (Goossens & Crain, 1992). Layering helps to initially reduce the cognitive, linguistic, and communicative load when training and building access skills. Using a layering approach, the initial training focuses on the motor components, and generally includes visual components. As the child becomes more skillful in managing the visual-motor aspects of the task, additional skills are systematically added to the training task in the following sequence:

1. Motor + visual components
2. Motor + visual + cognitive components
3. Motor + visual + cognitive + communicative components

For example, let's consider a child who is currently using automatic circular scanning with a Dial Scan and a Switch/Latch Timer as a communication device during morning circle time. Training on a voice output device is a next logical step for this child. Using a Macaw, the initial training would focus on the motor and visual aspects of automatic linear scanning; the child would need to shift from using a clock-like pointer to a moving light indicator. The child must then learn to anticipate the moving light indicator, rather than a moving pointer, and hit the switch at the appropriate moment. During this training phase, cognitive and communicative components of the task are minimized. Picture symbols selected for this training phase should be highly familiar to the child and can be used as requests for motivating toys or activities. Cognitive load is reduced when all activations of the device are equally acceptable, such as choosing among favorite songs.

Once the child's proficiency with the visual-motor aspects of the task has increased, then the cognitive load can be increased. Increasing the number of cells programmed for voice output from 4 to 8 or 16 cells, with empty cells between active cells, requires the child to be more careful with the timing of switch activation and adds a cognitive element. Changing the picture communication symbols from a less open-ended format to a more academic format would also increase the cognitive load. As the child achieves mastery at this level, then the communicative load can be increased. Picture symbol overlays can be designed to foster more initiations for social exchange, requesting, commenting, and asking questions.

The concept of layering is especially useful when attempting to teach the component skills for scanning; however, it can also be applied to direct selection skill development. For example, for a child who is being introduced to a headpointer, training will need to focus initially on the motor and visual components of pointing using large objects or pictures as targets. Gradually, the targets will become smaller and can be placed closer together. Later, the cognitive load will be increased when the targets include picture symbols for more academic activities, or if symbol sequencing is required. Focusing on the communicative component is the final layer.

Goossens and Crain (1992) believed that layering allows children to focus on gaining proficiency with one skill at a time, and that it allows trainers to isolate troublesome variables. When all components are presented simultaneously, the trainer cannot easily isolate the source of the problem. In the next section of this chapter, the layering of training components will be discussed relative to direct selection and scanning.

Some individuals will be able to move through the layers of training quite quickly; others may need more time to master the components. It is important to keep in mind that communication is the critical objective. Motor and cognitive elements are important to address, but the communicative use of an AAC system is the true objective. Too often children receive training and are given opportunities to use their AAC system to answer questions or participate in daily activities, but less training time and fewer opportunities are provided that focus on expanding the child's communicative competence.

Training for Direct Selection

Direct selection methods may need training that highlights only the motor and visual components. Individuals with visual-perceptual problems and lack of motor coordination may need training time to focus on the motor and visual aspects of pointing. Or, they may need time to adjust to the use of manual pointers or other adaptations, such as keyguards. Individuals who are being introduced to head pointers, mouthsticks, or optical pointers often need time to develop accuracy with this equipment. Experts feel that decisions regarding the use of light pointers are often made prematurely, in part due to lack of training (Blackstone, 1988). Children with cognitive impairments usually need structured training with eye gaze to learn how to direct and hold their gaze. Young children using single switches (BigMack or loop tapes) or multiple talking switches (ActionVoice, Switch Module, SpeakEasy, Lynx, AIPS Wolf, or the

AlphaTalker with the Remote Switch Adapter) may need time to practice coordinating eye and hand movement to access these switches.

Once motor and visual elements have improved, cognitive components can be added. Children with developmental delays must move beyond the activation of a single talking switch and learn how to make a choice between two or three switches by learning to discriminate among multiple switches that are paired with real objects, mini-objects, or pictures. Children using eye gaze must learn to sequence their gaze to look first at the communication partner to signal readiness, then look at the desired item, and then look back to the partner. Individuals using optical pointers must learn different features of the system, such as how to center the cursor.

Once the motor, visual, and cognitive aspects of the system have been addressed, then it is time to expand the use of the system to meet communication needs. Talking switches can be used to make choices and requests that are environmentally relevant, such as choosing a friend to sit beside at lunch. Eye gaze overlays might at first focus on open-ended play activities such as dressing a baby doll or coloring a picture, but as skills develop, overlays can address more specific communication functions, such as participation in board games, math, or reading activities. Pointing skills can progress from pointing to one symbol that represents a whole sentence, to learning to sequence two to three symbols to formulate a sentence.

Training for Scanning

Scanning skills vary with respect to visual-motor and cognitive skills requirements. Empirical data to help sort this out are sketchy at best. Decisions on how to train switch scanning skills depend upon the switch technique (step, automatic, or directed) that will be employed by the individual. AAC users who will use scanning do not need to learn all scanning techniques or all scanning patterns; training should focus on those scanning skills that appear most likely to lead to effective communication skills. Scanning training should be in line with communication goals. There is no set training hierarchy for scanning. What is important is to task analyze the skills needed for the method of scanning that has been identified as appropriate for that individual.

During the training stage that focuses on motor and visual skills, the emphasis initially is on learning switch control, that is, waiting, activating, holding, and releasing. The degree of switch control for each of these depends on the scanning technique selected. If the goal is to move a child toward automatic scanning, then it may be more important to use strategies that encourage switch activation and release. Adapted switch toys tend to reinforce holding skills and do not reinforce activation and release. Switch latch timers (Tash, Don Johnston, and AbleNet) can assist with this. Switch latch timers can be attached to switch-activated toys or appliances. They allow the item to be turned on by a single activation of the switch. The Don Johnston Switch/Latch Timer provides an audible beep when the child activates the switch to operate the toy. Hitting the switch a second time deactivates the toy. Using AbleNet's PowerLink 2 Control Unit, a radio or blender or other appliance is automatically deactivated after a preselected amount of time, which encourages the child to release and reactivate the switch in order to turn on the appliance again.

The next training stage adds a cognitive component to scanning. Here, the focus shifts to more complex scanning patterns. Training for scanning patterns can begin with low tech approaches. For example, the trainer can teach the individual to hit the switch when the trainer's finger touches the item he or she wants. The trainer slowly drags his or her finger across a row of objects or pictures until the child presses the switch. This is an effective way to introduce timed activations, because the trainer can adjust the speed of scanning according to the needs of the individual. When using low tech techniques to teach linear scanning, objects or pictures can be set up in a horizontal line. When working toward circular scanning, the trainer can arrange pictures in a circle on a bulletin board. The Orcca company has a line of products designed to introduce electronic scanning. Burkhart (1987) described early scanning training using toys that move in horizontal, vertical, and circular directions.

To introduce row column scanning, Goossens and Crain (1992) suggested first working on scanning item by item down a vertical column. Later, add a single horizontal row. Then, add a second vertical row to the scanning pattern. To introduce directional scanning, they suggested working in one direction at a time (i.e., up, down, left, or right). Then work on directed scanning in a cross-shaped pattern. For more information on teaching scanning patterns, the reader is referred to Goossens and Crain (1992).

Scanning training can take place using a dedicated AAC device or on a computer using scanning software. Some software is programmable to teach scanning patterns (Step by Step, Scan and Speak). There are also game-like software programs that reinforce switch control (Make It in Time, Motor Training Games). Interfaces such as Ke:nx allow for customization of scanning patterns on the computer. When focusing on scanning training, it is important to remember that speed and accuracy are relative; even able-bodied individuals cannot achieve 100 percent accuracy with row column scanning (Ratcliff, 1994; Szeto et al., 1993).

Auditory scanning training is critical for visually impaired individuals. Auditory scanning has elements of motor and auditory discrimination skills and is cognitively demanding. Training suggestions include initial low tech training using a live voice, where the trainer speaks the choices slowly with set 2 to 3 second pauses between each spoken choice. The sequence of choices is repeated two to three times. The AAC user hits his or her switch when he or she hears the desired item spoken. At first, it may be useful to pair a highly preferred item with a foil or nonpreferred item as a way to teach discrimination and switch control. For example, "cookie" could be paired with a less-preferred food choice, or "sing me a song" could be paired with "wash my face." At a later date, synthesized or digitized voice scanning using a tape recorder or other AAC device (e.g., Whisper Wolf, Action-Voice, DeltaTalker, Liberator, or DynaVox 2) can be introduced. Initially, auditory scanning training should give the child opportunities to select between concrete choices (e.g., juice/cookie or music/book). Over time, the goal is to expand the communication potential and move toward categories of choices (e.g., food options, playtime options) which then branch to specific choices.

Addressing Communication Needs

Using a layering approach, once the motor, visual, and cognitive training aspects of any scanning system have been addressed, it is important to expand the use of the system to address communication needs. Communication is the ultimate goal and it is important not to lose sight of this. Answering questions regarding numbers, colors, or science concepts is an important academic use of a communication device, but it does not address independent, everyday communication and the development of socialization and linguistic skills. There are numerous texts that describe functional and creative activities for the development of communication skills for children using direct selection, as well as scanning AAC systems (Burkhart, 1987, 1993; Culp & Carlisle, 1988; Elder and Goossens, 1994; Goossens, Crain and Elder, 1992). These texts promote the use of interactive communication strategies in natural environments, and the need for ready access to multiple communication systems within these environments.

Final Recommendations

Ultimately, information derived from the predictive feature match assessment process and training process contributes to the final recommendation for a specific AAC system. Critical paths of information across linguistic, cognitive, and motor domains must be carefully examined. The ability to use this information to make decisions regarding AAC is highly dependent on the skill of the professionals involved. Professionals with limited experience with AAC systems can still contribute needed information on language, cognitive, seating, positioning, visual, and motor issues, but should defer the final decision on a specific AAC system to professionals who specialize in AAC. Collaboration is greatly needed between the experts in AAC and the families and professionals who interact with the individual on a regular basis. Identifying the best AAC system often requires the input of many people in an effort to maximize the client's communication success.

SUMMARY

This chapter outlined the visual and motor access components of AAC assessment. Motor access assessment is combined with other areas of AAC assessment to help delineate the best overall system for communication. Motor access assessment identifies an individual's motor capabilities relative to AAC, while simultaneously factoring out those elements that will impede AAC. Prior to a motor access evaluation, issues of seating and positioning must be adequately addressed. Visual-perceptual issues must also be examined, as these will affect the type of AAC device selected, the types of symbol systems and their layout, as well as the positioning of the AAC system.

Motor access assessment is often an ongoing process. It may require multiple evaluation sessions. Periodic reevaluations are often necessary to monitor the accuracy and efficiency of motor access methods. This is especially true for children in the early developmental years, and for individuals with degenerative conditions. As part of the predictive feature match process, motor access evaluations must look at existing skills, while simultaneously considering long-term issues.

The MSIPT evaluation process described in this chapter is a sequential approach to motor access assessment. Movement patterns, sites of control, input methods, the positioning of devices and input methods, as well as targeting, must be addressed in turn. Direct selection methods are generally preferred because they are faster than scanning methods. However, when an individual's ability to use direct selection is too fatiguing, lacks accuracy, or results in limited access due to limited range of movement, then scanning methods are evaluated. Some individuals will use multiple methods of motor access, direct selection methods for some activities and scanning for others. This often depends on the nature of the activity and on the individual's endurance with different methods of selection. Once MSIPT options are identified, the overall communication effectiveness of these options must be examined relative to speed, accuracy, and reliability.

Motor access assessment, particularly for individuals with physical disabilities, is an essential component of AAC assessment. Logical, well thought out approaches to the evaluation of motor access contribute significantly to the total AAC assessment process, which seeks to maximize an individual's communication success.

REFERENCES

Angelo, J., & Smith, R. O. (1993). An analysis of computer-related articles in occupational therapy periodicals. *American Journal of Occupational Therapy, 47,* 25–29.

Anson, D. (1994). Finding your way in the maze of computer access technology. *American Journal of Occupational Therapy, 48,* 121–129.

Bailey, B. R., & Downing, J. (1994). Visual accents to enhance communication symbols. *RE:view, 26,* 101–117.

Bay, J. L. (1991). Positioning for head control to access an augmentative communication machine. *American Journal of Occupational Therapy, 45,* 544–549.

Bayer, D. M. (1984, June). Brochure on New Products from DU-IT. (Available from DU-IT Control Systems Group, Inc., 8765 Township Rd., #513, Shreve, OH 44676)

Blackstone, S. W. (1988). Upfront. *Augmentative Communication News, 1,* 1.

Blackstone, S. W. (1989). Visual Scanning: Training approaches. *Augmentative Communication News, 2,* 3–4.

Beukelman, D., & Mirenda, P. (1992). *Augmentative and alternative communication: Management of severe communication disorders in children and adults.* Baltimore: Paul H. Brookes.

Beukelman, S., Mirenda, P., Franklin, K., & Newman, K. (1992). Persons with visual and dual sensory impairments. In D. Beukelman & P. Mirenda, *Augmentative and alternative communication: Management of severe communication disorders in children and adults* (pp. 291–307). Baltimore: Paul H. Brookes.

Burkhart, L. J. (1987). *Using computers and speech synthesis to facilitate communicative interaction with young and/or severely physically handicapped children.* (Available from author, 6201 Candle Court, Eldersburg, MD 21784.)

Burkhart, L. J. (1993). *Total augmentative communication in the early childhood classroom.* (Available from author, 6201 Candle Court, Eldersburg, MD 21784.)

Church, G., & Glennen, S. (1992). *The handbook of assistive technology.* San Diego: Singular Publishing Group.

Culp, D. M., & Carlisle, M. (1988). *PACT: Partners in augmentative communication training.* Tucson, AZ: Communication Skill Builders.

Elder, P. S., & Goossens, C. (1994). *Engineering training environments for interactive augmentative communication.* Birmingham, AL: Southeast Augmentative Communication Conference Publications.

Everson, J. M., & Goodwyn, R. (1987). A comparison of the use of adaptive microswitches by students with cerebral palsy. *American Journal of Occupational Therapy, 41,* 739–744.

Fried-Oken, M. (1989). *Sentence recognition for auditory and visual scanning techniques in electronic augmentative communication devices.* Paper presented at the RESNA/USSAAC annual conference, New Orleans, LA.

Goossens, C., & Crain, S. (1986). *Augmentative communication assessment resource.* Wauconda, IL: Don Johnston Developmental Equipment.

Goossens, C., & Crain, S. S. (1992). *Utilizing switch interfaces with children who are severely physically challenged.* Austin, TX: Pro-Ed.

Goossens, C., Crain, S. S., & Elder, P. S. (1992). *Engineering the preschool environment for interactive symbolic communication.* Birmingham, AL: Southeast Augmentative Communication Conference Publications.

Harris, D. (1982). Communicative interaction processes involving nonvocal physically handicapped children. *Topics in Language Disorders, 2,* 21–37.

Jose, R. T. (Ed.) (1983). *Understanding low vision.* New York: American Foundation for the Blind.

Lee, K. S., & Thomas, D. J. (1990). *Control of computer-based technology for people with physical disabilities: An assessment manual.* Toronto: University of Toronto Press.

Levine, S. P., Gauger, J. R. D., Bowers, L. S., & Khan, K. J. (1986). A comparison of mouthstick and Morse code text inputs. *Augmentative and Alternative Communication, 2,* 51–55.

Light, J., Collier, B., Kelford Smith, A., Norris, L., Parnes, P., Rothschild, N., & Woodall, S. (1988, October). *Developing the foundations of communicative competence with users of augmentative and alternative communication systems.* Short course presented at the Fifth Biennial International Conference on Augmentative and Alternative Communication: Animations of the Mind, Anaheim, CA.

Mathy-Laikko, P., & Yoder, D. E. (1986). Future needs and directions. In S. W. Blackstone (Ed.), *Augmentative communication: An introduction* (pp. 471–494). Rockville, MD: American Speech-Language-Hearing Association.

Ratcliff, A. (1994). Comparison of relative demands implicated in direct selection and scanning: Consideration from normal children. *Augmentative and Alternative Communication, 10,* 67–74.

Smith, A. K., Thurston, S., Light, J., Parnes, P., & O'Keefe, B. (1989). The form and use of written communication produced by physically disabled individuals using microcomputers. *Augmentative and Alternative Communication, 5,* 115–124.

Swengel, K., & Varga, T. (1993, October). *Feature match: PennTech's AAC assessment process.* Paper presented at the Closing the Gap Conference, Minneapolis, MN.

Szeto, A. Y. J., Allen, E. J., & Littrell, M. C. (1993). Comparison of speed and accuracy for selected electronic communication devices and input methods. *Augmentative and Alternative Communication, 9,* 229–242.

Treviranus, J. & Tannock, R. (1987). A scanning computer access system for children with severe physical disabilities. *American Journal of Occupational Therapy, 41,* 733–738.

Weeks, C. D., Kelly, M., & Chapanis, A. (1974). Studies in interactive communication: Cooperative problem solving by skilled and unskilled typists in a teletypewriter mode. *Journal of Applied Psychology, 59,* 665–674.

Wright, C., & Nomura, M. (1985). *From toys to computers: Access for the physically disabled child.* (Available from the authors, P.O. Box 700242, San Jose, CA 95170.)

Yorkston, K., & Karlan, G. (1986). Assessment procedures. In S. W. Blackstone (Ed.), *Augmentative communication: An introduction.* (pp. 163–196). Rockville, MD: American Speech-Language-Hearing Association.

APPENDIX 7-A

MSIPT Assessment

Client:_____   Date: _____   Evaluator: _____

Date:	MSIPT # 1	MSIPT # 2	MSIPT # 3
Position of client			
Positioning adaptations			
Motivators			
M: **Movement**			
Movement concerns			
S: **Control Site**			
Site adaptations			
I: **Input method**			
Direct selection features: (Keyboard size and configuration, keyguards/grids, pressure sensitivity)			
Scanning features: (Scan method, scan pattern, scan speed, reactivation time, auditory scan, auditory feedback)			
P. **Position of input method** (Device/switch)			
T: **Targeting method** (Target size, number of keys/cells, number of active keys/cells)			
Speed of overall response			
Accuracy of overall method			
Reliability			
Overall quality			
Additional comments			

Training and Implementation Plan:

282

Chapter 8

THE ROLE OF LITERACY IN AUGMENTATIVE AND ALTERNATIVE COMMUNICATION

Denise C. DeCoste

The development of effective literacy learning programs for children who employ AAC systems due to severe speech and physical disabilities continues to present a monumental challenge to professionals. The reason is simple yet confounding: unable to speak or to manipulate pencil and paper, these children have difficulty developing and demonstrating their ability to read and write through conventional channels. As a result, educators cannot teach them using typical curriculum methods, nor can they evaluate their literacy through speaking or traditional orthography. There is a paucity of research on effective strategies for literacy instruction with this population, and consequently, there are few books which instruct professionals on how to teach literacy to these special individuals.

The first section of this chapter delineates literacy issues as they relate to individuals with severe speech and physical disabilities. The second section provides an overview of early literacy development,

and the final section describes instructional strategies specific to students with disabilities.

LITERACY ISSUES FOR INDIVIDUALS WHO USE AAC

The Importance of Literacy for Individuals Who Use AAC

Literacy for individuals with severe speech and physical disabilities is more than the ability to read a book or the ability to produce a written copy of thoughts; it is a link to information and a vital form of self-expression.

For individuals who are unable to speak, learning to read and to write is not just learning these skills. Literacy is a key to self-expression, a way to say exactly what is on your mind. Literacy provides access to language. (Blackstone & Poock, 1989, p. 1)

Smith, Thurston, Light, Parnes, and O'Keefe (1989) studied the written output generated on a microcomputer over a 4-week period by six individuals who were congenitally, physically disabled. Their results documented that written communication for these individuals was needed predominantly for homework, letter writing, and self-expression. Likewise, Vanderheiden and Lloyd (1986) identified writing, in addition to communicating messages, as important to individuals who are nonspeaking. Vanderheiden (1984) purported that there has been more emphasis on the use of technology for conversational communication for individuals with severe speech and physical disabilities and less emphasis on technology for writing. He stressed that it is critical that individuals learn to use technology that serves as the equivalent of "pencil and paper" to produce written work independently as do their able-bodied peers.

Effective literacy skills breed personal independence for individuals with severe speech and physical disabilities. Smith et al. (1989) stressed that greater independence with writing can decrease an individual's dependence upon an educational assistant to act as that person's scribe, and in the long run, can increase employment and recreational opportunities.

D. A. Koppenhaver, referring to nonspeaking individuals who rely on AAC, stated that writing and spelling are not given due instruction (personal communication, April, 1992). According to Koppenhaver, despite the fact that most AAC users communicate by composing, writing remains the single most neglected aspect of literacy instruction, research, and experience in the lives of most AAC users, especially those with physical impairments. He went on to state that few aspects of writing are more important to the AAC users than spelling, because of its power to expand communication potential.

The Prevalence of Literacy Difficulties in Children with Physical Disabilities

Although students with severe speech and physical disabilities represent a low-incidence population, the educational dilemmas for every one of these students presents a monumental challenge to educators. This challenge has not been met even though descriptive studies have documented the existence of literacy learning difficulties in children with cerebral palsy (CP) for more than 40 years. An excellent review of the literature on literacy issues in individuals with severe speech and physical disabilities was written by Koppenhaver and Yoder (1992).

Koppenhaver and Yoder's (1992) review of the literature indicates that between 50 to 100% of children with congenital CP, depending upon the degree of physical and speech impairment, cannot read. Results of studies examining literacy achievement relative to cognition are listed in Figure 8–1. The general finding of these studies—that about 50% of all students with CP with an average intelligence demonstrate literacy deficits—is a very broad estimate. This estimate actually may be understated among students who have severe physical impairments combined with severe speech impairments. Within this author's school district, students who are nonspeaking and physically disabled are followed by the assistive technology team, which notes their progress in acquiring literacy skills. Six students who are nonspeaking and physically disabled were identified between the ages of 5 and 15. These students attended general education classes with their able-bodied peers and were believed to have cognitive potential within average limits. None of these students was competitive with their peers in reading and writing abilities.

AUTHORS	STUDY SIZE	DESCRIPTION OF THE POPULATION	RESULTS
Barsch and Rudell, 1962	77	ages 5 to 16 attending a CP clinic	48% of the children with I.Q. scores between 90 and 110 scored below grade level in reading
Seidel, Chadwick and Rutter, 1975	23	ages 8 to 15 with CP or neurological dysfunction due to hydrocephalus with a mean I.Q. of 90	reading levels 2 or more years below chronological age
Danilova, 1983	240	ages 7 to 15 with CP receiving a standard public school curriculum in the Soviet Union	53% diagnosed as dysgraphic or dyslexic
Center and Ward, 1984	85	ages 6 to 16, mildly disabled with CP, integrated into regular schools in Australia	50% reported as marginal or unsuccessful with reading
Dorman, 1987	31	adolescents with CP	mean reading scores depressed relative to verbal I.Q. on the WISC-R or WAIS

Figure 8-1. Studies on literacy achievement relative to cognition.

Although it is difficult to administer a standard intelligence test to students with CP who can point, speak, or do both, it is even more difficult to test a student who is severely physically impaired and whose speech is unintelligible to unfamiliar listeners. Only a few studies have been done that specifically examine literacy for individuals with severe speech impairments, severe physical impairments, or both.

Schonell (1956) reexamined the Asher and Schonell (1950) data which suggested a positive correlation between CP and physical disability to reading performance; 75% of those students classified as severely physically handicapped and 100% of those listed as very severely physically handicapped were nonreaders. Of the students classified as quadriplegic, 81% were non-readers. The Barsch and Rudell (1962) study suggests a positive correlation between CP and speech involvement with reading performance. In this study of 77 children with CP, clinical judgment classified the students as articulate or inarticulate. Out of a sample of 19 children classified as inarticulate, 17 were below grade level in reading, 11 out of 19 could not read at all, and 18 out of 19 had limited sight word vocabularies. Smith (1990) compared the standard reading test scores of 10 nonspeaking children with CP, ages 7 to 10, to a group of 10 able-bodied children matched for gender, age, intelligence, and school. The study reported a significant difference between the two groups and found that 9 out of 10 nonspeaking students scored below average in reading.

Only a few studies have examined written literacy in individuals with severe speech and physical disabilities. In a descriptive case study, Berninger and Gans (1986) administered a set of standardized tests to measure the abilities of three males with CP, ages 9, 16, and 40, to process and produce written language. Spelling grade levels were 2, 4, and 6, respectively, and sentence comprehension grade levels were 2, 3, and 3, respectively.

In a 1987 comparative study, Koke and Neilson (as cited by Koppenhaver & Yoder, 1992) collected spelling data from the daily writings of three females with severe speech and physical disabilities, ages 16 to 22. Each individual demonstrated a high number of spelling and grammatical errors. Similar results were obtained in a descriptive case study by Smith et al. (1989). This study examined the written output of six individuals with congenital CP, ages 13 to 22. Writing produced over a 4-week period showed serious difficulty with grammatical morphemes and sentence structure for four of the six individuals.

In sum, literacy deficits among students with severe speech and physical disabilities are well documented. The causes of these literacy problems are less understood. The literature that explores the causes of these deficits is reviewed next.

Possible Reasons for Literacy Learning Difficulties

Koppenhaver and Yoder (1992), in their literature review, reported that:

Studies examining possible underlying reasons for the literacy learning difficulties observed in individuals with CP sort themselves into four categories: the relationship of cognition and literacy learning, concomitant impairments associated with CP, parental beliefs, and the nature of instruction provided to children with CP. (p. 159)

The first category of study, cognition and learning, has been discussed previously in this chapter as it relates to intelligence and CP. Reliable IQ scores are difficult to obtain with any assurance when standardized testing is adapted for young children who are physically handicapped and nonspeaking. At younger ages, motor skills and communication skills often have not reached their full developmental potential. As a result, standardized tests are often not reliable and do not offer valid predictive information regarding literacy potential (Koppenhaver & Yoder, 1992). IQ scores on young students with severe speech and physical disabilities are generally not conclusive at the preschool and early elementary school ages when literacy skills are developing. IQ scores, therefore, do not always provide useful information with which to make decisions regarding individualized teaching strategies for literacy learning. The three remaining categories of study will be described in the following section.

Impairments Associated with Cerebral Palsy

Studies that report on impairments associated with CP as they affect reading and writing focus on hearing and vision problems, including disordered eye movements, speed of writing, and dysarthria (poor articulation). In a descriptive study that looked at school achievement, Bowley (1967) reported that 15 out of 36 children with CP, ages 5 to 16, who did not progress with reading and math had hearing or speech defects. In a case study of an 18-year-old female with congenital quadriparetic CP, with normal hearing and corrected vision, standardized tests indicated reading and spelling scores at the grade 2 and 3 level (Dorman, in Koppenhaver & Yoder, 1992). Dorman reported that error analysis indicated that both visual and auditory deficits interfered with reading proficiency. Simpson (in Koppenhaver & Yoder, 1992), however, found no consistent relationship between perceptual adequacy and reading skill in 60 children with CP, ages 7 to 10, with a mean IQ of 83.

Problems with eye movements are often seen in children with CP. A few studies have explored the relationship of eye movement disorders with reading difficulties; however, no causal connection has been shown (Walsh, 1974). In a pilot study of 28 adults with CP and normal IQ, reading at the third-grade level or higher, disordered eye movements were found to impair reading speed but not the comprehension of text at a fifth-grade level (Jones et al., 1966).

Speed of writing via word processing can affect the quality of composition, as reported in a study of students with learning disabilities by MacArthur and Graham (1987). These researchers concluded that attention to the physical act of typing interferes with the higher order cognitive processes involved in composing. Motor incoordination not only slows the speed of typing, but can impede the quality of written composition.

Students with severe speech and physical disabilities often have very low word processing rates. Smith et al. (1989) reported that the speed of direct selection for their six subjects with CP ranged from 0.7 to 3.3 words per minute (WPM). Koke and Neilson (as cited in Koppenhaver & Yoder, 1992) reported the speed of direct selection to be 1.6 WPM for a subject using one finger, 1.2 WPM for a subject using a chin pointer, and 0.7 for a person using a head switch to scan. It took Christopher Nolan 50 hours spread over 24 days to complete a 2,000 word short story using a headstick (Wallace, in Nolan, 1981). In contrast, able-bodied individuals can usually achieve transcription rates from 40 to as fast as 80 words per minute, although motor demands combined with linguistic demands for purposes of written expression can also affect the speed of writing. In general, the written expression typing rates of able-bodied individuals are signifi-

cantly slower than transcription rates. In a study by Chapanis, Ochsman, and Parrish (1972), written expression typing rates were found to be 18 WPM for experienced typists and 10 WPM for inexperienced typists. Another study by Weeks, Kelly, and Chapanis (1974) obtained written expression rates of 27 WPM for experiences typists and 16 WPM for inexperienced typists. Even when taking into account written expression rates versus text copying rates, the rate of production by individuals with physical disabilities is markedly slower.

A question that is typically asked when young dysarthric students are presented with phonics instruction is whether children can learn letter-sound relationships when they cannot articulate the phonemes (speech sounds). Irwin (1972) found no significant correlation (.21) between articulation and sound discrimination in individuals with CP. Foley (1989) also found no significant correlation in a study of adults, ages 16 to 43, with dysarthria and anarthria. Foley (1993) suggested that linguistic ability may be a more important factor than articulation in the development of literacy skills in individuals with severe speech and physical impairments. Bishop (1985) compared seven adolescents with CP and dysarthria to individuals with physical disabilities and individuals with normal speech on the ability to spell words and found that the subjects with dysarthria had no more difficulty than the control subjects in using phoneme to grapheme relationships even when they could not correctly articulate English phonemes. In a later study, Bishop and Robson (1989) evaluated the spelling abilities of 48 individuals with CP between the ages of 10 and 18. Of this sample, 12 were anarthric and severely physically disabled, 12 were dysarthric, and the remaining 24 individuals had normal speech and served as controls. The researchers determined that the ability to spell words and nonwords (nonsense words) did not depend on speech. One anarthric individual performed perfectly on nonword spelling. However, as compared to the control group, their spelling abilities overall were generally lower. For more information on phonological awareness in nonspeaking individuals, the reader is directed to a review of the literature by Blischak (1994).

Richard Creech, an adult with severe speech and physical disabilities who is highly proficient in literacy skills, expressed the following:

I honestly can't imagine reading without phonetics. I couldn't say the words I read; therefore, my parents taught me to sound them out in my head; and this takes a mastery of phonetics. . . . Reading presents us with abnormal difficulties. Normally children learn to read by reading out loud. They learn the physical shape of sounds and words, which reinforces their reading. I have no idea what "can" feels like, its shape, its texture. To me, "can" is completely abstract. It is a combination of three phonemes that, combined form a morpheme. (1988, p. 12)

Home Environment and Literacy Experiences

The important influence of the home environment and parental support on literacy learning is well-documented in the literature on emergent literacy (Mason, 1980; Teale, 1986). Research on children without disabilities focuses on the importance of home environments that are rich in print and offer children access to printed materials (Stewart & Mason, 1989; Teale, 1978). It focuses on literacy props during play experiences (McGee & Richgels, 1990; Strickland & Morrow, 1989), and on the interactive nature of reading between a parent and a child (Strickland & Taylor, 1989; Sulzby & Teale, 1987). It also focuses on the importance of children having access to drawing and writing tools at home (Clay, 1987).

Only a few studies have investigated the role of the home environment on literacy learning for children with disabilities. Light and Smith (1993) indicated that preschool children with disabilities have a similar range of books and printed materials at home as compared to able-bodied peers; however, there were differences in the frequency and nature of their opportunities with books and printed materials. Whereas able-bodied children often were read to daily, children with disabilities were read to only two to three times per week. And whereas able-bodied children asked and answered questions about what was being read, children with severe speech and physical disabilities more often listened, looked, or pointed to pictures and did not or were unable to communicate interactively during reading opportunities.

Marvin and Mirenda (1993) conducted a survey and found that families of preschool children with disabilities placed a low priority on their children's literacy development and provided fewer experiences at home as compared to families of children in Head Start programs or families of typical preschoolers. In a follow-up study to determine the extent to which single or multiple disabilities may affect home-based literacy experiences, Marvin (1994) found that children with single disabilities were just as likely to have limited access to printed materials and infrequent reading and writing opportunities as children with multiple disabilities.

In a study that examined the quality of story reading interactions between preschoolers with SSPI who use AAC and their mothers, Light, Binger, and Smith (1994) found that mothers typically dominated the interactions and that the children had few means available to participate in the story reading interactions. Overall, studies on home-based literacy experiences suggest that children with disabilities have fewer literacy opportunities, and when literacy opportunities do take place, they are qualitatively different for children who are nonspeaking.

In a retrospective study, Koppenhaver, Evans, and Yoder (1991) conducted structured interviews with 22 literate adults with severe speech and physical disabilities about their childhood reading and writing experiences. Reports suggest that their homes often were rich in reading and writing materials and that they had many varied experiences with printed materials. Time was spent with reading in ways that they could see and follow the printed text. Individuals in this study often credited their parents with supporting them in learning to read. However, it was also found that there was limited access to writing materials. Opportunities to use writing tools were more often for drawing and making letters than for writing to communicate ideas.

Literacy Instruction at School

Although there is much research on reading and writing instruction with populations without disabilities, there is little research on behalf of students with disabilities. The focus of research has more often looked toward disabilities and accompanying deficits as the probable causes of literacy deficits. More studies have been conducted that link the nature of disabilities with literacy learning difficulties than with the nature of instruction. Richard Creech argued that many individuals with disabilities receive less instruction in reading and writing when compared with their peers (1988). The following three studies suggest that students with disabilities may receive quantitatively and qualitatively less literacy instruction, and more time may be provided on reading than on writing.

A descriptive case study by Wasson and Keeler (as cited in Koppenhaver & Yoder, 1992) conducted systematic classroom observations of 6-year-old twins of normal intelligence. One twin was able-bodied in a regular first-grade classroom with 22 students and one teacher. The other twin with severe speech and physical disabilities was in a special education class with eight students, a teacher, and two aides. Analysis of the observations indicated that, for the child with severe speech and physical disabilities, 50% of the school day was spent on noninstructional activities, such as moving in and between rooms, therapies, toileting, and feeding. The child with severe speech and physical disabilities had 20% of the opportunities to respond or ask questions as compared to his twin.

Mike (1987) conducted 63 two-hour observations over a 17-week period in a class of five students with CP, ages 10 to 14, reading below the third-grade level. Four students were severely physically impaired and one had severe speech impairments. Mike determined that actual time spent on reading was about 15 minutes per day and there was little interaction among students.

In a similar study, Koppenhaver and Yoder (1990a, 1990b) videotaped three teacher-student dyads in three states. With each dyad, all literacy instruction was recorded for 1 week during the fall, winter, and spring. All three students had severe speech and physical impairments due to CP, were 12 to 14 years of age, had hearing and vision within normal limits, and read 2 or more years below average for their chronological age. Each of the teachers had at least 5 years' experience teaching students with physical impairments. Between 30% and 42% of instructional time set aside for literacy instruction was lost to noninstructional activities such as fixing the computer, booting-up software, and toileting. More often, students focused on words and sentences in isolation in workbooks and on skill sheets, an activity that has been shown to be unrelated to improvement in reading in students without disabilities (Rosenshine & Stevens, 1984). Out of the 33 total instructional sessions analyzed for the study, there were only 9 occasions when students wrote text, and the students rarely read for more than 2 minutes per hour of instruction. Copying and spelling comprised 80% of the writing time; little time was spent on composing or editing. Writing was less often initiated by the students and more often guided by the teacher who asked questions to which the students could respond.

As part of a larger study, Smith et al. (1989) interviewed six adolescents and adults with severe speech and physical disabilities who demonstrated basic skills in reading and writing. When questioned on what had the greatest impact on learning to read and write, transferring to an integrated (inclusion) program, the efforts of a specific teacher, and access to technology were most often cited. M. Smith (1992) conducted case studies of two non-speaking children with cerebral palsy who have reading abilities in the normal range. The author suggested that the important factors that appeared to contribute to their reading success were good language skills, motivation for reading, the physical ability to point to words and turn pages without adult assistance, and reading support in the home environment. Factors that appeared to have less impact on reading success included visual and auditory memory, as both students scored below average when tested in these areas.

CHANGING VIEWS ON LITERACY

Today there are many books written on literacy development. Texts on emergent literacy in typically developing young children have been available to early childhood educators during the past 20 years. The extent to which special educators have been exposed to this field of study and its applications to special education is spo-

radic at best. Special educators often have little background in teaching reading and writing. When teachers have had coursework in teaching reading, they may not have had any exposure to the study of emergent literacy or that which comes before elementary school. There are few textbooks specific to literacy learning for students with disabilities that can guide teachers.

The section that follows has been written to help summarize the wealth of information that is available on literacy development. The purpose of this section is to promote the understanding that literacy develops early and that instruction in the early years has undergone radical change in response to research on how children acquire literacy skills. Reading and writing connections, as well as the roles of whole language and skill-based instruction, are better understood. Literacy instruction for educators working with students with disabilities must begin with a strong foundation in the basic tenets of early literacy learning.

Historical Influences on Literacy Instruction

Literacy was once viewed as the simple sum of two discrete areas: reading and writing. Today, in contrast, literacy is viewed as a multifaceted product of psycho-sociolinguistic factors, tied to language and cognitive development and to socio-cultural influences (K. Goodman, 1967; McGee & Richgels, 1990; Smith, 1982). Holdaway (1979) provided a framework for viewing literacy. He affirmed that literacy is a matter of language; it has many dimensions (physical, cognitive, and experiential); it is developmental (yet highly individualized and self-regulated); it is learned (in school and in the world at large); it is cultural (influenced by beliefs and attitudes); and, above all, it is highly complex. Holdaway's expanded definition of literacy is the result of an evolution of views: from the early 1900s to the present, there have been many influences on perspectives regarding reading and writing which, in turn, have shifted the ways in which reading and writing are taught. It is important to understand these changes in perspective because they help to explain the lack of instructional paradigms for individuals with disabilities who may not demonstrate the skills considered to be prerequisites for conventional reading and writing.

An understanding of this evolution begins in the early years of the 20th century, when the alphabetic method prevailed. This approach emphasized recognizing and naming letters while learning to read words (Ferreiro & Teberosky, 1982; Holdaway, 1979). Writing for younger children involved copying letters and words.

From the 1920s to the 1950s, gestalt and behaviorist research was dominant. If the whole was the sum of its parts, then it was reasonable to teach letters, then sounds, words, sentences, and paragraphs. Writing was directly taught as a set of individual subskills (encoding skills, sentence forming skills, composition skills, and so forth) in a carefully controlled, part-to-whole hierarchy (Edelsky, Altwerger, & Flores, 1991).

During this time, measurement and testing had a strong influence on educational theory. The maturational view was legitimized in a correlational study of IQ and reading by Morphett and Washburne (1931), who concluded that children with a mental age of 6 years, 6 months made better progress in reading than younger children, and that reading should be postponed until that time. The earliest use of the term "reading readiness" is found in the 1925 *Yearbook of the United States National Society for the Study of Education* (Coltheart, 1979). Tests such as the 1933 *Metropolitan Readiness Test* were designed to determine the skills that correlated with reading achievement. This set the stage for formalizing teaching practices and instructional methods, which

emphasized visual and auditory subskills and the sequenced mastery of prereading skills as a prerequisite to beginning basal readers (Teale & Sulzby, 1986).

By the latter half of the 20th century, the results of infant research by Bruner (1960), Brazelton (1969), and Kagan (1971) shifted the notion of reading readiness toward views on the importance of early intervention (Teale & Sulzby, 1986). The importance of early education took root when these and other studies showed that young children can learn many concepts. This led to the development of structured programs and materials to prepare kindergarten children for reading as soon as possible. With the exception of handwriting, writing to compose was introduced later after children could read. The civil rights activism of the 1960s helped to create early intervention programs such as Head Start, which provided highly structured reading readiness curriculums to minority and disadvantaged children (Teale & Sulzby, 1986). Thereafter, activism on behalf of the rights of individuals with disabilities led to the 1975 enactment of P.L. 94-142, the Education for All Handicapped Act. Reading readiness strategies were adopted into the special education curriculum which was individualized within a structured framework.

In the past decade, however, this approach to early literacy development has been undergoing a challenge. Opponents of reading readiness believe that it is "built upon a logical analysis of literacy skills from an adult perspective rather than upon a developmental perspective" (Teale & Sulzby, 1986, p. xiv). This change in conceptualization has been brought about by research in linguistics (Chomsky, 1957), studies on the metacognitive aspects of literacy learning, and by changes in research methodologies. Piaget, though he did not specifically address reading and writing, shifted the emphasis in educational research to learning from the child's perspective and to concepts of assimilation in learning (Ferreiro & Teberosky, 1982). Vygotsky (1962) made significant contributions to views of literacy as part of language learning, which involves social interaction as children and adults engage in literacy events. Dewey (1938) also emphasized the importance of the active engagement of the learner. M. Clay of New Zealand (1967), along with Durkin (1966), Y. Goodman (1967), and K. Goodman (1967) were among the first educators to investigate, from the child's perspective, how young children learn reading and writing, as opposed to how children are taught these skills.

Throughout this evolutionary period, the focus was more on how children learn to read than on how they learn to write. Graves (1978) observed that interest in reading research occurred before interest in writing research. For most of the century, student writing consisted of correct spelling using good handwriting. Spelling was a subject that had to be learned, and therefore, it was taught in a structured and sequential manner using workbooks and weekly tests.

Only in the past two decades has research on how children acquire written literacy indicated that spelling and writing develop naturally as children gradually make generalizations regarding conventional English (C. Chomsky, 1970; Henderson & Beers, 1980; Read, 1975) and that children's early writing approximations are legitimate attempts to convey meaning in written form (Bissex, 1980; Clay, 1975; Sulzby, 1983).

Emergent Literacy Research

More recently, considerable attention has been given to the study of emergent literacy. Emergent literacy literature focuses not only on instructional philosophies, but on the developmental processes by which children acquire literacy, in school as well as at home. A rapidly growing body of literature has grown out of a wealth of studies which propose that young children naturally develop literacy skills through various environmental influences. An understanding of emergent literacy is necessary to an understanding of literacy instruction for students who are nonspeaking and physically disabled. These students often demonstrate emerging literacy skills much later than their able-bodied peers, and their progress toward conventional reading and writing is often delayed.

Emergent literacy is a term that can be traced back to the 1960s, although the philosophy did not fully establish itself until the 1980s. Emergent literacy refers to children's reading and writing development in the early years (Clay, 1967; Hall, 1987; Mason & Allen, 1986; Teale & Sulzby, 1986). The term *emergent* denotes that development is ongoing (Sulzby, 1986), and *literacy* refers to the ability to find meaning in written symbols (McGee & Richgels, 1990). Sulzby and Teale (1991) delineated the following theoretical perspective:

Emergent Literacy is concerned with the earliest phases of literacy development, the period between birth and the time when children read and write conventionally. The term emergent literacy signals a belief that, in a literate society, young children—even 1- and 2-year-olds—are in the process of becoming literate. (p. 728)

As discussed earlier in this chapter, new lines of research with young children in the 1960s and 1970s (Clark, 1976; Clay, 1967; Durkin, 1966; Plessas & Oakes, 1964) significantly affected views of literacy learning. Emergent literacy research, which is intertwined with whole language research, made use of descriptive methodologies using naturalistic observation and suggested that young children are able to learn to read before the onset of formal schooling, a view that challenged the notion of reading readiness (Sulzby & Teale, 1991). Temple, Nathan, Temple, & Burris (1993, p. xv) referred to emergent literacy and whole language as "allied movements." Teale and Sulzby (1989) have delineated five dimensions to describe the emergent literacy perspective as seen in Table 8–1.

Research studies and detailed observations lend support to Teale and Sulzby's emergent literacy perspective. For example, descriptive studies show that children's interest in books often begins in the first year of life (Doake, 1986; Snow & Ninio, 1986). Though circumstances and events may differ, many children are exposed to a wide range of literacy events as they grow and observe adults pay bills, read the newspaper, check television listings, read recipes, write greeting cards and write shopping lists (Strickland & Morrow, 1989; Teale, 1986). In their play and in their drawings, many children scribble to imitate writing and use inventive spelling to add meaning to their pictures as shown by intensive comparative studies of individual children (Dyson, 1985; Ferreiro & Teberosky, 1982). Children often engage in pretend reading using their own words and yet they retain the meaning of the original story, as demonstrated in a descriptive developmental study by Sulzby (1985a). As they actively engage in these activities, children begin to form and test hypotheses about written language, such as how sounds relate to symbols and how symbols are combined in writing as exemplified in research by Clay (1975), Dyson (1985), Ferreiro & Teberosky (1982), Harste, Woodward & Burke (1984), and Read (1975).

Ferreiro and Teberosky (1982) conducted a well-known research study with 63 children ages four to six in Argentina and found that the children understood a great deal about print before participation in formal instruction in reading and writing. They maintained that reading is not deciphering and writing is not copying. Freeman and Whitesell (1985) conducted a similar study with children in Arizona, confirming the Ferreiro and Teberosky study. These studies demonstrate that children acquire literacy in the absence of formal instruction, the very thesis of emergent literacy.

Reading and Writing Connections

Overall, reading has received far more attention in the literature than writing (Birnbaum & Emig, 1983; Graves, 1978). However, in the last decade, research on reading and writing connections coupled with the research on emergent writing with young children has begun to redress the balance of attention toward the importance of writing instruction.

According to Birnbaum and Emig (1983), reading and writing are related but

Table 8–1. Five dimensions of the emergent literacy perspective.

- Reading and writing begin early.
- Literacy develops in real life settings to accomplish real goals.
- Reading and writing develop concurrently.
- Children learn through active encounters with written text.
- Adult-child interactions, especially in the home, influence literacy learning.

Source: Compiled from "Emergent Literacy: New Perspectives," by W. H. Teale and E. Sulzby, in D. S. Strickland and L. M. Morrow (Eds.), *Emerging Literacy: Young Children Learn to Read and Write,* 1989, Delaware: International Reading.

not "mirror images" of one another; "experiences in one may enhance growth in the other and their development may be intertwined" (p. 99). Tierney and Shanahan (1991) stated that reading and writing are influential to each other, especially in word-related knowledge in the early years. Reading and writing are also acts of composing and share similar, though not identical, underlying processes (Tierney & Pearson, 1983).

Certainly the work of C. Chomsky (1970) and Read (1971) demonstrated the relationship between phonics and writing. Chomsky asserted that writing for young children provides practice in letter-sound relationships and word analysis. Clay (1975) theorized that writing is a compliment to reading because it focuses the child's attention on the visual details of print. Dobson (1989) conducted systematic observations over a 2-year period of 18 children from the start of kindergarten to the end of first grade. Classrooms focused on reading and writing as part of language learning. Dobson found that the children first explored the mechanics of written language in their own writing and in the rereading of their own writing. Over time, the children refined their print strategies and applied this knowledge to storybook reading. But she also noted that the children composed more complex writing in response to story reading than on topics of their own choosing. She also found that children began at different levels of reading and writing abilities and developed at different rates. As a result of their research, Sulzby and Teale proposed that "reading and writing are not separate in a child's learning, nor do they develop sequentially. Instead, the two processes are mutually supportive and are intimately related to oral language" (1985, p. 11). In drawing conclusions from her research, Ehri (1989) described the interrelatedness of writing and reading as follows:

Writing draws learners' attention to sounds in words and to letters that might symbolize those sounds. This creates expectations about how spellings might be structured and makes learners more interested not only in the spellings of specific words, but also in how the general spelling system works. Reading exposes learners to the conventional spellings of words and declares which of the various possibilities are "correct." It provides the input learners need to store the correct spellings of specific words in memory and also to figure out how the general system works. (p. 65)

Dyson (1982) theorized that children must be actively involved in the writing process and that writing by dictation, common to the language experience approach, does not engage children directly. Dyson wrote that as children seek to solve the written language puzzle, "children must organize and put into action their conceptions of writing. In attempting to read or to have others read their writing, they must face the inevitable contradictions between what they thought they were doing and what they in fact did" (p. 833). Dyson stated that children must be given the opportunity to play with this puzzle in ways that are meaningful to them.

Shanahan (1988) outlined seven principles of instruction based upon research on reading and writing relationships. Aulls (1985) provided additional input on environmental factors that are important to reading and writing instruction (see Table 8–2).

A number of studies have demonstrated successful writing experiences with children (Haley-James, 1982; Hauser, 1982; Sowers, 1979). In a study on reluctant readers, Dobson (1985) conducted a ½ hour per day writing program with eight students who had shown little progress and interest in language arts during the first half of first grade. At the start, these students knew letter names, had a few sight words, knew some letter-sound correspondences, could write their names, and were inattentive during story reading. During daily writing sessions, the teacher's focus was on meaning and not on form. Children were en-

Table 8–2. Important principles of reading and writing instruction.

Shanahan:

- Reading and writing both need to be taught.
- They should be taught from the earliest grade levels.
- The reading-writing relationship should be emphasized in different ways at different developmental levels.
- Knowledge and process relations need to be emphasized.
- The connections between reading and writing should be made explicit to children.
- The communication aspects of reading and writing should be emphasized.
- Reading and writing should be taught in meaningful contexts.

Aulls:

- Continued opportunities to read and write meaningful text are needed.
- Collaboration and direct instruction are important.
- Strategies should include modeling the reading and writing process.
- It is important to encouraging risk taking and the use of inventive spelling.
- Varied opportunities for cooperative learning are beneficial.

Source: Compiled from "The Reading-Writing Relationships: Seven Instructional Principles," by T. Shanahan, 1988, *The Reading Teacher, 41;* and "Understanding the Relationship Between Reading and Writing," by M. W. Aulls, 1985, *Educational Horizons, 64.*

couraged to listen for the sounds in words and to experiment with inventive spelling. Dobson found that at first the children played it safe by writing familiar words and sentence patterns. But eventually they needed new words and new types of sentences to convey their thoughts. Gradually, the children became actively engaged in the writing process and their writing approximated adult forms. The students made progress in reading as well as writing and by the end of the year were writing stories that were more interesting and complex than their faster learning classmates.

Pinell (1989) conducted in-depth case studies of at-risk first-grade children participating in the Reading Recovery Program which used a holistic approach combining reading and writing activities. Results indicated this to be an effective approach when compared to an equivalent group of children participating in a more traditional compensatory program. C. Chomsky (1976) conducted detailed case studies

of five reluctant readers in the third grade who were 1 to 2 years below grade level in reading and who had already had 2 years of phonic skills and word analysis. The children engaged in daily rereadings of books while listening to the tape-recorded story and flash card games using words that the children had difficulty with when independently reading the stories. Chomsky asserted that the memorization of texts, which is a behavior common with preschool children, allowed the children to attend more to the printed text and to see the relationship of letters to sounds. After 4 months, the students were able to read the text in six or more books independently, and as the study progressed, the children began to make parallel progress with writing.

Current thinking dictates that reading and writing, though not identical, are mutually reinforcing and should be integrated instructionally. Tierney and Shanahan (1991) reviewed the recent research on reading-writing relationships and stated that research on reading-writing relationships is still in its infancy. They found that most research has been conducted with children under age 5, that few longitudinal studies exist, and that there is a paucity of research that examines individual differences or developmental issues. They concluded by stating that "reading and writing, to be understood and appreciated fully, should be viewed together, learned together, and used together" (p. 275). In a theoretical discussion, Kucer (1985) wrote that reading and writing run parallel and utilize many of the same mechanisms. For this reason, reading and writing should be integrated in the curriculum and not taught as separate subjects.

Research on the Development of Early Writing Behaviors

The emergent literacy proponents believe that children begin to show evidence of writing before the onset of formal schooling (Clay, 1975; Ferreiro & Teberosky, 1982; Harste et al., 1984; Temple et al., 1993). Case studies of young children by Bissex (1980), Cohn (1981), and Schickedanz (1990) depicted writing as a naturally occurring progression. Although Goodman's research review (1986) indicated that young children often do not perceive themselves as readers, they often do believe that they can write. About 50% of all 3-year-old children use scribble and letter-like forms and are able to converse about the purposes of writing.

The emergence of writing has received much less exposure than the emergence of reading (Hall, 1987). According to Sulzby and Teale (1985), it was previously believed that children's writing did not begin until age 6 or 7. It was not researched because their early attempts at writing were not considered readable.

The development of writing is likened to the natural development of speech (Halliday, 1989; Parker & Davis, 1983). Temple et al. (1993, p. 5) explained that "children do not trade in their immature speech for mature speech all at once. They always go through a sequence of stages of language use, moving from simple to complex." Learning to talk is not memorizing or practicing sentences but gradually understanding the rules of spoken language. This is also the case for learning to write in that children do not start to write using correct forms. They gradually come to understand the rules of spelling and composition. Infants begin to speak using "proto-language" which is refined over time in the context of language transactions with adults (Parker, 1983). Likewise, children use pretend or proto-writing and gradually refine this to adult standards.

Vygotsky (1978) saw writing as symbolic processing. He saw the gestures of infants as "writing in air" and a first attempt to communicate symbolically. He saw children's early scribbling as a motor act that then becomes representational as the child's lines and circles take on meaning. Children shift from drawing pictures to alphabetic writing when they understand that not only can you draw things, but you can also draw speech.

Although written language acquisition can be compared in development to speech, written language is also different from oral language. Oral language is transient and depends upon the context of the situation, whereas written language has permanence and is relatively decontextualized (Sulzby, 1986). In a study conducted by Purcell-Gates (1989), kindergartners were given two tasks: to tell a narrative orally about their last birthday and to pretend-read a story to a doll using a wordless picture book. The children perceived written language as different from oral language and used more formal "literary vocabulary" and "literary syntax" when pretend reading. Children's story retellings are considered an important link between speech and writing (King, 1989). It is through this experience that children gradually learn to write stories and learn that writing is not merely speech written down.

Children appear to enjoy writing long before formal schooling (Ferreiro & Teberosky, 1982). Hall, Moretz, and Statom (1976) identified 22 out of a sample of 79 children who used letters and words to communicate ideas in writing before formal instruction. In 17 out of 18 interviews conducted with parents of early writers, the parents reported that interest in writing preceded interest in reading.

There are numerous case studies (Bissex, 1980; Schickedanz, 1990) and longitudinal studies (Clay, 1975; Dyson, 1985; Ferreiro & Teberosky, 1982; Newkirk, 1989; Sulzby, Barnhart, & Hieshima, 1989) which show that writing does not necessarily begin with the alphabetic principle, but emerges out of drawing. Even after alphabetic writing emerges, drawing continues in association with writing and is used to compliment text and to support the writing by ensuring meaning (Ferreiro & Teberosky, 1982). McGee and Richgels (1990) wrote that, even when children are able to relate stories verbally and demonstrate a knowledge of story form, when they proceed to spell and write, they have difficulty remembering what they want to say. One strategy is to draw and talk, which helps them formulate what they want to say.

Graphic Forms of Writing

Young children informally experiment with writing. The graphic forms by which young children demonstrate early attempts at writing are categorized in similar ways by different researchers. There is general agreement, based upon observations of young children, that children write via "drawing, scribbling, letter-like forms, strings of well-learned elements, and various forms of invented spelling, as well as via conventional orthography" (Sulzby, 1985b, p. 193). There is less agreement on whether these behaviors develop in stages or at what age these graphic forms are dominant. In general, it is believed that patterns of development exist, but with individual variation (Sulzby, Teale, & Kamberelis, 1989.)

Clay's work in New Zealand (1975) provided some of the earliest characterizations of children's early writing development. Clay noted that children produced scribbles, mock linear writing, and mock letters. She observed strings of letters with no spaces. As a child began to understand words as discrete units, the child would insert dots or spaces to separate words.

Initially, children scribbled as a form of play with movement. Gradually, children discovered that scribbling could take different forms such as lines, circles, dots, and crosses. Then, children discovered that drawings could evolve out of these forms and represent objects and events. Finally, the children came to realize that writing is different from drawing and is represented by letter-like forms. Over time these letter-like forms were refined to look more like standard letters. Sometimes children used scribbles and mock letters as an act of pretend writing and later ascribed messages to their print. They eventually discovered that words could be segmented and that phonemes were represented by letters (Clay, 1975).

In their work with children between the ages of 4 to 6, Ferreiro and Teberosky (1982) identified five stages through which children learn to write. At level one, the children used graphic symbols in a linear fashion. They tended to see a connection between the visual aspects of words and the objects they represent, so that round symbols might represent a ball or long strings of symbols would represent a long object. At level two, the graphic forms were more refined to look like letters and were intended to convey information. At level three, a sound value was associated with each letter and each letter represented one syllable. At level four, the children no longer used the syllabic rule and instead understood that more letters were needed to construct a word. And at level five, the children had "broken the code" and understood a need to analyze the phonemes in words systematically.

Temple et al. (1993) also outlined discrete stages in spelling which have elements of all the previous classification studies. In the prephonemic stage, letter-like symbols or letters are strung together without any attempt to represent speech sounds. In the early phonemic stage, children attempt to represent one or two phonemes in words. In the letter-name stage, children use more letters which are "chosen to represent phonemes on the basis of the similarity between the sound of the letter name and the respective phoneme" (p. 103). In the transitional stage, words approximate English spelling and in the final stage, correct spelling is predominantly used and reflects knowledge of the rules of spelling. Ferrolli and Shanahan (1987) and Gentry (1982) have developed similar categorizations of spelling stages as seen in Figure 8–2.

Ferroli & Shanahan (1987)	Temple, Nathan, Temple & Burris (1993)	Gentry (1982)
Preliterate: RE (back) A (mail) TTT (peeked) F (stick)	**Prephonetic:** OIE (Lauren)	**Precommunicative:** MSOOE (Raisin Bran and doughnuts)
Initial Consonant: BET (back) MM (mail) PF (peeked) S (stick)	**Early Phonetic:** MBEWWMLNT (My baby was with me last night.)	**Semiphonetic:** BZR (buzzer) KR (car) BRZ (birds) OD (old)
Consonant Frame: BC (back) MOL (mail) PT (peeked) STC (stick)	**Letter-Name:** AMANROBSOSTHEPLESFONHEM (A man robs shoes. The police found him.)	
Phonetic: BAK (back) MAL (mail) PECT (peeked) SEK (stick)		**Phonetic:** IFU LEV AT THRD STRET IWEL KOM TO YOR HAWS (If you live at third street, I will come to your house.)
Transitional: BAQ (back) MAEL (mail) PEKED (peeked) STIK (stick)	**Transitional:** CAN WE GO SEE THE FORM WELL WE MITE GO LATER OHCAYE (Can we go see the farm? Well we might go later. Okay?)	**Transitional:** FAKTORES CAN NO LONGER OFORD MAKING PLAY DOW (Factories can no longer afford making play dough.)

Figure 8–2.   Three categorizations of developmental spelling stages.

Children experiment with writing long before they are formally taught writing. They progress naturally from unrefined scribbles to more conventional graphic letter-like forms. Their efforts indicate that written literacy behaviors more often emerge naturally, independent of formal instruction. Though children show individual variations and appear to move back and forth across different graphic forms, there is a general developmental trend toward higher level forms of writing over time (Allen et al., 1989).

Writing to Communicate

By the time children reach school age, most know that writing is used for the purpose of communicating messages, that it is composed of elements, and that it has certain forms and structures (Hall, 1987). Once children begin applying the alphabetic principle and using strings of letter-like symbols or letters of the alphabet, they convey an awareness of the desire to com municate using written symbols. The first piece of writing most children attempt to produce is their own name and this usually challenges their understanding of how written words are structured (Clay, 1975; Temple et al., 1993). When what they think they wrote does not match what was written, children must begin to alter their less mature notions for new hypotheses on how letters are combined to make words.

The first written text that is often seen usually accompanies a drawing and serves as a one word label (Hilliker, 1988). Clay (1975) and Dyson (1985) also saw list-making as a typical early writing style. Clay referred to this as the *inventory principle.* Children make lists of letters and numbers they can write, lists of inventive spellings, or lists of words they can write conventionally. Dyson (1985) was a daily participant observer in a classroom study of 22 children. The children wrote their names, wrote words to accompany pictures, and

wrote lists, especially of their friends' names. Talking was an important part of their writing. In 1982, Dyson and Genishi conducted a case study of two first graders' interactions while writing. They found that "composing was as much an oral activity as a writing activity" and that speech was a "frequent accompaniment to writing" (p. 126).

Word sequences become necessary when "writing bursts the confines of one word labels" (Hilliker, 1988). Narratives emerge when there is a need to express more than a one word label can convey. Two and three word phrases emerge to describe some element in their drawing (Clay, 1975). Even expository writing, when it emerges, is more of an organized list of attributes or descriptions or comments on a topic, such as lists of "I like" statements (McGee & Richgels, 1990).

Spelling

In the first half of the 20th century, spelling research was conducted to discover and design the most effective ways to learn the large numbers of words needed for writing. Emphasis was on perceptual processes and learning rates (Hodges, 1982). In 1919, Ernest Horn (as cited in Hodges, 1992) summarized what was needed on the subject of spelling: to know what words were needed for spelling, to affix grade levels to these words, to find the best ways of learning these words, and to find the means of measuring progress. During the second half of the 20th century, research by linguists such as C. Chomsky (1970) discovered that spelling was developmental. In the past decade, spelling has been taught under two different approaches which reflect divergent philosophies on language learning (Wilde, 1990). The traditional skills approach focuses on word lists, worksheets, and weekly tests, whereas the whole language approach focuses on spelling integrated into writing activities and de-emphasizes spelling accuracy on first drafts.

A study by Freyberg in 1964 found that there was little carryover from rote memorization of spelling lists unless the words were incorporated into writing. Johnson, Langford, and Quorn (1981) asserted that copying activities to reinforce spelling do not encourage children to use their knowledge related to written text.

Bissex (1980), based on her extensive case study of her son's spelling, wrote that "spelling ability grows from understanding a system and cannot be accounted for as the product of memorized lists of unpredictably spelled words" (p. 111). Beers and Beers (1980) conducted a study with 75 first-grade and 71 second-grade children. Using a list of 24 high and low frequency words, student test scores across the school year demonstrated that knowledge of how to construct these words changed systematically and sequentially over time. Bradley and Bryant's research (1983) confirmed that children from age 6 to 7 use phoneme to grapheme strategies when they spell words.

Inventive Spelling

Inventive spellings are the early spellings children produce on their own (Temple et al., 1993). Children use inventive spellings for writing in a manner similar to an infant's oral language inventions; they overextend the system of rules to meet communicative needs (Schwartz, 1988). According to Gentry (1981):

A writer selecting a spelling pattern must choose from available options, hypothesize a correct spelling, and test the hypothesis as a representation for conveying meaning in print. Hypothesis testing and generation of spelling patterns enable the writer to reorganize, restructure, and elaborate the options for spelling a word. (p. 380)

Sowers (1988) agreed that inventive spelling allows children to extend their knowledge of how words are constructed. Inventive spelling does not interfere with learning conventional spelling later. In the development of emergent writing, children first use random strings of letters, then beginning sounds, then beginning plus end sounds, then beginning plus end plus middle sounds. Generally, they use consonants at first and gradually, long vowels (long vowels say their letter name). Over time as their phonemic awareness develops, they begin to include short vowel sounds, digraphs (pairs of letters that represent single speech sounds, (e.g., *sh, ch, th, ck*), blends (e.g., *bl, str, sk*), and vowel combinations (e.g., *ae, ie*); these emerge in no particular order.

Certain error patterns are predictable (Chomsky, 1970; Henderson and Beers, 1980; Read, 1971, 1975; Sowers, 1988; Temple et al., 1993). Children frequently substitute *Y* for the sound of *W* because the letter name of *Y* is closer to the sound of *W* (Sowers, 1988). Children also tend not to include the nasal consonants *N* and *M* when they precede another consonant and are not clearly articulated, as in *lamp* or *kind*.

In a large scale study of writing compositions by 1,000 students in first through eighth grade, Taylor and Kidder (1988) found that spelling errors increase from first to fourth grade and then decline. The researchers noted that errors increase during this time because children's language is evolving, and they use more complicated word structure and vocabulary. The researchers proposed that spelling error is a sign of growth and that growth in spelling is impossible without error.

Various articles and studies have examined the role that inventive spelling plays in the emergence of literacy. Ehri and Wilce (1987) conducted a group comparison study with 12 matched pairs of children in kindergarten to determine whether children who are taught to produce phonic spellings have improved word reading ability. They concluded that phonetic spelling training contributed to reading scores and, therefore, spelling instruction should be linked to reading instruction. Schickedanz (1990) and Bissex (1980), in their respective longitudinal case studies of their sons' early literacy development, felt that reading provided input to spelling by providing opportunities to see conventionally spelled words.

Griffith (1991), in a study of 96 multiethnic first graders and 87 third graders with a wide range of socioeconomic status and abilities, found that phonemic awareness was an important predictor of spelling in the first grade where spelling is a sequential encoding process. In the third grade, spelling relied more on memorized orthographic units and word specific information. Numerous researchers have observed that young children articulate out loud as they are trying to spell phonetically, and that this behavior tapered off in later years as knowledge of spelling increased (Downing, DeStefano, Rich, & Bell, 1984; Sowers, 1988; Temple et al., 1993).

Clark (1988) conducted a study with 100 children from four first-grade classrooms, two of which used traditional spelling activities and two of which used inventive spelling. At the end of the study, more children from the inventive spelling classrooms were able to write on their own without assistance, produced longer units of writing and produced more spelling errors. Children from the traditional classrooms sought assistance, produced shorter units of writing, but had fewer spelling errors. Generally, the children in the inventive spelling classrooms wrote more from recall with less outside assistance and more of the classroom activities were child-centered. In contrast, children in the traditional skills classrooms used more writing aids and the activities were more teacher-centered. Juel (1992), in a longitudinal study of 54 children followed from first through fourth grades, found that, whereas in first grade spelling contributes most to writing, in higher grades ideas contribute more to writing. She also determined that poor writers were often poor spellers.

Spelling Instruction

Bissex (1980) stated that teachers should "regard errors as sources of information for instruction rather than mistakes" and that "instruction may be useful or crucial at only some stages of a learning process" (pp. 113–114). Sowers (1988) suggested teachers should "build on emerging competence" (p. 68) and that teachers should look for signs that a child is beginning to apply a spelling rule or principle inconsistently and teach to this rule.

Assessment is still a first step, however; qualitative assessment is recommended in addition to quantitative assessment, according to Bloodgood (1991). Marino (1981) and Furnas (1985) stated that careful observation is important to examine qualitatively the spelling errors or miscues in children's writing and that different spelling errors will warrant different approaches. Gentry (1981) suggested that children spelling at the phonetic stage may find formal instruction frustrating, but that formal spelling instruction will augment writing for children evolving from the transitional to the correct stage. Schickedanz (1990) suggested that children at the transitional level of spelling need more information and instruction, and that conventional spelling should be a focus in second drafts.

Gentry (1987) suggested the following guidelines for an effective spelling program: encourage writing and teach spelling as part of the total curriculum, encourage inventive spelling and de-emphasize correct spelling, and respond appropriately to students' writing efforts in ways that will help them build spelling skills. The latter requires teachers to understand how children learn to spell developmentally. Wilde (1990) also advocated a change in attitude toward spelling errors and suggested that children be taught spelling strategies and useful generalizations regarding English spelling patterns. Bloodgood (1991) concurred that spelling should be integrated into language arts and suggested the use of word studies that focus on orthographic patterns through the use of game-like activities, such as word hunts and concentration.

Temple et al. (1993) broke down strategies according to the student's writing level. At the *prephonetic* level, teachers should orient young children to the writing system by frequent exposure to books and other examples of writing. Children should be encouraged to take note of environmental print and be encouraged to write their names and label drawings. At the *early phonemic* level, children should also have access to lots of print in books and magazines and through choral reading with *big books* where the class reads with the teacher and the teacher gradually withdraws as the reader when the children are able to read passages and phrases on their own. A language experience approach that encourages children to dictate ideas and stories to the teacher who serves as scribe is appropriate at this stage and the previous stage because it allows the children to see word boundaries and relate sounds to words. Writing for meaningful purposes using inventive spelling should be encouraged and teachers should provide praise for what the children know. At the *letter name* stage, children are more aware of the details of spelling and should be encouraged to explore letter-sound rules. Books on tape, word banks, personal word lists, and lots of writing are recommended. When children produce more spelling at the *transitional* level, games and activities such as hangman and word sorting, which examine word features such as vowel patterns, digraphs, and word endings, are recommended.

McGee and Richgels (1990) provided a framework for teacher instruction that takes into account the children's developmental level in reading and writing. They described student behaviors and corresponding curriculum from the framework of novice readers and writers (around ages 3, 4, and 5), experimenting readers and writers (around ages 5 and 6), and accomplished readers and writers (around ages 6, 7, and 8). Classroom activities and supporting rationale are in keeping with a whole language orientation.

Templeton (1991b) strongly recommended grouping children for instruction according to developmental spelling levels. He urged teachers not to forego formal spelling instruction and suggested word studies that examine groups of words categorized according to common principles, and shared structural and semantic features. He even suggested using grade level spelling basals which are designed to assist with word studies.

Although some researchers report that young preschool children are not reluctant to write (Clay, 1975; Ferreiro & Teberosky, 1982), others report that children need to hear that inventive spelling is acceptable. Sulzby, Teale, and Kamberelis (1989) suggested telling children that "It doesn't have to be like grown up writing. Just do it your own way" (p. 70).

Based on her observations of young emergent writers, Schickedanz (1990) suggested that there are different styles of learning how to spell. She described children who attend to the visual aspects of how words look as well as children who attend to the auditory aspects and use more phonemic and syllabic strategies. Spelling development may also be guided in early writing stages by the questions children ask. Children ask for help in different ways; some just want help identifying a sound, some want help with a whole word, whereas others want to know if a word is correct after they have written it. Schickedanz cautioned that, when children begin to read conventionally, they may become reluctant to spell on their own. "Their visual knowledge is too great to allow sound based spellings to stand" (p. 103). She recommended that word banks, frequently used word lists, and dictionaries be introduced. She also cautioned that inventive spelling may not emerge when children are given a lot of information regarding the complexities of spelling. Gentry (1987) stated that not all children and hence, not all adults, learn to spell well. For these individuals it is important to learn how to proofread and to use dictionaries and electronic spell checkers.

Bissex (1980) provided a summarizing statement that addresses all children's capacity to learn spelling:

If children's learning of spelling is largely systematic, as is our orthography, then we would learn more instructionally from observing what a child knows about the system—what principles he can apply and what strategies he uses in his writings (as reflecting his concept of the spelling system)—than we would learn from asking what and how many words he knows. The same observations could be made of children with spelling difficulties as those progressing normally. (In our effort to understand disabilities, perhaps we have gone too far in putting such children in a separate category with separate questions asked about them.) (p. 116)

The Whole Language Versus Skills Instruction Debate

The debate over instructional philosophy often results in a debate over methods. F. Smith (1992, p. 432) referred to this as the "never-ending debate." Current debates focus on the "skills" or "basics" approach to teaching literacy versus the "whole language," "naturalistic," "emergent literacy" or "literature-based approach" (F. Smith, 1992, p. 432). Others have described this as the part-to-whole versus the whole-to-part debate (Weaver, 1990).

Generally, on one side there is instruction under a whole language paradigm, which is broad in concept and difficult to translate into instructional methods. Instruction under a whole language approach runs more to the informal, the transactional, and follows a psycho-sociolinguistic approach. On the other side is skills instruction, which is more traditional and formal in structure and follows the transmission model.

Whole Language Instruction

K. Goodman (1989) described whole language as a "dynamic evolving grass-roots movement" (p. 208). Watson (1989) wrote that "whole language is a label for mutually supportive beliefs and teaching strategies and experiences that have to do with kids learning to read, write, speak and listen in natural situations" (p. 133). Edelsky et al (1991) spoke of whole language as a professional theory in which the theory drives practice. Weaver (1990) emphasized that whole language is first a philosophy.

Edelsky et al. (1991) traced the theoretical basis for the theory of whole language back to the progressive education of the late 1800s to the early 1930s, a time in history when education was seen as the road to social reform. Like whole language, progressive education promoted the active engagement of the learner. Unlike whole language, reading and writing focused on whole-word learning and were not based upon literacy as language learning. Edelsky and her coauthors perceived that whole language has emerged out of language experience traditions as well as the open education movement, and that it incorporates process writing approaches. As described earlier in the section on historical influences on literacy instruction, whole language theory arose out of research in linguistics (N. Chomsky, 1957), theories on cognitive approaches to learning (Vygotsky, 1962), and by changes in research methodologies (Piaget, 1952). Whole language theory provided renewed interest in the nature of teaching and learning and provided an impetus to change classroom practices radically.

It is hardly surprising, given this varied collection of views, that the whole language paradigm is not easily defined, and not easily translated into instructional methods. Table 8–3 outlines the main tenets of the whole language paradigm, synthesized from the writings of Altwerger, Edelsky, and Flores (1987), K. Goodman, (1989), Teale (1982), Watson (1989), and Weaver (1990).

Whole language is a philosophy that applies to learners of all ages from infancy to adulthood (Altwerger et al., 1987; Newman, 1985). In the classroom, reading is learned by reading and writing is learned by writing across many subject areas such as literature, science, math, and social studies. The whole language approach proceeds from whole to part. Phonics and other skills, such as grammar and punctuation, are directly taught but in the context of reading and writing applications. Teachers are "kid watchers" (Y. Goodman, 1978), evaluating their progress as individuals and documenting change. Teachers do not expect students to learn the same things at the same time and reject scope and sequence curriculums. They structure their classrooms for purposeful activities and foster learning through social interaction. There is no uniform set of practices (Edelsky et al., 1991).

Skills Instruction

In contrast to the whole language approach, skills instruction is a theory as well as a more conventional set of practices. According to Templeton (1991a), "a skill is a coordinated set of cognitive and/or psychomotor behaviors that arise out of experience" (p. 590). Skills instruction has been a part of educational practice for most of the century. "It may be fair to say that in the early 20th century the notion of *skills* applied to the use or application of literacy, as well as to the means by which literacy was acquired" (p. 591). As described earlier in the section on historical influences on literacy instruction, skills instruction became firmly entrenched in American education as a result of experimental psychology, behavioral research, and educational measurement research, which led to part-to-whole skills hierarchies and formalized curriculum dominated by basal readers, phonic instruction, and spelling workbooks.

K. Goodman (1991) discussed the skills approach as viewing words as key units in learning to read and write. Textbooks sim-

Table 8-3. Main tenets of the whole language paradigm, synthesized from the writings of Altwerger, Edelsky, and Flores (1987), K. Goodman (1989), Teale (1982), Watson (1989), and Weaver (1990).

- Language is central to the whole language paradigm. Literacy development is likened to the ways in which oral language naturally develops. Children need to see and talk about written text and they need access to drawing and writing tools in order to explore language in written forms.

- Whole language is student-centered learning and teaching. The emphasis in reading and writing is on meaning; reading and writing approximations are accepted as part of the student's development.

- Whole language teachers are mediators and collaborators; classrooms are environments structured for meaningful learning. Teachers provide the scaffolding needed to support the ongoing development of individual learners.

- Whole language learning is essentially a social process mediated through language. Speech and discourse are important for interaction. Children need opportunities to observe literacy in everyday use and to talk about this at home and at school with adults and peers.

plified text by limiting sentence structure and vocabulary and by organizing them around phonic patterns. Phonic instruction was key to learning to read words and so phonic patterns were directly taught.

Although research in recent years has cast doubt on the constructs underlying the skills approach, the practices continue to be popular in classrooms. In an applied ethnographic study of kindergarten, first-grade and second-grade classrooms, Slaughter, Haussler, Franks, Jilbert, and Silentman (1987) derived the following description of "conventional classrooms" that use a skills approach: there is an emphasis on direct instruction and the use of basal readers.

Teacher-directed instruction is dominant. Skills are taught in isolation with the use of worksheets, workbooks, and copy writing. Independent work with an emphasis on correctness is stressed.

Unresolved Issues

The body of literature contrasting whole language and skills approaches indicates that, although the guiding philosophy of the skills paradigm has grown weak, the practices remain strong. In contrast, although the philosophy of whole language is powerful, the practices by which it should be implemented are vague. Paradigm shifts no doubt occur slowly as do changes in practice. As practitioners, we must sort through the theory as well as the practices to determine what works best for ourselves and our students.

Pearson (1989) spoke of his concern that whole language proponents want "revolution, not evolution" (p. 239). Yet, it is not clear that the answer is to compel teachers to choose between one paradigm or the other, rather than to extract and blend some good from each. Pearson pointed to some miscommunication that potentially serves to breed separatism. For one, whole language advocates de-

scribe the role of the teacher as an indirect facilitator. However, whole language teachers conduct short lessons and group demonstrations to their classes. Slaughter et al. (1987) conducted a descriptive study of whole language classrooms to gauge the extent of indirect teaching, which is advocated under the whole language approach, and direct teaching, which is more often associated with the skills approach. They reported that both direct and indirect instruction occurred in successful whole language classrooms; however, direct instruction was tied to the teacher's conception of the child's strengths and weaknesses. Pearson (1989) also criticized whole language advocates' strong bias against basals and tests, which he felt can still be important tools.

Advocates convey that whole language does not focus on skills. Yet it does not necessarily follow that whole language teachers should not teach skills. In fact, proponents of whole language do feel that skills such as phonics and spelling are important in literacy learning, but should be taught in the context of meaningful reading and writing activities and not in isolation (Hansen, 1985). Freppon and Dahl (1991) asserted that phonics should begin when the child has some basic understandings about written text and should be taught in the context of a literacy activity. "Our quibble isn't really with skills instruction at all but *how, when,* and *why* skills are taught" (Dudley-Marling & Dippo, 1991, p. 549). Templeton (1991a) stated: "We are coming to understand better which elements should be emphasized at different points in development, though there is still much to be learned here" (p. 593).

Basic Tenets of Written Literacy Instruction

In the 1980s instruction in the primary grades continued to focus on copying words and sentences with emphasis more on neatness, correct spelling, and hand-writing than on the expression of ideas (Dyson, 1985; Strickland & Morrow, 1989). A study by Bridge and Hiebert (1985) found that what little time was spent on writing in elementary school classrooms usually involved writing assignments that involved copying, and that less than 15% of the day in elementary school classrooms was devoted to writing instruction.

Adults play a key role in literacy instruction. Bruner (1978) introduced the term *scaffolding* to describe the type of support that mothers provide to children in the acquisition of language (Lehr, 1985). This term is often used to describe the role of the adult in the acquisition of literacy (Graves, 1983). Adults provide sufficient support to enable a child to participate in the learning process and gradually relinquish this support as the child's competence increases. Vygotsky (1962) referred to the *zone of proximal development* which is the potential area for growth where a child is dependent on adult assistance. He used this concept to describe the importance of teaching at the appropriate level in keeping with an individual child's needs.

Based upon his research, Graves (1991) stated that children need to write a minimum of 30 minutes per day, 4 days per week, in order to see changes in writing. And children with learning problems need even more time. Calkins (1986), McGee and Richgels (1990), Schwartz (1988), Strickland and Morrow (1989), and Temple et al. (1993) theorized that teachers must create an environment that is rich in literacy materials; they must model writing for children; they must encourage developmental spelling; and they must encourage children to share what they are writing. It is especially important to respond to the meaning expressed in beginners' writing and not only to the form of their writing. Calkins (1986) wrote that the job of teachers is to "respond to children's products in such a way that youngsters learn that

marks on the paper have the power to convey meaning" (p. 38).

Regarding topics, Hansen (1985) emphasized the importance of giving children choices. Teachers can help children generate options. Strickland and Morrow (1989) suggested writing as an extension of story reading. Other strategies include writing and publishing their own books, journal writing, and writing across the curriculum in areas of social studies, math, and science. Preschool and kindergarten children can use writing props in play areas, make signs, and have access to writing centers (Mills & Clyde, 1990; Routman, 1988).

INSTRUCTIONAL STRATEGIES FOR STUDENTS WITH DISABILITIES

Research on Instructional Strategies for Students with Disabilities

Despite the great body of literature on literacy learning for able-bodied children, scant attention has been paid to the ways in which children with multiple disabilities learn and can be taught literacy. Demographic studies and clinical experience indicates that literacy deficits are widespread and pervasive for students with severe speech and physical impairments, yet little has been done to apply theories of literacy learning to this population.

As described previously, a few descriptive studies suggest that classroom instruction may bear some responsibility for literacy learning delays. This does not indicate that teachers are shirking their responsibilities, but that there is little to guide teachers on effective strategies. Koppenhaver and Yoder (1990a) believed that teachers recognize the importance of literacy in the lives of students with disabilities, but that there is little information on how to instruct them in reading and writing. Courses and textbooks on how to teach reading or writing to students with disabilities are scant.

Overall, there is little research on effective intervention strategies to provide guidance to teachers of students with severe physical impairments and speech impairments. Intervention studies, thus far, have focused on improving the rate or accuracy of student response. Wasson and Keeler (as cited in Koppenhaver & Yoder, 1992) adapted worksheet materials and created an eye gaze response board which allowed a 6-year-old student with severe speech and physical disabilities to eye point to answers quickly rather than use her augmentative communication device. This adaptation tripled the number of response opportunities for written language activities. McNaughton and Drynan (1990) reported a case study of an 11-year-old student who typed with one thumb. By creating a keyboard overlay that allowed him to type high frequency words with one keystroke, his writing speed increased from three to eight words per minute. Harris (1978), in a study of three students who were 6 to 7 years of age with severe speech and physical disabilities, demonstrated that, when a teacher increased the wait time after asking a question, the frequency and length of student contributions increased.

In an investigation on the effects of repeated reading on word recognition (Koppenhaver & Yoder, 1988), a study was conducted with two young adolescents with severe speech and physical disabilities who were beginning readers. The researchers took slides of pages in easy-to-read books and recorded the text on audio tapes which enabled the students to re-read and listen to four stories. Both students showed improvement in word recognition for all four stories, with the most improvement occurring with the fourth and final story.

Two studies examined accuracy relative to spelling improvement. Koke and

Neilson (as cited in Koppenhaver & Yoder, 1992) conducted a single subject, B-A-B, withdrawal design to show that auditory feedback via speech synthesis improved the spelling of two out of three young adult females with severe speech and physical disabilities. Koppenhaver and Yoder (1989) conducted a multiple baseline, single subject design across three sets of words with two students age 13 with severe speech and physical disabilities, which investigated the effectiveness of the Horn (1920) spelling study strategy (look at the spelling word, visualize and verbalize the word, write the word). Their study indicated that this strategy was effective for both students on all three word sets. The student with the stronger phonemic discrimination skills appeared to have better retention over time. In a delayed posttest, both students scored better on the words learned via the Horn strategy than by traditional rote repetition and fill-in-the-blank workbook activities.

DeCoste (1993) employed a single subject design to evaluate the effectiveness of strategies under two instructional approaches, a skills-oriented approach and a whole language approach, to increase the spelling and writing skills of two girls and one boy ages 9 to 11 with severe speech and physical disabilities due to CP. All three students demonstrated literacy levels significantly below that of their elementary school peers. Over an 8 month period, all three students demonstrated an increase in spelling ability under the skills-oriented approach, as well as under the whole language-oriented approach. There were slightly higher increases under the skills-oriented conditions for all three students; however, students reported higher preferences for whole language-oriented activities. More important, all three students made gradual progress in spelling in a developmental progression similar to that of younger, able-bodied, emergent writers, as described by Temple et al. (1993). All three students also moved toward more mature levels of writing ability, but with more individual variation. One student progressed to generating sentences using conventional syntax (sentence structure) and showed an increase over the course of the study in sentence length and complexity (Table 8–4). Although the other two students demonstrated spelling and writing progress, they continued to have difficulty with syntax.

In a single subject study with two adults with CP and receptive language delays who use AAC, McNaughton and Tawney (1993) used an alternating treatment design over a 3- and 5-week period to investigate the effects of two skills-oriented instructional techniques to teach spelling: the copy-write-compare (CWC) method and the student-directed-cueing (SDC) method. Subjects improved their spelling performance using both instructional techniques. Posttest scores showed better retention for spelling using the SDC method for both individuals. Both the DeCoste study and the McNaughton and Tawney study demonstrated that individuals with severe speech and physical impairments can achieve changes in performance when provided with effective, individualized instruction. These studies support the premise that lack of individualized instruction or ineffective instruction may be a root cause of literacy deficits in individuals with severe speech and physical disabilities.

Overall, the literature on intervention strategies is scant, and has been written mostly within the last 5 years. The literature suggests that various intervention strategies can improve the literacy of students, but the dearth of intervention studies highlights the lack of definitive guidance in this area.

The Role of Technology in Literacy Instruction

Professionals working with individuals with CP are relying more on technology to provide "a means to pursue educational goals alongside their normal peers" (Ferrier & Shane, 1987, p. 107). According to Koppenhaver and Yoder (1992, p. 190), computers and other technology provide "a

Table 8–4. Changes in inventive spelling and writing over a 5-month period for a 9-year-old girl with severe speech and physical impairments using single switch scanning.

E IS H	He is home.
WE C GO T	We can go out.
I GIVE U A B CLAY	I give you a piece clay.
I PEEL THE ROJ	I peel the orange.
HER FRNS DINT WHAT TO HLP HR	Her friends didn't want to help her.
I WNT A PRPLE SILK DRS	I want a purple silk dress.
I GOT A BAB DL SE TOS.	I got a baby doll. She talks.
ROSCE KAM TU SCL TU SEE MI FRNS AND ME	Roxie came to school to see my friends and me.
PR SAM MILK IN TO THE BLNDR	Pour some milk into the blender.

Note: Underlined words were copied as part of a skills-oriented spelling lesson. (The student was asked to put a targeted spelling word in a sentence.) Non-underlined words were produced independently.

vital prosthetic function" for individuals with impaired speech and physical abilities. Vanderheiden (1984) saw greater emphasis on using assistive technology to meet spoken communication needs and less emphasis on written communication. He stressed the importance of providing children with physical disabilities with the equivalent of "paper and pencil" in the form of assistive technology in order that they may have "a chance at a meaningful education" (p. 61). Meyers (1984) used case study reports to demonstrate the necessity of using computers as literacy tools for school-aged children with disabilities.

Garner and Campbell (1987) reminded professionals that "technology is not an end in itself" (p. 129). They emphasized that there must be a guiding philosophy when applying technology and that effective instructional practices are "always a prerequisite to the use of technology" (p. 129). Putting assistive technology research that focuses on the effectiveness of hardware and software before research on the nature of literacy learning for individuals with disabilities may be like putting the cart before the horse. At this time, it is equally important to investigate how students with disabilities acquire literacy rather than focusing only on what tools work best.

Assessment and Instructional Strategies for Developing Literacy

Achieving literacy is an ongoing, developmental process. As described earlier in this chapter, typical children are on a literacy continuum from infancy. Likewise, individuals with disabilities should have access to literacy learning opportunities. An individual's access to literacy learning should not be denied because of his or her disability, nor should literacy learning be aborted if that individual has not achieved conventional reading and writing skills by the end of elementary school. Farrell and Elkins (1995) referred to the "learn early or never attitude" that is applied to students with disabilities. They perceived that students with disabilities, particularly those with intellectual disabilities, are moved into vocational or daily living curriculums just when they are beginning to achieve concepts of literacy. They stressed that language and literacy should be integrated across the curriculum at all ages, including adolescence, and that literacy should be viewed as part of a lifelong learning process. This position does not reflect a "back to basics" education which focuses exclusively on reading, writing and arithmetic, but the idea that literacy learning can be integrated quite naturally into the everyday activities of individuals with developmental disabilities.

Profiles of Emergent Literacy Learners

The following section provides basic strategies in areas of emergent literacy assessment and instruction to guide educators working with students who use AAC. Assessment and instructional strategies must take into consideration the unique needs and abilities of the individual learner. In the sections that follow, strategies will be presented at three general levels: literacy beginners, novice readers and writers, and experimenting readers and writers. These levels were coined by McGee and Richgels (1990) in describing literacy development in typical children, but the same terms can be applied just as easily to students with disabilities of all ages, hence avoiding traditional grade or age levels to describe appropriate instructional strategies. These instructional levels should act as a general guide to educators; teachers must add to this their knowledge of the student's individual learning style.

Literacy Beginners. Literacy beginners are individuals who are in the process of understanding that books are pleasurable and involve interaction between a reader and a listener, that books are handled in particular ways (e.g., right-side-up and left-to-right), and most important, that pictures are symbols that convey information about objects and actions.

Novice Readers and Writers. Novice readers and writers are individuals who are in the process of learning that printed text carries the message and conveys information. Novices are beginning to attend to words in text and pay more attention to identifying individual letters, especially to those in their names. They may string letters together to signify words, but have not yet mastered phonemic principles of sound-symbol correspondence. Novices are aware of environmental print and can identify signs and labels in and out of context. They demonstrate an understanding of how events tie together to make a story.

Experimenting Readers and Writers. Experimenting readers and writers are more aware of the effort it takes to read and write. They know most of the letters of the alphabet and are beginning to associate letter names with the letter sounds. They understand that words are made up of combinations of letters and use inventive spelling, sometimes combined with familiar conventionally spelled words, to write in a way that conveys a message. Their writing demonstrates that they differentiate written language from spoken language.

The end stage of emergent literacy learning is the transition to conventional reading and writing. During this time, children may overgeneralize spelling rules. Their skill with reading and writing tasks depends upon the demand of the task at hand. It is at this stage that traditional approaches to reading and writing instruction can be utilized, such as emphasis on sight word vocabulary, spelling rules, and word study. For the purposes of this chapter on literacy learning for individuals using AAC, instructional strategies will focus on the earlier emergent stages where there is a lack of practical information on instruction for students with severe speech and physical disabilities.

Reading Assessment Strategies

Individuals with speech that is somewhat intelligible to familiar listeners can be assessed in more traditional ways using standardized, graded reading passages. Individuals with severely limited or no intelligible speech output present more of a challenge. In Chapter 5, direct selection methods for screening literacy with individuals who are nonspeaking using manual pointing, head pointing, eye gaze, or yes/no question formats are described. Letter name knowledge, letter sound knowledge, sight word recognition, spelling for words, phrases, and sentences, and general reading comprehension can be evaluated in this way. It is more difficult, however, to know with certainty if a student who is nonspeaking can read each word in a passage in order to determine a level of reading proficiency. One option is to use a maze procedure to adapt reading passages (Koppenhaver & Yoder, 1988). Guthrie, Seifert, Burnham, and Caplan (1974) used the maze procedure to modify text by deleting approximately every fifth word in the story. For every word deleted, three choices are provided, including two alternative words and the one correct word. A individual who is nonspeaking would indicate which one of the three words fits the passage using pointing or eye gaze. For example:

only
The brown bear went over the mountain.
after

The alternatives should include an incorrect word that is the same part of speech as the correct word (e.g., *after*), and an incorrect word that is a different part of speech (e.g., *only*). A percentage of accuracy can be obtained by dividing the number of correct responses by the total number of responses. Guthrie et al. (1974) indicated that the optimal instructional level is 60 to 70 percent accuracy. An accuracy level of 85 to 100 percent indicates that it is time to move to a higher reading level.

Guthrie et al. suggested that reading passages selected for the maze procedure should be about 120 words long. The maze technique as described works well when evaluating students who are reading at a first-grade level or above. Passages of 120 words are generally too long to present to students at emergent literacy levels. However, this author has used the maze strategy as a pretest and posttest to guide weekly instruction with passages with as few as 50 words. It is important to systematically delete words (such as every fifth word) and not just delete major content words. The reading proficiency of prepositions, articles, and conjunctions is as significant as the reading of nouns, verbs, and modifiers. The maze procedure provides a systematic way to assess and monitor paragraph reading informally.

Reading Instruction Strategies

The most important ingredient for literacy learning is daily input. Daily reading is important for young children using AAC, and is still important for older students at emergent literacy levels. For young children, there are many picture books, predictive books, and easy-to-read publications available. For older students at emergent literacy levels, there are fewer appropriate fiction titles available. Some early elementary fiction books with subject matter that is less juvenile may be appropriate (See Table 8–5). For older students, there are more easy-to-read, nonfiction publications (See Table 8–6).

For Literacy Beginners. At the beginning stages, reading should be integrated into everyday experiences. Communication boards utilizing aided language stimulation strategies as outlined by Goossens, Crain, and Elder (1992) and Elder and Goossens (1994) promote the knowledge that pictures are symbols that convey meaning. Aided language stimulation uses communication displays as a way to build receptive language and provide a means of communication. These communication strategies reinforce language development, as well as early literacy concepts. Low tech and high tech communication overlays should retain the word labels with the picture communication symbols.

Daily schedules that combine pictures and key words, as well as labeling objects in the student's environment are popular strategies that call attention to pictures and words. Weekly messages to be sent home to parents can be written in a rebus format which combines pictures and words to convey the message.

Even individuals who do not demonstrate an awareness of text forms can still enjoy story reading. For older students at the secondary level, teacher-made books that use pictures (and some text to guide the adult reader) to tell stories about students' everyday activities promote the concept that reading is pleasurable and a source of communication interaction.

For beginner and novice readers, story reading, combined with picture communication symbols that relate directly to the story, is a way to foster an interest in reading (Figure 8–3). It provides a means for individuals who are nonspeaking to participate in story reading by enabling them to answer questions, ask questions, and make comments about the story. At times it may also be useful to simplify the original text and adapt it using picture communication symbols (Figure 8–4). Recently there has been an increase in commercial products that promote the reading of text combined with picture communication symbols (Kelly & Friend, 1993; King-DeBaun, 1990; Musselwhite, 1993). However,

Table 8–5. Easy-to-read fiction titles appropriate for older students at early literacy levels.

Author	Publication Date	Title	Publisher
Blos, W.	1987	Old Henry	William Morrow
Brett, J.	1988	The First Dog	Harcourt Brace Jovanovich
Bunting, E.	1990	The Wall	Clarion Books
Bunting, E.	1991	Fly Away Home	Clarion Books
Cleary, B.	1984	Lucy Chuck	William Morrow
Cole, J.	1985	Doctor Change	William Morrow
Day, D.	1991	The Walking Catfish	Macmillan
DeFelice, C.	1989	The Dancing Skeleton	Macmillan
Dragonwagon, C.	1990	Home Place	Macmillan
Fisher, L.	1991	Cyclops	Holiday House
Fleischman, S.	1988	The Scarebird	Greenwillow Books
French, F.	1991	Anancy and Mr. Dry-Bone	Little, Brown
Goble, P.	1993	The Lost Children	Bradbury Press
Griffith, H.	1987	Grandaddy's Place	Greenwillow
Griffith, H.	1980	Georgia Music	Greenwillow
Hartley, D.	1986	Up North in Winter	E. P. Dutton
Herriot, J.	1986	The Christmas Day Kitten	St. Martin's Press
Herriot, J.	1985	Only One Woof	St. Martin's Press
Leaf, M.	1987	Eyes of the Dragon	Lothrop, Lee, & Shepard
Locker, T.	1985	The Mare on the Hill	Dial Books
Lyon, G. W.	1992	Who Came Down that Road	Orchard Books
Melville, H.	1991	Catskill Eagle	Philomel Books
Pryor, B.	1987	The House on Maple Street	William Morrow
Rylant, C.	1985	The Relatives Came	Bradbury Press
San Souci, R.	1984	The Boy and the Ghost	Simon & Schuster, Inc.
Stevens, J.	1989	Androcles and the Lion	Holiday House
Turkle, B.	1981	Do Not Open	E. P. Dutton
Van Allsburg, C.	1986	The Stranger	Houghton Mifflin Co.
Van Allsburg, C.	1991	The Wretched Stone	Houghton Mifflin Co.
Van Allsburg, C.	1992	The Widow's Broom	Houghton Mifflin Co.
Zemach, Harve	1971	A Penny a Look	Farrar, Straus & Giro

using software such as Boardmaker or Speaking Dynamically or by cutting and pasting picture symbols, the instructor can create story boards that correspond to a child's favorite stories. Separate communication boards can be created or the picture symbols can be pasted directly on the pages of the individual's favorite book.

Table 8–6. Nonfiction publications for older students at emergent literacy levels.

Titles	Publishers
General topics:	
New True Books	Chicago Press
Science:	
Seymour Simon Series	Macmillan Publishing
Eyewitness Juniors	Alfred A. Knopf
The Child's World Series	Encyclopedia Britannica
Large as Life Series	Alfred Knopf
Books for Young Explorers	National Geographic Society
Eye Opener Series	Macmillan Publishing
Biographies:	
Picture Book Biographies	Holiday House
Art:	
Museum of Modern Art Series	Delacorte Press
Photography Books	Dutton Children's Books

Note: List compiled by Edward Tamulevich, Media Specialist, Montgomery County Public Schools, Rockville, MD.

For Novice Readers. At the novice stage, the goal of story reading is to call the individual's attention to the text. By linking key words or phrases in the written text with pictures from the story or with picture communication symbols, a teacher builds the understanding that print carries the message. Another way to introduce text to children or older students in a meaningful way is to create personalized albums of familiar environmental print such as favorite restaurant logos (McDonalds, Pizza Hut), favorite food labels (Coke, Kix cereal), and favorite stores (nearby drugstores and banks). Environmental print can be cut directly out of newspaper and magazine advertisements or from the products themselves (box tops, restaurant napkins). For older students, this can be a way to increase awareness of environmental print, and to build useful community-based skills, such as food shopping.

For Experimenting Readers. Experimenting readers are beginning to recognize letters and associate letter names with their corresponding sounds. It is not critical for a student to be able to name all the letters of the alphabet or identify phonemes in isolation before actively engaging in story reading. The objective at this stage is not to drill students on the alphabet, phonetic decoding, or sound blending, but to call their attention to how initial letters have sounds that say their names. Even for older students who are developmentally disabled, the ability to relate letter names to initial letter sounds is a functional skill. For example, it can help them differentiate words on a shopping list or find a phone number on the family's speed dial.

The traditional language experience approach is useful at this stage because it focuses on the one-to-one correspondence

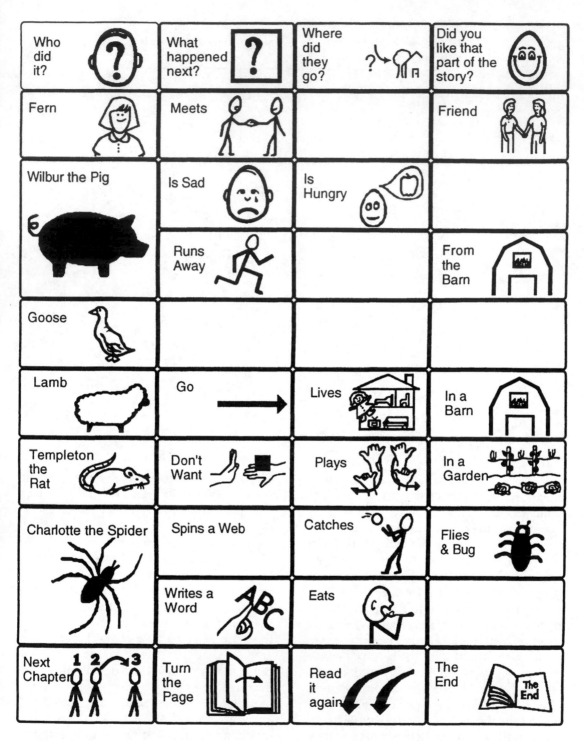

Who did it?	What happened next?	Where did they go?	Did you like that part of the story?
Fern	Meets		Friend
Wilbur the Pig	Is Sad	Is Hungry	
	Runs Away		From the Barn
Goose			
Lamb	Go	Lives	In a Barn
Templeton the Rat	Don't Want	Plays	In a Garden
Charlotte the Spider	Spins a Web	Catches	Flies & Bug
	Writes a Word	Eats	
Next Chapter	Turn the Page	Read it again	The End

Figure 8–3. A story board using Picture Communication Symbols. Courtesy of Boardmaker (Mayer-Johnson Co., Solana Beach, CA.).

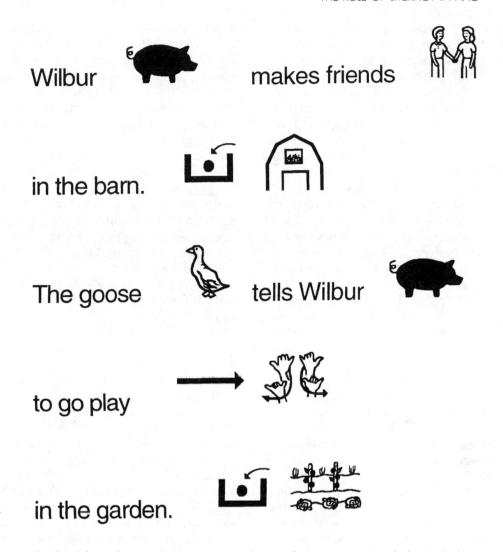

Wilbur   makes friends

in the barn.

The goose   tells Wilbur

to go play

in the garden.

Figure 8–4. Adapted story text incorporating Picture Communication Symbols. Symbols courtesy of Boardmaker (Mayer-Johnson Co.., Solana Beach, CA.).

of speech to text and because it provides a way to call attention to the initial letter sounds of key words. In the language experience approach, the teacher writes on large sheets of paper what the students contribute verbally, then the students practice reading what was written. Language experience lessons are easily integrated into a curriculum and often revolve around science activities, cooking activities, or how-to themes (e.g., how to make a bird feeder). For nonspeaking students, overlays using picture communication symbols and key words can be used in conjunction with language experience lessons to enable the student using AAC to participate in the activity.

Commercially made predictive, repetitive, early childhood books, as well as teacher-made books that combine simple written text with pictures encourage proto-reading and build the emergent literacy concept that print can be "read." Teacher-made books are useful because they can be geared to student ability levels and can build on the individualized interests of the student. Simple "listing" books start out with an unfinished statement on the first page (*For breakfast, I like*) and then have one or two words on each successive page (*pancakes, orange juice*). "Repeated sentence" books have a main theme (*Things I like about school*) and then a repeating sentence starter on each successive page (*I like my teachers, I like music*).

As the experimenting reader's literacy skills increase, reading materials must be adapted to keep pace with new abilities. At the experimenting stage, individuals gradually become aware that words have distinct beginning and ending consonant sounds. Gradually, they begin to discriminate medial consonant sounds and long vowel sounds. With these skills, children can experiment with reading and try to "figure out" written words. Choral reading is useful at this stage even with individuals who have limited speaking abilities. Together, students can practice reading simple poems, familiar songs and even jokes. Overhead projectors are useful for this.

It is often difficult to find easy reading passages that are appropriate for older students. This author has found it is best to copy and enlarge passages from children's magazines (e.g., *Sports Illustrated for Kids*) and easy-to-read nonfiction series. Another way to encourage experimenting readers to read is for the teacher to compose a daily personalized message on the computer. Using talking word processors such as IntelliTalk, Talking Text Writer, or Macintosh's Simple Text to speak the text of the written message.

Recently there has been a rapid increase in the number of CD ROM interactive books available. These are often an excellent way to provide reading experiences to children with physical disabili-ties. CD ROM features that highlight words as they are read and allow the speed of the text being read to be slowed are helpful for emergent literacy readers. The CD ROM interactive story topics published thus far are generally more appropriate to younger students. It is hoped that there will be more CD ROM interactive books in the future that are appropriate material for older emergent literacy students. CD ROMs by Queue, Inc., offer a wide range of fiction and nonfiction titles which are noninteractive, but provide simple reading passages accompanied by pictures and voice output, which are appropriate for older experimenting readers.

Using software such as HyperStudio and KidPix with its slide show features is an excellent way to write stories for students. This easy-to-use software allows teachers to design stories which match the interest and reading level of their students. Click It by Intellitools allows students with physical disabilities using a single switch to control on-screen page turning. Photographing pages of a book or story and developing slide shows to be used with the Ablenet Slide Projector Control is another way that an individual who is a single switch user can control page turning. This can be a costly and time-consuming process, so it is important to choose stories that have a lot of appeal and can be used again and again. Video cameras, digitized cameras, and scanners are another way that books can be adapted for an individual with physical disabilities who cannot hold a traditional book or turn its pages.

Audio book recordings can be used to promote reading skills when accompanied by a written text and when the recorded reading is read somewhat slowly with pauses between pages. If necessary, the instructor can retape the book using a peer's voice. Audio books-on-tape recordings, when used exclusively as an adaptation for poor readers, allow the individual to hear the story and build listening comprehension skills, but they do not develop the individual's abilities to read written text. Audio book recordings without accompanying written text should be used when the content of what is being presented is the central concern, rather than the reinforcement of reading skills. To reinforce reading skills, students must have opportunities to match speech to text.

The same also applies to reading machines such as the Bookwise Reading Edge. This technology provides a way for individuals to listen to text, but alone, it does not reinforce the reading of written text. However, when combined with a computer and dedicated software, it allows the individual to see the text as it is being read. This technology is quite costly and requires skill to operate the hardware and software components.

Reading with Nonspeaking Students. What about reading aloud for individuals who are completely nonverbal? This author has had success with a method that combines gestures, eye gaze, and pictures. Eric is a nonspeaking high school student with physical disabilities who can only produce open vowel sounds. Although Eric is nonverbal, he is still very motivated to participate in the reading process. The following method referred to as interactive-cued reading was designed to allow Eric to engage actively in reading aloud.

Reading passages, consisting of one or two paragraphs, are copied and enlarged and placed where Eric can easily read the text. Initially, the teacher slowly reads the passage aloud pointing to each word. During the second reading, Eric and the teacher assign a picture or a gesture to target words in the sentences. For example, for the word *out* Eric looks out the window; for the word *throw* Eric swings his arm to the side; for the word *sound*, he looks at a picture of an ear placed on his wheelchair tray. During the third reading, the teacher silently points to each word in the passage. When the teacher points to a designated target word, Eric makes the agreed upon gesture or eye gazes to the appropriate picture or referent for that word. Interactive-cued reading allows the student who is nonspeaking to participate actively in the reading process. It is often best to repeat the reading passage for a few days to give the student time to master the written text. It is also useful to use the maze procedure described previously as a pretest and posttest for this reading activity as a way to collect data on a student's reading skills and as a way to know when it is time to move to higher level reading passages.

Above all, daily exposure to reading is important for literacy learning for students with special needs of all ages. It is especially important that reading opportunities be geared to a student's particular literacy learning stage and be integrated into ongoing daily activities. For students demonstrating literacy learning potential at the experimenting level and beyond, especially those who are nonspeaking and severely physically disabled, daily one-on-one time is often needed to allow for active participation and to develop conventional reading skills. Actual time on task is the critical ingredient for demonstrating improvement in reading skills.

Spelling and Writing Assessment Strategies

Reading and writing instruction for individuals with special needs requires ongoing diagnostic teaching. Assessment strategies should focus more on the process of literacy learning and be used for formative purposes to formulate and plan teaching activities and to monitor progress. Process-oriented assessments are best achieved through careful observation or "kid watching" (Goodman, 1991), combined with ongoing recordkeeping. It is important to observe the efforts of students as they write and interact with books. Much can be learned about how and what students understand relative to literacy by analyzing their reading and writing efforts. Individual reading and writing portfolios are a good way to keep track of progress over time. Keep dated samples of students' independent writing, sentence dictation, and spelling test results in a folder. Audio or video tape book interactions and reading efforts. Multiple measures on multiple occasions provide a better record of progress over time than do single measurements at the start and end of the year.

Letter Name and Phoneme Knowledge. Writing assessment should begin with letter name and phoneme knowledge. As a starting point, it is important to gauge a student's level of mastery for naming all the upper and lower case letters of the alphabet, as well as identifying their corresponding sounds. For individuals who are nonspeaking, assessing letter name and phoneme knowledge can be accomplished using eye gaze or pointing as appropriate. Consonant sounds, long vowels, short vowels, and digraphs should be assessed.

At this point, it is also important to check that the student understands common teacher terminology such as "letter," "first sound," "last sound," "word," and "sentence." Clay (1985) has developed a method of assessment to evaluate a student's understanding of concepts of print.

Spelling and Writing Assessment. Spelling can be assessed in a variety of ways. To begin, ask an individual to spell as many words as he or she can. Stop after the student has produced about 10 words. This will provide an overview of the individual's approach to spelling. Students with little phonemic awareness will produce strings of random letters; however, students with a growing understanding that letters are combined in certain ways to make words will produce familiar names, high frequency words, and may make inventive spelling attempts.

Another way to gauge a student's level of spelling is to give a developmental spelling test (Koppenhaver, 1990). The student's spelling performance provides a general developmental framework for writing instruction. For example, a student whose overall approach to spelling is represented at the Initial Consonant level (based on Ferroli and Shanahan's 1987 categorizations as outlined in Figure 8–2), should be encouraged to begin discriminating final consonant sounds. A student at the Consonant Frame level should be given instruction in discriminating voiced medial consonants and vowel sounds, beginning with long vowels. Students at the Phonetic level should begin to focus on blends, digraphs, and vowel combinations, whereas students at the Transitional level are ready for more traditional spelling rules and word study. These represent general instructional guidelines, as the best approach to diagnostic teaching is through a careful analysis of each student's work. By analyzing a student's spelling and writing, it is possible to gain a great deal of insight for the purpose of designing individualized spelling and writing instruction.

Developmental spelling levels are highly correlated with early reading levels and can predict reading achievement (Morris & Perney, 1984; Zutell & Rasinski, 1989). Richgels (1995) stated that inventive spelling demonstrates a student's understanding of phoneme-grapheme relationships which is critical to successful reading. Analyzing children's inventive spellings can inform teachers of when to teach what as part of written language instruction (Invernizzi, Abouzeid, & Gill, 1994). Because individuals who rely on AAC often cannot read aloud for the teacher to easily determine a reading level, developmental spelling test results can provide a window on where to start with reading activities, as well as with writing activities.

Dictated sentences such as those provided by Clay (1985) and Kemp (1987) are another good method for demonstrating spelling improvement over time (Table 8–7). This method has been used successfully by this author with students who are nonspeaking by first reading the sentence to the student and then asking them to try their best to spell each word on the computer. Each word in the sentence should be spoken slowly by the evaluator one word at a time, but not stretched or over-articulated so that the word becomes phonetically disassembled.

Once students are spelling more at the Consonant Frame level, it is useful to get a baseline on high frequency words and sight words. There are a variety of word lists as seen in Table 8–8. Some are based on reading frequency or writing frequency and some are based on the needs of individuals who use AAC. There is considerable overlap among these lists.

Writing samples are another way to assess ongoing writing progress. However, simply asking a student to write something is often too daunting a task, and if the student is spelling at an Initial Consonant or Consonant Frame level, the teacher may not be able to discern what the student wrote. It is best to establish a topic with the individual who is nonspeaking to obtain a prompted writing sample. Ask yes/no or multiple choice questions to help narrow down a topic for the sample sentence. With young students, it is often useful to read a story or look at pictures to help them establish a writing topic. Prompted writing also provides insight into a student's ability to formulate written language. Although some students using various forms of developmental spelling will produce sentences using standard syntax, others may have significant difficulty with this, indicating a need for additional language assessment.

Spelling and Writing Instruction Strategies. Individuals who rely on AAC often have multiple disabilities. Consequently, their early developmental years are characterized by a prolonged focus on motor development and activities of daily living. Liter-

Table 8–7. Dictation sentences.

Clay's Dictation Sentences:

I have a big dog at home. Today I am going to take him to school.

I can see the red boat that we are going to have a ride in.

The bus is coming. It will stop here to let me get on.

The boy is riding his bike. He can go very fast on it.

Kemp's Dictation Sentences:

My name is (student's name). I'm going to be a _____.

(Choose a word with the student for sentence two and rehearse before the dictation task.)

My mom goes to work. She brings me to school in the car.

I'm going to get _____ for my birthday. I'm going to be _____.

Source: Compiled from *The Early Detection of Reading Difficulties* (p. 39), by M. M. Clay, 1990 (revised edition), Portsmouth, NH: Heinemann; and from *Watching Children Read and Write* (p. 210), by M. Kemp, 1987, Portsmouth, NH: Heinemann.

Table 8-8. Sources of frequently used written and spoken words.

Types of Word Lists	Sources
The 1,000 most common words in written English material	Fry, E., Polk, J., & Fountoukidis, D. (1988). *Reading teacher's book of lists.* Englewood Cliffs, NJ: Prentice Hall.
The most frequently found words in written material	Dolch, B. W. (1936). *Dolch basic sight words.* Champaign, IL: Garrard Press.
The most common words found in selected written assignments of nondisabled students from second through sixth grade	McGinnis, J. S., & Beukelman, D. R. (1989). Vocabulary requirements for writing activities for the academically mainstreamed student with disabilities. *Augmentative and Alternative Communication, 5*(3), 183-191.
The first 2,500 words of spoken English	Stemach, G., & Williams, W. (1988). *Word express: The first 2500 words of spoken English.* Novato, CA: Academic Therapy Press.
The most commonly spoken words by nondisabled young children	Beukelman, D. R., Jones, R. S., & Rowan, M. (1989). Frequency of word usage by nondisabled peers in integrated preschool classrooms. *Augmentative and Alternative Communication, 5*(4), 243-247.
The 500 most frequently used words by five adult augmentative communication system users	Beukelman, D. R., Yorkston, K. M., Poblete, M., & Naranjo, C. (1984). Frequency of word occurrence in communication samples produced by adult communcation aid users. *Journal of Speech and Hearing Disorders, 49,* 360-367.

acy skills often take a back seat in those early years to the day-to-day demands of feeding, toileting, and therapies. Literacy learning may be delayed or it may have less emphasis in the academic day because less actual time is spent on literacy learning. As a result, students may begin to develop literacy skills at older ages as compared to typical peers. This can be problematic in that older students are more aware of what conventional reading and writing looks like, and therefore, may be more reluctant to take risks and experiment in their reading and writing efforts. Risk taking, experimentation, and persistence are important ingredients for literacy learning, as it is through the process of hypothesis testing that children begin to sort out the rules by which words are formed. Initially, the young girl whose spelling and writing progress was depicted in Table 8–4 was reluctant to write. As a 9-year-old, she was aware of how words

and sentences look and knew that her writing efforts would not appear to be "correct." However, with encouragement to use inventive spelling (i.e., spelling approximations) to get her ideas out, the focus was shifted toward meaningful communication exchange and away from any concern over "correctness."

This author has found that older students at the novice and experimenting level need frequent encouragement and positive feedback which legitimizes their attempts at writing. It is important to let these individuals know that initial writing attempts do not have to look like "grown-up" or dictionary spelling; this is how everyone first learns to write. Encourage them to get their ideas out. Focus more on meaning than on product. Gentle editing should focus on what the student is ready to master. Final copies should be shared with others and pride expressed for their efforts in conveying their ideas.

Literacy learning by itself is not a curriculum. Literacy is not 30 minutes three times per week. Literacy needs to be integrated into learning activities throughout a student's day. A thematic approach to literacy learning through curriculum integration can be utilized at many different age levels and developmental levels (Figure 8–5). Using this approach, reading and writing activities can be developed within the context of science or social studies themes. Students in an inclusion setting who are operating at younger literacy levels as compared to their typical peers can participate in parallel activities that address their particular reading and writing skills. For older students in more self-contained classrooms with a focus on functional life skills, reading and writing activities for authentic and meaningful purposes can still be incorporated into daily routines. Table 8–9 presents examples of func-

Adapted and Parrallel Curriculum

GENERAL EDUCATION TOPIC	ADAPTED CURRICULUM	PARALLEL CURRICULUM
SCIENCE THEME: Living Things Characteristics of Animals	Read adapted passages from nonfiction books about animals Make a book "All About Animals" and write a new page each day about an interesting animal	Sort pictures to discriminate animals from that which is not an animal Make a "flap book" called "What am I". Put pictures and labels under the cut-out flap
SOCIAL STUDIES THEME: State History Topography	Identify mountains and lakes on a State map Read an adapted travel brochure about the State Imagine you are traveling and write a postcard about the scenery	Spin off from the "Brown Bear, Brown Bear" book by and write a picture book using the student's name, e.g., "Brian, Brian, What Do You See?" "On land, I see grass and trees. In the water, I see boats and fish..."
WORLD STUDIES THEME: Industrial Revolution	Read adapted passages about the history of machines and create a book about old and new machines to read at school and at home. Write advertisements about modern day or old fashioned appliances	Find pictures of machines in a store catalogue or a newspaper advertising insert Make a scrapbook of "Machines that Help Us" Use pictures and label each picture.

Figure 8–5. Reading and writing activities which are adapted or run parallel to the general education curriculum.

tional IEP objectives for older students at emergent literacy levels.

For some students at experimenting levels, there is more of a need for daily, one-on-one, direct teaching, in addition to reading and writing activities incorporated throughout the school day. This is especially so for AAC communicators with severe speech and physical impairments who rely on single switch scanning to operate word processing software. These students often benefit from having a minimum of one period per day to focus directly on reading and writing. These students need more time and more individualized instruction because of the nature of their disabilities combined with the complexity of their assistive technology.

Beginner and Novice Writers. Students at beginner levels are in the process of understanding that pictures convey meaning. These students may not be aware of letters and words. At this level, students should be encouraged to create pictures using drawing programs. For example, the "rubber stamp" feature of KidPix software allows students to stamp pictures on the screen. To call their attention to printed text, it is useful to label the pictures they've chosen. In this way, you are combining pictures and words to increase awareness of printed text. Children typically first experiment with writing when drawing, including words to label parts of their drawings. They begin to insert words in their pictures when the pictures alone are insufficient to convey their intended messages and when written text is recognized as an extension of speech.

Students at novice levels are beginning to attend to words in text and pay more attention to individual letters, especially those in their name. These students may make marks on paper to indicate they are "writing." They may scribble their names or make strings of letters on the computer to represent a written message.

Table 8–9. Functional IEP objectives for older students at emergent literacy levels.

The student will recognize his or her name in different contexts.

The student uses a book's pictures to help retell a story.

The student identifies grocery story environmental print in context and uses this to find items on a shopping list.

The student uses initial phonemes to discriminate among movie or television listings.

The student locates names on a telephone speed dial list using phonetic strategies.

The student uses phonetic strategies to sort and deliver in-house mail.

The student locates food items and prices on a menu using phonetic and sight word strategies.

The student uses phonetic "consonant frame" strategies to identify items on a shopping list.

The student uses knowledge of functional sight words and phonetic strategies to read a short message.

The student uses one-to-one speech-to-text correspondence when reading a simple recipe.

The student reads simplified versions of news articles.

Their pretend or proto-writing attempts indicate that they understand that writing is something people do to convey information. Their attempts may indicate an understanding that words are made up of letters; however, there is a lack of an awareness that words are made up of letters that correspond to individual sounds. At this level, proto-writing should be encouraged. Students should be given opportunities to use pencils or markers or write on the computer. Scribble writing or strings of letters should be legitimized and praised as meaningful writing attempts. It is acceptable to write the dictionary spelling of their intended message at the bottom of their paper. In center-based programs, writing tables or areas can be set up in the classroom which are outfitted with an old typewriter, paper, writing utensils, letter stamps, and magnetic letters. Writing for different purposes can be encouraged by providing stationary and envelopes, shopping list pads, note pads, prescription pads, restaurant order pads, sales pads, or phone message pads. Picture dictionaries, picture communication symbols, word banks, and environmental print albums are also useful to have on hand to encourage writing.

Writing for typical children usually begins with the writing of their name. Writing their name to "sign in" in the morning, sign their artwork, sign a card, or sign up for a classroom job gives students opportunities to see that writing is important. A student who cannot handwrite can use a rubber stamp customized with that student's name to sign in. Students who rely on eye gaze can eye point to their name or the individual letters of their name written on small adhesive notes positioned around the eye gaze board or frame. As the student gazes at the whole name or letters in sequence, the note is removed from the frame and positioned on the sign-up chart. Students who use scanning can use a computer to write their name and print it on adhesive labels.

Children often begin to focus on the beginning letter in their name and the sound associated with the letter name. With the exception of some letters like c, w, and y, the names of most letters can be associated with their sounds. For example, the f sound is evident when you say its letter name. Calling attention to the first letters and beginning sounds of students' names and other key words is one way to call attention to letter-sound relationships.

Not all students with special needs will move out of these early stages of literacy learning. However, the teacher cannot know this unless many varied opportunities have been provided to explore these early literacy concepts. What is most important is to provide a supportive learning environment that accepts nonconventional writing efforts; an environment that supports experimentation and risk taking where reading and writing are integrated into functional and meaningful activities for authentic purposes.

Experimenting Writers. Experimenting writers are beginning to associate letter names with letter sounds. They understand that words are combinations of letters, and they experiment with spelling and writing in an effort to "break the code" and discover just how letters are combined to form words. It is this experimentation that is critical for students at this level. It is not a matter of encoding or sound blending letter sounds sequentially from left to right. Children demonstrate that they first pay attention to first-letter consonant sounds, then to end-letter consonant sounds. Thereafter, they begin to discriminate medial consonant sounds, and they begin to hear long vowel sounds, as long vowels are letters that say their names. These skills are the rudiments of "inventive" spelling and give students the power to begin conveying information in written form. Although their writing is not yet conventional, in this way they are learning to break the written code. Students at the experimenting level are demonstrating spelling at Initial Consonant, Consonant Frame, and Phonetic levels (as described in Figure 8–2). As students move from phonetic levels to transitional levels of spelling, more traditional spelling and writing approaches are appropriate, with emphasis on consonant blends, short vowels, digraphs, word families, and word study emphasis on word endings, prefixes, and suffixes. Use student writing samples to make teaching decisions as to what a student is ready to absorb. Mini-lessons tied to the editing of their written work are often more meaningful than a singular emphasis on spelling rules.

At this level, it is still more important to focus on the meaning that underlies what they are writing, rather than just focusing on its "correctness." An overemphasis on correcting spelling and syntax errors causes students to be reluctant to experiment with writing, which slows their concept development on how words are constructed and combined to produce meaningful writing. Edit gently, focusing on one or two features the student seems ready to learn.

When writing with students who are nonspeaking and employing inventive spelling, it can be difficult to interpret what they wrote. Asking a student to write about an undefined topic can be frustrating to both the student and the teacher if the intended message is indiscernible. The best way to avoid this is to use an activity or book as a starting place for writing. Talk with the student about the book or activity and jointly agree on a writing topic. Further define this topic so that two or three ideas are discussed with the student. The student can then choose among these ideas and begin to write. With students who are very reluctant to write and are spelling at the initial consonant level, even more support may be needed initially. For these students, it is necessary to

jointly agree on the words or sentence to be written. Over time, when confidence and spelling approximations improve, this level of support can be phased out.

Writing activities should center on authentic and meaningful purposes. Additional functional writing ideas include making signs, writing invitations, writing on the classroom calendar, writing shopping lists, recipes, or birthday cards. More formal writing activities can include writing friendly letters, postcards, letters of complaint, how-to books, or all-about books. It is useful to build writing activities around student interests or to write on themes generated by the curriculum. Themes that emerge from books can serve as a springboard into writing. For example, students reading a story about a wishing well can write about what they would wish for. Students reading *The Carrot Seed* by Krauss and Johnson (1945) can plant flower seeds and then write a how-to book on how to grow flowers.

Initially, children often generate word lists or phrases, rather than narratives in sentence form. Writing activities at this level can be simplified. For example, after reading *The Hungry Caterpillar* (Carle, 1969), children can create a book about their favorite foods with one word to a page accompanied by magazine pictures or picture communication symbols. Or, students can start with a title page such as "When I'm a teenager, I will" and write a short phrase per page to make a short book on the theme of growing older. Irrespective of the writing activity, it is important to validate writing efforts. Table 8–10 presents examples of writing by students at the experimenting level. Phrases or sentences written by the students were printed out on separate pages, placed in plastic page protectors, and formed "books" which the students could take home to read with their families. Exact translations, conventionally spelled, were written at the bottom of each page of the student's

Table 8-10. Examples of students writing (in italics) at the experimenting level.

Title page:	My Favorite Foods	
Page 1:	My favorite foods are	
Page 2:	*is kem*	ice cream
Page 3:	*pez*	pizza
Page 4:	*cnde*	candy
Page 5:	*ht dgs*	hot dogs
Title page:	If I Had a Magic Lamp	
Page 1:	*I go t jmaca*	I go to Jamaica.
Page 2:	*I by Carrie gld ring*	I buy Carrie a gold ring.
Page 3:	*I by jgwr cr*	I buy a Jaguar car.
Title page:	I Can	
Page 1:	*I can dv mi wljr*	I can drive my wheelchair.
Page 2:	*I can mak pkjrs*	I can make pictures.
Page 3:	*I can reed*	I can read.
Page 4:	*I can rit*	I can write.

work. This allowed the families to read each page and provided opportunities for students to see conventionally spelled words. Displaying students' work and giving them opportunities to have their work read aloud using the student's AAC device also served to encourage future writing efforts.

CONCLUSION

There is abundant research with typical young children without disabilities over the past 20 years demonstrating that the literacy continuum begins in infancy and develops throughout early childhood. However, the lack of comparable data on literacy achievement for children with special needs using AAC is deplorable. Current research indicates that students with disabilities lack adequate literacy learning experiences, however, there are no studies that suggest that children with disabilities cannot begin to develop literacy skills in early childhood.

Too often the nature of a student's disability is used as the exclusive cause for delayed literacy skills. Recent research suggests that home literacy experiences and school instruction are elements that must be reexamined relative to delays in literacy learning. No longer can special education professionals assume that literacy instruction should be reserved only for students who demonstrate the potential for conventional reading and writing abilities. The all-or-nothing approach to literacy instruction in special education is no longer acceptable. Although not all children with disabilities will achieve conventional reading and writing skills, there are many achievements along the literacy continuum that are applicable to the education of students with disabilities. Home-school partnerships and instructional changes are needed to promote literacy learning for students with disabilities.

For nonspeaking individuals, literacy is more than just learning to read and write; it expands the individual's potential to actively communicate on any subject. But literacy instruction is not simply a matter of adapting or downsizing the regular kindergarten or first-grade curriculum. The "how" of literacy instruction depends on the ability of educators to match strategies to the student's present level of skill and learning style. The role of the educator is to understand how literacy develops and to custom fit meaningful strategies that facilitate on a daily basis the student's progress toward literacy development. Special educators need a strong foundation in emergent literacy learning and an equally strong commitment toward individualized literacy learning for all.

REFERENCES

Allen, J. B., Clark, W., Cook, M., Crane, P., Fallon, I., Hoffman, L., Jennings, K. S., & Sours, M. A. (1989). Reading and writing development in whole language kindergartens. In J. M. Mason (Ed.), *Reading and writing connections* (pp. 121–146). Boston: Allyn & Bacon.

Altwerger, B., Edelsky, C., & Flores, B. (1987). Whole language: What's new? *Reading Teacher, 41,* 144–154.

Asher, P., & Schonell, F. E. (1950). A survey of 400 cases of cerebral palsy in childhood. *Archives of Disease in Childhood, 25,* 360–379.

Aulls, M. W. (1985). Understanding the relationship between reading and writing. *Educational Horizons, 64,* 39–44.

Barsch, R. H., & Rudell, B. (1962). A study of reading development among 77 children with cerebral palsy. *Cerebral Palsy Review, 23,* 3–12.

Beers, J. W., & Beers, C. S. (1980). Vowel spelling strategies among first and second graders: A growing awareness of written words. *Language Arts, 57*(2), 166–177.

Berninger V. W., & Gans B. M. (1986). Assessing word processing capability of the nonvocal,

nonwriting. *Augmentative and Alternative Communication, 2,* 56–63.

Beukelman, D. R., Jones, R. S., & Rowan, M. (1989). Frequency of word usage by nondisabled peers in integrated preschool classrooms. *Augmentative and Alternative Communication, 5,* 243–248.

Beukelman, D. R., Yorkston, K. M., Poblete, M., & Naranjo, C. (1984). Frequency of word occurrence in communication samples produced by adult communication aid users. *Journal of Speech and Hearing Disorders, 49,* 360–367.

Birnbaum, J., & Emig, J. (1983). Creating minds, created texts: Writing and reading. In R. P. Parker & F. A. Davis, (Eds.), *Developing literacy: Young children's use of language* (pp. 87–104). Newark, DE: International Reading Association.

Bishop, D. V. M. (1985). Spelling ability in congenital dysarthria: Evidence against articulatory coding in translating between phonemes and graphemes. *Cognitive Neuropsychology, 2,* 229–251.

Bishop, D. V. M., & Robson, J. (1989). Accurate non-word spelling despite congenital inability to speak: Phoneme-grapheme conversion does not require subvocal articulation. *British Journal of Psychology, 80,* 1–13.

Bissex, G. L. (1980). *GYNS AT WRK: A child learns to write and read.* Cambridge, MA: Harvard University Press.

Blackstone, S. W., & Poock, G. K. (1989, January). Upfront. *Augmentative Communication News, 2,* 1–3.

Blischak, D. M. (1994). Phonological awareness: Implications for individuals with little or no functional speech. *Augmentative and Alternative Communication, 10,* 245–254.

Bloodgood, J. (1991). A new approach to spelling instruction in language arts programs. *The Elementary School Journal, 92,* 199–207.

Bowley, A. H. (1967). A follow up study of 64 children with cerebral palsy. *Developmental Medicine and Child Neurology, 9,* 172-182.

Bradley, L., & Bryant, P. E. (1983). Categorizing sounds and learning to read: A causal connection. *Nature, 301,* 419–421.

Brazelton, T. B. (1969). *Infants and mothers: Differences in development.* NY: Delacorte Press.

Bridge, C. A., & Hiebert, E. H., (1985). A comparison of classroom writing practices, teachers' perception of their writing instruction, and textbook recommendations on writing practices. *The Elementary School Journal, 86,* 152–172.

Bruner, J. S. (1960). *The process of education.* Cambridge, MA: Harvard University Press.

Bruner, J. S. (1978). The role of dialogue in language acquisition. In A. Sinclair, R. J. Jarvelle, & W. J. M. Levelt, (Eds.), *The child's conception of language.* New York: Springer-Verlag.

Calkins, L. M., (1986). *The art of teaching writing.* Portsmouth, NH: Heinemann.

Carle, E. (1969). *The hungry caterpillar.* New York: World Publishing.

Carle, E. (1983). *Brown bear, brown bear, what do you see?* New York: Holt

Center, Y., & Ward, J. (1984). Integration of mildly handicapped cerebral palsied children into regular schools. *Exceptional Child, 31,* 104–113.

Chapanis, A., Ochsman, R. B., Parrish, R. N., & Weeks G. D. (1972). Studies in interactive communication modes on the behavior of teams during cooperative problem solving. *Human Factors, 14,* 487–509.

Chomsky, C. (1970). Reading, writing, and phonology. *Harvard Educational Review, 40,* 284–309.

Chomsky, C. (1976). After decoding: What? *Language Arts, 53,* 288–296.

Chomsky, N. (1957). *Syntactic structures.* The Hague: Mouton.

Clark, L. K. (1988). Invented versus traditional spelling in first graders' writing: Effects on learning to spell and read. *Research in the Teaching of English, 22,* 281–308.

Clark, M. M. (1976). *Young fluent readers: What can they teach us?* Portsmouth, NH: Heinemann Educational.

Clay, M. M. (1967). The reading behavior of five-year-old children: A research report. *New Zealand Journal of Educational Studies, 2,* 11–31.

Clay, M. M. (1975). *What did I write?* Auckland, NZ: Heinemann Educational.

Clay, M. M. (1985). *The early detection of reading difficulties* (rev. ed.). Portsmouth, NH: Heinemann.

Clay, M. M. (1987). *Writing begins at home.* Portsmouth, NH: Heinemann.

Cohn, M. (1981). Observations of learning to read and write naturally. *Language Arts, 58,*

549–555.

Coltheart, M. (1979). When can children learn to read—And when should they be taught. In T. G. Waller & G. E. MacKinnon (Eds.), *Reading research: Advances in theory and practice* (Vol. 1). New York: Academic Press.

Creech, R. (1988, October). Paravocal communicators speak out. *Aug-Communique: North Carolina Augmentative Communication Association Newsletter, 6*(3), 12.

Danilova, L. A. (1983). *Methods of improving the cognitive and verbal development of children with cerebral palsy* (R. H. Silverman, Trans., Monograph No. 23). New York: World Rehabilitative Fund.

DeCoste, D. C. (1993). Effects of intervention on the writing and spelling skills of elementary school students with severe speech and physical impairments. *University Microfilms International,* (University Microfilms No. 9318049).

Dewey, J. (1938). *Experience and education.* New York: Collier Books.

Doake, D. B. (1986). Learning to Read: It starts in the home. In D. R. Tovey & J. E. Kerber (Eds.), *Roles in literacy learning* (pp. 2–9). Newark, DE: International Reading Association.

Dobson, L. N. (1985). Learning to read by writing: A practical program for reluctant readers. *Teaching Exceptional Children, 18,* 30–36.

Dobson, L. N. (1989). Connections in learning to write and read: A study of children's development through kindergarten and first grade. In J. M. Mason, (Ed.), *Reading and writing connections* (pp. 83–103). Boston: Allyn & Bacon.

Dolch, B. W. (1936). *Dolch basic sight words.* Champaign, IL: Garrard Press.

Dorman, C. (1987). Verbal, perceptual and intellectual factors associated with reading achievement in adolescents with CP. *Perceptual and Motor Skills, 64,* 671–678.

Downing, J., DeStefano, J., Rich, G., Bell, A. (1984). Children's views of spelling. *Elementary School Journal, 85*(2), 184–198.

Dudley-Marling, C., & Dippo, D. (1991). The language of whole language. *Language Arts, 68,* 548–554.

Durkin, D. (1966). *Children who read early.* New York: Teachers College Press.

Dyson, A. H. (1982). Reading, writing and language: Young children solving the written language puzzle. *Language Arts, 59,* 839–839.

Dyson, A. H. (1985). Individual differences in emerging writing. In M. Farr (Ed.), *Advances in writing research: Vol. 1. Children's early writing development* (pp. 59–125). Norwood, NJ: Ablex.

Dyson, A. H., & Genishi, C. (1982). Whatta ya tryin' to write?: Writing as an interactive process. *Language Arts, 59,* 126–133.

Edelsky, C., Altwerger, B., & Flores, B. (1991). *Whole language: What's the difference?* Portsmouth, NH: Heinemann.

Ehri, L. C. (1989). Movement into word reading and spelling: How spelling contributes to reading. In J. M. Mason (Ed.), *Reading and writing connections* (pp. 65-79). Boston: Allyn & Bacon

Ehri, L. C., & Wilce, L. S. (1987). Does learning to spell help beginners learn to read words? *Reading Research Quarterly, 22,* 47–65.

Elder, P. S., & Goossens, C. (1994). *Engineering training environments for interactive augmentative communication: Strategies for adolescents and adults who are moderately/severely developmentally delayed.* Birmingham, AL: Southeast Augmentative Communication Conference Publications.

Farrell, M., & Elkins, J. (1995). Literacy for all? The case of Down Syndrome. *Journal of Reading, 38*(4), 270–280.

Ferreiro, E., & Teberosky, A. (1982). *Literacy before schooling.* Portsmouth, NH: Heinemann.

Ferrier, M. S., & Shane, H. C. (1987). Computer based communication aids for the nonspeaking child with cerebral palsy. *Seminars in Speech and Language, 8,* 107–122.

Ferroli, L., & Shanahan, T. (1987). Kindergarten spelling: Explaining its relationship to first-grade reading. In J. E. Readence & R. S. Baldwin (Eds.), *Research in literacy: Merging perspectives* (36th Yearbook of the National Reading Conference). Rochester, NY: NRC.

Foley, B. E. (1989). *Phonological recoding and congenital dysarthria.* Unpublished doctoral dissertation, University of Massachusetts, Amherst, MA.

Foley B. E. (1993). The development of literacy in individuals with severe congenital speech and motor impairments. *Topics in Language Disorders, 13*(2), 16-32.

Freeman, Y. S., & Whitesell, L. R. (1985). What preschoolers already know about print. *Educational Horizons, 64,* 22–24.

Freppon, P. A., & Dahl, K. L. (1991). Learning about phonics in a whole language classroom. *Language Arts, 68,* 190–197.

Freyberg, P. (1964). Comparison of two approaches to the teaching of spelling. *British Journal of Educational Psychology, 34,* 178–186.

Fry, E., Polk, J., & Fountoukidis, D. (1988). *Reading teacher's book of lists.* Englewood Cliffs, NJ: Prentice Hall.

Furnas, A. (1985). Watch me. In J. Hansen, T. Newkirk, & D. Graves, (Eds.), *Breaking ground: Teachers relate reading and writing in the elementary school* (pp. 37–44). Portsmouth, NH: Heinemann.

Garner, J. B, & Campbell, P. H. (1987). Technology for persons with severe disabilities: Practical and ethical considerations. *Journal of Special Education, 21*(3), 122–132.

Gentry, J. R. (1981). Learning to spell developmentally. *The Reading Teacher, 34,* 378–381.

Gentry, J. R. (1982). An analysis of developmental spelling in GNYS AT WRK. *The Reading Teacher, 36,* 192-200.

Gentry, J. R. (1987). *SPEL . . . is a four letter word.* Portsmouth NH: Heinemann.

Goodman, K. S. (1967). Reading: A psycholinguistic guessing game. *Journal of the Reading Specialist, 4,* 126–135.

Goodman, K. S. (1986). *What's whole in whole language?* Portsmouth, NH: Heinemann.

Goodman, K. S. (1989). Whole-language research: Foundations and development. *The Elementary School Journal, 90*(2), 207-221.

Goodman, K. S. (1991). Whole language: What makes it whole? In B. M. Power & R. Hubbard (Eds.), *Literacy in process* (pp. 88–95). Portsmouth, NH: Heinemann.

Goodman, Y. M. (1967). *A psycholinguistic description of observed oral reading phenomena in selected young beginning readers.* Unpublished doctoral dissertation, Wayne State University, Detroit.

Goodman, Y. M. (1978). Kidwatching: Observing children in the classroom. In A. Jaggar & M. T. Smith-Burke (Eds.), *Observing the language learner* (pp. 9–18). Urbana, IL: National Council of Teachers of English; Newark, DE: International Reading Association.

Goossens, C., Crain, S. S., & Elder, P. S. (1992). *Engineering the preschool environment for in-*

teractive, symbolic communication. Birmingham, AL: Southeast Augmentative Conference Publications.

Graves, D. H. (1978). *Balance the basics: Let them write.* A report to the Ford Foundation. New York: Ford Foundation.

Graves, D. H. (1983). *Writing: Teachers and children at work.* Portsmouth, NH: Heinemann.

Graves, D. H. (1991). All children can write. In B. M. Power & R. Hubbard (Eds.), *Literacy in process* (pp. 67–78). Portsmouth, NH: Heinemann.

Griffith, P. L. (1991). Phonemic awareness helps first graders invent spellings and third graders remember correct spellings. *Journal of Reading Behavior, 23*(2), 215–233.

Guthrie, J., Seifert, M., Burnham, N. ,& Caplan, R. (1974). The maze technique to assess, monitor reading comprehension. *Reading Teacher, 28*(2), 161–168.

Haley-James, S. M. (1982). When are children ready to write? *Language Arts, 59,* 458—463.

Hall, M. A., Moretz, S. A., & Statom, J. (1976). Writing before grade one: A study of early writers. *Language Arts, 53,* 582–585.

Hall, N. (1987). *The emergence of literacy.* Portsmouth, NH: Heinemann Educational.

Halliday, M. (1989). *Spoken and written language.* NY: Oxford University Press.

Hansen, J. (1985). Skills. In J. Hansen, T. Newkirk, & D. Graves (Eds.), *Breaking ground: Teachers relate reading and writing in the elementary school* (pp. 183–191). Portsmouth, NH: Heinemann.

Harris, D. (1978). *Descriptive analysis of communicative interaction processes involving nonvocal severely physically handicapped children.* Unpublished doctoral dissertation, University of Wisconsin at Madison.

Harste, J. E., Woodward, V. A., & Burke, C. L. (1984). *Language stories and literacy lessons.* Portsmouth, NH: Heinemann.

Hauser, C. M. (1982). Encouraging beginner writers. *Language Arts, 59,* 681–686.

Henderson, E. H., & Beers, J. (Eds.). (1980). *Developmental and cognitive aspects of learning to spell.* Newark, DE: International Reading Association.

Hilliker, J. (1988). Labeling to beginning narrative: Four kindergarten children learn to write. In T. Newkirk & N. Atwell (Eds.), *Understanding writing* (2nd ed., pp. 14–22).

Portsmouth, NH: Heinemann.

Hodges, R. E. (1982). Research update: On the development of spelling ability. *Language Arts, 59,* 284–291.

Holdaway, D. (1979). *The foundations of literacy.* New York: Ashton Scholastic.

Horn, E. (1920). Principles of method in teaching spelling as derived from scientific investigations. *The 18th Yearbook of the National Society for the Study of Education* (pp. 52–77). Bloomington, IL: Public School Publishing.

Invernizzi, M., Abouzeid, M., & Gill, J. T. (1994). Using students' invented spellings as a guide for spelling instruction that emphasizes word study. *The Elementary School Journal, 95*(2), 156–167.

Irwin, O. C. (1972). *Communication variables of cerebral palsied and mentally retarded children.* Springfield, IL: Charles C. Thomas.

Johnson, T. D., Langford, K. G., & Quorn, K. C. (1981). Characteristics of an effective spelling program. *Language Arts, 58,* 581–588.

Jones, M. H., Dayton, G. O., Bernstein, L., Strommen, E. A., Osborne, M., & Watanbe, K. (1966). Pilot study of reading problems in cerebral palsied adults. *Developmental Medicine and Child Neurology, 8,* 417–427.

Juel, C. (1992). Longitudinal research on learning to read and write with at-risk students. In M. J. Freher & W. H. Slater (Eds.), *Elementary school literacy: Critical issues* (pp. 73–96). Norwood, MA: Christopher-Gordon.

Kagan, J. (1971). *Change and continuity in infancy.* NY: Wiley.

Kelly, J., & Friend, T. (1993). *Hands-on reading.* Solana Beach, CA: Mayer-Johnson.

Kemp, M. (1987). *Watching children read and write.* Portsmouth, NH: Heinemann.

King, M. L. (1989). Speech to writing. In J. M. Mason (Ed.), *Reading and writing connections* (pp. 7–29). Boston: Allyn & Bacon.

King-DeBaun, P. (1990). *Storytime: Stories, symbols and emergent literacy activities for young, special needs children.* Park City, UT: Creative Communicating.

Koppenhaver, D. A. (1990, February). Literacy instruction and nonspeaking students with cerebral palsy. *Assistive Device News.* (Available from the Pennsylvania Assistive Device Center, 150 South Progress Ave., Harrisburg, PA 17109).

Koppenhaver, D. A., Evans, D. A., & Yoder, D. E. (1991). Childhood reading and writing experiences of literate adults with severe speech and motor impairments. *Augmentative and Alternative Communication. 7,* 20-33.

Koppenhaver, D. A., & Yoder, D. E. (1988, October). Independent reading practice. *Aug-Communique, North Carolina Augmentative Communication Association Newsletter, 6*(3), 9-11.

Koppenhaver, D. A., & Yoder, D. E. (1989). Study of a spelling strategy for physically disabled augmentative communication users. *Communication Outlook, 10*(3), 10–12.

Koppenhaver, D. A., & Yoder, D. E. (1990a, July). *A descriptive analysis of classroom reading and writing instruction for adolescents with severe speech and physical impairments.* Paper presented at the International Special Education Congress, Cardiff, Wales.

Koppenhaver, D. A., & Yoder, D. E. (1990b, August). *Classroom interaction, literacy acquisition, and nonspeaking children with physical impairments.* Paper presented at the biennial meeting of the International Society for Augmentative and Alternative Communication, Stockholm, Sweden.

Koppenhaver, D. A., & Yoder, D. E. (1992). Literacy issues in persons with severe speech and physical impairments. In R. Gaylord-Ross (Ed.), *Issues and research in special education* (pp. 156–201). NY: Teachers College Press.

Krauss, R, & Johnson, C. (1945). *The carrot seed.* NY: Scholastic.

Kucer, S. L. (1985). The making of meaning: Reading and writing as parallel processes. *Written Communication, 2,* 317–336.

Lehr, F. (1985). Instructional scaffolding. *Language Arts, 62,* 667–672.

Light, J., Binger, C., & Smith, A. K. (1994). Story reading interactions between preschoolers who use AAC and their mothers. *Augmentative and Alternative Communication, 10,* 255–268.

Light, J., & Smith, A. K. (1993). The home literacy experiences of preschoolers who use augmentative communication systems and of their nondisabled peers. *Augmentative and Alternative Communication, 9,* 10–25.

MacArthur, C. A., & Graham, S. (1987). Learning disabled students composing under three methods of text production: Handwriting, word processing and dictation. *Journal of Special Education, 21*(3), 22–42.

Marino, J. (1981). Spelling errors: From analysis to instruction. *Language Arts, 58,* 567-572.

Marvin, C. (1994). Home literacy experiences of preschool children with single and multiple disabilities. *Topics in Early Childhood Special Education, 14,* 436–454.

Marvin, C., & Mirenda, P. (1993). Home literacy experiences of preschoolers enrolled in Head Start and special education programs. *Journal of Early Intervention, 17,* 351–367.

Mason, J. M. (1980). When do children begin to read: An exploration of four-year-old children's letter and word reading competencies. *Reading Research Quarterly, 15,* 203–227.

Mason, J. M., & Allen, J. B. (1986). Prereading: A developmental perspective. In P. D. Pearson et al. (Eds.), *Handbook of reading research* (Vol. 1, pp. 505–543). New York: Longman.

McGee, L. M., & Richgels, D. J. (1990). *Literacy's beginnings: Supporting young readers and writers.* Boston: Allyn & Bacon.

McGinnis, J. S., & Beukelman, D. R. (1989). Vocabulary requirements for writing activities for the academically mainstreamed student with disabilities. *Augmentative and Alternative Communication, 5,* 183–191.

McNaughton, D., & Drynan, D. (1990, August). *Assessment and intervention issues for written communication: A case study.* Paper presented at the biennial meeting of the International Society for Augmentative and Alternative Communication, Stolkholm, Sweden.

McNaughton, D., & Tawney, J. (1992). Comparison of two spelling instruction techniques for adults who use augmentative and alternative communication. *Augmentative and Alternative Communication, 9,* 72–82.

Meyers, L. F. (1984). Unique contributions of microcomputers to language intervention with handicapped children. *Seminars in Speech and Language, 5,* 23–34.

Mike, D. G. (1987, December). *Literacy, technology, and the multiply disabled: An ethnography of classroom interaction.* Paper presented at the meeting of the National Reading Conference, St. Petersburg, FL.

Mills, H., & Clyde, J. A. (1990). *Portraits of whole language classrooms: Learning for all ages.* Portsmouth, NH: Heinemann.

Morphett, M. V., & Washburne, C. (1931). When should children begin to read? *Elementary School Journal, 31,* 496–508.

Morris, D., & Perney, J. (1984). Developmental spelling as a predictor of first-grade reading achievement. *The Elementary School Journal, 84,* 441–457.

Musselwhite, C. (1993). *RAPS: Reading activity projects for older students.* Phoenix, AZ: Southwest Human Development.

Newkirk, T. (1989). *More than stories: The range of children's writing.* Portsmouth, NH: Heinemann Educational Books.

Newman, J. M. (Ed.). (1985). *Whole language: Theory in use.* Portsmouth, NH: Heinemann Educational.

Nolan, C. (1981). *Dam-burst of dreams.* London: Pan Books.

Parker, R. P. (1983). Language development and learning to write: Theory and research findings. In R. P. Parker & F. A. Davis (Eds.), *Developing literacy: Young children's use of language* (pp. 38–54), Newark, DE: International Reading Association.

Parker, R. P., & Davis, F. A. (Eds.). (1983). *Developing literacy: Young children's use of language.* Newark, DE: International Reading Association.

Pearson, P. D. (1989). Reading the whole language movement. *The Elementary School Journal, 90,* 231–241.

Piaget, J. (1952). *The origins of intelligence in children* (M. Cook, Trans.). New York: International University Press.

Pinell, G. S. (1989). Success of at-risk children in a program that combines writing and reading. In J. M. Mason, (Ed.), *Reading and writing connections* (pp. 237–260). Needham Heights, MA: Allyn & Bacon.

Plessas, G. P., & Oakes, C. R. (1964). Prereading experiences of selected early readers. *The Reading Teacher, 17,* 241–245.

Purcell-Gates, V. (1989). What oral/written language differences can tell us about beginning instruction. *The Reading Teacher, 42,* 290–294.

Read, C. (1971). Pre-school children's knowledge of English phonology. *Harvard Educational Review, 41,* 1–34.

Read, C. (1975). *Children's categorization of speech sounds in English.* Urbana, IL: National Council of Teachers of English.

Richgels, D. J. (1995). Invented spelling ability and printed word learning in kindergarten. *Reading Research Quarterly, 30*(1), 96–109.

Rosenshine, B., & Stevens, R. (1984). Classroom instruction in reading. In P. D. Pearson (Ed.), *Handbook of reading research* (pp. 745–798). New York: Longman.

Routman, R. (1988). *Transitions: From literature to literacy.* Portsmouth, NH: Heinemann.

Schickedanz, J. A. (1990). *Adam's righting revolutions.* Portsmouth, NH: Heinemann.

Schonell, F. E. (1956). *Educating spastic children: The education and guidance of the cerebral palsied child.* London: Oliver & Boyd.

Schwartz, J. I. (1988). *Encouraging early literacy.* Portsmouth, NH: Heinemann.

Seidel, U. P., Chadwick. O. F. D., & Rutter, M. (1975). Psychological disorders in crippled children. A comparative study of children with and without brain damage. *Developmental Medicine and Child Neurology, 17,* 563–573.

Shanahan, T. (1988). The reading-writing relationship: Seven instructional principles. *The Reading Teacher, 41,* 636–647.

Slaughter, H. S., Haussler, M. M., Franks, A. S., Jilbert, K.A., & Silentman, I. J. (1987, April). *A fieldwork study of the instructional and social contexts of learning to read and write in Chapter 1 and regular classrooms.* Paper presented at the American Educational Research Association annual meeting, Washington, DC.

Smith, A. K., Thurston, S., Light, J., Parnes, P., & O'Keefe, B. (1989). The form and use of written communication produced by physically disabled individuals using microcomputers. *Augmentative and Alternative Communication, 5,*(4), 115–124.

Smith, F. (1982). *Understanding reading* (3rd ed.). New York: Holt, Rinehart & Winston.

Smith, F. (1992). Learning to read: The never-ending debate. *Phi Delta Kappan, 73* (6), 432–441.

Smith, M. (1990, August). *Reading achievement in non-speaking children: A comparative study.* Paper presented at the biennial meeting of the International Society for Augmentative and Alternative Communication, Stolkholm, Sweden.

Smith, M. M. (1992). Reading abilities of non-speaking students: Two case studies. *Augmentative and Alternative Communication, 8*(1), 57–65.

Snow, C. E., & Ninio, A. (1986). The contracts of literacy: What children learn from learning to read books. In W. H. Teale & E. Sulzby (Eds.), *Emergent literacy: Writing and reading* (pp. 116–138). Norwood, NJ: Ablex.

Sowers, S. (1979). Research update: A six-year-old's writing process: The first half of first grade. *Language Arts, 56,* 829–835.

Sowers, S. (1988). Six questions teachers ask about invented spelling. In T. Newkirk & N. Atwell (Eds.), *Understanding writing: Ways of observing, learning and teaching* (2nd ed., pp. 62–70). Portsmouth, NH: Heinemann.

Stemach, G., & Williams, W. (1988). *Word express: The first 2500 words of spoken English.* Novato, CA: Academic Therapy Press.

Stewart, J., & Mason, J. M. (1989). Preschool children's reading and writing awareness. In J. M. Mason (Ed.), *Reading and writing connections* (pp. 219—236). Boston, MA: Allyn & Bacon.

Strickland, D. S., & Morrow, L. M. (Eds.). (1989). *Emerging literacy: Young children learn to read and write.* Newark, Delaware: International Reading Association.

Strickland, D. S., & Taylor, D. (1989). Family storybook reading: Implications for children, families and curriculum. In D. S. Strickland & L. M. Morrow (Eds.), *Young children learn to read and write* (pp. 27–34). Newark, DE: International Reading Association.

Sulzby, E. (1983). *Beginning readers' developing knowledges about written language project.* Final report to the National Institute of Education (NIE-G-80-0176). Evanston, IL: Northwestern University.

Sulzby, E. (1985a). Children's emergent reading of favorite storybooks: A developmental study. *Reading Research Quarterly, 20,* 458–481.

Sulzby, E. (1985b). Kindergartners as writers and readers. In M. Farr (Ed.), *Advances in writing research: Vol. 1. Children's early writing development* (pp. 127–199). Norwood, NJ: Ablex.

Sulzby, E. (1986). Writing and reading: Signs of oral and written language organization in the young child. In W. H. Teale & E. Sulzby (Eds.), *Emergent literacy: Writing and reading* (pp. 50–89). Norwood, NJ: Ablex.

Sulzby, E., Barnhart, J., & Hieshima, J. A. (1989). Forms of writing and rereading from writing: A preliminary report. In J. M. Mason (Ed.), *Reading and writing connections* (pp. 31–50). Boston, MA: Allyn & Bacon.

Sulzby, E., & Teale, W. H. (1985). Writing development in early childhood. *Educational Horizons, 64,* 8–12.

Sulzby, E., & Teale, W. H. (1987, November). *Young children's storybook reading: Longitu-dinal study of parent-child interaction and children's independent functioning* (Final report to the Spencer Foundation). Ann Arbor: University of Michigan.

Sulzby, E., & Teale, W. H. (1991). Emergent literacy. In R. Barr, M. L. Kamil, P. B. Mosenthal, & P. D. Pearson, (Eds.), *Handbook of reading research* (Vol. 2, pp. 727–757). New York: Longman.

Sulzby, E., Teale, W. H., & Kamberelis, G. (1989). Emergent writing in the classroom: Home and school connections. In D. S. Strickland & L. M. Morrow (Eds.), *Emerging literacy: Young children learn to read and write* (pp. 63–79). Newark, DE: International Reading Association.

Taylor, K. K., & Kidder, E. B. (1988). The development of spelling skills: From first through eighth grade. *Written Communication, 5,* 222–244.

Teale, H. T. (1978). Positive environments for learning to read: What studies of early readers tell us. *Language Arts, 55,* 922–932.

Teale, H. T. (1982). Toward a theory of how children learn to read and write naturally. *Language Arts, 59,* 555–570.

Teale, H. T. (1986). Home background and young children's literacy development in early childhood. In W. H. Teale & E. Sulzby (Eds.), *Emergent literacy: Writing and reading* (pp. 173–206). Norwood, NJ: Ablex.

Teale, W. H., & Sulzby, E. (Eds.). (1986). *Emergent literacy: Writing and reading.* Norwood, NJ: Ablex.

Teale, W. H., & Sulzby, E. (1989). In D. S. Strickland & L. M. Morrow (Eds.), *Emerging literacy: Young children learn to read and write.* Newark, Delaware: International Reading Association.

Temple, C., Nathan, R. G., Temple, F., & Burris, N. A. (1993). *The beginnings of writing* (3rd ed.). Boston: Allyn & Bacon.

Templeton, S. (1991a). New trends in an historical perspective: The "what" and "why" of skills instruction in literacy. *Language Arts, 68,* 590–595.

Templeton, S. (1991b). Teaching and learning the English spelling system: Reconceptualizing method and purpose. *The Elementary School Journal, 92*(2), 185–201.

Tierney, R. J., & Pearson, P. D. (1983). Toward a composing model of reading. *Language Arts, 60,* 568–580.

Tierney, R. J., & Shanahan, T. (1991). Research on the reading-writing relationship: Interactions, transactions, and outcomes. In R. Barr, M. L. Kamil, & P. Mosenthal, (Eds.), *Handbook of reading research* (Vol. 2, pp. 246–280). New York: Longman.

Vanderheiden, G. C. (1984). Technology needs of individuals with communication impairments. *Seminars in Speech and Language, 5,* 59–67.

Vanderheiden, G. C., & Lloyd, L. L. (1986). Communication systems and their components. In S. W. Blackstone (Ed.), *Augmentative communication: An introduction* (pp. 49–161). Rockville, MD: American Speech-Language-Hearing Association.

Vygotsky, L. S. (1962). *Thought and language.* Cambridge, MA: MIT Press.

Vygotsky, L. S. (1978). *Mind in society.* Cambridge, MA: Harvard University Press.

Walsh, L. E. (1974). Measuring ocular motor performance of cerebral palsied children. *American Journal of Occupational Therapy, 28,* 265–271.

Watson, D. J. (1989). Defining and describing whole language. *The Elementary School Journal, 90*(2), 129–141.

Weaver, C. (1990). *Understanding whole language: From principles to practice.* Portsmouth, NH: Heinemann Educational.

Weeks, C. D., Kelly, M. & Chapanis, A. (1974). Studies in interactive communication: Cooperative problem solving by skilled and unskilled typists in a teletypewriter mode. *Journal of Applied Psychology, 59,* 665–674.

Wilde, S. (1990). A proposal for a new spelling curriculum. *The Elementary School Journal, 90*(3), 275–289.

Zutell, J., & Rasinski, T. (1989). Reading and spelling connections in third and fifth grade students. *Reading Psychology, 10,* 137–155.

Chapter 9

FUNDING AND LEGAL ISSUES IN AUGMENTATIVE AND ALTERNATIVE COMMUNICATION

Patricia R. Ourand and Sylvia Gray

Prior to the 1970s, there was little in the way of federal legislation that directly addressed the rights of individuals with disabilities in society at large. Individuals with severe communication disorders and their families fended for themselves or relied on private or religious charities for assistance. There was no overarching national program, set of requirements, or source of assistance.

Beginning in 1975, Congress embarked on an ambitious legislative program to establish national rights for individuals with disabilities. The Education for All Handicapped Children Act, P.L. 94-142, made public schools responsible and accountable for the education of children with disabilities. Subsequent legislation addressed educational services for preschool children. Other enactments emphasized the provision of technology to assist adults with disabilities in entering and maintaining employment and provided grants to states to fund equipment and services.

The provisions of these federal statutes vary. In some instances, Congress has established requirements that states must follow. Some requirements direct the states to provide services at no cost to the individual. In other instances, federal law seeks to bring about change by making funds available, either through grants to the state or through tax deductions and credits to businesses and individuals. Congress has also funded a number of work incentive programs through the Social Security Administration. Federal and state laws are overlapping and are implemented by a host of federal, state, and local agencies. Particularly for the individual seeking funding for an augmentative and alternative communication (AAC) device or service, finding the correct path through the maze can be a daunting process.

Many professionals who provide services to individuals who are nonspeaking feel uncomfortable discussing funding and tend to avoid this component of service delivery. It is a topic that does not appear in many university training programs or continuing education seminars. AAC funding is a time-consuming effort. The hours spent pursuing funding options are usually not built into a professional's or family's weekly schedule. Although there is a history of successful AAC funding precedents, the funding process is not getting easier. In fact, in today's environment of managed health care and stretched educational dollars, funding for AAC devices and services has grown more difficult.

With tightened funding resources, professionals need to move toward documenting the efficacy of AAC services in terms of customer satisfaction, value, quality, and cost (DeRuyter, 1995). That is, professionals will need to document the dollars required to provide AAC services and equipment and compare those dollars against cost savings and quality outcomes that can be achieved if the consumer has improved communication abilities. For example, funding an AAC system and related therapy services may cost a school system $8,000 to implement for a single student. If the student's improved communication abilities enable him or her to work independently with less need for a one-to-one teaching assistant, the school system could potentially save the same amount of money in personnel costs within a year. If the student's functional communication abilities improve when using the AAC system, the long-term outcome for future employment and educational opportunities also increases. This movement toward outcome-based decisions for funding AAC services is just beginning, and will potentially change the funding picture in the near and distant future (DeRuyter, 1995).

Despite these difficulties, there is funding available for AAC devices and services. Obtaining funding requires perseverance, salesmanship, and will power, along with a good working knowledge of funding options. AAC funding is available for those professionals and consumers willing to spend the time and effort to obtain the dollars. Although this chapter cannot instill character traits of perseverance or salesmanship, it can provide professionals and consumers with knowledge regarding funding streams and legal issues related to AAC.

This chapter reviews the significant federal laws as they relate to the provision of AAC services. Particular emphasis is placed on federal laws that have an impact on sources of funding for AAC services and devices. This chapter also addresses public and private medical assistance and insurance, federal work incentive programs, tax deductions and credits, and alternative sources of funding, such as public and private organizations. Finally, the chapter presents a basic plan for seeking funds for AAC devices and services.

FUNDING RESPONSIBILITIES

In order to successfully identify and leverage sufficient funding, pertinent AAC services must be identified and subsequently provided. These actions will ensure that the consumer is receiving the most appropriate AAC device while limiting underuse and abandonment of equipment. Additionally, such an approach ensures that the funder will not be asked for additional services and devices to prematurely replace those provided previously. To ensure success, these services cannot be provided in isolation. The topic of funding for AAC devices and services requires input from numerous sources. There is often oversight regarding who is responsible for this aspect of services delivery. A collaborative team must be assembled to guarantee that an individual receives the appropriate device and services. This team may include the consumer, parents or other family members, educator, rehabilitation counselor, rehabilitation technologist, speech-language pathologist, occupational therapist, physician, equipment vendor, and other service providers and professionals.

Once the team has been established, each member contributes knowledge of his or her individual expertise in funding. In most circumstances, the process of funding equipment and services will be assumed by more than one individual on the team. The purpose of relying on more than one individual is to expand the base of knowledge and resources brought to the funding process. Together, the combined skills of a team will be able to successfully identify and access appropriate funding sources. The team should strive to seek collaboration between funding sources. Many times more than one funding source is available to share in the responsibility of providing recommended AAC devices and services. Such solutions allow the consumer access to appropriate AAC equipment, while allowing each funding source to serve an increased number of consumers. Without collaboration, many funding alternatives will begin to deplete funds as the result of the enormity of AAC fiscal responsibilities.

OVERVIEW OF FUNDING RESOURCES

Morris & Golinker (1991) noted that there are

- over twenty federal funding streams that could pay for assistive technology devices and services,
- situations where more than one funding stream will reimburse for assistive technology needs for an infant, child, teenager, or adult with a disability,
- gaps in the funding picture for individuals of a certain age, with different types of disability, certain types of technology, and length of time support will be provided. (p. 41)

There are numerous funding resources available for the coverage of AAC services and devices. Figure 9–1 categorizes various funding alternatives by resource category and ages served. Funding resources include federal entitlement programs, health insurance programs, Social Security Administration work incentive programs, Internal Revenue Code deductions, and alternative sources.

FEDERAL STATUTES

Individuals with Disabilities Education Act (IDEA)

For children in need of AAC services and equipment, the focus is very often on the delivery of services and the provision of equipment within the educational system, and the primary federal law that requires the provision of services and equipment is the Individuals with Disabilities Education Act (IDEA). As originally enacted in 1975, the law was called the Education for All Handicapped Children Act, P.L. 94-142. Prior to 1975, children with disabilities were not guaranteed the right to a free, appropriate, public education. The education of children with disabilities was customarily viewed as the responsibility of the parents—not the schools. The more severe the disability, the more likely that the child would not receive an education in the public school. It was common practice to institutionalize children with disabilities or to create private schools that were separate from the public schools. In 1975, with the passage of the Education for All Handicapped Children Act, P.L. 94-142, the education of children with disabilities became the responsibility of the public schools.

The Education for All Handicapped Children Act, P.L. 94-142, established the foundation for educational services for all children with disabilities. This law guarantees (a) the right to a free, appropriate,

AAC FUNDING RESOURCES	Age of Eligibility			
	0 to 3	3 to 21	16 to 65	65+
FEDERAL ENTITLEMENT PROGRAMS				
Individuals with Disabilities Education Act (IDEA)				
IDEA, Part H, Early Intervention Grants	x			
IDEA, Part B, State Grant Programs	x	x		
Rehabilitation Act Amendments of 1992				
Basic State Grants, Title I			x	
Supported Employment, Title VI - C			x	
Independent Living, Title VII - A			x	x
Section 504	x	x	x	x
Section 508			x	
HEALTH INSURANCE PROGRAMS				
Medical Assistance (Medicaid, MA)				
EPSDT - Children's Services	x	x		
Adult Services			x	x
Waiver Programs	x	x	x	x
Medicare Part B			x	x
Private Insurance	x	x	x	x
SSA WORK INCENTIVE PROGRAMS				
Plan for Achieving Self Support (PASS)			x	x
Impairment Related Work Expenses (IRWEs)			x	x
Continued Medicaid Eligibility (Section 1619(b))			x	x
Continuation of Medicare Coverage			x	
Medicare for People with Disabilities Who Work			x	
INTERNAL REVENUE CODE (IRS)				
Medical and Dental Expense Deductions	x	x	x	x
Depreciation of Capital Equipment	x	x	x	x
Section 44: Disabled Access Credit (DAC)			x	x
Section 51: Targeted Jobs Tax Credit			x	x
State Sales Tax	x	x	x	x
Charitable Contributions	x	x	x	x
Impairment Related Work Expenses (IRWE's)			x	x
ALTERNATIVE FUNDING SOURCES				
Technology Related Assistance Programs	x	x	x	x
Monetary Loan Programs	x	x	x	x
Equipment Loan Programs	x	x	x	x
Disability Organizations	x	x	x	x
Service Clubs	x	x	x	x
Private Funds or Foundations	x	x	x	x

Figure 9–1. AAC funding resources.

public education to all children with disabilities; (b) the provision of educational services to the maximum extent appropriate in the least restrictive environment; (c) the participation of parents in the educational process; (d) due process procedures for challenging and appealing decisions; (e) the right to related services necessary to benefit from special education instruction; and (f) an Individualized Education Plan (IEP) to be developed for every child who is eligible for special education

IDEA Eligibility Requirements

Infants and Toddlers. Early intervention services are provided to infants and toddlers who meet the eligibility criteria as defined by IDEA (part H). Eligibility is determined by age (birth to 3) and evidence of a developmental delay, as measured by appropriate diagnostic instrument(s), in one or more of the following areas: cognitive, physical, communication, social or emotional, and adaptive development. Infants and toddlers may also be eligible for service if they have a diagnosed condition that results in a high probability for a developmental delay.

Preschool. In order to be eligible for special education services at age 3, it must be determined that the child meets the eligibility criteria for one of the disabilities identified in IDEA. Although federal law does not identify a developmental delay as an IDEA-eligible disability, a state at its discretion may determine that the diagnosis of developmental delay will be included in the eligibility criteria for providing services to children at age 3.

School Age. Under IDEA, eligibility for school age services is determined according to 13 disability areas: autism, deaf-blindness, deafness, hearing impairment, mental retardation, multiple disabilities, orthopedic impairment, other health impaired, serious emo-

tional disturbance, learning disability, speech or language impairment, traumatic brain injury, and visual impairment.

Implementation of IDEA

IDEA is a federal mandate directed at the states, which are required to implement its requirements. Each state and local education agency (LEA) or intermediate unit (IU) has some discretion with regard to how dollars are allocated and appropriated for assistive technology. This includes AAC devices and services. In some states, separate line item assistive technology budgets exist within the state department of education for these purposes. These budgets are frequently a combination of federal funds and, in some cases, state dollars. It is a good idea for professionals and parents of children with disabilities to be aware of existing access to funding for AAC devices and services available in their own local school system, as well as other communities within the same state and other states (D. Wolfenden-Parker, personal communication, 1995).

The law was amended in 1986, and a new Part H was added, the Handicapped Infants and Toddlers Act, P.L. 99-457.

The amendments established an early intervention program that provides services for children with disabilities from birth through age 2 and for their families. The goals of this program are to coordinate the many service programs that currently exist, to ensure that infants, toddlers, and their families who need these services actually receive them, and, where gaps in services exist, to provide them directly. A complete listing of state programs for infants and toddlers with disabilities can be found in Appendix C at the end of this book. These programs can be contacted for more specific information regarding available services.

The regulations implementing Part H note that the need for assistive technology must be determined on a case-by-case basis along with the development of the required Individualized Family Services Plan (IFSP). P.L. 99-457 increased the emphasis on family involvement, resulting in service delivery models that stress family-focused approaches.

Generally, the Part H program is the "payer of last resort." This means that professionals must exhaust all other funding options prior to using Part H dollars to purchase equipment or services. Even so, the program must take whatever steps are necessary to ensure that services and equipment identified in the IFSP are provided "without delay." The key to effective funding of AAC services and equipment under Part H is to specifically write the need for AAC into the IFSP.

In 1990, Congress reauthorized and again amended the Education for All Handicapped Children Act. The name of the act was changed to the Individuals with Disabilities Education Act (IDEA, P.L. 101-476). Also, the authorization of the provision of assistive technology devices and services was included in IDEA. Assistive technology devices and services were defined in this amendment utilizing the definition from the Technology-Related Assistance for Individuals with Disabilities Act of 1988. In more recent legislation, the 1991 amendments to IDEA, Congress added provisions to strengthen the transition from infant and toddler programs to existing preschool programs, and to increase parental participation in decision making.

Table 9–1 lists the assistive technology components of IDEA. The assistive technology components (devices and services) will be discussed as they relate to the provision of AAC.

Assistive Technology Devices

An augmentative communication system, whether low tech or high tech, is considered an "assistive technology device" as

the use of an AAC system will increase, maintain, or improve the functional communication capabilities of students with communication disabilities. As such, if an IEP committee determines that an AAC device is required in order for a student to receive a free, appropriate, public education, a school district is obligated to provide an appropriate communication system for that child. Most school districts will recognize their legal responsibility in providing an AAC device and comply; however, some school districts may not initially be willing to provide an AAC device. In this event, the family may need to seek outside assistance or legal counsel.

Assistive Technology Services

The law also recognizes that the mere provision of an AAC device is not sufficient for ensuring that a student will be able to benefit from the device. Six assistive technology services are identified in IDEA (see Table 9–1). Each will be discussed in turn.

AAC Evaluation. Recommendations for an augmentative communication system should be based on an evaluation. The school district is responsible for providing an AAC evaluation for students with severe communication disorders. School districts may have identified and trained a local district assessment team that can provide this service. If local district personnel lack the expertise to conduct this evaluation, then the district may have to contract with a consultant or an evaluation facility in order to provide this service.

AAC Device Acquisition. The law is clear that, if an AAC device is required, the school district must provide the device. Public schools providing special education services to students with disabilities receive federal funds to assist with the cost of the education of those students. These federal funds can be used to purchase special-

Table 9–1. Assistive technology requirements of IDEA.

---

§300.308

"Each public agency shall ensure that assistive technology devices or assistive technology services, or both, as those terms are defined in §300.5–300.6, are made available to a child with a disability if required as part of the child's

(a) Special education under ff300. 17;

(b) Related services under ff300. 16; or

(c) Supplementary aids and services under ff300.550(b)(2)."

§300.5 Assistive Technology Devices

"As used in this part, 'assistive technology device' means any item, piece of equipment, or product system, whether acquired commercially off the shelf, modified, or customized, that is used to increase, maintain, or improve the functional capabilities of children with disabilities."

§300.6 Assistive Technology Services

"As used in this part, 'assistive technology service' means any service that directly assists a child with a disability in the selection, acquisition, or use of an assistive technology device. The term includes"

(a) The evaluation of the needs of a child with a disability, including a functional evaluation of the child in the child's customary environment;

(b) Purchasing, leasing, or otherwise providing for the acquisition of assistive technology devices by children with disabilities;

(c) Selecting, designing, fitting, customizing, adapting, applying, retaining, repairing, or replacing assistive technology devices,

(d) Coordinating and using other therapies, interventions, or services with assistive technology devices, such as those associated with existing education and rehabilitation plans and programs;

(e) Training or technical assistance for a child with a disability or if appropriate, that child's family; and

(f) Training or technical assistance for professionals: (including individuals providing education or rehabilitation services), employers, or other individuals who provide services to, employ, or are otherwise substantially involved in the major life functions of children with disabilities.

---

ized equipment that is necessary for the student's education. However, it should be cautioned that if the communication system is purchased by the school, then the school owns the device. Problems with this funding source occur when the student moves out of the boundaries of the school district, or when the student graduates or "ages-out" of the public schools, because the device remains the property of the district. Therefore, even though the public schools must provide AAC, it is still important to assist the student in obtaining a personal communication device that belongs to him or her.

The law does permit school districts to coordinate the funding of AAC with other agencies. Vocational Rehabilitation has funds available to assist with the employment process for people with disabilities. Medicaid may fund communication devices. These and other funding sources are discussed in greater detail later in this chapter.

Technical Support of the AAC Device. This service addresses the need of continuing support beyond the acquisition of an AAC device. Once an AAC device is provided, the school district will be responsible for keeping the device in functioning condition. School districts should budget a certain percentage of monies for this purpose. Most students with AAC needs will require support in customizing the device to meet their unique needs. This may include customizing vocabulary which may involve programming the device, creating overlays, or redesigning low tech systems. Customizing access methods may also be required. This might involve adjusting the input rate, adjusting scan rate, or the mounting of a switch. This service could also address the issue of designing or customizing a mounting system for the communication device.

Coordination of Support Services. The issues and needs of students with AAC requirements are very complex. It is common for these students to need the services of many professionals. It will be important for the school to coordinate the efforts of the physical therapist, occupational therapist, vision specialist, speech-language pathologist, educators, and other team members in regard to the student's AAC system.

AAC Training: Student and Family. Students will often need intensive training in the use of their AAC systems. Lack of training and the type of training strategies implemented are identified as major contributing factors when a student is not a successful communication device user (Goossens, Crain, & Elder, 1992). As a result, this service is considered paramount to the success of the device. Parent training is also an important service that schools need to provide. The communication system needs to be supported in the home environment as well as the school environment.

AAC Training: Other Communication Partners. This service addresses the need for the communication system to be supported in all environments. In the educational environment, this means that general edu-

cation teachers, special education teachers, and paraprofessional staff will need training in the management and use of the communication system. This will help ensure that the communication system will be supported in the classroom environment and will be integrated into classroom routines. This training will need to occur prior to classroom transitions or whenever a change of staff is involved.

For students who are transitioning to work, the training will need to extend to the vocational environment. Training for employers should occur prior to community-based instruction or work-site placement. For students who are living in group homes or in other nontraditional living arrangements, training should be provided to the staff so that the system can be supported in this environment.

Evolving Legal Issues Under IDEA

Because the provision of assistive technology is a relatively new area in the law, legal issues related to its implementation are in the process of being tested in the courts. At this time, the parameters of the law have not been fully established. Issues such as cost, providing "appropriate" versus "best" dedicated devices, home use of devices, and liability for repair are under scrutiny, but remain "gray" areas of interpretation.

Cost. Cost is always a concern when providing services to students. School districts do not have unlimited budgets, and strive to provide needed services to students in a fiscally responsible manner. An emerging issue is whether the school district is required to provide the "best" device for a student, or a device that is merely "appropriate." According to IDEA, schools are ex-pected to limit the provision of assistive technology to educational relevance. Device recommendations and decisions should be based on functional AAC evaluations of the child in the natural environment. When making decisions regarding AAC device selection, cost cannot be a determining factor. Despite the controversy over "appropriate" versus "best," the recommendation for equipment based on feature selection issues has been upheld in court cases. For example, if one of the device features recommended for the student was abbreviation/expansion, then a device that did not provide this feature could not be considered simply because it costs less.

Dedicated Devices. Generally, school districts have not been responsible for providing personal devices such as eyeglasses or hearing aids. Some districts have been reluctant to provide a dedicated AAC system for a student because it was viewed as a personal device. In a letter dated November 19, 1993, the Office of Special Education Programs (OSEP) ruled that if an IEP committee determines that the provision of a device (e.g., hearing aid or AAC system) is needed In order for a student to receive a free appropriate, public education, then the school district is obligated to provide the device (Hehir, l993).

Home Use. In the past, school districts assumed that if the district owned the device then the district could make the rules governing its use. Many districts did not permit augmentative communication devices owned by the school to go home with the student. In a letter dated November 27, 1991, OSEP ruled that if an IEP committee determined that a student needed access to a device in the home environment in order to receive a free, appropriate, public education, then the school must provide access to the device in the home environment (Schrag, 1991).

Repair of Personal Devices. In a letter dated August 9, 1994, OSEP determined that the school district could be responsible for the repair or replacement of a person-

ally owned device. The letter concluded that if the AAC device was necessary and utilized to implement the student's IEP, then the school was responsible for repairing the device or otherwise obtaining another AAC device so that the IEP could be implemented (Hehir, 1994).

The Rehabilitation Act Amendments Of 1992

The 1986 reauthorization of the Rehabilitation Act placed considerable emphasis on the provision of technology to assist individuals with disabilities in entering and maintaining employment. In order to gain as much information as possible on the provision of rehabilitation technology, the Act was amended in 1992 to add four new state plan requirements in the area of the state Vocational Rehabilitation plan. According to Button (1993), states are now required to:

- Describe how a broad range of rehabilitation technology services will be provided at each stage of the rehabilitation process. [Sec. 101(a)(5)(C)(i)]
- Describe how a broad range of rehabilitation technology services will be provided on a statewide basis. [Sec. 101(a)(5)(C)(ii)]
- Describe the training that will be provided to vocational rehabilitation counselors, client assistance personnel, and other related services personnel. [Sec. 101(a)(5)(C)(iii)]
- Describe the manner in which assistive technology devices and services will be provided, or worksite assessments will be made, as part of the assessment for determining eligibility and vocational rehabilitation needs of an individual. [Sec. 101(a)(31)]

These amendments include numerous statements related to rehabilitation technology, which encompass AAC devices as well as services. It is of critical importance that specific assistive technology equipment and services be included in the Individualized Written Rehabilitation Program (IWRP). The IWRP is a rehabilitation plan for adults receiving services within the Vocational Rehabilitation system. It describes specific services and equipment that will be provided, with vocational goals tied to the provision of assistive technology. Without a written signed IWRP, no AAC services or equipment can be provided.

It should be noted that rehabilitation technology is exempt from comparable service and benefit requirements. Stated simply, this means that the Vocational Rehabilitation program must readily provide necessary AAC services and devices to individuals who require them to attain vocational goals and objectives. Individuals do not need to show proof that other payers were researched and approached prior to requesting these services from Vocational Rehabilitation.

Many students with disabilities will require assistance from the rehabilitation system upon leaving public education programs. In recognition of this need, the 1992 Amendments include numerous amendments related to transition planning and programming (L. Golinker, personal communication, 1994). A definition of transition services has been added into the law. Transition services "that promote or facilitate the accomplishment of long-term rehabilitation goals and intermediate rehabilitation objectives" also have been added to the scope of rehabilitation services [29 USC Section 723(a)(14)].

Programs funded under this transition mandate may begin providing services to children ages 14 and older. Transition services will most likely be offered in the form of AAC evaluations, treatment, and devices being provided in collaboration with the local school system. These provisions do not in any way shift the burden of re-

sponsibility for transition planning from the education system to the rehabilitation system. Rather, they will force coordination and collaboration between the systems. For students ages 14 to 21, transitional services, as well as traditional services of vocational rehabilitation, supported employment, and independent living can be pursued.

Section 504 of The Rehabilitation Act of 1973

Additional sections of the Rehabilitation Act of 1973 may offer direct or indirect procurement of AAC. Section 504 of the Rehabilitation Act of 1973 requires recipients of federal funding to make programs and activities accessible to people with disabilities. These regulations are designed to eliminate discrimination on the basis of disability in programs and activities that receive federal financial assistance. Section 504 denies federal funds to any institution whose practices or policies discriminate against individuals with disabilities.

This program protects children and adults with disabilities against discrimination in many settings. In specific circumstances, Section 504 has been invoked in an effort to compel an institution to accommodate the need for services and devices. This legislation has resulted in a number of outcomes, including various actions to remove physical barriers to education and employment. In a small number of cases, the acquisition of AAC devices, or specific portions of a device, may be available through this mandate.

Section 508 of The Rehabilitation Act of 1973

The 1992 Amendments update Section 508 of the Rehabilitation Act which deals with electronic accessibility. The revised Section 508 requires the General Services Administration of the United States Government to develop and establish guidelines for federal agencies for electronic accessibility, regardless of the medium. Although Section 508, if invoked, may not be available to provide an entire AAC system, certain features of the entire configuration, such as a printer, may become available for the user through this alternative.

The processes for accessing AAC services and devices through Vocational Rehabilitation programs differ in each state, and must be identified and researched individually. A listing of State Vocational Rehabilitation Agencies can be found in Appendix C of this book.

The Americans with Disabilities Act (ADA)

The Americans with Disabilities Act (P.L. 101-476) was modeled after the major civil rights statutes. Major provisions of the law provide comprehensive civil rights protection to persons with disabilities, and prohibit state and local governments from refusing to allow a person with a disability to participate in a service, program, or activity simply because the person has a disability. The ADA contains a broad definition of individuals with disabilities, including individuals with physical or mental impairments that substantially limit a "major life activity." Examples include speech and hearing impairments, as well as specific learning disabilities. The law is designed to guarantee access to public facilities, government services, transportation, and communication.

The focus of the act is not on federal funding, nor on the direct provision of services. However, there are requirements in the law that pertain to AAC users. The ADA prevents an employer from denying a job to an individual who can perform the work required, but uses AAC. Employers with more than 15 employees are required to provide reasonable accommodations

for employees with disabilities to enable qualified employees to carry out their jobs, unless the accommodations cause undue hardship to the employer. (As discussed later in this chapter, tax deductions may be available to the small business to ease the burden of these expenses.) Reasonable accommodations can also include assistive technology and technology access. The ADA is enforced by the U.S. Department of Justice.

The Technology-related Assistance for Individuals with Disabilities Act Amendments of 1994 (Tech Act)

The Tech Act, P.L. 103-218, is a federal competitive grants program which provides monies for states to establish a statewide, consumer-responsive service delivery system designed to effect systems change regarding assistive technology. As it was first enacted in 1988, the Tech Act contains a definition of assistive technology devices that is sufficiently broad to encompass high tech, low tech, and no tech devices. The law was reauthorized and expanded in 1994.

Tech Act programs do not necessarily provide direct funding for AAC equipment or services. In fact, most states use Tech Act grants to fund broad programs to disseminate information and provide referrals to increase access to assistive technology. Most Tech Act programs have a funding or assistive technology policy specialist on staff. These staff members should be able to direct consumers, advocates, professionals and others in identifying the most appropriate sources of equipment, services, and funding. Additionally, several Tech Act states do operate financial loan services or equipment loan programs to help with the purchase of devices and services. A complete listing of Tech Act programs can be found in Appendix C.

HEALTH INSURANCE PROGRAMS AS A SOURCE OF FUNDING

Medical Assistance

Medical Assistance (e.g., Medicaid, MA) can be an appropriate funding mechanism for AAC services and devices for many individuals. However, before this option can be considered, an individual's eligibility for the program and medical need for services must be determined. The most critical questions surrounding this funding source are: In what state does the individual reside? How old is the individual? What is the medical necessity for AAC? The answers to these questions will be critical in ascertaining whether or not this funding stream is available and appropriate.

Some background information is necessary in order to understand the Medical Assistance funding system. Medical Assistance is a program that is administered at the state level with oversight at the federal level. The federal administrating agency, the Health Care Financing Administration (HCFA), mandates that each state must develop a plan that identifies specific services offered within that state. The services identified in each state are a combination of services that are required by federal guidelines, and optional services that can be selected from a schedule also provided in federal guidelines. Because each state has the option of choosing specific, yet different, combinations of services, each state offers a different Medicaid program. Given this design, coverage for AAC services and devices occurs for some individuals in some states, yet does not in other locales. For example, some states have opted to provide Medical Assistance coverage for all individuals with physical disabilities, regardless of income or age. Other states use specific financial eligibility guidelines to determine who can receive benefits through the program. A listing of state Medical Assistance Agencies appears in Appendix C. These agencies should be contacted to determine which services are provided and their eligibility criteria.

According to Golinker (1993), "Medicaid funding for AAC devices and services is well-established as a legal matter, although in many states, not as a practical matter. AAC devices clearly satisfy the three substantive standards all Medicaid programs impose as preconditions to funding. These general characteristics of AAC devices are common to every state in the Medicaid program" (p. 24). These three standards are:

- AAC devices are within the scope of a variety of Medicaid services provided in every state.
- AAC devices are a form of treatment.
- AAC devices are medically necessary.

All states participating in the Medical Assistance program operate with a definition of "medically necessary" as a criterion for providing AAC coverage. Consumers should be familiar with the definition of "medically necessary" used within their state to determine potential coverage for AAC services and devices. Additionally, each state pens a separate definition for durable medical equipment (DME). The basic components of DME incorporate the following parameters:

- DME can withstand repeated use.
- DME is primarily and customarily used to serve a medical purpose.
- DME is not useful in the absence of illness or injury.
- DME is appropriate for use in the home.

Medical Assistance Services for Children

The children's component of Medical Assistance is known as Early Periodic Screening, Diagnosis, and Treatment (EPSDT). These services are mandated by the Omnibus Reconciliation Act of 1989 (OBRA, 1989), requiring that as of April 1, 1990, states must provide "treatment for which federal reimbursement is available, whether or not such services are covered under the State plan" (42 USC Section 1396d(r)(5)). Simply stated, this mandate requires all states to offer all federally mandated treatments for Medical Assistance eligible recipients under 21 years of age.

The EPSDT program offers the following treatment services which may cover AAC evaluation and treatment services and devices.

- Home health services
- Inpatient hospital care
- Outpatient hospital care
- Rehabilitation services
- Speech, language, and hearing
- Prosthetics
- Community supported living arrangements for persons with developmental disabilities
- Other diagnostic, screening, preventive, and medical or remedial services (provided in a facility, a home, or other setting) recommended by a physician or other licensed practitioner of the healing arts, for the maximum reduction of a physical or mental disability.

Because AAC services are within the scope of speech and language treatment options, many states are funding AAC services and equipment under EPSDT guidelines. In addition, AAC devices can sometimes qualify as prosthetic durable medical equipment. Appendix C lists coordinators of EPSDT programs in each state. These individuals can be contacted to obtain information and guidelines regarding the provision of AAC services and equipment.

Medical Assistance Services for Adults

Because each state offers a different selection of Medicaid optional services, individuals over age 21 are only covered by the services defined in the state plan. Careful review of the state plan can identify which of the following optional services are covered under the state plan and which of these can be targeted for the provision of AAC services and devices.

- Home health services (42 USC Section 1396d(a)(7))
- Outpatient hospital services, a required service
- Rehabilitative services (42 USC Section 1396d(a)(13)) which provide "for maximum reduction of physical or mental disability and restoration of a recipient to his best possible functional level" (42 CFR Section 440.130(d))
- Speech, language and hearing services (42 USC Section 1396d(a)(11)) defined as "diagnostic, screening, preventive and corrective services provided or under the direction of a speech pathologist or audiologist, for which a patient is referred by a physician. It includes any necessary supplies and equipment" (42 CFR Section 440.110(c)(1)).
- Durable Medical Equipment (DME) as a required service for individuals eligible for nursing home care (42 CFR Section 440.70(b))
- Prosthetic devices (42 USC Section 1396d(a)(12)) defined as "replacement, corrective, or supportive devices prescribed by a physician or other licensed practitioner of the healing arts within the scope of his practice as defined by the law to: 1) artificially replace a missing portion of the body; 2) prevent or correct physical deformity or malfunction; or 3) support a weak or deformed portion of the body" (42 CFR Section 440.120 (c))

Consumers, professionals and advocates can locate this information in the Medical Assistance state plan and provider manuals. If any one or more of the above services are offered through the state plan, then AAC services and devices may be covered for adults in that state.

Medical Assistance Waiver Services

Medicaid's most flexible eligibility option is a waiver (Morris & Golinker, 1991). With this option, the federal government allows a state to design specific Medicaid programs to meet the needs of a subset of the population in that state. Historically, certain populations of individuals in need of Medicaid services could not receive them because they did not meet one or more of the program's eligibility requirements. Individuals were frequently institutionalized because appropriate community-based care was unavailable under existing health insurance options. In order to address this growing problem, federal guidelines were written that authorize states to request a waiver of certain federal requirements, usually income eligibility, for certain populations. These programs are known as waivers. Waiver programs are designed in each state so that individuals can receive cost-effective, community-based services instead of more expensive, less appropriate institutional care. Waiver programs are written for a specific population of persons with disabilities (e.g., physically disabled children, medically fragile individuals, respirator dependent individuals, the elderly). In many states, these programs include the provision of assistive technology services and devices as part of the waiver guidelines. On a practical level, service providers and consumers must ascertain which waiver services are covered in their state and proceed from that point. Appendix C lists state contacts for Medical Assistance that can be contacted for information on waiver programs.

Medicare

The Medicare program, Title XVIII of the Social Security Act, covers health care services for the elderly age 65 and over; persons receiving Social Security disability payments more than 2 years; and all citizens who have end stage renal disease (Kander & White, 1994). There are two parts to Medicare. The first part, Hospital Insurance (Part A Medicare) is automatic for all Medicare beneficiaries. The optional Part B, Supplemental Medical Insurance (SMI), is financed by monthly premiums paid by individuals who choose to enroll. Part B covers related medical services and supplies, and durable medical equipment (DME). Additionally, Part B covers physical therapy, occupational therapy, and speech-language pathology services in a doctor's office, as an outpatient, or in the home.

When Part B benefits are used, the consumer is required to pay an annual deductible for each calendar year. After meeting the deductible, Part B generally pays 80% of the Medicare approved amount for covered services received during the rest of the year. Medicare will only pay for equipment if the prescribing physician can certify in writing that the equipment is needed to help the person reduce or manage problems associated with a diagnosed medical condition.

In one case, an administrative law judge ruled that Medicare must reimburse a claimant for an AAC device and supplies. The judge also ruled that the AAC device replaced damaged communication-related functions of the claimant's brain and restored his capacity to communicate. It was found that the AAC device constituted a prosthetic device. The justification was that use of an AAC device allowed the individual to communicate, become much more functional, and maintain greater independent living. It was noted that an AAC device essentially replaces the malfunctioning part of the claimant's body (e.g., the brain, mouth, or larynx) and thus met the criteria that Medicare recognizes to improve the functioning of a malformed body member pursuant to 42 USC Section

1395(y)(a)(1)(A). Moreover, it was found that the computer satisfied the statutory definition of a prosthetic device under 42 USC Section 1395x(s)(A) in that it replaced part of the function of an impaired body organ. At the same time, this ruling noted that AAC devices do not qualify as DME. (*The Clearinghouse Review,* 1993).

Given this information, clinicians must be aware that intermediaries do have discretion in individual AAC decisions. It should also be noted that Medicare has historically reimbursed for artificial larynxes. The use of an AAC device to replace an impaired body organ may be analogous to the justification that has been used to fund artificial larynges. Clinicians should be careful to investigate whether it is more prudent to submit an AAC claim under guidelines for DME or under guidelines for prosthetic devices. Additionally, new codes have been adopted for the Physician's Current Procedural Terminology (1996). These new codes cover "evaluation for use and/or fitting of a voice prosthetic or augmentative/alternative communication device to supplement oral speech" (92597) and "modification of a voice prosthetic or augmentative/alternative communication device to supplement oral speech" (92598). These current and timely additions to the coding may suggest progress in favorable coverage of AAC devices for individuals with Medicare as health insurance.

As with any funding source, requests and approvals are not harmonious unless the mission, purpose, and program guidelines are the same. For this reason, it is of critical importance that individuals pursuing funding from any source become familiar with the policies, regulations, and practices of that program.

Private Health Insurance

The use of private health insurance for coverage of AAC devices and services is dependent on the individual policy. Many individuals with disabilities may secure reimbursement for assistive technology services and devices through health insurance coverage. A standard health insurance plan provides parameters for payment decisions regarding specific types of services. It is unlikely that an insurance policy will list specific services (e.g., assistive technology, rehabilitation technology); however, coverage for DME, prosthetics, rehabilitation, speech-language pathology, and occupational therapy services may include AAC devices and services. In most instances, a fair amount of discretion is allowed the claims adjuster and supervisors with regard to interpreting the intent of the policy and the scope of services rendered (Morris & Golinker, 1991). This discretion has allowed coverage of devices and services in many instances.

As with all funding options, whenever a private health insurance policy is being considered the consumer or advocate should review the specifics of that policy to assure that assistive technology devices or evaluation and treatment services are covered. For example, some insurance companies require preauthorization (preapproval) for all services, whereas others may require submitting requests for DME to a different address than regular claims. Once an individual policy has been reviewed, a request should be submitted for services rendered or equipment recommended, as covered by that policy. It is helpful to have one or more letters from physicians documenting the medical need for AAC services and devices. Managed care health insurance agencies such as health maintenance organizations typically will require the approval of the individual's primary physician.

If a denial is received, an appeal should be pursued immediately. Frequently, the timelines allowed for appealing a decision from a private insurance carrier are also outlined in the policy and guidelines. This timeline can be as brief as 30 days. In some cases, once additional documentation and justification are provided by the physician or clinician, a positive decision is rendered on appeal. In other cases, an appeal will need to be pursued through to the insurance medical review board.

SOCIAL SECURITY ADMINISTRATION (SSA) WORK INCENTIVE PROGRAMS

It can be documented that most people, including those with disabilities, want to work, but may require specific equipment to accomplish this goal. The Social Security Administration (SSA) offers programs known as work incentive programs which enable individuals to purchase services and equipment needed to gain, return to, or maintain employment. It is important for disability beneficiaries to understand that they can still receive cash benefits from the SSA while they purchase AAC devices and services necessary to work. These programs have been in effect since the early 1970s and are becoming widely used since they are more flexible and generous than in previous eras.

In order to take advantage of work incentive programs as a funding resource, an individual must be eligible to receive SSA benefits. These beneficiaries include individuals receiving Social Security Disability Insurance (SSDI), as well as those receiving Supplemental Security Income (SSI). To be eligible for SSDI, a person must meet the following criteria:

- Have worked and paid Social Security taxes for enough years to be covered under Social Security. The size of the SSDI benefit is based on the amount paid into FICA.
- Be considered medically disabled.
- Not be working, or working but earning less than the substantial gainful activity level.

To be eligible for SSI based on a medical condition, a person must meet the following guidelines:

- Have little or no income or resources.
- Be considered medically disabled.
- Initially not be working, or working but earning less than the substantial gainful activity level.

Once an individual is receiving one or both of these benefits and has a vocational objective or job, accessing one or more work incentive programs may enable the consumer to purchase AAC devices or services. A description of specific work incentive programs that may assist with the purchase of AAC services and devices are reviewed in the next section of this chapter.

Plan for Achieving Self-Support (PASS)

This program allows a person with a disability to set aside income and resources toward a work goal for a specified period of time. Resources set aside under a plan are not counted toward SSA resource limits, thereby enabling an individual to maintain eligibility for SSA benefits (i.e., cash and health insurance). This specific work incentive program enables an individual to prepare to pursue a vocational goal. This preparation may require an AAC device and services. If so, SSA will authorize an individual to allocate resources to save for or purchase an AAC device or services, while maintaining eligibility to receive SSA benefits.

To become eligible for this work incentive program, an individual or advocate must design a "plan" that outlines the individual's work goal and all costs the individual would like to cover using this program (e.g., purchase of an AAC device, training, maintenance). This plan must be submitted in writing and should include pertinent information describing the individual's plan for allocating funds. The SSA evaluates the plan and determines its acceptability. Once approved, the PASS will be reviewed periodically to assure compliance. A PASS can be designed for a period of time up to 48 months. Once a PASS becomes effective, an individual receiving SSDI may become eligible for additional cash benefits under the SSI program. An individual receiving SSI, but with resources above SSA limits, can continue to receive SSI cash benefits that may have been discontinued had the PASS not been in effect.

Impairment-Related Work Expenses (IRWEs)

This program provides continuing SSI or SSDI benefits to offset the unique expenses associated with working with a disability. The program enables a consumer to start working while collecting a salary and continue to receive benefits in order to pay for personal care, medical costs, mobility aids, adaptive equipment, and other "impairment-related" costs. These expenses are deductible when (1) the expense enables a person to work; (2) the person, because of a severe physical or mental impairment, needs the item or service for which the expense is incurred in order to work; (3) the cost is paid by the person with a disability and is not reimbursed by another source; and (4) the expense is "reasonable," that is, it represents the standard charge for the item or service in the person's community.

An individual who is working and requires an AAC device or services can consider this program as a means of "writing off" against salary which is used to pay for these expenses. If the individual "writes off" a sufficient amount of salary, he or she may maintain eligibility for SSA benefits, such as continued monthly pay

Continued Medicaid Eligibility (Section 1619(b))

This incentive continues Medicaid coverage for most working SSI beneficiaries under age 65 until earnings reach a specific level, as identified in each state. This work incentive program is designed to ensure that SSA beneficiaries do not lose medical insurance as a result of entering or maintaining employment. The effect of this program is that MA covered services, available under the state plan, remain available to an individual, even while maintaining employment. A consumer may wish to consider this program to maintain eligibility for MA if the state Medicaid program covers AAC services and devices.

Continuation of Medicare Coverage

This provision allows SSDI beneficiaries to receive at least 39 months of hospital and medical insurance after initiating employment. A consumer may wish to consider this SSA program as a strategy for maintaining eligibility for Medicare. As noted in the section describing Medicare, once the individual is covered through Medicare, coverage for AAC services and devices may become available to the consumer.

Medicare for People with Disabilities Who Work

This SSDI Work Incentive, created by Congress in 1990, allows certain people who have returned to work to purchase continued Medicare coverage after premium-free Medicare ends due to work. This program can enable a consumer to maintain eligibility for Medicare. Continuation of Medicare coverage may allow the consumer to access coverage for AAC devices through this health insurance program.

These programs are only a sampling of the numerous and varied options available. For additional information regarding the various work incentive programs of the SSA, professionals or consumers can call the SSA (1-800-772-1213) to request a copy of the *Red Book on Work Incentives.* A listing of Social Security Administration Regional Offices can be found in Appendix C.

INTERNAL REVENUE CODE

The federal income tax laws provide numerous and varied tax credits and deductions which are available to individuals, or their families, when purchasing AAC devices and services.

The deductibility of goods and services interact in several ways. Sometimes goods will only be deductible if recommended by a physician. Other times, a health professional's diagnosis and recommendations, while not a legal prerequisite to deductibility, constitute powerful evidence of the nature and purpose of the expense. (Mendelsohn, 1993, p. 57)

Internal Revenue Code credits and deductions that may be accessed for the purchase of AAC services and devices may fall into several categories, described in the next section of this chapter.

Medical Deductions

All disability-related medical care expenses are tax deductible, although the amount of the deduction is limited as personal income increases. In appropriate circumstances, the cost of AAC devices is deductible. Disability-related items may be divided into three groups: (1) items designed or modified specifically for use by an individual with a disability; (2) items in common use that acquire their significance through some unique functional

capacity they confer on the user with a disability; and (3) items that combine common use and specially designed components (Mendelsohn, 1993). If AAC services or devices are purchased by an individual or family, a tax accountant should be consulted to determine the right to deduct the expenses.

Depreciation of Capital Equipment

Technology, whether assistive or not, can be categorized as capital equipment for taxation purposes if it is expected to remain in service for more than 1 year. The cost of purchasing capital equipment can be depreciated over a period of several years depending on the category of equipment purchased. For computers, the time frame for equipment depreciation is typically either 5 or 7 years, depending on accounting decisions. Most individuals would prefer to list AAC equipment as a medical deduction in the year of purchase, however it may be more financially advantageous to opt for capital depreciation of the equipment over the 5 to 7 year period (Mendelsohn, 1993). Consideration of such an expenditure under applicable IRS rulings must be discussed with a tax accountant, well versed in the tax law and recent rulings.

Disabled Access Credit (DAC)

This tax credit was enacted on November 5, 1990, and is frequently referred to as Title 26, Internal Revenue Code, Section 44. The purpose of the credit is to allay fears of small businesses with respect to ADA compliance, as well as to provide encouragement for compliance through tax subsidization. This credit is available to "eligible small businesses." A qualifying small business is defined as one that in the preceding year had gross receipts of one million dollars or less, or employed no more than 30 fulltime employees (Mendelsohn, 1993). The credit is in the amount of 50% of "eligible access expenditures" that exceed $250 but do not exceed $10,250 for a taxable year. A business may take the credit each year that it makes eligible access expenditures for an employee or customers.

The Internal Revenue Code defines four major categories of eligible expenses. These include removal of architectural, physical, communication, and transportation barriers that prevent access to or use of the business by persons with disabilities; provision of services such as qualified readers, taped texts, and other "appropriate methods" for making materials available to people with sensory impairments; acquisition or modification of equipment or devices for individuals with disabilities; and provision of other similar services, modifications, materials, or equipment.

Where appropriate, this credit may be available to a business to provide AAC devices for a specific individual who is an employee. In many instances, this alternative provides an indirect subsidy to the individual.

The credit can be used to meet the needs of established workers who encounter disabilities and want to continue working, or who reveal hidden disability after being employed for a period of time. It is almost always preferable for a business to keep an employee working rather than incurring costs of disability retirement. (Mendelsohn, 1993, p. 151) IRS Form 8826 is necessary to claim this credit.

Targeted Jobs Tax Credit (TJTC)

This credit is found in Title 26, Internal Revenue Code, Section 51. As similarly illustrated before, this credit may provide an indirect means of funding for AAC services and devices by providing an employer with a credit that may subsequently be used to pay for an employee's AAC needs. Using this program, an employer is eligible to receive a tax credit of up to 40% of the first $6,000 of first-year wages of a new employee with a disability. The employee must be referred by state or local vocational rehabilitation agencies, a State Commission on the Blind, or the U.S. Department of Veterans Affairs, and be certified by a State Employment Service. In order to access this credit, it is critical that the worker belong to one of the targeted populations identified by the law. These populations include individuals with disabilities who are Supplemental Security Income (SSI) recipients and persons referred by the Vocational Rehabilitation agency (Mendelsohn, 1993).

There is no credit after the first year of employment. For an employer to qualify for the credit, a worker must have completed at least 120 hours of work for the employer. The TJTC is an incentive specifically tailored to new hiring, as the purpose of the program is to bring people from underemployed groups into the work force. This tax credit is not available for hiring anyone who has ever previously worked for the company. IRS Form 5884 is necessary to claim this credit.

State Sales Tax

Consumers purchasing AAC devices may be able to save a small percentage of the cost of a device by inquiring if state sales tax on the product is exempted. "States vary enormously in what they exempt from sales tax and in the procedures for obtaining the exemptions. In some cases, devices ordered through the mail allow the buyer to save the cost of sales tax" (Mendelsohn, 1993, p. 215). Some states provide specific special exemptions for individuals with disabilities. If an exemption is not available, advocacy could lead to legislation to create an exemption.

Charitable Contributions

The Internal Revenue Code allows for a deduction, up to certain limits, of that amount that an individual or business contributes to an organization that qualifies as a 501(c) nonprofit charitable corporation. In some instances this option can be incorporated when individuals choose to contribute to the purchase of an AAC device. For example, a grandparent might make a charitable donation to a nonprofit agency, and the agency can use the donation to purchase AAC equipment for the grandchild, who is a client of the agency. This strategy can only be accessed in certain situations. Check with a tax accountant before considering this approach.

Impairment-Related Work Expenses (IRWEs)

IRWEs were added to the Internal Revenue Code in 1986. This program is very similar to a program described in the Social Security Administration section of this chapter. The Code defines IRWE as "expenses of a handicapped individual as defined in Section 190(b)(3) for attendant care services at the individual's place of employment and other expenses in connection with such place of employment which are necessary for such individual to be able to work, and with respect to which deduction is allowable under Section 162 determined without regard to the section."

This program allows tax deductions for expenses an individual must pay in order to hold a job, as long as they are related to the individual's disability. Unlike other employee business expenses, IRWEs are not limited to 2 percent of adjusted gross income. This can make the IRWE one of the most effective and far-reaching of all the Federal Work Incentives allowed by the IRS.

ALTERNATIVE FUNDING SOURCES

Monetary and Equipment Loan Programs

Monetary loan programs provide individuals with disabilities and their families with an alternative funding source that can be used for the purchase of AAC services and devices. These programs do not directly fund AAC equipment. Instead, families can receive no interest or low interest loans to assist in the purchase of equipment. In some states, these loan programs are operated through Tech Act funded programs or other local disability organizations. In other states, the programs are administered by commercial lending institutions. Most of these loan programs have only been in operation since 1990 and the programs vary with regard to private, state, and federal funding. In many of these programs a degree of flexibility can be provided by offering co-signers, technical assistance, credit counseling, and repayment flexibility.

Another example of a loan program is an equipment loan closet. With this model, an organization or government agency maintains an inventory of equipment that is available to consumers for loan or rental. AAC devices are among the preferred pieces of equipment for many of these programs. As with most programs, policies and procedures vary from program to program. In some cases, loans are allowed for extended periods of time, with no fee assumed. In other programs, a nominal fee is required for administrative purposes. In still other programs, loans are permitted for a short period of no more than 2–4 weeks.

The Amyotrophic Lateral Sclerosis (ALS) Society in many locales offers an equipment loan closet for its members. Many other disability groups and service organizations (e.g., Lions Club, Paralyzed Veterans of America) offer similar programs. Being aware of these various loan programs may enable a consumer to take advantage of one or both of these strategies for the successful procurement of AAC devices and services. Information about these programs can be obtained by calling the state Tech Act program (see Appendix C in this text).

Community, Service and Disability Organizations

Every state, county, and local jurisdiction has numerous service and disability organizations. Some examples would be the ALS Society, Muscular Dystrophy Association (MDA), United Cerebral Palsy (UCP), Kiwanis Club, Rotary International, Jack and Jill Club, and many others. Frequently, it is within the mission of these organizations to assist individuals with disabilities in the purchase of assistive technology services and devices.

The process for accessing these funds varies with each organization, but there is usually some relationship between the organization and the requester (e.g., membership by a family member, disability type). In many cases, written justification and documentation is requested. Depending on the organization, requests are reviewed on a scheduled basis (monthly, quarterly, or annually). If this option is to be considered, a consumer, family member, or advocate should investigate the most appropriate organization to match the needs of the individual. For example, the MDA may provide funding for an AAC device or services, but the individual must present with diagnoses served by MDA. In other cases, a community organization such as

the Lion's Club will consider a request for funding, but would want the request to be made on behalf of the individual by a member of that organization. As noted before, contact the state Tech Act project for information on these organizations.

Private Funds and Foundations

This final funding source is important to the provision of loans and grants for the purchase of AAC services and devices. In most cases, as noted previously, there must be some similarity between the purpose and mission of the fund or foundation and the individual's needs. Frequently, a letter of intent or a short proposal is needed in order to access foundation dollars. The documentation should note the goals and objectives for AAC, as well as the purpose of the equipment in question. If a match is made and funds are available, equipment or services can be purchased with the donated funds.

DEVELOPING A FUNDING STRATEGY

Developing a funding plan is an important component of AAC services. Once the assessment process has delineated an appropriate AAC device for an individual, and a trial period has successfully reinforced the assessment results, then it is time to identify potential funding sources (ABLEDATA, 1992). Once an array of potential sources has been identified, then the team needs to determine which of the identified funding sources is a match for the client. Because different sources of funding have different eligibility requirements and rules regarding equipment purchasing, the task is to determine which funding source fits the circumstances of the individual seeking funding. This will depend on factors such as age, disability, employment status, insurance coverage, geographic location, and even the availability of community service organizations. Preparing justification statements is another critical step in the process. The identification of potential funding sources, matching sources to the individual's circumstances, and the preparation of justification statements will be discussed herein.

Identifying Potential Funding Sources

As discussed previously in this chapter, locating funding can be a time-consuming process, which is why a collaborative approach is often best. It is beneficial to the client and certainly less overwhelming to any one person when the search for funding is shared among members of the team, which includes family members.

To begin, it is useful for the team to schedule a funding planning meeting. The purpose of this meeting would be to discuss the steps involved in locating funding and to secure the investment of multiple members of the team to pursue funding. Figure 9–2 provides a format for devising a funding plan.

The first step in the creation of a funding plan is to itemize the equipment for which funding is needed to be sure that there is final agreement among all team members. The team should feel sure that the device is appropriate to the educational or vocational needs of the individual, and that it is what the client and his or her family want. Another factor to consider in the final analysis is whether there will be sufficient training and ongoing services to support the use of the recommended device. In addition to the AAC device, other items related to the AAC system such as special communication software, mounting systems, carrying cases, batteries, cables, and printers may also be needed. At some point, the cost of these items and the companies that produce or supply such items will need to be specified.

Thereafter, organizations to be contacted in regard to funding should be identified. This list may include agencies and organizations which provide information on funding such as federal, state, and local advocacy groups, as well as potential funding sources such as LEAs, private health insurance companies, Medical Assistance programs, or vocational rehabilitation services. The list can also include community service organizations, foundations, banks, and other potential sources described previously in this chapter. Individual team members who volunteer to contact these organizations should be identified on the Funding Plan.

As organizations are contacted, it is important to keep track of information such as phone numbers and the names of persons contacted at the various organizations. If, at some point, a team member exits to a new job and is no longer involved, then the information is preserved for others. This information is also vital when making follow-up calls. Because the funding process can take many months, it is important to keep ongoing documentation on who was contacted, how organizational contacts can best be reached, as well as the actual information obtained as a result of phone calls, meetings, or written materials. Periodic team meetings to update information and progress are useful to keep the process moving along. It is also helpful to maintain separate files on each of the funding organizations or agencies contacted. For each funding source, it is important to log phone calls, dates on which justification letters, forms, or other reports were sent, and dates on which responses were received.

Once appropriate organizations have been contacted and information relative to funding is obtained, then the process of sorting through the information to delineate probable funding sources begins. At this point, it is important to tie the requirements of selected funding sources to the

AAC Funding Plan

Client: _____Date:_____

Disability: _____

RECOMMENDED EQUIPMENT:

Item	Company	Cost

FUNDING RESOURCES:

Organization	Responsible Team Member	Contact & Phone No.	Information Obtained	Follow Up Steps

JUSTIFICATION STRATEGIES:
(e.g., letters, reports, and other documentation to be submitted by doctors, therapists, school staff, parents, vocational staff, others)

Type of Documentation: Submitted by:

_____

_____

_____

_____

_____

Figure 9–2. AAC funding plan.

individual's needs and circumstances. If an individual is Medicaid eligible, then funding strategies in line with Medicaid regulations can be outlined. If the child is approaching transition age, then steps for obtaining funding through vocational services can be defined. If private health insurance coverage looks promising, then strategies for this can be outlined.

Again, it is important to pursue multiple sources of funding. An 18-year-old who is currently receiving AAC services in school, but is planning to pursue a postsecondary education toward a goal of employment, may be eligible for AAC funding through more than one federal entitlement program and his or her health insurance plan. He or she may also want to pursue a monetary loan through a disability organization to obtain funds for items not covered under one or more of the funding sources. One parent who actively pursued funding for her son obtained his communication device through medical health insurance, and his printer from a service organization. A grandparent purchased computer peripherals and the mother arranged to purchase software at cost from a local computer store. Letters and reports justifying funding through these sources were vital throughout her search.

Funding Justification Strategies

Letters or reports are usually needed to justify that the AAC device in question is appropriate. The content of letters and reports should be geared to the requirements of the targeted funding source. If the consumer pursues funding through private health insurance, then medical necessity must be addressed. If services and an AAC device are being pursued through vocational rehabilitation, then letters or reports should tie this to the individual's enhanced independence and his or her ability to prepare, obtain, or keep a job. Letters written to seek procurement of an AAC device through a school system will need to address LRE and appropriate education.

According to Morris and Golinker (1991), reimbursement for assistive technology from public funding sources and private insurers will most often succeed or fail depending upon the ability of the applicant to prove essential need according to the agency standard and write an acceptable justification. Table 9–2 presents examples of funding justifications and how the justification for the need for AAC varies across different funding programs.

Although the creation of a funding plan will not guarantee funding, it serves

Table 9–2. Examples of AAC funding justifications.

AAC Funding Program	Funding Justification
Special Education:	The student requires an AAC device and support services in order to participate in and take advantage of the educational curriculum.
Vocational Rehabilitation:	The individual needs AAC services and equipment to gain, maintain, or return to employment.
Medical Insurance: (Medical Assistance, Medicare, Private)	The patient requires an AAC service and/or device due to significant medical need. AAC services and devices provide the patient with the ability to manage personal care and access emergency, routine and preventive medical care.

as a road map for pursuing funding. Identifying a range of potential sources of funding assistance increases the chances that appropriate sources will be located. As phone contacts are made and team members, including family members, collaborate to pool information, funding requirements and eligibility issues come into focus. No one source may meet all of the funding needs, but sources are available. Accessing these sources requires perseverance above all else.

SUMMARY

Funding AAC equipment and services is an important component to the service delivery process. As stated in the introduction, funding can be a frustrating and lengthy process. However, the joy of obtaining a successful funding outcome on behalf of an AAC consumer more than outweighs most of the frustrations. This chapter reviewed several major programs that mandate or provide AAC services and categories of funding sources. Professionals, consumers, and families should use this information as an introductory outline of available options. Further investigation of specific funding regulations and resources within each individual's state and community will be needed. A good place to begin the funding process is to contact the funding or policy specialist employed by the Tech Act program in each state. Appendix C of this book lists state contacts for each Tech Act program.

Readers of this chapter are cautioned that the funding process is likely to become more difficult in the near future. Professionals and consumers may be forced to compete for funding by demonstrating the benefits that AAC services and equipment can achieve for a given individual (DeRuyter, 1995). These benefits will encompass quality of life issues, customer satisfaction, and actual cost savings that can be gained through the provision of AAC. Viewing service delivery as a dollars and cents decision is difficult for most AAC professionals, consumers, and families. It will require us to rethink our justifications for expensive AAC systems and lengthy ongoing services. Careful documentation of outcomes that are achieved when AAC is implemented successfully needs to be gathered by professionals (DeRuyter, 1995). Outcome data can be used to document the efficacy of particular AAC interventions and can generate information that can be used to make informed decisions regarding funding and service delivery.

REFERENCES

ABLEDATA. (1992, July). *ABLEDATA Database of Assistive Technology: Funding assistive technology.* (ABLEDATA Fact Sheet, No. 14). Silver Spring, MD: National Rehabilitation Information Center.

Americans with disabilities act. (1990), P.L. 101–336.

Button, C. (1993). Reauthorization of the rehabilitation act increases access to assistive technology. *A.T. Quarterly, 2,* 1.

The Clearinghouse Review. (1993, November), *1,* 1.

DeRuyter, F. (1995). Evaluating outcomes in assistive technology: Do we understand the commitment? *Assistive Technology, 7,* 3–8.

Education for all handicapped children act. (1975), P.L. 94–142.

Golinker, L. (1993, March). Freedom of speech. *Team Rehab Report, 3,* 24–29.

Goosens, C., Crain, S. S., & Elder, P. S. (1992). *Engineering the preschool environment for interactive, symbolic communication.* Birmingham, AL: Southeast Augmentative Conference Publications.

Handicapped infants and toddlers act. (1986). P.L. 99–57.

Hehir, T. (1993). November 19, 1993 letter to Dr. Peter Seiler, Superintendent of Illinois School for the Deaf, 20 IDELR 1216.

Hehir, T. (1994). August 9, 1994 letter to Anonymous, 21 IDELR 1057.

Individuals with disabilities education act. (1990). P.L. 101-476.

Kander, M. L., & White, S. C. (1994). *Medicare handbook for speech-language pathology and audiology services*. Rockville, MD: ASHA.

Schrag, J. (1991). November 27, 1991 letter to Anonymous, 18 IDELR 627.

Mendelsohn, S. B. (1993). *Tax options and strategies for people with disabilities*. New York: Demos.

Morris, M. W., & Golinker, L. (1991). *Assistive technology: A funding workbook*. Arlington, VA: RESNA Press.

Omnibus reconcilation act. (1989). P.L. 101–239.

Physician's Current Procedural Terminology—CPT 1996. (1996). Chicago: American Medical Association.

Rehabilitation act. (1973). P.L. 93–112.

Rehabilitation act amendments. (1992). P.L. 102–569.

Social security act, Title XVIII. (1965). P.L. 89–97, codified in 42 U.S.C. § 1395, et seq. (1996 ed.).

Technology-related assistance for individuals with disabilities act. (1988). P.L. 100–407.

Technology-related assistance for individuals with disabilities act amendments. (1994). P.L. 103–218.

Section 2

USE OF AAC WITH SPECIFIC POPULATIONS

Chapter 10

AAC AND INDIVIDUALS WITH PHYSICAL DISABILITIES

Denise C. DeCoste

Individuals with physical disabilities face multiple challenges which often include the lack of ability to communicate effectively in spoken or written form. Problems with communication interaction often begin early in the lives of children with physical disabilities when caregivers and school staff fail to recognize their communicative signals (Houghton, Bronicki, & Guess, 1987; Wilcox, Kouri, & Caswell, 1990). Early intervention AAC is critical for the development of communication and social interaction skills in children with physical disabilities in order to facilitate active communication exchange and to prevent passivity (Light, Collier, & Parnes, 1985). The range of low tech and high tech options for interactive communication has increased significantly and the benefits of AAC to this population are widely recognized today.

In a historical account of the development of AAC, Zangari, Lloyd, and Vicker (1994) indicated that the existence of communication strategies for individuals with physical disabilities dates back to the 1950s and 1960s. During this period, the strategies used were generally nontechnical and included the use of signing, communication boards, Morse code, and typewriter controls. With the advent of the microprocessor and the development of speech synthesis, technical advances in hardware and software significantly increased AAC options in the 1970s and 1980s. As a result, today's generation of individuals with physical disabilities has a much greater array of communication options. In the 1990s and beyond, we can expect a continued emphasis on refinement in AAC devices in areas of speed, sophistication, miniaturization, and affordability (Zangari et al., 1994).

Although there have been marked improvements in AAC devices over the past two decades, now there is more of a need to focus on the effective use of these devices and on everyday strategies—technical and nontechnical—which will enhance the implementation of AAC practices in the home, school, vocational, and community settings. To ensure the best use of AAC systems for individuals with physical disabilities, we must look comprehensively at all the elements that create communication competence across the life span of each individual.

This chapter begins by discussing AAC issues for individuals with cerebral palsy, a nonprogressive disorder of movement, and early onset diseases including rare gene mutations and metabolic diseases. Current concerns as well as assessment and communication strategies specific to individuals with physical disabilities are explored. Training strategies and other issues related to the implementation of AAC in home, school, community, and work environments are also addressed. Whereas this chapter deals with the overall topic of AAC for individuals with physical disabilities, issues pertaining to this population are embedded throughout this book, including Chapter 5 on assessment principles, Chapter 6 on seating and positioning, and Chapter 7 on motor access. For more information on adults with acquired physical disabilities, the reader is referred to Chapter 13.

PHYSICALLY DISABLED POPULATIONS WHO MAY BENEFIT FROM AAC

Cerebral Palsy

Cerebral palsy (CP) is not a disease in the usual medical sense, as it has no single cause nor a consistent set of symptoms. Batshaw and Perret (1992, p. 191) defined CP as a "disorder of movement and posture that results from a nonprogressive abnormality of the immature brain." Damage associated with CP generally occurs during intrauterine development (44%), during labor and delivery (19%), or during the first month of life (8%; Batshaw & Perret, 1992). Damage that occurs during intrauterine development can be caused by genetic and chromosomal abnormalities, exposure to teratogenic drugs, intrauterine infections, and developmental brain malformations. Labor and delivery complications and pre-eclampsia can also result in CP, though this is not as common as

once thought (Nelson & Ellenberg, 1986). Perinatal causes of CP can include sepsis, asphyxia, and prematurity. In over 40% of diagnosed cases of CP there is no known cause. Some individuals who have physical impairments similar to CP acquire the condition later in life. Acquired causes of physical disabilities in adults and children such as meningitis and head injuries are discussed in Chapter 13.

According to Lipkin (1991), CP continues to occur in 1 to 3 per 1,000 live births in industrialized nations. There has been little overall decrease in the numbers of CP cases, in spite of improved medical neonatal care (Hagberg, Hagberg, & Zetterstrom, 1989). Estimates of the incidence of school-age children with CP is around 400,000 (Erenberg, 1984; Lord, 1984). In addition to motor deficits, individuals with CP often have cognitive, vision, hearing, or seizure problems (Batshaw & Perret, 1992).

Motor Problems

Motor problems associated with the different types of CP must be taken into consideration during AAC assessment and intervention. CP motor characteristics are associated with the location in the brain where the damage occurred. The type of CP often predicts the need for AAC. There are four major classifications: spastic, dyskinetic, ataxic, and mixed (Lipkin, 1991; see Table 10–1). Estimates of the incidence of the different types of CP vary from study to study. Although the overall number of CP cases has remained about the same for the past 20 years, there have been some shifts in the incidence of specific types of CP. Increases in the number of surviving low birth weight infants resulting in spastic diplegia account for the rise in spastic types of CP; at the same time, there has been a decrease in the incidence of athetoid CP as a result of improvements in the treatment of hyperbilirubinemia (Batshaw & Perret, 1992).

Table 10–1. CP motor problem classifications and resulting AAC issues.

Classification	Affected Area of the Brain	Estimates of the Percentage of the CP Population	AAC Issues
Spastic type	Motor cortex of the cerebrum (Pyramidal Tract)	63–94% of all CP cases identified	
Subtypes:			
Diplegic (all 4 limbs involved with the legs more involved)		25% of spastic types	Oral musculature not involved; may need computer for written communication needs
Hemiplegia (one side of the body)		45% of spastic types	Oral musculature usually not involved; may need computer for written communication needs
Quadriplegia (all 4 limbs involved)		30% of spastic types	AAC commonly needed due to involvement of speech musculature
Ataxic type	Cerebellum	10–15% of CP cases identified	Speech intelligibility is a problem; AAC may be needed to repair communication breakdowns
Dyskinetic type	Basal ganglion in the cerebrum (Extrapyramidal tract)	6–37% of CP cases identified	Variability of muscle tone affects total body movement and speech musculature; AAC usually needed
Subtypes:			
Athetoid type: Choreoathetoid			Extreme high tone or low tone affects total body and speech musculature; AAC commonly needed
Dystonic type: Rigid			
Mixed type	Motor cortex and basal ganglion	12% of CP cases	Extensive brain damage; total body involvement; AAC commonly needed

Source: Compiled from *Children with Disabilities: A Medical Primer* by M. L. Batshaw and Y. M. Peret, 1992. Baltimore, MD: Paul H. Brookes Publishing Company; and from "Epidemiology of the Developmental Disabilities" by P. Lipkin in A. J. Capute and F. J. Accardo (Eds.), *Developmental Disabilities in Infancy and Childhood*, 1991, Baltimore, MD: Paul H. Brookes Publishing Company.

Prevalence of AAC Issues in Individuals with Cerebral Palsy

The Bureau of Education for the Handicapped (BEH; 1976) estimated that there were 581,600 children under the age of 16 in the United States who were cognitively able but could not talk. Lafontaine and DeRuyter (1987) conducted a database study specifically on individuals with CP who were nonspeaking, ages 2 to 60 years, referred to the Nonoral Center at Ranchos Los Amigos Medical Center in Downey, California. This study indicated that 31.5% of the nonspeaking patients had a primary medical diagnosis of CP. Of these, 37.9% were age 21 and younger, with females accounting for 40.9% of the total population and males accounting for 59.1% of the population.

Aiello (as cited in Matas, Mathy-Laikko, Beukelman, & Legresley, 1985) conducted a demographic study in 1980 of nonspeaking students in Orange County, California, and found their number to be 0.2% of the total school-age population. (Aiello defined *nonspeaking* as persons who have a severe speech problem due to neuromuscular or physical deficits, and who cannot, at the present time, use speech independently as their primary means of communication.) Aiello reported that the majority of these nonspeaking students were multiply handicapped or severely and profoundly handicapped.

Matas et al. (1985) conducted a study in 12 counties in the state of Washington. (Matas et al. used the term *nonspeaking* to refer to persons who have a severe speech problem due to physical, neuromuscular, cognitive, or emotional deficits and not due primarily to hearing impairment, and who cannot, at the present time, use speech independently as their primary means of communication.) They found that nonspeaking students comprised 0.6% of the total 1981 school enrollment and 6% of the total special education enrollment. Matas et al. reported that 47.3% of the nonspeaking students were multiply handicapped, 28.2% were classified as mild to moderately retarded, and 13.6% had severe to profound mental retardation. The total percentage of nonspeaking students by handicapping condition was 100% for the multiply handicapped students, 100% for students with severe to profound mental retardation, and 12.3% for students with mild to moderate retardation. This study reflects the commonly used estimate of nonspeaking students in the U.S., that is, nonspeaking students comprise less than 1% of the total school age population and between 4% to 6% of the special education population.

In a demographic study conducted throughout Scotland that focused specifically on AAC systems and persons with CP, information was obtained on the types of AAC systems used, the communication abilities of individuals using AAC, and the circumstances in which the AAC systems were used. Murphy, Markova, Moodie, Scott, and Boa (1995) surveyed individuals who use AAC, including 72 children, 37 adolescents, and 107 adults. Although 15% did not know or did not provide diagnostic information, 47% were identified as having spastic CP, 23% had athetoid CP, 3% had ataxic CP, and 15% had mixed type CP. Low tech systems represented more than 50% of all AAC systems in use and most of the individuals had more than one type of aided AAC system. In addition to aided systems, respondents indicated that they also used yes/no indications, facial expressions, gestures, and eye pointing to communicate. Of those using high tech systems, 11 systems were text output only, 80 systems were used with voice output only, and 34 systems were used with text and speech output. Eighty percent of the individuals using AAC had their current system for 3 years or less and 22% reported that they had plans to change to another system, more often another high tech system.

Early Onset Diseases

Early onset diseases are relatively uncommon and they may be misdiagnosed (e.g., attributed to CP) or go unrecognized in the early years. Inborn errors of metabolism and rare gene mutations are often the cause of early onset diseases, resulting in progressive neurologic disorders and pervasive developmental delay. One statewide demographic survey of over 5,000 nonspeaking individuals conducted in Victoria, Australia, provided a general ranking of the causes of severe communication disorders (Bloomberg & Johnson, 1990). Many of the causes were listed as unknown; however, between the ages of 2 and 21, the predominant number of cases were CP (442), developmental delay (273), genetic/congenital (236), autism (183), trauma (65), and progressive neurological diseases (38).

Unlike children with CP, children with early onset disorders may make slow progress or get worse over time. The extent to which AAC intervention is useful depends on the age of onset, the course of the disease, whether language was initially intact, and the presence of associated conditions such as cognitive, visual, or auditory impairments.

CHARGE Association is a rare mutant gene disorder characterized by retarded growth and potentially severe visual and auditory impairments. Low tech AAC strategies and sign language can be used to promote language development and build communication skills over time.

Angelman syndrome is a genetic disorder characterized by ataxic movement resulting in unsteady ambulation, fine motor problems, cognitive deficits, severely limited speech, oral-motor problems, and behaviors such as hyperactivity, short atten-

tion span, and inappropriate laughter. Individuals with Angelman syndrome often have higher receptive than expressive language skills, and because few individuals acquire functional speech, AAC techniques are an important consideration from infancy through the adult years (Blackstone, 1995). As presented by Blackstone, AAC techniques in the early years should focus on interactive turn taking, adapted switch toys, and using objects to teach choice-making skills. As the child progresses, the shift to symbolic understanding using picture communication boards and simple voice output communication devices is emphasized. Miller (1995), in a parent guide to Angelman syndrome which was based on a survey of 179 families who have children with the syndrome, reported that most individuals use manual signs and gestures, 40% use picture communication boards, and only about 20% use voice output devices.

Inborn errors of metabolism such as adrenoleukodystrophy and Lesch-Nyhan disease can cause progressive neurologic degeneration. Adrenoleukodystrophy is an enzyme deficiency resulting in a toxic build-up. Unless treated early, the disease is characterized by a very gradual loss of motor control, loss of sensory functions, and mental retardation. Speech and language skills may develop in the early years and then slowly decline. AAC strategies can be utilized for communication; however, these strategies must be continually reassessed and readjusted as the individual's cognitive abilities and associated conditions deteriorate. Lesch-Nyhan disease is another rare progressive neurologic disorder caused by a deficient enzyme. This disease is characterized by choreoathetoid movement, mental retardation, and speech and language problems.

Duchenne muscular dystrophy is a progressive muscle disease caused by a mutant gene on the X chromosome. It occurs in approximately 2 out of every 10,000 males (Buyse, 1990). The onset of Duchenne muscular dystrophy occurs in early childhood and survival does not occur beyond adolescence or young adulthood, however, language skills are usually well developed prior to onset. Written communication problems arise before spoken communication becomes an issue. Because proximal shoulder movement declines prior to distal wrist and finger control, adapted keyboards, manual pointers, and on-screen keyboarding using a mouse or trackball are options that allow the individual a means of written communication. High tech written communication strategies using scanning and rate enhancement techniques may become necessary as upper extremity strength and range of motion decline. Low tech AAC such as eye gaze techniques may be necessary later in the course of the disease when respiratory functions and oral muscles are insufficient to support speech.

AAC strategies can be useful intervention methods with early onset diseases, such as those just described. When the onset of a disease occurs in late childhood and language skills have had an opportunity to develop, AAC is used to support existing communication skills. When the course of the disease is slow and associated losses in hearing and vision are on a gradual decline, the AAC specialist must reassess the child's communication status on a regular basis in order to plan for revisions to the AAC system. When cognitive deterioration is slow to occur, it is important to provide a range of communication strategies with the understanding that simpler, more concrete strategies will be most useful in the long term. In situations where degeneration does not occur, but progress is slow, AAC strategies will need to be reevaluated on an ongoing basis with emphasis on helping the individual achieve his or her communicative potential.

CURRENT ISSUES CONCERNING THE USE OF AAC FOR INDIVIDUALS WITH PHYSICAL DISABILITIES

Today, current issues in AAC go beyond the problems of system mechanics and address concerns from a broader perspective. For the individual using AAC, a variety of AAC issues can arise over the course of that person's life. AAC systems must be constantly updated to keep pace with the needs of the individual and the demands of changing environments. Suffice it to say, AAC systems are rarely stable because of ever changing events. AAC problems and concerns are a rule rather than an exception. Devices need repair, AAC vocabulary needs to be regularly updated and programmed, and new persons in contact with individuals using AAC need training. AAC teams, as well as individuals who use AAC and their families, must develop a flexible attitude and expect that changes are ongoing. AAC systems can take many years to develop so that they are individualized to the needs and abilities of the user. They are never "finished"; they are always "in process."

Changing Developmental Needs Affecting AAC Use

Children with CP and early onset degenerative diseases need frequent reassessment due to changes in the status of motor, language, and cognitive abilities. For a child with CP, AAC needs must be frequently evaluated to determine whether the strategies are keeping pace with the child's growth and development. Is more vocabulary needed? Is the child ready for a more sophisticated system? Is it time for the young child with limited upper extremity use to learn scanning skills? Is the child with Angelman syndrome who exhibits limited attention ready to learn two symbol sequencing? These questions and others must be addressed as the child's physical and cognitive needs change and grow.

Children with early onset degenerative diseases eventually have the opposite problem. Professionals must be aware of possible decreases in skills and adjust AAC strategies accordingly. Children with adrenoleukodystrophy who have lost the ability to speak may also lose hearing or vision skills and this will affect communication strategies. A child with muscular dystrophy may lose proximal shoulder movement while retaining distal finger movement, resulting in diminished keyboarding abilities and making the shift to thumb-activated single switch scanning necessary. At some point, he or she may have diminished breath support and need to shift gradually to an eye gaze system of communication. To keep up with developmental as well as degenerative changes, AAC professionals and the family must keep an eye toward the future and provide ongoing assessment.

Training Issues

AAC training for the individual who uses AAC systems and for his or her communication partners is ongoing because of changing circumstances. When new communication situations arise, communication needs can change, requiring alterations to AAC strategies and equipment. When this occurs, reassessment followed by additional training is necessary. When physical abilities improve or decline, training to teach the use of a new method of motor access is needed. For example, when a boy with muscular dystrophy begins to show increased difficulty moving his arm to access all the keys on a keyboard using the end of a pencil or an adapted manual pointer, then it may be time to explore the use of on-screen keyboarding software

such as ScreenDoors or HandiKEY. This allows the individual to use a mouse or trackball to click on letters displayed on the screen and it provides rate enhancement through word prediction and abbreviation-expansion strategies.

Changes in communication settings often require additional training to new communication partners. When a child who uses AAC changes to a new class or to a new school or when an individual who uses AAC makes the transition to a new vocational setting, the communication partners change and therefore additional training is needed. Communication partners may need training on how to read an individual's eye gaze and yes/no eye movements. Training may be needed on how to set up, turn on, and troubleshoot the AAC device. Or training may be needed on how to adapt educational or work-related activities for nonspeaking individuals.

Meeting ongoing training needs is a major responsibility. This is especially so for individuals with severe speech and physical disabilities, for they have fewer ways to explain their needs. For example, a nonspeaking girl in a power wheelchair was delivered by bus to her new elementary school. Inadvertently, a staff member shifted the lever on one side of her power wheelchair so that it was no longer in gear on that side. As a result, the student, using her joystick control, could only drive in circles. A staff member unfamiliar with power wheelchair operation repeatedly warned her to stop fooling around and drive to her classroom, reducing the child to tears. Because her voice output communication device was not mounted on her chair during the bus ride, she had no readily available means of explaining the cause of the wheelchair problem, and her first day at school was a disaster. Prior training to staff on wheelchair operation, as well as on communication strategies, could have prevented this.

In the early years, educators and therapists or AAC teams may take on much of the responsibility for staff training. Training needs must be anticipated each time the child moves to a new classroom, to a new school, and even to a new summer program. As the child grows older and becomes involved in community activities, the family often carries the responsibility of familiarizing friends, caretakers, and extended family on how to utilize aided and unaided communication strategies.

When individuals using AAC move into adulthood, they may have learned to advocate for themselves, or they may still need to depend on others to explain communication techniques. Some individuals who use AAC will carry instruction cards or affix them to the tray of the wheelchair. These cards can explain how to read their yes/no signals (e.g., *Hi, my name is Karen, I communicate with my eyes . . .*) or even how to set up and troubleshoot their AAC system. In the adult years, more so than in the school years, there is often less coordination across communication environments. Establishing who is responsible for providing training for work settings, or group homes, or recreation centers is not always easy to manage. The reader is referred to Chapter 17 for issues related to training in adult settings.

Hardware and Software AAC Issues

Although there have been many improvements in the AAC hardware and software options available to individuals with physical disabilities, issues that often surface revolve around systems integration and durability. The more integrated a user's system is, the more independent that person will be. Can the user independently turn on and off his or her electronic communication and mobility systems? Can the AAC device be powered through the battery of the electric wheelchair, or must the user be ever conscious of running out of speaking time? Can the user drive his or her power wheelchair and conveniently stop to talk with a friend using the AAC device or must he or she opt for use of one over the other? Can the individual use the AAC system while writing, or does he or she have to shut down the word processing software in order to boot up the communication software? Independence is greatly enhanced for individuals with physical disabilities when systems integration is taken into consideration; when the sum of the parts is given as much attention as the individual parts.

Durability is another common problem. Technology breakdowns are not uncommon. Individuals with physical disabilities, unlike able-bodied nonspeaking persons, rely heavily on their equipment. A voice output device that is not working properly is a catastrophe for an individual who uses AAC; his or her ability to participate actively in social, educational, and work-related situations is severely hampered. And with each equipment breakdown, who is available to diagnose the source of the problem? If the breakdown requires repair, who is responsible for funding the repair and how long will the individual be without his or her communication system? Equipment breakdowns are inevitable and AAC teams must have plans in place which outline the steps to take when problems occur. Technical súpport for maintenance is critical to reduce the time in which individuals who use AAC are without their primary communication devices. Also, back-up communication systems must be readily available when communication devices break down.

Funding Issues

Funding is a bigger problem for individuals with physical disabilities because they generally require more equipment support. It is not unusual for AAC communicators with physical disabilities to need a power chair, a van equipped with a wheelchair lift, a manual wheelchair, a bath chair, a bath lift, and an adapted commode. To support them educationally, a computer with multiple adaptations, as well as an electric page turner or reading machine, may be necessary. High tech communication devices may cost thousands of dollars. The overall cost can be enormous. No single funding source can often bear the cost of these very expensive items. Funding sources including health insurance, local school system resources, family resources, and charitable funds must be combined. For a more complete discussion of funding issues and for more specific information on funding resources, see Chapter 9.

Abandonment of AAC Systems

AAC professionals recognize that ongoing change is an essential element of the AAC process. However, when change involves the rejection of implemented strategies and devices, there is bound to be disappointment on the part of all the team members who helped design the AAC system. Abandonment of AAC devices and other types of assistive technology is not uncommon. Phillips (1991) reported that almost one third of assistive technology devices are abandoned. The reasons for this included (a) the device did not increase functional independence; (b) service and repair was difficult to obtain and costly; and (c) the device was too hard to use, required too much assistance from others, or was unreliable (Batavia, Dillard, & Phillips, 1990). Reasons why AAC devices may be abandoned include (a) the device is too difficult for caretakers to program and set up; (b) the access method is inefficient or fatiguing; (c) unaided methods are faster or more efficient; and (d) there is not enough room or time to set up all the equipment and so it is left behind.

When professionals make recommendations regarding AAC devices, the needs of the individual must be measured against the practicalities of communication settings. A great deal of time goes into the assessment process in order to design the best system possible. However, the "best" system may not be the most practical system in all communication settings. In order to reduce the possibility of device abandonment, it is important that team members realistically address the individual's needs, abilities, and expectations. This can be done by carefully surveying the opinions of all who are involved (e.g., individuals using AAC, the family, and representatives from community, school, and work settings), and to the extent possible, anticipating communication needs across upcoming life transitions. For example, a young man with severe speech and physical disabilities who is about to graduate from high school with limited vocational options may opt to focus on using the Internet to maintain communication with friends and access to information. A high tech voice output device may not really be needed by the individual and his family at home, but an AAC system that has modem capabilities may be an enhancement to communication with the world at large.

AAC devices may cease to be used regularly due to changes in other aspects of the user's daily life. For example, a new wheelchair may be constructed of wider diameter metal tubing, making it impossible to attach the mounting bar for the AAC device to the wheelchair frame. A new seating system may affect the person's method of access so that it becomes difficult to activate his or her head switch as before. When physical or situational changes occur for an individual with physical disabilities, without addressing resulting changes to the AAC system, then the likelihood of abandonment, intentional or otherwise, is increased. It is imperative for AAC teams to coordinate services and to provide ongoing holistic support to individuals with physical disabilities. Ongoing training and technical support helps to prevent device abandonment (Galvin & Toonstra, 1991).

Research Issues

There is very little literature, especially research-based studies, on AAC relative to individuals with physical disabilities. The literature generally includes anecdotal records, case studies, demographic surveys, and studies on intervention effectiveness. Most empirical studies involve single subject design or have a small sample size. Comparative group design is often impractical with individuals with complex disabilities and complex histories.

There is certainly merit to anecdotal accounts. Chedd (1995), a parent of a child who is nonspeaking, offers practical advice to parents who are getting started with AAC, such as how to get started, how to set realistic goals, and how to integrate pictures into everyday conversations with a child. Case study research moves beyond the anecdotal to offer in-depth analyses of individual situations. Goossens (1989) provided a detailed description of a child with CP and her progress as a result of AAC assessment and intervention. A case study by Letto, Bedrosian, & Skarakis-Doyle (1994) investigated the development of communicative functions over a 10-month period in a young preschool child with CP. McGregor, Young, Gerak, Thomas, and Vogelsberg (1992) used preinstruction, natural environment teaching techniques, and sequential withdrawal of preinstruction to instruct a young man with CP and moderate mental retardation to use a customized overlay on a Touch Talker. These case studies paint individual pictures of the effects of AAC intervention.

Group studies demonstrate trends over a larger sample of individuals. Mar and Sall (1994) conducted a study of 26 students with dual sensory impairments, many with CP and a few with syndromes such as CHARGE Association and congenital rubella, to examine the effectiveness of AAC interventions. The authors concluded that microcomputer technology can facilitate critical communication skills in students with severe and profound mental retardation.

Communication interaction studies have included young children with physical disabilities and their caregivers. Hanzlik and Stevenson (1986) compared the ability of mothers to respond positively to their children. They found no difference when comparing mothers and children with CP to mothers and children with mental retardation, or mothers and able-bodied children. Wilcox et al. (1990) looked at the consistency of mothers, educators, and speech-language pathologists to recognize the communicative cues of children with physical disabilities and found a high degree of variability. The authors concluded that interaction sensitivity was partner-child specific. Light et al. (1985) found that caregivers, mostly mothers, of children with physical disabilities who were nonspeaking tended to dominate communication interactions and that the children tended to forfeit turntaking opportunities unless required to respond.

Clearly, more research is needed on a wide variety of issues related to AAC and individuals with physical impairments. In the last few years, there has been a significant increase in the number of studies that examine literacy learning in individuals who are nonspeaking and physically disabled. The reader is referred to Chapter 8 for descriptions of studies on literacy.

ASSESSMENT STRATEGIES SPECIFIC TO INDIVIDUALS WITH PHYSICAL DISABILITIES

AAC assessment is often referred to as predictive evaluation, because professionals must make practical predictions based on their knowledge of development and plan AAC strategies accordingly. AAC assessment is also a multistepped process. First the contributing members of the assessment team must be identified. AAC needs and expectations must be examined. Assessment of the individual's abilities with various types of high and low technology systems must be conducted. Information and funding resources must be explored, and an implementation plan must be devised. AAC evaluation strategies are discussed at length in Chapters 5, 6, and 7, thus, the following sections will reflect on evaluation strategies specific to individuals with physical disabilities who are nonspeaking .

Identifying AAC Assessment Team Members

There are a number of important steps that should precede an AAC assessment of an individual who is physically disabled. Identifying the team members who will play a role in the assessment process is important. It is critical to get input from the individual, his or her family, and caregivers. In addition to the speech-language pathologist, input from physical and occupational therapists is generally a must because of expertise with seating, positioning, motor access, and spatial perceptual issues. The educator and vocational counselor are usually essential members of the team, providing input on school and work issues. Because of the complexity of equipment issues for some individuals with physical disabilities, it may be necessary to include a rehabilitation engineer who can examine the compatibility of various electronic components and integrate them (e.g., powered mobility, computer, AAC system, and environmental controls). For more information on AAC team development, refer to Chapter 2.

Obtain Background Information

Another step in the initial process is to obtain appropriate background information. Prior to assessing individuals with physical disabilities, medical information relative to diagnosis, prognosis, and associated conditions is important. Information on associated conditions such as hearing and visual acuity, as well as seizures, is essential. Information on cognitive, memory, and language functioning is needed along with information on learning style and literacy levels. AAC strategies that are presently in use and those that have been previously attempted should be identified. When preparing to evaluate children, it is useful to know about behavioral issues and activities that are motivating to the child. Motivating topics and activities will help team members prepare evaluation materials.

Often it is helpful to observe or obtain a video of the child in his or her natural environments. Seeing how the child moves is especially useful for delineating the range of options for the motor access part of the evaluation; seeing how the child interacts in his or her communication environments helps to set the stage for assessing communication functions.

Information on the individual's daily routines is helpful in sorting out the types of communication systems that should be included in the upcoming assessment. Individuals with physical disabilities usually change positions throughout their day—a factor that must be considered when developing communication strategies. In addition to needing an AAC system mounted to his or her wheelchair, a child may need a system that is accessible when he or she is seated in a beanbag chair or in a prone stander. A young person with a degenerative disease may need a system that is accessible from both a wheelchair and a bed. This information can be obtained through a questionnaire that is sent to key informants from the primary communication environments such as school, home, and work.

Evaluation Settings

Assessment for the purposes of delineating effective AAC systems can take place in a variety of settings. In the educational environment, it may take place at the student's school, or it may take place in a more central or regional education center where the AAC team is housed. It can also take place in the child's home. This is often the case for infants and toddlers. Going directly to the child's school or home is beneficial when you want to evaluate the use of AAC in the context of the child's natural environments. On the other hand, assessment in a central location is beneficial when there is a great deal of equipment that needs to be used as part of the evaluation.

AAC departments in hospital settings or regional clinics usually have the benefit of a central equipment library and a team of in-house experts. They do not always have the benefit of evaluating communication in the everyday contexts in which it occurs. Hospital and regional centers can often arrange off-site visits to local schools, homes, or work sites for this reason. This is also beneficial to the family. Transporting individuals with physical disabilities and degenerative conditions is often complicated, and multiple appointments for the purpose of assessment can be stressful to families when long distance travel is involved.

Seating and Positioning Issues

Given the many steps involved, it is unusual to complete an AAC assessment for an individual with severe physical disabilities in one appointment. The first appointment usually begins with a review of the individual's seating and positioning. This must be addressed prior to any evaluation of how the individual will physically access a communication device. Optimal motor access is dependent upon optimal seating and positioning. If an individual's positioning is less than optimal, then additional appointments are needed to address this. In the interim, the physical and occupational therapist can create a mock-up of the most likely seating position and continue with the evaluation with the understanding that final decisions on AAC options may be dependent upon resolving the seating and positioning problems. In some cases, it can take weeks or months to optimize a seating system. Temporary AAC systems will need to be developed during this period of time. For more detailed information on seating and positioning, see Chapter 6.

Incorporating Meaningful Activities

The course of the assessment process depends upon many variables, such as the degree of motor impairment and the age of the child. AAC evaluations with babies often have a more informal, playful approach than those conducted with older students. Initial AAC assessments for children with significant motor impairment can take time in order to sort out the child's best method of motor access. The young child's cognitive level and interests will guide the choice of activities that are employed as part of the evaluation process. It is possible to conduct a comprehensive and sequential assessment and yet incorporate activities that will be of interest to the child. This will help obtain the child's optimal performance. For example, if the child is interested in books or likes music, use story reading and musical instruments as part of assessment to evaluate theuse of a headpointer to make choices. If a young girl likes having her nails done, or an adult enjoys sporting events, program vocabulary for this on a voice output device to evaluate direct selection skills versus scanning abilities.

Informal Observation

At the start of the first assessment session, it is helpful to talk informally with the individual and family. During this warm-up period, AAC team members have an opportunity to observe an individual's movements and communication style. Does the individual point to indicate what he or she wants, or does he or she use eye gaze to direct others? Does upper extremity movement appear functional for communication? Are there reliable movements that could be used to access a switch? Does the individual use vocalizations, and for what pragmatic functions? Does the individual seem attuned to text as well as pictures? It is also helpful to note the individual's energy level at the start of the assessment so that this can be compared to performance later in the session to gain a sense of whether fatigue is major issue. This is also a time to observe the communication strategies used by the individual's family, school staff, vocational staff, or other communication partners. The first few minutes of the initial assessment session can provide critical pieces of information on where to begin the more formal part of the assessment process.

Evaluating Motor Access

Guidelines rather than standardized tests exist for conducting motor access assessment (Beukelman & Mirenda, 1992; Goossens & Crain, 1986, 1992; Lee & Thomas, 1990). The critical aspects of the motor access evaluation that are specific to individuals with physical disabilities involve (a) determining the best possible movement pattern and body site for direct or indirect selection; (b) delineating the best arrangement for symbol selection; (c) noting critical features of the AAC system; and (d) identifying the best position of the AAC system relative to the position of the individual. These components are discussed in detail in Chapter 7.

By the conclusion of the motor access assessment, the therapist should be able to outline one to three possible methods for accessing communication. Often, a primary method of motor access is clear. For example, if the individual can point using an index finger, this may be the fastest and most direct method of access. However, if the individual's quality of movement is slow and laborious and fatigue is often an issue, then a secondary, back-up method involving single switch scanning may be needed. This is often the situation for in-dividuals with muscular dystrophy. For children with physical as well as developmental disabilities, it is important to understand the extent to which the physical disability is interacting with the cognitive disability. The child may be able to point to pictures, thereby demonstrating good physical access skills, but have difficulty understanding that symbols are representations of actions, objects, or events. The opposite can also occur. The child may understand the underlying meaning of symbol representations, but be unable to physically control the movements to reach for these symbols. With very young children, there is a need to identify not only what is the current best method of access, but also to identify emerging methods of access. Parallel training on two or three methods of motor access may be needed until the child matures.

Parallel training (Goossens & Crain, 1992) involves training on a higher, more difficult method of motor access concurrent with the child's everyday use of an easier method of communication. With young children, especially, there is a need to separate communication from motor access development. To facilitate communication, children require an easier, less taxing method of motor access. However to facilitate motor access development, parallel training on a higher level of motor access is needed. For example, a therapist may feel a young child has the potential to learn direct selection through pointing, but at this stage, communication needs to occur through the easiest motor modality, for example, eye gaze. Training on direct selection may take place during one-on-one therapy sessions or it can be incorporated into daily activities when communication is not as critical an element. The communicative importance of an activity dictates the method of access.

Parallel training concepts can also be applied to individuals with degenerative diseases. Although the individual may be currently successful when pointing to letters, the course of the disease may require parallel training on eye gaze strategies or auditory scanning. Motor access evaluation in cases of degenerative disease must be ongoing and forward thinking in order to provide for the future communication needs of the individual.

Evaluating Visual Perceptual Skills

Visual as well as spatial perceptual problems are often of concern in individuals with physical disabilities. Background information on visual acuity is very important prior to any evaluation of AAC. During the AAC assessment process, it is important to examine the individual's ability to scan and localize to visual stimuli. Communication systems with fixed overlays, as opposed to dynamic screen overlays, may be less disorienting to individuals who have difficulty with visual scanning and localizing.

Some individuals with physical disabilities due to early brain damage have significant difficulty processing visual symbols. Acuity is not the central problem, but the ability to interpret visual information is severely hampered. These individuals often demonstrate decreased visual attention, and they respond more quickly to auditory stimuli. Their ability to discriminate information from pictures is significantly less than their ability to process information received auditorily. For example, a young child with CP with only mild visual acuity problems was able to talk about cows, what they do, and what noises they make, but was unable to identify a cow in picture form. Other individuals with severe visual processing deficits use phonemic strategies to attempt to spell words, but cannot accurately identify letters when presented visually. In cases such as this, where the individual has ample visual acuity but severe visual processing deficits, it is important to investigate logically and sequentially his or her ability to process visually based information. Can he or she interpret photos, illustrations, black and white drawings, letters, or numerals? Is visual discrimination aided by simplifying or enlarging picture communication symbols, or by separating symbols, or by adding color or highlighting cues? Is the individual more successful when auditory cues are combined with visual symbols?

Individuals with severe visual processing deficits who use direct selection often will learn to use color and location cues to memorize communication overlays. For these individuals, it is imperative to avoid changing the locations of symbols. When upgrading communication overlays, it is important to keep commonly used symbols in the same relative locations; it is also helpful to group and color code symbols. Individuals with physical disabilities who rely on single switch scanning often do best with auditory scanning or auditory cueing combined with visual scanning. The degree to which these strategies will assist the individual with severe visual processing deficits will need to be carefully examined. The reader is referred to Chapter 7 for more information on the assessment of visual-motor and visual perceptual skills.

Additional Areas of Testing

In addition to the evaluation of motor access, there is often a need for additional testing to assess receptive language skills, symbol systems, spelling and writing abilities, and so forth. Testing methods need careful consideration when assessing an individual with physical disabilities who is nonspeaking. Test materials may need adaptation and nonstandard approaches may be necessary. Test materials, such as pictures, letters, or words, may need to be enlarged and spaced apart to accommodate an individual who has only gross movement for pointing. Eye gaze strategies combined with multiple choice test formats may be needed for the individual with severely limited upper extremity use. Evaluation strategies to determine literacy levels, language abilities, and symbol systems are described in Chapter 5.

Feature Match

"Feature match," a phrase coined by Penn-Tech (Swengel & Varga, 1993) is the process of matching the individual's needs and abilities to the many features of various high and low tech AAC and assistive technology systems. It represents the intended outcome for the AAC assessment process. It is the sum total of a great deal of information which must be sorted through in order to arrive at recommendations that will meet the needs and expectations of individuals using AAC and enhance communication with communication partners in a variety of environments. For individuals with physical disabilities, more so than other populations, determining motor access is of primary importance in the feature match process. Once background information and current assessment information is gathered, reviewed, and summarized, then AAC team members can match the needs and abilities of individuals using AAC to a wide range of high and low tech devices and strategies. Team members must use the expertise they have developed over time with regard to AAC and combine this with up-to-date knowledge of available AAC devices and other equipment, such as mounting systems, switches, interfaces, and software.

Systems integration, the degree to which technologies work together for the user, is another important element that is not always an issue with populations who are not physically disabled. A young man who relies on AAC and a power wheelchair will need to be able to independently access the controls for both. For example, the position of the joystick that controls the wheelchair should not interfere with the positioning of the AAC device. Computer access should also be compatible with AAC access whenever possible. If the AAC device is designed to be used as a computer interface, then the individual should access the computer via the AAC device, rather than having to master two separate systems of motor access. The process for determining feature match relative to motor access is discussed in Chapter 7. To ensure the staying power of the feature match process, trial periods for the use of AAC devices need to be scheduled and strategies for effective use must be clearly articulated.

Trial Periods

Once the formal testing has been completed, the team will need to assemble to discuss all the data and to determine future steps. Because it is not always possible to accomplish feature match in one or two sessions, and because AAC teams need to have a high degree of confidence in their AAC recommendations before requesting funding, it is usually best to set up a trial period with an AAC system. This gives the individual, the family, and school or work personnel an opportunity to be sure the system meets their combined needs and expectations. It gives the AAC team additional information with which they can refine their recommendations.

For individuals with physical disabilities, the learning component of motor access is an issue that needs time before final decisions are made. Learning a new or adapted method of access takes time and practice. A child may need practice with a new scanning method before a decision is made to implement a scanning system. An individual may need practice with an optical pointer before this equipment is purchased. An adult may need practice time with the use of Morse code to determine if this is a faster method of input. Short-term equipment loans are often necessary during trial periods. Trial periods can be as short as a week or take place over many months. Trial periods need to be viewed as a normal part of the assessment process and should include specific monitoring plans to keep track of data and system revisions. Persons responsible for monitoring the trial period should be identified.

Implementation Plans

Once the total AAC team, including the individual and his or her family, make a final decision on an AAC system, the process does not stop. Locating sources of funding for AAC devices is very much a part of the process. In addition, the AAC team should outline implementation plans that deal with family, staff, and AAC user training, physical management of the device, and transportation of the device. It is also practical to begin identifying the communication environments in which the device will be introduced initially and begin planning the vocabulary for these communication environments. Again, it is important to identify and plan for the implementation of multiple communication systems. Low tech systems for some communication functions to serve as a backup to high tech systems need to be included in the implementation plan. For example, a young woman may use a wallet-sized picture communication system in the community and use a voice output communication device at work. A child may use a communication board out on the playground and use a voice output AAC device in the classroom.

COMMUNICATION STRATEGIES SPECIFIC TO INDIVIDUALS WITH PHYSICAL DISABILITIES

Multiple communication strategies are the general rule, especially for individuals with physical disabilities. Strategies can be "aided" through the use of equipment, including no tech, low tech, and high tech equipment options, or they can be unaided, in the case of signing, eye pointing, and gestures. Aided and unaided strategies are discussed in more detail in Chapter 3. The following strategies are more commonly employed with individuals with severe physical disabilities.

Unaided Strategies

Unaided strategies are communication techniques that are always available to the individual. They need no special equipment, no special set up or mounting systems. They are the unique methods by which a person has learned to communicate nonverbally. They are a powerful and valid means of communication. It is often amazing how much a person with severe physical disabilities can communicate just using eye gaze; she looks at you, she stares at the clock on the wall, and she looks back at you. In that brief moment, she has secured your attention, made a reference to the time, and shifted the communicative turn-taking back to you. Using contextual cues, you know she wants to know how long you are staying.

Unaided techniques do, however, require a knowledgeable communication partner who is familiar with these communication strategies. In the case of sign language, the listener must possess, at least receptively, a signing vocabulary. Gestural communication involves shared referents; the nonspeaking individual and the communication partner need to have a common understanding of the significance of certain gestures. For example, when the nonverbal individual turns his head to the side, the partner must know from past experience that this means "no more." Eye movements for yes and no are a common unaided communication strategy. Upward eye movements often signify "yes," whereas side-to-side or downward eye movements signify "no." Nodding and shaking one's head, smiling and frowning, or eye blinking can also serve this function; it all depends on what has been established with the nonspeaking individual.

For individuals with severe physical disabilities, eye movements, head movements, and gross movement gestures are a way to call for attention, indicate needs, and make choices. The strength of these techniques lies in their portability. The weakness of these techniques is that they are often left to interpretation or are dependent upon the skill of the partner to interpret the message and ask pertinent questions to confirm the message. To acquaint people who are unfamiliar with such techniques, some individuals who use AAC will tape a communication instruction card to their tray which explains the unaided methods by which they communicate. The user calls attention to the card using eye gaze. This strategy provides the individual with physical disabilities who is nonspeaking a measure of control when unaided strategies are a primary means of communication.

Aided Strategies

Aided strategies involve some method of interface or equipment or communication technique to make them work. No tech strategies involve no equipment, low tech strategies involve simple equipment, and high tech strategies involve more sophisticated, usually programmable, types of equipment.

No Tech Communication Strategies

No tech strategies, like unaided techniques, are generally portable and accessible. However, they often require more of an active, facilitative role on the part of the communication partner. For some people, the techniques used with individuals who are nonspeaking, and physically disabled come naturally, but training is often needed for others. Pointing to picture symbols or objects is a no tech method of communication for individuals who have sufficient upper extremity range of motion and dexterity. When this is absent, headpointers or chinsticks can also be used for direct selection through pointing. If pointing is not an option, three or four pictures or objects in the environment can be placed on the individual's tray or on a table. Individuals using AAC can eye gaze to the desired item, or the communication partner can point to each of the items and await a yes response from the user, indicating the desired item.

Hand signals are a quick way of communicating choices. Using this technique, the communication partner pairs his left hand with one choice and his right hand with the other. For example, the partner will ask, "Do you want a Coke or a Sprite?" He then shakes his left hand in the air while saying, "Coke?" and shakes his right hand while saying, "Sprite?" The individual using AAC then looks at the hand that is associated with his choice of drink. With some training, this technique works well even with young children.

Auditory scanning is another technique used with individuals who are nonspeaking and physically disabled. It is somewhat less concrete, involves careful listening, and is used generally in situations when there are more than two choices. With this strategy, the communication partner asks a question and then verbally presents three to four choices with brief pauses between each choice, repeating the choices until the individual responds. When the individual using AAC hears her preferred choice, she can hit a switch or use "yes" eye movements to convey her choice.

The 20 questions technique is often used as a communication strategy with AAC communicators who have severe physical disabilities, but have a distinct yes and no response. The communication partner asks a series of questions moving from the general to the specific in order to narrow down the communication topic. It requires the communication partner to ask logical, sequential questions that lead to a choice or an idea or a concern that the nonspeaking individual is attempting to communicate. This technique can be risky, especially when the partner is unable to determine the exact nature of what the individual is attempting to convey. This is especially true with individuals with severe physical disabilities who cannot repair the communication breakdown because they do not have a readily available, alternate means of communication that they can reach for or move to obtain.

All of these techniques are easy to use, require no equipment, and can be employed at almost any time. However, these techniques require a dominant communi-

cation partner. An individual relying on no tech AAC is highly dependent upon the skill of the partner and has less control over the direction of the conversation. These techniques alone do not promote active, independent communication and must be used in balance with other communication strategies which give individuals using AAC more opportunity to initiate and control the direction of the conversation.

No tech strategies can get very sophisticated for individuals who are functioning at a higher level. Some individuals who use AAC work out ingenious no tech systems of communication with familiar communication partners. For example, verbal scanning of the alphabet can be combined with word prediction and yes/no questions to spell words and express ideas. The communication partner verbally scans through the letters of the alphabet until the individual using AAC indicates the desired first letter. This is repeated for the second letter and continues until the communication partner is able to predict the word that is being spelled. For some communication dyads, this is a faster technique than their aided system provides, because the adult partner can predict faster or can respond faster than single switch scanning allows.

Another sophisticated technique involves a simulation of group-item scanning and branching. The communication partner first asks, "Is it A to L or M to Z?" When the user indicates "A to L," this narrows the field of choices and the partner then asks, "A to G or H to L?" If the user indicates "A to G," the partner then recites "A . . . B . . . C . . . D" until the user indicates that "D" is the chosen letter. Because a vowel is a likely next letter, the partner then verbally scans throughout the vowels, "A . . . E . . . I . . . O . . . " until the user indicates that "O" is the desired vowel. The partner uses word prediction and asks whether "dog" is the intended word. Primary caregivers and AAC communicators can achieve high rates of speed, accuracy, and reliability with these sophisticated no tech methods.

Low Tech Communication Strategies

Eye gaze boards, often called "E-Trans," are a common low tech communication strategy used with individuals who have difficulty pointing and, instead, rely on eye gaze to indicate choices. See Chapter 3 for a description of eye gaze boards and methods of use. The user fixes her eye gaze on a symbol to communicate her choice and then looks back at the communication partner for acknowledgment of her choice. Young children can start out with two symbols placed in the top corners of the eye gaze frame, and can gradually increase this to four, eight, or more symbols. Eye gaze strategies combined with encoding strategies as described in Chapter 3 can further increase communication options.

Clock scanners are another low tech method of communication. Communication symbols are placed in a circular pattern on the face of the clock scanner and the individual using AAC depresses a switch until the dial is pointing to the preferred symbol.

Simple voice output technologies with which individuals who are physically disabled can communicate by using gross body movements include the BigMack by Ablenet, a large switch with built-in digitized speech, or the Switch Module by Toys for Special Children. Using one to four switches, these and other simple technologies add the element of "voice" to the communication interchange. These devices are easy to use and quick to program. They are appropriate for individuals who have gross unilateral or bilateral arm movements, and are relatively inexpensive equipment. For example, a single voice output switch can be used to allow a child to participate in a story reading activity by recording a frequently repeated phrase from the story (e.g., "and he was still hungry" from *The Hungry Caterpillar* by Eric Carle). At the end of the school day, it can be used to send a message home that conveys what the child did at school that day. For an older individual with physical disabilities, a single voice output switch can communicate a frequently needed phrase such as "please turn the page" or it can be used to order lunch at a nearby restaurant.

The benefits of low tech strategies are that they are generally low cost and easy to use. They are often combined with high tech strategies to provide an alternate means of communication in different positions or activities. Whereas high tech devices have generic, preprogrammed vocabulary, low tech strategies can offer a means of providing supplemental vocabulary. For example, a high tech device may provide the vocabulary needed for participation in the morning opening activities, whereas the low tech clock scanner provides words or picture communication symbols that are specific to the day's activities (e.g., topic vocabulary for a school assembly on fire prevention). The drawbacks to low tech devices and strategies are that they have limited vocabulary, and therefore, limited communication power.

High Tech Communication Strategies

Individuals who can point with good accuracy at one- to two-inch targets have high tech options that store larger amounts of vocabulary (AlphaTalker, Touch Talker, Liberator, Hawk, Macaw, DigiVox, Action-Voice, and DynaVox). Individuals with more severe physical impairments often cannot point accurately or efficiently; these individuals may need scanning systems or optical pointing technologies. Many of the AAC devices just listed have scanning options built in, or the manufacturers produce dedicated versions of the device which provide scanning options.

There are optical pointing systems which are built in (Liberator) or dedicated optical pointing systems (FreeWheel or HeadMaster). These high tech devices and others are discussed in more detail in Chapter 3.

For individuals with physical disabilities, high tech AAC systems offer the most communication power. They provide a means to initiate "voiced" communication, and they allow storage of large amounts of vocabulary which gives the individual more topics on which to communicate. AAC systems that include text-to-speech as well as picture-based communication such as the Liberator, DeltaTalker, and DynaVox provide a literate individual with the ability to spell out words and phrases not preprogrammed into the device. This gives the individual even more control over everyday communication. High tech voice output systems allow an individual to initiate communication. It is hard to initiate communication using a no tech, eye gaze system when a student is confined to a wheelchair and the teacher is across the room. Although communication via an electronic device will never replace the ability to speak, it is a promising substitute in the absence of speech. The drawback of these devices is that they are expensive, take time to program, and are often heavy. For ambulatory individuals who use AAC, especially children, these devices are cumbersome to carry around. For individuals in wheelchairs, there are mounting and transporting issues to consider. Nonetheless, high tech devices represent a means of communication that was not possible 20 years ago.

Matching the needs and abilities of the individual to the features of various communication systems, whether low tech or high tech, is a complicated process. It requires skill and experience on the part of AAC specialists. These specialists must have a thorough understanding of a wide variety of communication strategies and they must have in-depth knowledge of a broad range of AAC devices. Feature match recommendations should not be based on what device the specialist knows or likes best. Feature match should be linked to the communication needs of the individual.

TRAINING STRATEGIES SPECIFIC TO THE POPULATION

Although multiple communication strategies are the general rule for individuals with physical disabilities, it is how these strategies are used that ensures successful communication outcomes. Training is a critical component of the AAC intervention process. Training can be examined from two perspectives: training the user and training his or her communication partners, which can include family members, teachers, peers, co-workers, and even members of the community.

Training Individuals Using AAC

Training the user is often an ongoing process, especially in situations where a child's skills are continuing to develop, and conversely, in situations where an individual's skills are declining. It is important to task analyze the skills that the individual needs to obtain to communicate effectively. In all cases, it is important to focus initially on communication strategies that will be successful and of functional daily use. In the case of children, ongoing training is often carried out by school staff with consultation from local AAC teams. Communication training is best when integrated into natural, daily activities. Isolated or pull-out training (when a child is removed from the classroom for one-on-one or small group training) is sometimes needed when initially introducing a new AAC communication strategy.

In the case of adults with physical disabilities, it is important to gear training to everyday needs and incorporate training into real world environments. Training strategies should be prioritized based on identified critical life skills, and training should be structured to ensure incremental success.

Although training may begin in a more clinical one-on-one setting, skills will need to be generalized to natural settings such as the grocery store, the hair salon, and work settings.

At times, it is necessary to focus training on more than one communication approach. A toddler who is physically disabled may be learning to refine his arm movement to activate two to three large switches to activate a voice output device. At the same time, staff may decide, because the child has sufficient head control, that it is time to try a headpointer as a way to provide the youngster with an increased number of symbol selections. In the future, staff may want to introduce switch-operated visual scanning techniques.

Although it may seem practical to teach one method at a time, parallel training is often essential in order to keep pace with a child's development. This is also the case for individuals with degenerative diseases. Although the individual may be working to maintain his ability to communicate by pointing to picture communication symbols, staff may need to begin parallel training on auditory scanning, knowing that the individual is gradually losing visual acuity.

It has been this therapist's experience that we often underestimate the number of motor access strategies children can learn to use simultaneously. Nonetheless, to reduce confusion with multiple training strategies, it is often helpful to keep training activities distinctly separate. For example, using the previous example of the toddler, it might be best to focus on the direct selection of switches during snack time, and practice the use of the headpointer during play time with a bubble blowing activity. It is important to emphasize, once again, that easy methods of motor access should be the method of choice for communicatively important activities so that the individual can focus on language expression. Motor access training should not interfere with activities where communication and language development are at stake.

Training Communication Partners

In addition to providing training to individuals using AAC, it is also important to provide ongoing training to the communication partners who are significant in the life of the child. Family members, caregivers, peers, teachers, and work coaches are principal trainees; however, it is also helpful to identify others who are important in the life of the individual, such as cafeteria workers and bus drivers.

Training to potential communication partners can be delivered in two different ways, specific or general. Specific training delivers training on communication strategies that are unique to that AAC communicator. General training provides instruction on generic topics to groups of people. General training on topics such as "integrating AAC into the classroom" or "designing communication overlays" can be delivered at the classroom level or local school team level. General training on "designing overlays for vocational settings" or "strategies for integrating AAC into community settings" can be delivered to interested stakeholders through local workshops or through professional conferences.

Specific training to individuals using AAC and significant others can be provided in one-on-one or small group situations. The method in which training is delivered depends upon the needs of individual using AAC. Following an AAC assessment, it may be necessary to provide training on multiple issues. For example, training will undoubtedly be provided directly to an adolescent using a new AAC device on how to use the device effectively in different settings for different purposes. Training on how to set up, mount, and troubleshoot the individual's communication system may need to be conducted with the instructional assistant and the teacher, whereas training on how to program the new AAC device is provided to the family and school team. Instruction on how to communicate with the individual who is using a new device may be a topic of interest to the entire school, including peers.

Handouts, written directions, set-up diagrams, troubleshooting information, phone numbers for technical support, and so forth should be reviewed, organized in a file or a notebook and kept in a convenient location. Videotapes are useful for providing training on complex systems. These are often available through the manufacturer or you can make training tapes that demonstrate the actual user and his or her system. This is especially useful when a student is transitioning to a new school setting. Training should cover every conceivable situation no matter how trivial (e.g., battery recharging, cable attachment, checking the tightness of screws and other maintenance issues) as the nonspeaking individual may not be able to guide the caregivers in how to set up and implement the system. Effective training is a time-consuming process; nevertheless it is essential to the success of individuals using AAC.

PROMOTING EFFECTIVE AAC ACROSS ENVIRONMENTS

Communication interactions between two speaking individuals, when analyzed, are highly complex. It is no less complex between a nonspeaking individual using AAC and his or her myriad communication partners across multiple environments.

One of the most troublesome aspects of communication interaction for individuals with physical disabilities is whether they have opportunities to be active rather than merely passive participants in communication interactions across multiple settings.

When an AAC device is set up primarily to respond to questions, then an individual using AAC is relegated to a passive role where he or she must wait for others to ask questions. Individuals with physical disabilities in fixed positions or in manual wheelchairs are more at risk for this because, unlike nonspeaking individuals who are ambulatory, they cannot independently move about to direct the action of another person, or actively greet others and initiate a social interaction. It is only to the degree that we sensitize others to these daily issues that we can lessen the risk of severely narrowing communication interactions for individuals with physical disabilities who use AAC. For example, it is helpful to provide an individual who is physically disabled with a quick means of calling attention to initiate a conversation. By using a BigMack or other low tech device which is programmed to say "I've got something I'd like to tell you," the individual can actively engage the attention of a communication partner. The individual using AAC can then shift to his or her communication device to write a new message or access a prestored message. In light of the current emphasis on inclusion of persons with disabilities in general education, vocational, and community settings, it is important to design AAC systems that promote active communication interactions across multiple environments.

AAC Integration Issues in the Home

At home, families have set daily routines. These routines may or may not include a broad range of communication interactions. Families have their own ways of communicating and may not have a need to use multiple high and low tech devices at home. On the other hand, families may not be aware when their communication interactions are limiting the user's opportunities to communicate in more active ways. Implementation within the home needs to examine these issues without treading on the family's right to maintain a home atmosphere that does not imitate all day therapy. Professionals must keep in mind that families of individuals with physical disabilities have complicated and busy days. Implementation strategies for the home must balance the communication needs of the individual against the needs of the total family. Chapter 14 provides more information on issues related to AAC in the family and home.

Integrating AAC strategies into the home must be prefaced by permission to examine communication interactions within the home setting. It is one thing to instruct a family in the use of new AAC strategies; it is another to cast judgment on the extent to which these strategies are integrated into the home. However, once a family is comfortable with a few communication strategies, they are often ready to expand these strategies. Determining a family's readiness to integrate additional communication strategies into the home can be done through an occasional meeting to discuss current communications means, including the need for additional vocabulary or new strategies that could increase communication opportunities. Meetings to specifically discuss current AAC use should be regularly scheduled with families, and should not be limited to annual educational reviews, or crisis situations. Preventing AAC device abandonment depends on proactive rather than reactive implementation plans.

AAC Integration Issues in School Settings

Schools also have set routines. By their very nature, schools require communica-
tion; teachers ask questions as part of instruction and students respond. Integrating AAC into the classroom presents a real challenge to teachers. Keeping up with educationally relevant AAC vocabulary is one ongoing challenge, and finding appropriate ways to actively include students who use AAC in classroom activities is another. Evaluating the extent to which AAC use is effectively integrated into daily educational experiences is a continuing need. When left to chance, there is a greater likelihood that students with physical disabilities will use their devices primarily for answering questions. Although this will serve to "include" the student in classroom activities, it seriously limits the ability of individuals using AAC to develop a wide range of communication skills to meet a wide range of communication functions. In addition to answering who, what, where, and why questions, students need to be able to initiate questions, to comment on activities, to express ideas, to make exclamations in socially appropriate contexts, to call attention to their successes, to convey their dislikes, to request help, and to interact successfully with peers. Meeting these everyday communication needs goes well beyond merely plugging next week's vocabulary into the student's AAC device.

Meeting the full range of communication needs is a daunting task for any one person. In the educational mainstream, it certainly cannot be the sole responsibility of the general education teacher, nor can the general educator fully abdicate this to others. It also cannot be the sole responsibility of the special education teacher, the instructional assistant, the speech-language pathologist, or the AAC specialist. When only one professional addresses these issues, then only one side of the communication equation is addressed. Integrating communication into the school setting is a team approach and should be addressed collaboratively. It requires the combined perspectives of the different team members. Teachers provide input on classroom communication needs and on vocabulary related to upcoming teaching units. Instructional assistants provide information on the effectiveness of daily AAC strategies. The speech-language pathologist provides perspective on broadening communication functions. AAC specialists provide expertise on how AAC systems can best address school-based needs.

Obviously, although AAC communication needs must be met on a daily basis, teams cannot meet daily to plan for this. The first step in integrating communication strategies into the classroom is to delineate clearly the communication needs of the school environment. It is helpful for the school team to meet at the beginning of the school year to outline the daily school schedule of individuals who use AAC and to determine what types of AAC strategies will best address daily school activities. The team must also look at the types of communication interactions that will occur as part of this daily schedule and identify additional strategies that will foster the broad development of communication skills. Scheduled meetings to discuss the effectiveness of current strategies are needed throughout the year. It is a failure on the part of the school team when communication issues are not discovered until the end-of-year review. The reader is referred to Chapter 15 for additional information on AAC in the educational setting.

AAC Issues in the Work Setting

The transition to work is a big step for an individual who uses AAC, his or her family, for the professionals setting up vocational placements, and often for the people who work alongside an AAC communicator. It is especially difficult to locate jobs for individuals who are physically disabled, even more so when the individual uses AAC. Nonetheless, AAC teams can help ease the transition for AAC students taking part in vocational training. The integration of AAC into the work setting has many of the same issues previously described, including limited communication opportunities. Because the focus is on training job skills, communication opportunities may be limited to answers to work-related questions, requests for help, or requests for more work. There may be less attention paid to facilitating conversation between co-workers, or few opportunities to ask clarifying questions or comment about work tasks.

Similar to that of the school setting, communication in the work setting must be examined across the day's events. AAC vocabulary must take into consideration not only the vocabulary related to the work task, but also consider social greetings upon entry to work, small talk and coffee break conversation, cafeteria needs, and daily care concerns such as feeding and bathrooming. Engineering the environment for communication interaction is critical (Elder & Goossens, 1994). Training must be aimed not only at individuals using AAC, but also at the job coach, supervisors, and co-workers who will need to learn how to communicate with nonspeaking individuals. For additional information on AAC in adult program settings, the reader is referred to Chapter 17.

Beukelman and Mirenda's (1992) work on identifying potential participation barriers is particularly helpful when considering AAC in the work setting. The authors discussed methods to identify opportunity barriers as well as access barriers. In the work place, opportunity barriers may be the result of a lack of knowledge on the part of co-workers, or it may be an attitudinal problem. Access barriers at work may be due to a need for environmental adaptations, or it may be that the individual's AAC system is not appropriate to the work environment. For example, a sophisticated voice output device may not be appropriate for an individual who serves food in a cafeteria.

To identify critical AAC issues for staff working with nonspeaking secondary students, a small AAC survey was recently conducted with six high school special education teachers in a large suburban school system. These teachers reportedly had one, two, or three high school students with cognitive impairments who used AAC on a daily basis in community and job training settings. Although five out of six teachers rated AAC use at the job site as "very important," they also indicated that there were barriers to effective AAC use on the job site. Reasons included (a) the equipment was unwieldy, too difficult to program, and too large or too heavy; (b) there was insufficient time to program vocabulary or create communication boards; and (c) more job site training was needed with co-workers. Although this survey was small in sample size, it illustrates some important AAC issues in vocational settings: more portable, lightweight AAC equipment which is easy to program is needed, and more time is needed for creating communication overlays and for training co-workers.

Communication and literacy is very important to higher functioning, nonspeaking individuals with physical disabilities in the workplace. Because of their motor impairments, work assignments will be geared toward tasks that require communication and literacy skills, rather than physical skills. Text editing and computer programming are options for individuals who are high functioning. Copying text, delivering instructions to co-workers, messenger, and museum guide roles are appropriate jobs for some individuals who use AAC, but they often require higher level communication and literacy skills. The degree to which these skills have been developed will influence the types of jobs that can be sought.

AAC Issues in the Community

In light of efforts to include individuals with disabilities into the mainstream, including general education classrooms, camp settings, and other recreational and community settings, there is a pressing need to coordinate efforts to promote the use of AAC in community-based activities. The prime difficulty is who should take on the responsibility for this. In school settings, it is easier to identify responsible staff, but in community settings such as public recreation centers, church groups, scouting groups, and local store and restaurant settings it is much harder to coordinate AAC issues. Once the individual is age 21 and no longer enrolled in an educational setting, interagency service coordination is also a problem.

To prepare for these situations, it is often helpful to teach individuals using AAC to self-advocate by including phrases in their communication systems that will explain how they best communicate. For example, an AAC device might say "I communicate with my eyes. Eyes up means 'yes' and eyes down means 'no.'" Because the family is often responsible for explaining AAC strategies to members of the community, it may be helpful to work with the family to outline the best strategies for this. Principal strategies should be simple and easy to learn for those who are not familiar with AAC. It can also be beneficial to help families identify different strategies for different situations. Voice output communication devices might be fine at church, but a waterproof communication board will be best at the community pool.

The portability of devices is a critical component in community settings. If a device is too heavy to carry around, it is unlikely that it will be used out in the community. More portable AAC systems are now on the market such as the Parrot by Zygo and the MessageMate by Words Plus. The WalkerTalker by Prentke Romich is a voice output system that is worn around the waist. Currently, there are more lightweight, text-based portable AAC devices than lightweight, picture communication systems with voice output. Text-based systems such as the LightWriter and the Q.E.D. Scribe by Zygo Industries offer more open-ended communication as it only takes 26 keys to create any word or phrase. Picture-based systems are not as open-ended and the memory requirements of the device increase with the number of words or phrases needed. In the future, as more AAC devices are developed that are lighter, more compact, and therefore easier to transport, AAC use in the community will be greatly enhanced.

CONCLUSION

The road to effective AAC use is long and uneven. Individuals develop at different rates and life circumstances change. AAC assessment is a sequential process that requires a structured trial and error approach. By its very nature, the diagnostic process is slow and solutions evolve over time. Vocabulary needs are ever changing and there is always a new person who needs training in how to be a good communication partner. For individuals with physical disabilities who do not speak, AAC provides a means of expression and a way to interact with others. It allows the person behind the physical disability to be recognized and respected.

AAC technologies for individuals with physical disabilities only date back about 20 years. In a relatively short period of time, AAC has come a long way in providing a voice to persons with severe motor impairments. The commitment to AAC technologies for persons with physical disabilities is presently strong and the push for improvement needs to focus on refining and expanding what we currently know. Research is urgently needed to demonstrate best strategies in the assessment and use of AAC from the broader perspective of AAC use in the home, at school, at the job site, and in community settings. Although today individuals who are physically disabled have more options for AAC use, there is much that professionals still need to know to improve service delivery to a statistically small, but nonetheless important, group of people.

REFERENCES

Batshaw, M. L., & Perret, Y. M. (1992). *Children with disabilities: A medical primer.* Baltimore, MD: Paul H. Brookes.

Batvia, A., Dillard, D., & Phillips, B. (1990). How to avoid technology abandonment. *Proceedings of the 5th annual conference: Technology and persons with disabilities,* Los Angeles, CA pp. 43–52.

Bureau of Education for the Handicapped (1976, December). *Conference on communication aids for non-vocal severely physically handicapped persons.* Alexandra, VA.

Beukelman, D., & Mirenda, P. (1992). *Augmentative and alternative communication: Management of severe communication disorders in children and adults.* Baltimore: Paul H. Brookes.

Blackstone, S. (1995). Angelman syndrome and AAC. *Augmentative Communication News, 8*(3), 1–8.

Bloomberg, K., & Johnson, H. (1990). A statewide demographic survey of people with severe communication impairments. *Augmentative and Alternative Communication, 5*(1), 50–60.

Buyse, M. L. (Ed.). (1990). *Birth defects encyclopedia.* Dover, MA: Center for Birth Defects Information Services.

Chedd, N. A. (1995). Getting started with augmentative communication. *Exceptional Parent, 25*(5), 34–39.

Elder, P. S., & Goossens, C. (1994). *Engineering training environments for interactive augmentative communication: Strategies for adolescents and adults who are moderately/severely developmentally delayed.* Birmingham, AL: Southeast Augmentative Communication Conference Publications.

Erenberg, G. (1984). Cerebral palsy. *Postgraduate Medicine, 75*(7), 87–93.

Galvin, J., & Toonstra, M. (1991). Adjusting technology to meet your needs. *Proceedings of the 6th annual conference on technology and persons with disabilities,* pp. 267–273. Los Angeles, CA.

Goossens, C. (1989). Aided communication intervention before assessment: A case study of a child with cerebral palsy. *Augmentative and Alternative Communication, 5*(1), 14–26.

Goossens, C., & Crain, S. (1986). *Augmentative communication assessment resource.* Wauconda, IL: Don Johnston Developmental Equipment.

Goossens, C., & Crain, S. S. (1992). *Utilizing switch interfaces with children who are severely physically challenged.* Austin, TX: Pro-Ed.

Hagberg, B., Hagberg, G., & Zetterstrom, R. (1989). Decreasing perinatal mortality—Increase in cerebral palsy morbidity. *Acta Paediatrica Scandinavica, 78,* 664–670.

Hanzlik, J., & Stevenson, M. (1986). Interaction of mothers and their infants who are mentally retarded, retarded with cerebral palsy, or nonretarded. *American Journal of Mental Deficiency, 90,* 513–520.

Houghton, J., Bronicki, G., & Guess, D. (1987). Opportunities to express preferences and make choices among students with severe disabilities in classroom settings. *Journal of the Association for Persons with Severe Handicaps, 12,* 18–27.

Lafontaine, L. M., & DeRuyter, F. (1987). The nonspeaking cerebral palsied: A clinical and demographic database report. *Augmentative and Alternative Communication, 3*(2), 153–162.

Lee, K. S., & Thomas, D. J. (1990). *Control of computer-based technology for people with physical disabilities: An assessment manual.* Toronto: University of Toronto Press.

Letto, M., Bedrosian, J. L., & Skarakis-Doyle, E. (1994). Applications of Vygotskian developmental theory to language acquisition in a young child with cerebral palsy. *Augmentative and Alternative Communication, 10,* 151–160.

Light, J., Collier, B., & Parnes, P. (1985). Communicative interaction between young nonspeaking physically disabled children and their primary caregivers: Part I. discourse patterns. *Augmentative and Alternative Communication, 1*(2), 74–83.

Lipkin, P. (1991). Epidemiology of the developmental disabilities. In A. J. Capute & P. J. Accardo, (Eds.). *Developmental disabilities in infancy and childhood* (pp. 43–68). Baltimore, MD: Paul H. Brookes.

Lord, J. (1984). Cerebral palsy: A clinical approach. *Archives of Physical Medicine and Rehabilitation, 65,* 542–548.

Mar, H. H., & Sall, N. (1994). Programmatic approach to use of technology in communication instruction for children with dual sensory impairments. *Augmentative and Alternative Communication, 10,* 138–150.

Matas, J. A., Mathy-Laikkko, P., Beukelman, D. R., & Legresley, K. (1985). Identifying the nonspeaking population: A demographic study. *Augmentative and Alternative Communication, 1,* 17–31.

McGregor, G., Young, J., Gerak, J., Thomas, B., & Vogelsberg, R. T. (1992). Increasing functional use of an assistive communication device by a student with severe disabilities. *Augmentative and Alternative Communication, 8*(3), 243–250.

Miller, L. W. (1995). *Angelman syndrome: A parent's guide.* Gainesville, FL: Angelman Syndrome Foundation.

Mirenda, P., & Mathy-Laikko, P. (1989). Augmentative and alternative communication applications for persons with severe congenital communication disorders: An introduction. *Augmentative and Alternative Communication, 5,* 3–13.

Murphy, J., Markova, I., Moodie, E., Scott, J., & Boa, S. (1995). Augmentative and alternative communication systems used by people with cerebral palsy in Scotland: Demographic survey. *Augmentative and Alternative Communication, 11*(1), 26–35.

Nelson, K. B., & Ellenberg, J. H. (1986). Antecedents of cerebral palsy: Multivariate analysis of risk. *The New England Journal of Medicine, 315,* 81–86.

Phillips, B. (1991). *Technology abandonment: From the consumer point of view.* Washington, DC: REquest Publication

Swengel, K., & Varga, T. (1993, October). *Feature match: PennTech's AAC assessment process.* Paper presented at the Closing the Gap Conference, Minneapolis, MN.

Wilcox, M. J., Kouri, T. A., & Caswell, S. (1990). Partner sensitivity to communication behavior of young children with developmental disabilities. *Journal of Speech and Hearing Disorders, 55*(4), 679–693.

Zangari, C., Lloyd, L. L., & Vicker, B. (1994). Augmentative and alternative communication: An historic perspective. *Augmentative and Alternative Communication, 10,* 27–59.

Tom's AAC Story: Transitions and Change

Denise C. DeCoste

Tom is 16 years old and attends high school. Tom has congenital cerebral palsy (CP), cannot speak, and has voluntary control of eye and head movements only. With these limited movements, he can move about in an electric wheelchair and communicate quite effectively. Despite his many physical disabilities, he is highly personable, well liked, and well adjusted. Recently, for the homecoming football game, he participated in pep rallies, accompanied the football team onto the field, and had a front row seat for the game. It was a great day for Tom and his family, who have watched him struggle over many hurdles to be accepted as just one of the guys.

Tom's assistive technology story began when he was a preschooler and will continue throughout his life. His long path to this point is a living illustration that assistive technology is not static, but must constantly change and adapt to meet new situations—some of them foreseeable, and others not.

By age 4, it was clearly apparent that Tom was unable to use his arms to point and could not verbalize sounds other than to laugh or cry. His first AAC system involved eye gaze and an acrylic board; Tom would gaze at the desired picture and then back to his communication partner on the opposite side of the transparent board. At age 6, Tom was introduced to linear scanning on an Apple II computer using a head switch and an Adaptive Firmware Card. The cursor would highlight one letter at a time and Tom would hit the switch when the cursor got to the desired letter. Considering that there are 26 letters in the alphabet, this type of communication was painfully slow. Because of difficulty keeping his head erect for long periods and due to distractibility, he would frequently miss the desired letter and have to start all over again. It took many years and lots of in-school training support for Tom to master scanning. Over time, he learned group item scanning and by age 10 he had memorized a group item scanning array and knew by the number of auditory beeps when the cursor was approaching the desired letter. But because his ability to spell and write independently was very limited, Tom primarily used scanning on the computer to write spelling words or to copy short sentences. During the early elementary years, Tom also had trial periods with optical pointing and Morse code, however, head control was never sufficient to use either access method.

At age 7, a Light Talker was introduced to provide Tom with voice output. The Light Talker used row column scanning.

Tom started with the 32 location overlay and gradually progressed to 128 locations. Because of Tom's limited literacy skills, he used Minspeak picture symbols to communicate whole phrases and rarely used the Light Talker's spell mode.

For Tom, the mastery of technology preceded literacy, and his academic timeline differed from his able-bodied peers. Whereas typical children experiment with writing by kindergarten, Tom did not have effective access to writing until he was able to manage the complex task of scanning. Whereas other children had access to books and could experiment with reading aloud, Tom could not hold a book, turn its pages, or sound out words. Where other children build words into phrases and learn syntax, Tom used Minspeak to communicate whole phrases, which made the act of communication more efficient, but did not build syntax skills.

As a result, it was not until age 11 that Tom mastered initial consonants and long vowel sounds and could finally communicate novel ideas through inventive spelling. It was not until this point that educators discovered the extent of Tom's language learning disabilities. Using inventive spelling, Tom was finally able to express his thoughts independently via the computer. His sentences revealed significant difficulties with syntax and sentence structure. For example, one day Tom wrote "may happy birthe me tv." This sentence clearly conveyed a meaningful thought; that his birthday was in May and that he wanted a television. However, it was typical of his unconventional approach to written communication. Although Tom clearly understood what was said to him verbally, he was unable to produce normal language structures on his own. His writing was telegraphic in style. The meaning was clear, but the grammatical structures were atypical. Because Tom could not speak or write, grammar instruction had not been a consideration. Yet for Tom, writing was more

than just an academic goal; it was and continues to be critical to his ability to communicate what's on his mind.

At the same time that Tom was being introduced to scanning and the Light Talker, he was also learning to maneuver a motorized wheelchair. A wheelchair with multiple directional head switches was his first method of independent mobility, though the ride was anything but smooth due to the nature of unidirectional switches. Next, Tom was outfitted with a headpointer which he used to operate an adapted joystick control. This provided a smoother ride, but the joystick had to be positioned at midline, which interfered with the Light Talker mount. The headpointer itself interfered with Tom's ability to activate the head switch used to operate his Light Talker. Now Tom could "walk but not talk" or vice versa.

Toward the end of elementary school, more changes were in store. Tom acquired an IBM compatible laptop computer with a Multivoice synthesizer and the SoftKey switch adapter to allow for Scanning using Scanning WSKE II and Talking Screens software. This multiple component system was assembled to serve his spoken and written communication needs both at school and at home. The word prediction features of Scanning WSKE II combined with the Multivoice synthesizer helped Tom compensate for his poor spelling skills, reinforced word recognition skills, and enhanced his rate of writing. But the drawback to multicomponent AAC systems is the sheer number of pieces that have to be recharged, assembled, turned on, and packaged for transport each time Tom wants to make use of his system.

To further complicate matters, Tom transitioned to middle school where he changed classes every 45 minutes, and the race to get him to class and get his system set up often fell short. The need to get him to class via crowded hallways also affected his independent mobility; Tom stopped using his motorized chair. In the push to inclusion, Tom's assistive technology goals took a back seat. More often, he relied on low tech strategies to respond to assignments. Individual instruction to develop literacy skills focusing on reading, spelling, and writing was at a minimum and no longer was a priority at the middle school level. In this environment, the pressure was intense and Tom was clearly unhappy. To make matters worse, Tom underwent hip surgery, and the following year broke his femur in a bus accident. When he was released from the hospital, he returned home for 2 months and received educational tutoring at home. Once he returned to school, he had difficulty sitting in his wheelchair for more than a few hours at a time. No one could foresee these setbacks, but setbacks of one sort or another are almost inevitable.

When the next major transition to high school was about to occur, the assistive technology team that had followed Tom since kindergarten took a more active role in placement decisions. Together with Tom's mother, a placement was sought that would allow for more of a balance between inclusion opportunities and scheduled time to continue to develop mobility, communication, and literacy skills. A high school situation was located that would allow for a daily combination of mainstream/inclusion classes, functional English and math classes, and independent study time to work with his instructional assistant on mobility, communication, and literacy skills.

Overall, this arrangement has been much more satisfactory, but unpredicted disruptions of another sort have broken the continuity of Tom's progress. In a year and a half Tom has had three different instructional assistants and a period of 2 months with no instructional assistant. Although the transitions from grade to grade are predictable, the transition to a new instructional assistant every few months has been difficult for all involved. Tom, who has to be lifted, catheted, and fed, has had to learn to trust the physical handling skills of three new assistants. Extensive training for Tom's computer, his low and high tech methods of communication, his positioning and wheelchair issues, and his learning needs are barely completed before having to start again with a new assistant. In short, although his high school situation is a significant improvement over middle school, real life changes beyond Tom's or his team's control have kept it from being all it could be.

Currently, Tom's school situation is stable; he enjoys his mainstream classes and the socialization opportunities they provide. Tom continues to improve in the use of his technology to communicate. His reading has improved, his spelling is stronger, his sentences are longer and more grammatically correct, and he more often uses text as a way to communicate. He even uses Quicken software to keep his personal finances organized. For the time being, all is well. Well . . . perhaps not; Tom's motorized chair is malfunctioning, his seating no longer supports him effectively, and his computer hard drive is dying. There is seemingly no end to transitions and change in the life of a young man who is technology dependent.

Key Points to Remember

- For individuals with severe physical disabilities, reliable motor access often lags significantly behind the individual's cognitive ability to use complex AAC systems. Motor access must be addressed early.
- Multiple methods of access will be tried in the early years of development. Specified periods of parallel access training should be provided until the degree of success with each method can be gauged.

- It can take many years for individuals with severe physical disabilities to master all the elements of scanning.
- Literacy skills are often compromised by limited motor access, resulting in limited opportunities for active reading and writing. Daily opportunities are needed using low and high tech strategies.
- Syntax development should be closely monitored with students who are nonverbal. Opportunities to use typical grammatical structures are important for eventual written communication development.
- Integrated communication and mobility systems are needed to allow individuals who are physically disabled and non-speaking the ability to "walk and talk." During the early years, it may be less feasible to integrate these systems, however, systems integration should be the long-term objective.
- Inclusion opportunities are socially beneficial, but time spent in inclusion settings should be balanced by the need for time to address individualized academic, communication, and mobility goals. School situations must have the flexibility to provide this.
- Although low tech as well as high tech communication strategies are needed, decisions to rely on low tech strategies should not be driven by environmental barriers.
- Technology-dependent individuals do not benefit from frequent changes in personnel, especially instructional assistants. Constant training for new staff is not cost-beneficial in the long run.
- Assistive technology is never static, but must change and adapt to meet real life situations—some foreseeable and some that cannot be predicted. The need for change is often situational, accidental, equipment related, or people related. Change and transitions are the rule, not the exception. Plan ahead to the extent possible.

Chapter 11

AAC AND CHILDREN WITH DEVELOPMENTAL DISABILITIES

Cynthia Weitz, Mark Dexter, and Jacquelyn Moore

C hildren with developmental language or speech disorders frequently benefit from augmentative and alternative communication (AAC) strategies. These children have severe expressive or receptive communication disorders or both which sometimes occur in isolation, or as part of a global developmental disability. Children with specific language impairment, pervasive developmental disorder, developmental apraxia of speech, autism, Down syndrome, or other types of developmental disabilities may need to use AAC strategies to supplement or enhance their language development. These children offer challenges to professionals, especially during the early years of language development. In the very young child, it is often difficult to determine the nature and degree of language impairment, to accurately diagnose the presence of other factors such as cognitive disabilities, and to predict the child's future prognosis for language or speech development.

In the past, young children diagnosed with severe language and speech disorders would have received years of traditional speech therapy focused on developing spo-

ken communication skills (Silverman, 1995). AAC would have been recommended only after traditional therapy techniques had failed. Today, professionals realize that AAC strategies can provide children who have developmental delays with an immediate means of communication; can facilitate expressive and receptive language development until other communication modalities improve (i.e., speech); and can serve as a bridge to future spoken language development (Kangas & Lloyd, 1988; Silverman 1995). AAC provides an expressive method of communication to facilitate language development in children who, in all likelihood, will eventually use speech to communicate. The focus of this chapter is on children with developmental disabilities who have the potential to use AAC strategies to develop receptive and expressive language skills, including speech. The chapter begins by presenting an overview of using AAC as a tool to enhance language and speech development. Specific AAC assessment and intervention issues are then presented in two separate sections for children with developmental apraxia of speech and for children with pervasive developmental disorders, including autism.

DEVELOPMENTAL COMMUNICATION DISORDERS

Children with developmental language and speech disorders are often more dissimilar than similar. A simplistic method of categorizing these children is to look at development across the domains of nonverbal cognitive abilities, receptive language, expressive language, and speech. These four domains are interrelated, yet can develop at different rates in different children. Children can have delayed or disordered abilities in one, two, three, or all four domains. For example, some children have normal cognitive and receptive language abilities with impaired expressive communication and speech skills. Others have normal language and cognitive skills with severe oral motor speech difficulties. Still others may have receptive and expressive language abilities that are below other cognitive abilities, or might have speech articulation skills that are superior to receptive and expressive language levels.

Detailed language and speech characteristics cannot be easily listed for individuals who have developmental disabilities because of the numerous diagnoses that are included under this label. In addition, children with the same diagnosis can have dissimilar patterns of language development. Many parents will hear about other children with the same medical diagnosis as their child and make developmental comparisons. Although parent networks can be helpful sources of information, a medical diagnosis is not always a good predictor of future speech or language development (Romski & Sevcik, 1988). For example, one of the authors is currently providing services to three 6-year-old children with Down syndrome. Their language abilities fall on a continuum. One child uses jargon, speaks in one to two word phrases using a telegraphic style, and has poor articulation, which results in unintelligible speech.

A second child uses three to four word incomplete sentences to describe concrete immediate events with 70% intelligibility in familiar listening contexts. The third child uses complete four to six word sentences, is able to discuss past and future events, and is 95% intelligible even in unfamiliar listening environments. In summary, each child presents with a unique set of communication characteristics. The decision to implement AAC strategies and the selection of appropriate interventions has to be determined individually by professionals and family members.

THE DECISION TO IMPLEMENT AAC

The American Speech-Language-Hearing Association (ASHA, 1991) defined an AAC system as "an integrated group of components, including the symbols, aids, strategies, and techniques used by individuals to enhance communication. The system serves to supplement any gestural, spoken, and/or written communication abilities" (p. 10). Augmentative systems are not intended to be substitutes for, but are to be used in conjunction with, the residual abilities to speak and write (Silverman, 1995). AAC intervention commences at the individual's existing language level versus waiting for him or her to attain a certain skill; more of a "try and see" rather than a "wait and see" strategy (Goossens, 1989; McGregor, Young, Gerak, Thomas, & Vogelsberg 1992; Romski & Sevcik, 1988).

The decision to implement AAC requires extensive speech and language evaluation, periods of trial therapy, and frequent reevaluations of progress to integrate AAC methods into an overall communication intervention plan. AAC can be combined with traditional speech and language training techniques or can be presented as an alternative to traditional therapy. The course of AAC intervention may be supplementary, short term, or adopted as a long-term strategy to be used across the child's life span. Multiple AAC strategies can be sampled separately or concurrently. AAC can also be implemented in one or across all communication environments. The goal is to provide the child with communication skills that go beyond simple requests, rejections, and identification of wants and needs. It also involves developing the ability to share information, to achieve social closeness, and to learn social etiquette along with other higher level cultural and communication abilities (Beukelman & Mirenda, 1992).

Integrating AAC with Speech

Parents of children with developmental disabilities often want speech to be the primary means of communication for their child. It is often the fear of both the older child and his or her parents that shifting the attention from the speech output mode to AAC systems will deemphasize the importance of developing and improving verbal output, reduce motivation for speech communication, and even cause the individual to stop talking. At this time, there is no documentation to support the notion that AAC reduces an individual's motivation to verbally communicate or the development of speech. On the contrary, Silverman (1995) reviewed more than 100 published and unpublished reports that indicated that at least 40% of AAC users increased their spoken output in conjunction with the use of AAC. Possible reasons for the increase in verbal output relate to the reduced pressure to perform verbally, the use of graphic symbols, and the development of alternate input and output channels, taking the pressure off of the traditional auditory-vocal channels (Kangas & Lloyd, 1988).

Jamie is an example of how communication skills can evolve over time. At age 3, Jamie exhibited generalized hypotonia and was nonverbal. He was introduced to a Touch Talker, but it was not used often. At the age of 4, his family moved and he entered a school for children with developmental disabilities and also received private speech therapy. In private therapy, he worked jointly on vocal production and the use of the Touch Talker. In kindergarten, Jamie increased his verbal output, but was only intelligible 20% of the time. He used the Touch Talker in functional ways to make requests and communicate responses. He was motivated to not only model the speech of people with whom he interacted, but also to talk along with his device. During his first-grade year, he often initially produced his messages verbally and if they were not understood, he would then use the Touch Talker to repair the communication exchange. Once a printer was purchased, he also began to use the device more for written output than for verbal output. As his literacy and his understanding of letter-sound relationships improved, Jamie's articulation skills also improved. By the time Jamie entered the second grade, he would not use the Touch Talker as an expressive means of communication; instead he saw himself as a "speaker." The Touch Talker was housed in the closet most of his third-grade year and when he was in the fourth grade, the family donated the device to another child. His intelligibility continued to improve so that he was understood 75% to 85% of the time by his communication partners. In Jamie's case, speech training and AAC strategies were combined to support his ongoing communication development.

Children with developmental disabilities have a variety of spoken language skills, ranging from very delayed speech and language to mild degrees of speech unintelligibility. Nonetheless, it has been found that many of these children continue to think of themselves as functional "speakers." From their viewpoint, the fact that family members and consistent communication partners are able to understand

and translate their communication messages overrides the fact that the majority of people they come in contact with are unable to decipher their communication attempts. For example, Anne was a bright middle school student with a severe speech impairment. When confronted with the fact that listeners often did not understand her, she stated "If people are around me long enough, they begin to understand what I am saying . . . if not, a friend can tell them what I said." Although this strategy satisfies her at this time, it will become less acceptable as she approaches her adult years and must address independence issues to meet vocational and recreational goals.

The type of situation and the communication partners tend to dictate the particular AAC modes or combinations of modes to be used during a communication interaction. Anne, the student previously discussed, was less than 30% to 40% intelligible in fluid, connected speech with unfamiliar communication partners. Her family understood her most of the time, so this allowed her to comfortably use verbal speech at home, as well as at school with familiar classmates and staff members. At school, Anne's primary mode of communication was speech, but her verbal responses were often misunderstood, much to the frustration of her teachers, classmates, and eventually, to herself. She reduced the length of her responses, and augmented the exchange with nonsymbolic expressions (e.g., eye gaze, gestures). Anne finally admitted that there were times when she knew the answer or had something to contribute and simply did not because of the effort involved. She occasionally used an alphabet board that gave the listener the option of seeing the first letter (and more, if necessary) of the word she was saying. When the context was known, seeing the first letter was often enough for the listener to figure out the word. However, when presented with the task of participating in a speech contest, Anne wrote the speech and then programmed it into a voice output AAC device. Anne not only participated in the contest, but became one of the semifinalists (because of the content of her speech, not the mode of delivery). Anne was thrilled that the voice output AAC system had afforded her the opportunity to participate, something she could not have done using her natural speech.

Clearly, speech is looked upon as the preferred method of communication, even for speakers with limited speech. Articulation therapy is especially important in the early years of development when speech potential is difficult to predict. However, AAC can be used as a method to enhance speech, as well as a method of augmenting communication. AAC, as part of a multimodal communication system, may be a short-term strategy until speech reaches an acceptable level of intelligibility, or it may be a long-term strategy to build and maintain effective communication. AAC can also be a supplementary option for situations when it is imperative for a person with speech impairment to be understood. AAC does not impede the development of speech; in fact, AAC can serve as a form of scaffolding to support the use of speech in the early years of development.

Using AAC to Facilitate Language Development

Over the past 20 years in the area of speech and language intervention the focus has shifted from "teaching people to speak, to giving students language, and now to helping students communicate" (Ferguson, 1994, p. 7). In many cases, a disorder in language may not be fixable, but possibly by "facilitating the attainment of socially effective communication, interactions can become more effective for an individual with developmental disabilities and associated communication impairments as they interact in their community" (National Joint Committee for the Communicative Needs of Persons with Severe Disabilities, 1992, p. 4). In the area of augmentative and alternative communication, the challenge is "to determine how non-speaking individuals can best facilitate their daily interactions in educational, vocational, community, and home environments. The communication aids employed are the tools in the process; the central issue is the effectiveness of the interaction" (Light, 1988, p. 66).

Symbolic communication in any modality can be used to build receptive language, as well as to convey expressive messages. Symbolic communication can include verbal expressions, sign language, photographs, line drawings, objects, and graphic symbols. Again, the use of these systems goes beyond simply giving the individual a means to "talk." It must be remembered that symbol systems have unique properties and performance capabilities that will, in and of themselves, affect language development and conversational competence (Gerber & Kraat, 1992).

For the individual with severe communication impairments, augmentative communication strategies and systems can compliment the acquisition of functional communication and language skills. Some of the reasons for this relate to the systems themselves; augmentative communication strategies can act as a key to accessing the natural speech and language skills of an individual with developmental disabilities. Because individuals who are nonspeaking and limited speaking are in the process of acquiring linguistic abilities, AAC systems can help an individual structure the communication message (Nelson, 1992). This fact was evidenced in the expressive language development of Edward. Edward was a limited speaker with Down syndrome and mild mental retardation. Edward's academic environment was structured as a multimodal communication environment. His spontaneous speech consisted of three to four word sentences. When using a picture communication display to augment his speech, his expressions consistently increased to five to six word sentences without outside prompting. His verbal expressions were clearer because his rate of speech was slower. Edward openly demonstrated that he was aware of his increased skills with the communication system. He would purposely search for specific communication displays to help him make particular requests or participate in particular activities. Edward seemed pleased with both his AAC system and the responses and reinforcement received from his communication partners when he used the picture displays.

AAC can also be used to enhance language comprehension. Many children with receptive language delays have difficulty following conversational communication exchanges or understanding directions or questions. Augmenting spoken messages with a visual representation can increase a child's ability to comprehend communication. Visual cues can be in the form of manual sign languages, natural gestures, facial expressions, and graphic picture communication symbols including photographs and line drawings. When teachers pair speech with manual signs or with visual symbols, it provides comprehension support, slows down the delivery of the message, and often results in favorable completion of the communication exchange. For example, a 5-year-old student was asked to sit down, a message the staff knew she understood. After several attempts to get her to comply, the direction was repeated and paired with signs. The student immediately imitated the signs and oral directions, as if solidifying her understanding of the message, and then followed the direction by sitting and staying in her seat. In another example, a student was given directions to get materials out of his mailbox and place them in his book bag, get his coat and hat, and sit at his desk and wait for a snack. When only oral directions were given, the student required one-step directions and several repetitions, sometimes with physical prompting to complete the task. When directions were paired with an AAC picture communication board, the student was able to follow two to three step directions. It was also useful to have the student verbally repeat the directions using the picture board. Although both of these examples involved giving specific directions (not at a conversational level), the augmentation of a message with visual cues can assist language comprehension at any level. In the classroom, it is critical for the child to follow routines and directions; therefore, if tools exist that can add to a student's success, they should be explored and used.

For individuals with language disabilities and severe speech impairments, AAC systems and strategies can be used as a bridge to higher levels of communication interaction, enabling children with developmental disabilities to actively participate in home, school, and community environments. AAC is neither a crutch nor a single solution to speech and language impairments. To further illustrate this point, the next two sections of this chapter will focus on implementing AAC strategies with specific diagnostic categories of children. As stated previously, children with developmental disabilities are often more dissimilar than similar. The degree and nature of communication impairment varies widely from individual to individual. However, these two diagnostic populations have unique characteristics that can be used as a framework to discuss AAC assessment and intervention issues. The first section will focus on children with developmental apraxia of speech. Children with this disorder have severely impaired speech motor abilities with relatively intact receptive language skills. AAC is fre-

quently used to facilitate speech and expressive language development until speech intelligibility improves. In contrast, children with pervasive developmental disorders and autism have underlying global language difficulties with relatively normal speech motor skills. These children frequently require AAC strategies to enhance language understanding and expression.

DEVELOPMENTAL APRAXIA OF SPEECH

Definition and Demographics

Developmental apraxia of speech (DAS) has been given many labels, including developmental verbal dyspraxia, childhood verbal dyspraxia, apraxic dysarthria, and cortical dysarthria (Marquardt & Sussman, 1991). No matter what the label, the very existence of the disorder is often questioned in the literature (Blackstone 1989; Crary, 1993). A recent point-counterpoint by Robin (1992) and Hall (1992) indicated that researchers appear to be accepting its existence. Square (1994) indicated that clinical researchers were converging on a "consistent definition of the disorder as one in which the central control mechanism for the temporal sequencing of complex volitional speech movements is disrupted in the absence of other, observable muscular function abnormalities" (p. 151). She further stated that the basis for the disorder is an impairment of sensorimotor integration.

Professionals who work with individuals with DAS must be sensitive to the need for parents and other professionals to understand the terms that are used. A recent edition of *Communicating Together*, a parent newsletter, gave an excellent definition of DAS. It explained that some children have difficulty producing speech sounds due to strength or weakness of the muscles used for articulation. It went on to note that for children with DAS, the strength or weakness of the speech musculature is not the issue. The problem lies in planning the motor movements for speech (Kumin, 1994).

Communication Characteristics in DAS Populations

If DAS exists, then what are its characteristics? Many researchers have indicated that DAS is a complex of symptoms (Crary, 1993; Hall, 1992; Marquardt & Sussman, 1991). Individual children will display a different symptom complex, depending on individual differences. Cumley and Jones (1992) suggested the following commonly agreed upon characteristics:

1. Difficulty in imitating both nonspeech movements and speech sounds in the absence of abnormalities of the tongue, lips or palate.
2. Difficulty in initiating speech movements.
3. Unawareness of articulator positions, resulting in prominent phonemic errors.
4. Impairment in production of sound sequences.
5. Occasional telegraphic speech.
6. Disturbances in repetition of speech and in conversation, with frequent prosodic disturbances (e.g., slowed rate, uneven stress).
7. Inconsistency of articulator output and errors. (p. 230)

Another characteristic of DAS that is commonly noted is better proficiency in receptive language as compared to expressive language (Hall, 1992; Marquardt & Sussman, 1991; Robin, 1992; Rosenbek & Wertz, 1972). Rosenbek and Wertz suggested four characteristics to distinguish DAS from a functional articulation disorder. DAS includes vowel errors, oral nonverbal apraxia, groping trial and error be-

havior, and increased errors on longer responses.

If it is accepted that DAS exists, how many children have this disorder? Shriberg (1994) has been working on a classification system for developmental phonological disorders based on the DSM model (*Diagnostic and Statistical Manual of Mental Disorders—IV*, American Psychiatric Association, 1994). He proposed five subgroups of children with developmental phonological disorders: (1) Speech Delay (SD) without associated involvement; (2) Speech Delay + Otitis Media with Effusion (SD+OME); (3) Speech Delay + Developmental Apraxia (SD+DAS); (4) Speech Delay + Developmental Psychosocial Involvement (SD+DPI); and (5) Residual Errors (RE). Shriberg estimated the incidence of SD+DAS at 1 to 2 children per 1,000 and the gender ratio as 80% to 90% male. In addition, he felt there is a familial connection but that "limited subject descriptions . . . do not allow percentage estimates" (p. 28).

Hodge (1994) took exception with researchers' attempts to narrow the subject group to those with (1) normal hearing, cognition, and receptive language; (2) the absence of obvious sensorimotor or structural impairments; (3) moderate to severe speech intelligibility; and (4) speech characteristics of DAS. Hodge pointed out that speech characteristics of DAS can be present in a variety of other conditions, including mental retardation, developmental delay, and attention deficit disorder, among others.

In contrast, Hayden (1994) suggested that DAS should be diagnosed only after the exclusion of sensory, cognitive, and language components that could result in the disruption of speech movement sequencing. This limits the population she would recognize as having DAS to a very small number. She also stated that "DAS does not have the same root cause as autism" (p. 121) and that disorders that are primarily of an emotional or pragmatic nature should be ruled out. Apraxic-like symptoms may be a result of one or more additional sensory or processing disruptions or the interactions among them. Overall, although there appears to be more agreement that DAS exists, there is not yet a consensus on the characteristics of the DAS population.

Intervention Strategies Specific to the Population

Whether one accepts a broad or narrow definition of DAS and its population, training issues remain. Ferry, Hall, and Hicks (1975) stated that if intelligible speech has not developed by age 6 in a child with DAS it is "unlikely to develop" (p. 751). Hodge (1994) stated that for some children DAS was a chronic condition for whom "normal speech production is not a realistic expectation" (p. 99). Acquisition of intelligible speech is often a long process. The child with DAS needs practice in improving verbal skills as well as in some augmentative means of communicating until speech becomes the primary communication mode.

When planning an intervention program for the child with DAS, it is critical to offer multimodal communication from the onset. Crary (1993) stressed that in planning intervention the program must fit the child and not the reverse. When reviewing both speech training as well as AAC strategies, the speech-language pathologist must remember that each child presents unique challenges. One child may require an emphasis on strategies for building speech, another may require intensive AAC techniques, and others may require a program that equally emphasizes both strategies.

Speech Training Techniques

Strategies for intervention naturally include those that stress intensive speech training.

Crary (1993) suggested that the failure for improvement in speech production after prolonged therapy, often cited as a characteristic of DAS, may be partially due to a "mismatch between the child's performance capabilities and the nature of the therapy program" (pp. 208–209). He emphasized that the treatment program must fit the child, rather than fitting the child into a program based on one theoretical construct of DAS. Crary pointed out the differences between "bottom up" and "top down" programs. Programs that build speech from the "bottom up" start with individual movements, sounds, coarticulatory sound sequences, and so forth. Programs that build speech from the "top down" focus on words, phrases, or sentence level productions. Crary emphasized the need for a multifocal intervention program, addressing motor speech (executive) issues, phonologic (planning) issues, as well as the syntactic deficits commonly seen in children with motor speech disorders. According to Crary, all three elements should be addressed in each session, rather than in a hierarchical structure.

Many speech treatment approaches have been described in the literature. The problem facing the clinician is choosing an approach that will work for each child and building an appropriate program for that individual. As the focus of this book is AAC strategies, specific speech training programs will not be reviewed in depth. The reader is referred to Cumley and Jones (1992) for a summary of natural speech intervention recommendations. Also, in a review of the literature, Pannbacker (1988) discusses selected therapy approaches to DAS and their general effectiveness. Readers interested in an updated discussion of therapy techniques should refer to Klick (1994) for the Adapted Cueing Technique, Hayden and Square (1994) for the PROMPT System, and Helfrich-Miller (1994) for Melodic Intonation Therapy. In addition, readers should investigate some of the available commercial apraxia programs such as *Easy Does It for Apraxia and Motor Planning* (Strode & Chamberlain, 1993) and *Easy Does It for Apraxia—Preschool* (Strode & Chamberlain, 1994).

Augmentative and Alternative Communication (AAC) Strategies

When suggesting AAC techniques to parents of a child with DAS, it is important for speech-language pathologists to remember the strong desire and expectation of parents that their children will speak. Family folklore often includes stories about a child's first words, and stories of the "darndest things" that the child said. In contrast, parents of children with DAS are hoping to hear their child's first word approximation or first intelligible word or sentence. When professionals first suggest using AAC methods, parents often feel that we have "given up" on speech or that by introducing AAC techniques their child will never speak (Blackstone, 1989).

Parent counseling is often an important first step to the introduction of AAC techniques. Blackstone (1989) presented nine steps for gaining family acceptance of AAC in a therapy program for the child with DAS. Her suggestions emphasized both education about DAS and AAC, and the presentation of videotapes of successful AAC users. Table 11–1 summarizes her suggestions.

Parents sometimes seek confirmation that AAC is an accepted technique in the treatment of DAS. Researchers and experts such as Crary (1993), Hall, Jordan, and Robin (1993), Cumley and Jones (1992), Blackstone (1989), Hodge and Hancock (1994), and Mirenda and Mathy-Laikko (1989) among others have suggested AAC techniques as part of an overall therapy plan for the child with DAS. However, there is a paucity of research studies on the efficacy of AAC techniques with this population. Culp (1989) presented a case example of the use of a multimodal communication system with an 8-year-old girl with DAS. Strategies included natural speech, gestures, sign language, and communication boards. An important component was training in the Partners in Augmentative Communication Training (PACT) program (Culp & Carlisle, 1988). This program attempts to develop functional and positive communicative interactions be-

Table 11–1. Strategies for promoting family acceptance of AAC for the child with developmental apraxia of speech.

1. Provide discussion and demonstration of how speech is produced and clearly explain the child's speech problem.
2. Clearly explain the benefits of multiple communication systems, including speech, sign language, and aided AAC techniques.
3. Have the child use a particular AAC technique in an activity to demonstrate what the child can do and the value of AAC.
4. Offer written information about DAS and AAC and follow up with a family discussion.
5. Have the family talk with other families whose children have been successful using AAC strategies.
6. Show videotapes of other children with similar problems communicating successfully with AAC.
7. Show videotapes demonstrating improvements in speech, language, and communication skills over time.
8. Begin AAC at school or in other environments if the family does not want to use AAC strategies at home.
9. If the family rejects implementation of AAC procedures, work on speech, gestures, conversational repair strategies, letter cueing, etc. Periodically reintroduce aided AAC approaches.

Source: From "Individuals with Developmental Apraxia of Speech" by S. Blackstone, 1989, *Augmentative Communication News*, 2(2), p. 2. Copyright 1989 by Sunset Enterprises. Adapted with permission.

tween children who are AAC users and their communication partners. Results indicated that there was a positive increase in communication from inclusion in the program. Culp suggested that work on speech alone may not ensure success for the DAS population and that further research is needed on the "role and timing of the introduction of AAC" (p. 32).

There are several elements intrinsic to the nature of AAC techniques that make it a natural component of a therapy program for the child with developmental apraxia of speech. As noted previously, a common characteristic of DAS is a discrepancy between receptive and expressive language skills. AAC techniques allow children to continue to build receptive language skills while giving them access to an alternative expressive language modality. Expressive syntactic skills can be built through AAC, with the expectation that, when speech develops, carryover to the oral mode of communication will be easier. These authors' clinical experience has found that, for children who are just beginning to put oral words together into longer utterances, AAC techniques can be very powerful in organizing words into semantically and syntactically correct sentences. AAC systems also include a strong visual component. Visual cueing is a constituent of many of the speech training strategies mentioned previously, such as the Adapted Cueing Technique, which provides a visual cue for speech sounds. The picture overlays typical of AAC systems require pointing to picture cues to represent words or phrases. Pointing to picture symbols in conjunction with verbal output slows the rate of speech production. Slowing the rate is another technique for speech training that is included in the literature for DAS. Use of AAC systems also involves the use of a motor response, again a component of some speech training programs. Thus, it appears that AAC techniques inherently include many of the components that have been found to be effective in speech training therapy for children with DAS.

Characteristics of AAC Systems. Available AAC techniques include both unaided and aided systems. Unaided techniques would include natural gestures and manual signs. Aided techniques would include the use of picture symbol communication boards in various formats as well as voice output devices. There are advantages and disadvantages to both systems and clinicians should remember the importance of finding a system that suits the unique needs of each child. Blackstone (1989) pointed out that use of unaided versus aided approaches is not an either/or question, but a matter of emphasis. She suggested that clinicians should consider the advantages of a multimodal approach. Sign language may work well in some contexts, whereas in other situations the use of voice output AAC devices or picture symbol boards may lead to more successful communication.

Before looking more closely at the important elements of unaided and aided AAC systems, it is important to consider several critical factors when evaluating any AAC system in relation to the DAS population. These include portability, vocabulary size, and costs. As Hall et al. (1993), Blackstone (1989), Cumley and Jones (1992), Culp (1989), and Mirenda and Mathy-Laikko (1989) pointed out, the child with DAS is typically ambulatory and requires a system that is portable and accessible in all environments. Vocabulary selection is affected by the need to have sufficient vocabulary for the many different activities the child will participate in, hence, vocabulary size can be large and unpredictable. The issue of cost, critical in the selection of an AAC system for any individual, is particularly challenging with the DAS population. Many parents may view the AAC system as a bridge or transitional system until their child develops functional oral speech. Because of that position, investment in an expensive system is often viewed as not cost effective. Clinicians and parents may need to do a very careful needs analysis of the child before settling on the communication system that will best serve the child while still remaining within the economic resources of the family.

Unaided Gesture/Sign Systems. Children with DAS frequently develop their own system of natural gestures that are understood by those who know the child (Hall et al., 1993). The use of gestures does not always mean that a child is a good candidate for using sign language. As Hall et al. stated, children with DAS may have overall fine or gross motor apraxia affecting their ability to produce signs as well. As a result, clinicians need to determine the presence and degree of hand and limb apraxia before introducing a manual sign language system. An evaluation by an occupational therapist may be a critical component of the decision-making process. If it is determined that sign language is an option for a child with DAS, parents often need reassurance that the use of signs will not impede the development of oral language. Hall et al. found that, as oral skills improved, sign language use spontaneously faded.

Advantages of Unaided Systems. One obvious advantage of sign language is its portability. Like natural speech, the child or parent can never leave the system at home or in the car. In the school environment, sign language is always available in the many different locations that a typical child might access, including the art and music rooms, assembly halls, and outdoor play areas. Vocabulary size is potentially unlimited with a manual signing system. New words can be added without regard to the size of a picture board or the memory limits of a voice output device. The cost is limited only to the number of sign language classes and books the parents, school staff, and child may need to become proficient signers.

Disadvantages of Unaided Systems. Although sign language is readily available to the child in a variety of environments, imprecise signing is often an issue with the child with DAS. As mentioned previously, these children often exhibit some degree of fine and gross motor apraxia in addition to apraxia of speech. Parents often have to translate their children's sign as well as their speech, and children may develop a dependence on adult interaction and support for communication.

Although vocabulary size may be unlimited, Blackstone (1989) pointed out that most of the world does not understand or use sign language. Most children with DAS live in the hearing world. Reliance solely on sign language as an AAC system limits the child's communication partners to those family members and school personnel who have sign language knowledge and familiarity with the idiosyncrasy of that child's signing. Blackstone further cautioned that family and school staff need to have a strong commitment to total communication for it to work. Cumley and Jones (1992) pointed out that family, school, and friends often need considerable learning time to be fluent signers. This learning time limits the child's ability to immediately communicate in a variety of contexts. Blackstone also suggested that individuals and their communication partners often don't remember to use the signs they have been taught. Instead, a small number of easily recognizable signs should be taught and aided approaches should be stressed (Blackstone, 1989).

Implementation of Unaided Systems. The use of gesture and sign language as a component of an AAC system will only be effective if the family, school team, and therapists are consistent in its use. As mentioned previously, there are hindrances to using unaided systems with the child with DAS.

What strategies are effective in increasing the use of sign language in environments that are typically for the hearing? Adults committed to using a signing system should enroll in a sign language course. Although learning signs from a book can be done, it is very difficult to rely solely on static illustrations for mastering a dynamic manual system. For those living in urban areas, universities, colleges, and community colleges frequently offer sign language courses, both as credit and noncredit courses. Large county school systems also may offer sign language as part of an evening adult education program. In smaller communities, religious or service institutions may be willing to offer a sign language course if there is sufficient interest.

The number of sign language books appearing in bookstores has been increasing as interest in this topic has risen in the mainstream population. Most bookstore chains now offer a few selections. For those interested in a larger selection, the Gallaudet University bookstore is a good resource. A CD-ROM program, The American Sign Language Dictionary on CD-ROM (Sternberg, 1994), is now available. It features video clips of over 2,000 words being signed as well as traditional sign illustrations.

A strategy that the authors have found effective in the preschool classroom is to choose five to six signs that correspond with each preschool unit's vocabulary. Sign illustrations are photocopied and shared with family and school staff. These signs are emphasized during group and individual language activities. Therapists or teachers can also videotape themselves signing each new unit's vocabulary and send videotapes home to interested families. Parents must also share new signs that have been taught and used at home with school staff. Signs from home and school can then be reinforced in all environments.

Aided Systems. Aided systems include low tech systems, such as nonelectronic picture and text based systems including communication books, wallets, boards, and miniboards, and high tech systems such as voice output communication aids (VOCA, Blackstone, 1989). Many low and high tech systems are picture based. Picture symbol communication is more transparent and easily understood than sign language, making communication more accessible across environments. Blackstone considered this to be a significant factor in choosing aided approaches over unaided approaches.

Attitudes of communication partners toward the child with DAS may have a significant impact on the use of different communication systems. Gorenflo and Gorenflo (1991) studied the attitudes of persons without disabilities toward persons with physical disabilities who were nonspeaking using different augmentative communication systems. They found attitudes to be "significantly more favorable toward an individual using a technological augmentative communication technique such as a VOCA" (p. 23). Use of such devices should be considered in therapy protocols for the child with DAS.

Unfortunately, picture-based systems are not always readily accepted by families and school. Culp (1989) reported that signing was preferred by the 8-year-old with DAS in her study. However, the child's mother found that revision of the picture-based communication system resulted in more frequent use in a variety of situations. Kravitz and Littman (1990) suggested that when a communication system is not being used, change and expansion of vocabulary might increase success.

Advantages of Aided Systems. Clearly, aided systems will not be as portable as unaided systems. However, there are a variety of formats available in aided systems, including wallet systems and mini-boards that can be carried in waist packs or attached by key holders to belt loops. As technology allows greater miniaturization of voice output systems, new devices have been introduced that offer digitized voice yet are lightweight (see Chapter 3).

A number of different picture symbol systems are available for aided communication systems. Picture symbols will vary from those that are concrete to those that are more abstract. This allows greater flexibility in finding a match between the child and a symbol system. See Chapter 4 for a description of different symbol systems. Once a system has been chosen, picture systems are easily understood by communication partners in the environment. Adding voice output to the system further increases the likelihood of completing communication attempts. Once vocabulary has been accessed, voice output en-sures that a child will be heard, even if a parent, teacher, or peer is not directly attending to the child. This is an important safety issue as well, as a child with a "voice" is more likely to be attended to than one who is silent.

Disadvantages of Aided Systems. The portability of a nonelectronic system will be influenced by its size. Although a three-ring notebook system allows for an expanded vocabulary, it is cumbersome to walk and access vocabulary simultaneously. When the child wants to communicate, the interaction stops while the notebook is retrieved and the appropriate vocabulary found. Tabbing pages with some type of picture cue or text can speed the process of moving through the communication book. This makes accessing vocabulary somewhat faster.

The playoff between issues of portability and vocabulary size is important for the child with DAS. When a wallet or mini-board is chosen, vocabulary size is re-duced. Although electronic voice output AAC devices continue to be revised, the systems that have the greatest potential for large picture vocabularies continue to be unwieldy for the ambulatory child. There are walkers available in which the heavier devices can be placed and then pushed (see Chapter 3). Some parents reject these systems because they feel it draws attention to their child and makes them look more disabled.

Costs of producing both low and high tech systems will vary. Whether one chooses to produce picture boards with stickers, or by copying symbols from a picture symbol book and then cutting and pasting to construct a display, or with a computer program, the cost can be prohibitive in time or money. Blackstone (1989) reported on an unpublished finding from Kravitz that the process of developing a picture miniboard from start to finish may be up to 12 hours. The workload can be reduced if school, therapists, and families labor together to produce picture symbol boards. When school and family coordinate efforts, the finished product can be available sooner. Computer programs can be used to create picture displays (e.g., Boardmaker, DynaVox for the Macintosh). These programs reduce the time outlay, but they are expensive and require easy access to computers and printers. The cost of AAC voice output devices continues to make their purchase problematic for the child with DAS. The devices that offer the most vocabulary may be considered too expensive for the child with DAS, especially if the expectation is that the child will eventually use speech to communicate. Devices should be field-tested to ensure that they are appropriate and will be used effectively and safely by the child in a variety of environments before purchasing.

Compromise, after careful consideration of all the individual issues, may be necessary. Families and professional staff should decide which issue dominates, be it portability, vocabulary size, or cost, and seek to maximize that issue while still maintaining benefits in the other areas as well. For those children with limited or no previous exposure to AAC techniques, a "go slow" approach may be appropriate. Begin with a variety of low tech approaches and, if successful, then consider the introduction of high tech systems.

Implementation of Aided Systems. Although aided systems can be quite effective in increasing communication options for the child with DAS, implementation is often a problem. Goossens, Crain, and Elder (1992) noted some of the problems in implementing AAC systems. They found that aided systems were used infrequently by students, were limited in communicative intents, and often were used in response to adult cueing, rather than spontaneous communication. Boards were often created as choice making rather than conversation making boards. Goossens et al. suggested that in the school environment, it is important to build systems based on the communication needs of the classroom as a whole and then work to individualize the system according to the needs of the student. This of course would apply to the home environment as well. Professionals need to recognize that communication is not the curriculum. Instead, communication should be integrated into the curriculum. Goossens et al. suggested the use of Aided Language Stimulation as a training strategy for increasing the use of aided AAC systems. Aided Language Stimulation simply means that the verbal partner points to the symbols on the communication display while speaking to the child. Just as we would not expect children to learn sign language if we never signed to them, we cannot expect children to become proficient at using their aided systems if we don't use them simultaneously when speaking.

In implementing this system in the home, families should inventory the activities of the household, prioritize which are the most frustrating with regard to communication, and begin slowly adding communication displays. Vocabulary should be carefully chosen to offer communication and not just question answering and choice making. Communication displays need to be kept close to the activity. (The spontaneity of sign language may be why it is preferred by some children over aided language systems.) Communication displays can be placed in toy boxes, in the book corner, on the refrigerator, in the dresser and bathroom. These displays can be larger versions of those in a wallet system or used in addition to the wallet. Parents should point to the communication displays as they speak to their child. Modeling increases the appropriate use of the system by the child.

In the classroom, a similar tack should be taken. Communication displays or voice output communication systems should be available in the different activities of the classroom, in the bathroom, and at snack time. A strategy these authors have found effective in the preschool is to provide communication boards corresponding to weekly curriculum themes. The sign language vocabulary of the week is depicted on one side; the other side is the picture communication display. Additionally, displays are developed that correspond to the children's favorite books and nursery rhymes. One therapist has sent an AAC device home with kindergarten books programmed on it. The child's homework was to "read" the book to his parents. This of course proved to be an extremely effective strategy, so much so that the child insisted on sleeping with the AAC device!

Creating Conditions for Effective Use of Unaided and Aided Systems

In order for an AAC system to be effective, the child with DAS will need to possess certain pragmatic language skills. Cumley and Jones (1992) pointed out the importance of topic-setting strategies, clarification and repair strategies, and decision-making strategies regarding when to use which communication modality. Problems often arise when a child with DAS introduces a new topic that is unintelligible to the listener. Topic-setting strategies might include a list of frequently used topics on a topic picture board (Blackstone, 1989). Clarification and repair strategies include repetition, rephrasing, changing or adding communication modes, gesturing, body language/pantomime, and pointing to cues in the environment (Blackstone, 1989). Cumley and Jones also pointed out that communication partners can be taught prompts to facilitate repair strategies.

The child with DAS may need to role-play communication breakdowns and work through decision-making strategies. If the child's initial and repeated verbal messages are not understood, what system will he or she try next? Will the communication partner make a difference in the system used? A child may sign with a parent or teacher, but perhaps use a picture communication system or voice output device with a peer. Direct teaching of these strategies may make an important difference in the child's ability to communicate across situations and increase his or her comfort level with the AAC system.

Whether AAC is viewed as a supplement to natural voice or whether AAC is viewed as the primary means of communication for the child with DAS, it is important to remember the importance of a multimodal communication system for these children (Blackstone, 1989; Cumley & Jones, 1992; Mirenda & Mathy-Laikko, 1989). Therapy should provide opportunities for intensive speech training, gestural or sign language communication, as well as aided AAC. The use of multiple communication systems increases the opportunities for children with DAS to interact with a variety of individuals across a wide array of environments.

AUTISM AND PERVASIVE DEVELOPMENTAL DISORDERS

Children with pervasive developmental disorders (PDD) including autism have historically been identified as demonstrating profound language communication deficits. In fact, communication is often considered to be the central disability associated with this syndrome. Parents and professionals are increasingly recognizing the need for program interventions to address functional communication needs within all aspects of a child's life. This recognition includes the use of AAC for individuals with autism. However, augmentative and alternative forms of communication have not always yielded success with individuals with autism. The failure of many intervention programs to build a solid communicative foundation for functional AAC may be limiting its success with this population. The introduction of any augmentative communication system is jeopardized if training is not adequately drawn from the child's preexisting forms of communication. "A common mistake in teaching communication skills to children with autism is neglecting to build a strong communicative basis for these skills" (Beukelman & Mirenda, 1992, p. 279).

This section presents a practical overview of general communication characteristics associated with pervasive developmental disorders, including autism. Current AAC training strategies are presented with regard to creating the conditions for effective communication. In addition, a theoretical discussion concerning the efficacy of stimulus-response and naturalistic language communication training methods is delineated for children with autism. This section outlines the basis for using AAC with children with pervasive developmental disorders.

Definition and Demographics

Autism is a developmental disorder that often results in serious deficits in social, language, and cognitive functioning (Kanner, 1943; Rimland, 1964; Rutter, 1978). Most epidemiological studies report a prevalence of autism in approximately 4 to 5 persons per 10,000 (Volkmar & Cohen, 1988). Other studies, using a broader definition of pervasive developmental disorders (PDD), which includes autism, report 10 to 15 individuals per 10,000 (Bryson, Clark & Smith, 1988; Burd & Kerbeshian, 1983; Denckla, 1986; Zahner & Pauls, 1987). The ratio of male to female cases is 4 : 1. It is estimated that 25% (Paluszny, 1979) to 61% (Fish, Shapiro, & Campbell, 1966) of individuals with autism are functionally nonverbal and will not develop gestural or other nonverbal means to communicate without systematic AAC intervention.

Within the broad continuum of PDD, approximately 60% of individuals with autism have IQ scores below 50; 20% between 50 and 70; and 20% greater than 70 (Ritvo & Freeman, 1978). A sizable minority of individuals with autism often have uneven intellectual development characterized by isolated splinter skills that go beyond what might be expected from their functioning in other areas (Rimland & Fein, 1988; Treffert, 1988). Sometimes splinter skills are noted in general visual perceptual performance, mathematical calculations, hyperlexic word recognition, music, and various attentional idiosyncrasies. These solitary skills are not often understood when viewed from a traditional developmental perspective. It is not uncommon to see these savant-like abilities as having little functional pragmatic value unless specific interventions can be used to shape them into something more meaningful.

Most researchers in the field of autism agree that autism is a behaviorally defined syndrome that is reflected in some type of developmental dysfunction in the central nervous system within the areas responsible for social and communication development (Gillberg, 1989; Volkmar & Cohen, 1988). In recent years researchers have made significant gains in the identification of various biological factors associated with autism; however, the precise neurobiological process that causes autism is yet to be identified (Gillberg, 1990).

The *Diagnostic and Statistical Manual of Mental Disorders* (DSM-IV; American Psychiatric Association [APA], 1994) defines autism as a severe form of a pervasive developmental disorder characterized by qualitative impairments in social interaction, communication, and the manifestation of restricted repetitive and stereotyped patterns of behavior, interest, and activities. Pervasive developmental disorder (PDD) is a term that is used in DSM-IV to describe a continuum of disorders that includes autism. DSM-IV provides a list of classified behaviors from which a minimum of six behaviors have to be identified to obtain a diagnosis of autism (see Table 11–2). Many children who do not meet the necessary criteria for autistic disorder are typically identified as having PDD, not otherwise specified (see Table 11–3). This category is used when a child's behavior does not meet the set criteria established for autism. Other DSM-IV categories of PDD similar to autism are identified as Rett Syndrome, Childhood Disintegrative, and Asperger Disorders (APA, 1994; Gillberg, 1990).

Communication Characteristics of Autism

It is within the broad continuum of PDD that one can identify a variety of communication characteristics in individuals with autism. The communicative profiles of autism generally range from persons who are nonverbal to those who use speech as their primary means of communication. It is difficult to understand why some indi-

Table 11–2. DSM-IV Diagnostic criteria for Autistic Disorder (299.00).

A total of six (or more) items from (1), (2), and (3), with at least two from (1), and one each from (2) and (3):

Qualitative impairment in social interaction, as manifested by at least two of the following:

- marked impairment in the use of multiple nonverbal behaviors such as eye-to-eye gaze, facial expression, body postures, and gestures to regulate social interaction.
- failure to develop peer relationships appropriate to developmental level.
- a lack of spontaneous seeking to share enjoyment, interests, or achievements with other people (e.g., by a lack of showing, bringing, or pointing out objects of interest).
- lack of social or emotional reciprocity.

Qualitative impairments in communication as manifested by at least one of the following:

- delay in, or total lack of, the development of spoken language (not accompanied by an attempt to compensate through alternative modes of communication such as gestures or mime.
- in individuals with adequate speech, marked impairment in the ability to initiate or sustain a conversation with others
- stereotyped and repetitive use of language or idiosyncratic language.
- lack of varied, spontaneous make-believe play or social imitative play appropriate to developmental level.

Restricted repetitive and stereotyped patterns of behavior, interests, and activities, as manifested by at least one of the following:

- encompassing preoccupation with one or more stereotyped and restricted patterns of interest that is abnormal either in intensity or focus.
- apparently inflexible adherence to specific, nonfunctional routines or rituals.
- stereotyped and repetitive motor mannerism (e.g., hand or finger flapping or twisting, or complex whole-body movements).
- persistent preoccupation with parts of objects.

Delays or abnormal functioning in at least one of the following areas, with onset prior to age 3 years: (1) social interaction, (2) language as used in social communication, or (3) symbolic or imaginative play.

The disturbance is not better accounted for by Rett's Disorder or Childhood Disintegrative Disorder.

Source: Diagnostic and Statistical Manual of Mental Disorders (pp. 70-71), by the American Psychiatric Association, 4th edition, 1994, Washington DC: Author. Copyright 1994 by the American Psychiatric Association. Reprinted with permission.

Table 11–3. Pervasive developmental disorder, not otherwise specified (299.80).

This category should be used when there is a severe and pervasive impairment in the development of reciprocal social interaction or verbal and nonverbal communication skills, or when stereotyped behavior, interests, and activities are present, but the criteria are not met for a specific Pervasive Developmental Disorder, Schizophrenia, Schizotypal Personality Disorder, or Avoidant Personality Disorder. For example, this category includes "atypical autism: presentations that do not meet the criteria for Autistic Disorder because of late age at onset, atypical symptomatology, or subthreshold symptomatology, or all of these.

Source: Diagnostic and Statistical Manual of Mental Disorders (pp. 77-78) by the American Psychiatric Association, 4th edition, 1994, Washington DC: Author. Copyright 1994 by the American Psychiatric Association. Reprinted with permission.

viduals learn to speak and others do not. One might speculate that the absence of many critical prelinguistic skills in the earlier years could be one possible reason. It is also hypothesized that neuromotor issues related to apraxia of speech may account for some of the nonverbal and limited speech profiles seen in developmental disabilities (Marquardt, Dunn, & Davis, 1985) and autism (Biklen, 1990).

Atypical Speech

Many children with autism demonstrate atypical speech production that is difficult to understand. General speech characteristics may include stereotypic expressions that can involve varying degrees of echolalia. Prizant's (1983) review of autism theorized that individuals with autism often process visual and auditory information in a *gestalt* fashion as opposed to an analytical one. This means that large chunks of auditory or visual information are remembered holistically and reproduced in various forms of echolalic speech (Prizant, 1983). To the individual with autism, a lengthy utterance may be perceived as a single unit with little recognition of the individual words produced. These echolalic expressions can be remarkably complex in production, as seen with exact echolalia or delayed echolalic forms. It is important to recognize that deficits in receptive language can sometimes be masked by more advanced echolalic expressions. It is common to hear a wide spectrum of echolalic behaviors that range from noncommunicative to communicative. The echolalic individual may be heard to parrot back words and phrases immediately after their occurrence or repeat them hundreds of times in a self-stimulatory manner. Self-stimulatory speech usually holds little communicative value. Delayed echolalia can often be heard in the repetition of commercial jingles or a caregiver's reprimand long after its occurrence.

It has been suggested that the use of echolalia by children with autism can represent various stages of communication development and should be viewed as a normal transition toward communicative language (Prizant & Wetherby, 1988). For example, a child with autism who echoes the *Price Is Right* television show expression "Come on down!" may later echo it to tell a sibling who is standing at the top of the stairs to come down. This example demonstrates how echolalic speech can typically evolve from exact repetitions to echolalic forms of communication. Prizant and Wetherby (1988) further suggested that those individuals who are echolalic may have a favorable prognosis toward the eventual use of functional speech, primarily because the mechanism of echolalia is often increasingly used to communicate with others.

Most individuals with autism who do speak rarely demonstrate any phonological difficulties. Intelligibility is not often affected with those who use stereotypic speech (Tager-Flusberg, 1981). What is affected is the qualitative aspects of speech communication. The speech production of individuals with autism is often seen as severely limited if not self-stimulatory in nature. Many individuals who are able to produce or reproduce speech are not always able to use their utterances to manipulate functional outcomes in the environment. The use of speech by individuals with autism does not preclude the use of augmentative communication intervention, primarily because the quality and function of their speech can be very limiting (Bebko, 1990; Mirenda & Schuler 1988).

Practitioners in the field report that for individuals with autism there is a significant difference in the mean length of utterance calculated between echolalic and spontaneous utterances. Nonecholalic spontaneous speech is often a truer reflection of receptive and expressive language abilities. It is important to understand that individuals with autism will use a variety of echolalic and spontaneous speech behaviors to communicate. An understanding of how these various forms of speech communication behaviors are used can indicate the direction of intervention and the role of supplemental AAC. As with most individuals with limited speech, there is an important link between verbal and nonverbal forms of communication and AAC interventions can be used to support both (Reichle & Karlan, 1985; Ricks & Wing, 1976).

Nonverbal Communication

Individuals with autism who are limited speakers or nonverbal are good candidates for augmentative communication (Bebko, 1990; Berkowitz, 1990; Kiernan, 1983; Mirenda & Schuler, 1988). As with all persons with developmental disabilities, it is critically important that an adequate analysis of communication behaviors be conducted before making any specific recommendations concerning augmentative communication. Prelinguistic communication issues related to communicative intent and means-end causality are often a starting point for exploring potential uses of nonsymbolic or symbolic communication forms (Carr, 1989; Siegel-Causey & Guess, 1989).

Unaided Nonsymbolic Communication

For many individuals with autism, nonsymbolic forms of communication, such as vocalizations, eye contact, facial expressions, gestures, body movements, postures, and touch can be critically important in supporting functional communication. The listener often uses these nonsymbolic forms of communication to interpret the behaviors of the individual with autism. These prelinguistic behaviors are often the foundation from which symbolic communication can be built. It is not difficult to understand that a child's tantrum is communicating something. What can be difficult to understand is the exact relationship between the behavior and the child's communicative intent (Carr, 1989; Prizant, 1987; Siegel-Causey & Guess, 1989).

When an individual's communication is primarily preintentional and occurs infrequently it may be premature to set up any formal symbolic communication system (Prizant & Wetherby, 1988; Schuler & Prizant, 1987). The initial focus of intervention for these individuals should be to attempt to facilitate existing nonsymbolic forms of communication in preparation for a more formalized system later (Mirenda & Schuler, 1988).

For some individuals with autism, it is quite possible that critical nonsymbolic forms of communication are not adequately developed for interpretation. Practitioners may want to identify a specific nonsymbolic form of communication to be trained further. For example, if eye contact during interactions was targeted as a desired nonsymbolic communication skill, the training program might systematically reinforce eye contact as it occurs during a motivational activity. This activity could be centered around the desire of the child to hold a favorite toy. The toy would be given to the child when direct eye contact was made, thus the favorite toy is used naturally to reinforce eye contact. This simple procedure can be used in any situation when the child wants something.

Another example of facilitating nonsymbolic communication might involve placing a desired item just out of the reach of the child to elicit a reaching response. The child's reaching for the desired item is naturally reinforced when the facilitator gives the desired item to the child. This reaching response can be further developed by placing the desired item in a clear container that cannot be opened by the child. The targeted behavior might be to have the child touch the facilitator's hand before opening the container with the desired item. This behavior is reinforced by opening the container and giving the child access to the desired item.

Every attempt should be made to extend current nonsymbolic means of communication in a way that diversifies existing communicative functions of individuals with autism. AAC interventions that systematically target the development of nonsymbolic and symbolic communication are based on the recognition that individuals with autism possess a continuum of communication abilities.

Intervention Strategies Specific to Autism

Parents and professionals are often faced with a smorgasbord of treatment options to choose from as they attempt to find the program that best addresses the educational needs of a child with autism. This process can often be overwhelming for parents and warrants careful consideration and support. Today, there is more consensus on interventions that emphasize the important role of communication in the educational treatment of children with autism. Given the broad array of AAC techniques and strategies used with children with autism, it is critical that parents and professionals understand that AAC training needs to be systematically linked to the ecological needs of school, community, and home. No one AAC system can adequately address all communication needs across multiple environments. AAC is multimodal and should be trained as the environment dictates. Multimodal communication allows the child to develop his or her expressive language skills, while allowing for alternatives to support communication in a variety of settings. It is likely that the majority of individuals with autism will use a variety of AAC skills that fall along the continuum of nonsymbolic and symbolic forms of expression.

It has long been recognized that the optimum time for beginning communication intervention for autism is when the child is preschool age or younger (Hoyson, Jamieson & Strain, 1984; Lovaas, 1987; Simeonnson, Olley, & Rosenthal, 1987;

Wetherby, 1985). Advances in early identification and in the diagnosis of autism have promoted a variety of services provided to children with autism at home and in their school settings (Prizant & Wetherby, 1988). Initial steps in providing intervention for children with autism typically occur between the ages of 2 and 3. School systems today are increasingly providing a variety of services for preschool-age children with autism that are tailored for both the home and school settings.

Many young children with autism initially come into preschool programs with serious dysfunctional behaviors that can camouflage their communication abilities. Many demonstrate no functional communication skills; however, an analysis of behavior may help to provide insights into the development of various prelinguistic concepts such as cause and effect relationships, means-end causality, and communicative intent (Wetherby & Prizant, 1990). These critical skills are the basis for building a communication foundation from which both speech and AAC skills can be built. It is important to recognize that individuals with autism who do not possess many prelinguistic communication skills remain candidates for AAC intervention. It is often through the use of AAC interventions that individuals with autism can concurrently learn critical prelinguistic skills associated with functional communication.

An initial assessment of a young child's nonsymbolic and symbolic forms of communication is essential to identify a starting place for AAC intervention. Chapter 4 in this text presents information on AAC symbols ranging from real objects to abstract graphic symbols such as the written word. The child's learning style and cognitive level dictates what communication symbol system works best. It is important to note that a combination of these symbol systems is often appropriate for children with autism. Many children with autism who are beginning to use symbols have different strategies for symbol recognition. They may cue into small details, colors, or other portions of a symbol without truly processing the symbol as a whole. Children often memorize the location of a symbol without visually regarding the symbol itself. Children with autism can learn to use a specific symbol, in a specific location, within a specific context, yet are unable to use the symbol communicatively if the symbol is changed slightly, moved to a new location, or introduced into a novel context. For children who are just beginning to associate pictures with communication, maximum symbol cues (e.g., colored backgrounds, consistent symbol locations, tactile differences) should be used to facilitate discrimination between symbol choices. As the child's ability to discriminate symbols improves, these cues can be systematically faded in small steps.

Picture Exchange Communication System

Although many young children with autism have little or no functional communication, most of these children have a basic understanding of cause and effect. This can frequently be seen by the way a child uses tantrum behaviors to manipulate outcomes. Other simple examples of cause and effect behavior might include the child turning on and off the classroom lights or the repeated flushing of the restroom toilet. Even though a child can physically manipulate certain outcomes, it is sometimes difficult to establish the communicative intent associated with means-end causality. Practitioners must determine if the child can use more conventional means to communicate. For instance, a child who enjoys activating a switch to move a toy train can sometimes be taught to use a symbolic method to request the desired item. A picture exchange setup is appropriate for this type of situation even when a child has yet to demonstrate symbolic means-end causality.

The Picture Exchange Communication System (PECS) is one training approach that has been used successfully to promote symbolic communication with individuals with autism (Bondy & Frost, 1993). The picture exchange technique teaches children to initiate a communicative act to receive a concrete outcome. Because children with autism are not highly reinforced by typical social rewards associated with the act of communication, the use of a picture exchange setup can provide for immediate and concrete reinforcement while teaching the social interaction necessary for communication. This type of communication training is excellent for those who are demonstrating emerging intentional communication.

Many children who have difficulty pointing to pictured symbols may find it easier to use a velcro-based system where the child directly removes a symbol from a velcro communication board. The picture symbol is then handed to an adult in exchange for a desired item or action. The PECS setup initially teaches the concept of how to use an object (the symbol) to obtain a desired item or outcome. At first, the child pays little attention to the actual picture symbol used. The child simply learns that if he or she gives something to another person he or she will get something in return. In other words, the PECS user gives a symbol to a listener, who then gives back the desired item. It is through this exchange format that the PECS user can begin to learn how to use symbols as objects to manipulate specific outcomes in the environment. This format also helps promote the idea of communication as a social exchange. As the individual learns to exchange specific symbols for desired items or actions, he or she can potentially learn the critical communication skills that move him or her toward more conventional forms of augmentative communication.

Many young children with autism use PECS as a transitional system to the use of traditional two-dimensional communication displays. Communication displays are typically used when it can be demonstrated that the individual has a working knowledge of means-end causality and can make a choice between picture symbols by pointing with his or her finger to the desired symbol.

Aided Language Stimulation

Aided Language Stimulation strategies that were first introduced by Goossens (1989) have been used successfully within a wide spectrum of developmental disabilities including autism. Aided Language Stimulation is a receptive and expressive teaching strategy in which a facilitator points to an array of symbols on a communication display as he or she verbally interacts with the child (Goossens et al., 1992; Romski & Sevcik, 1992). This is a departure from past practices in which the teaching of symbols was conducted within a noninteractive receptive training format (Goossens et al., 1992). This type of training was characterized by asking a child to point to a specified picture in the hope that this alone would train the new vocabulary. It was once thought that a child needed to demonstrate an isolated knowledge of select vocabularies before using them on a communication display; however, in recent years, research has shown this not to be a reliable practice (Goossens et al., 1992). Reductionistic instructional strategies that teach AAC skills in stilted, stimulus-response training modes have done little to promote functional augmentative communication (Light, Collier, & Parnes, 1985). The use of more naturalized holistic training strategies such as Aided Language Stimulation have been effective in teaching functional communication with individuals with autism (Cafiero, 1995). The dynamic use of Aided Language Stimulation strategies can provide the context in which individuals with autism

can learn to comprehend and express language in a way that is similar to children who can speak (Goossens et al., 1992).

If a child is to become a functional user of an AAC system, the facilitator must learn to use the child's AAC system to communicate with the child (Goossens, 1989; Goossens et al., 1992). When using Aided Language Stimulation strategies, the facilitator attempts to simulate the natural modeling of verbal language skills typically provided for children who can speak. In doing so, the facilitator employs various semantic contingency techniques involving the recasting and expansion of the child's expressions as he or she points to various pictured symbols on a communication display. For example, a child eating pancakes for breakfast may point to a picture symbol of *pancakes* to make a request for "more." The facilitator, in turn, could choose to repeat the child's expression by pointing to *pancakes* or choose to expand it by pointing to a two symbol sequence of *more + pancakes*. The facilitator may also consider recasting the child's expression by modeling additional content in sequencing *hungry + more + pancakes*. These semantic contingencies refer to the facilitator's continuation of a child's expressed interest by repeating, expanding, or extending the semantic content of the child's expression. Aided Language Stimulation strategies allow the facilitator to shape the child's communications into longer, more complete, or more correct forms of expression. By placing the child's expression into a longer or more complete context, the facilitator provides the child with an opportunity to understand more complex utterances while using child directed information. The facilitator can use Aided Language Stimulation strategies to model more effective forms of communication for the child using an AAC system.

It is well recognized that the comprehension of spoken language can be challenging for most individuals with autism

(Fay & Schuler, 1980; Prizant, 1982). Recent research conducted by Peterson, Bondy, Vincent, & Finnegan (1995) investigated the effects of altering communicative input using picture symbols for nonverbal students with autism. The results of this study showed that the augmented use of picture symbols improved the comprehension of spoken language significantly. Peterson et al. (1995) further demonstrated that the visual preferences of many individuals with autism can serve to support language comprehension and functional communication for individuals with autism. Aided Language Stimulation attempts to use these principles by pairing picture symbols with speech to promote comprehension of spoken language while modeling functional augmentative communication use.

Aided Language Stimulation provides interactive receptive and expressive symbol training by modeling interactive communication display use. The graphic symbols used on a communication display allow for repeated examination. This closely matches the visual processing preference common to most individuals with autism (Beukelman & Mirenda, 1992). If a child is to learn to use a communication display frequently and interactively, he or she must be provided with continual models of interactive use. It is the facilitator's consistent use of augmented input that is central to the use of Aided Language Stimulation for the promotion of functional communication skills (Beukelman & Garrett, 1988; Goossens et al., 1992; Romski & Sevcik, 1992). Aided Language Stimulation has done much to expand the notion that augmentative communication training techniques can be used in a more naturalistic, meaningful manner to promote communication skills that go beyond making simple requests.

Orthographic Communication Systems

AAC systems that use written words are useful for many individuals with autism (Mirenda & Schuler, 1988). Many individuals with PDD or autism demonstrate hyperlexic reading abilities (Burd, Fisher, Knowlton, & Kerbeshian, 1987; Goldberg, 1987; Silberberg & Silberberg, 1967). Hyperlexia refers to the precocious ability of an individual to recognize written words far above his or her language and cognitive capabilities. Although word recognition is high, actual reading comprehension is often poor; however, comprehension is thought to be at least equal to overall intellectual and receptive language levels (Pennington, Rogers, & Welsh, 1987). The majority of individuals who are hyperlexic use speech as their primary means of communication, yet often demonstrate serious expressive difficulties associated with the pragmatic use of language. Hyperlexic individuals with autism can be remarkable decoders of words and have been known to use the written word to cue speech and formulate verbal output. Low tech setups using the written word or a combination of words and pictures can be used to supplement general communication needs across various settings.

Computer-Assisted Technologies

The use of computers and other adaptive technologies can be helpful in further accessing and understanding the internalized language of many individuals with autism. The visual presentation routes provided by computer technologies seem to match more closely the visual processing learning styles of hyperlexic individuals.

Very little research to date has been conducted to investigate the specific use of computers with autism. However, practitioners in the field report that many individuals with autism are highly motivated by computers and peripheral technologies. Some studies have reported language gains in children with autism when involved with computer-assisted instruction (e.g., Colby & Smith, 1971; Frost, 1984;

Hedbring, 1985; Panyan, 1984). The data from these investigations suggest that applications of computer technology may stimulate the development of language communication with these children. Panyan (1984) reported that the use of computers with individuals with autism is promising and warrants further research. Microcomputer presentations can be reliable and consistent without the many idiosyncratic and incidental behaviors that accompany adult or peer teaching (Panyan, 1984). It appears that the use of computers is consistent with autistic cognitive styles and processing preferences as evidenced by the fact that many individuals with autism are remarkably interactive with educational and entertainment software. Computers are increasingly being considered for integrative use within many intervention programs designed for PDD and autism. The much sought-after joint attention between instructor and student can more frequently be achieved when using computer technologies.

Adaptive hardware technologies such as Discover:Board, IntelliKeys, and the Touch Window have been successful in providing alternative and adaptive keyboard access to computers. These technologies give the practitioner an opportunity to simplify the operations of the computer while maintaining full access to software applications. It is this type of assistive technology that can provide both the practitioner and the individual with autism the opportunity to explore the many possibilities consistent with the individual's unique learning style.

Voice Output Communication Aids

Voice output communication aids (VOCA) have often been a logical extension of the successful use of computers. Devices such as the AlphaTalker, DynaVox, Macaw, SpeakEasy, WalkerTalker, Hawk, and Wolf are a few of the VOCA systems that have

been known to provide voice to many individuals with autism. AAC devices that provide voice output can enhance communication through an organized storage of vocabularies which can be quickly accessed as the situation dictates. It is difficult to predict which individuals will respond positively to voice output. One must be careful not to assume that those who are able to operate the classroom computer will automatically be appropriate users of voice output AAC devices. This must be investigated on a case-by-case basis.

Because most individuals with autism are ambulatory, issues related to device portability are a concern. This issue must be analyzed with the understanding that no single AAC setup is appropriate for all environments. A multimodal approach to AAC that involves the combined use of nonsymbolic and symbolic communication systems and both low and high tech setups is preferred.

Creating the Conditions for Effective Use of AAC Systems

Finding a Balance: Stimulus Response Versus Naturalistic Training

In the 1980s researchers made significant contributions in language communication interventions for individuals with autism (Goldstein, 1991). Many autism programs use interventions that incorporate a highly structured behavioral approach (Hoyson et al., 1984; Lovaas, 1987). More recently, educational programs for children with autism are reevaluating their approach to training functional communication skills. Attention has been directed toward finding a balance between stimulus-response behavioral methods and naturalistic language training technologies.

Stimulus Response Training. Much of the language instruction in programs for individuals with autism is teacher directed, involving mass trials of stimulus response training. For example, an intervention may train selected vocabularies by having the child point to an object or picture when told "show me shoe" or "point to ball." This target behavior would be taught to a preset criteria level over numerous trials. Other stimulus response training examples might involve correctly matching a pictured item to the correct corresponding object or training the discrimination of picture symbols by having the child point to the correct item from an array of symbols. The difficulty with these types of practices is that they have little to do with real communication.

One could argue that many of the targeted behaviors selected for this type of training are important for the development of future communication skills; however, there is little evidence that skills learned in an isolated stimulus response paradigm will concurrently generalize into something useful or meaningful (Stokes & Baer, 1977). It has been well-documented that generalization can be difficult to achieve in individuals with autism (Koegel & Rincover, 1977). Most practitioners who use behavioral technologies understand that the generalization of a learned skill is not usually a passive phenomenon, but an active one requiring substantial programming. The generalization of learned skills is without a doubt the greatest challenge that behavioral intervention programs face today when teaching functional communication skills to individuals with autism.

Increasingly, researchers have highlighted the need for communication intervention to be integrated into the student's total environment. Instructional designs used in special education are frequently not consistent with the Low Inference theory originally introduced by Brown, Nietupski, and Hamre-Nietupski (1976), which recognizes that students with severe disabilities have significant difficulty generalizing information. Teachers cannot assume that the criterion performance trained in one situation will result in the criterion performance in a similar but different situation (Brown et al., 1976). Low inference abilities may contribute to a lack of generalization across cues, modalities, persons, and settings for individuals with severe developmental disabilities. Teachers of students with autism cannot assume that a skill trained in one setting will spontaneously generalize to other settings.

Goossens, Crain, and Elder (1992) stated, "There is a pervasive tendency to teach communication in stilted, stimulus-response paradigms . . . as opposed to teaching AAC use in contexts that allow students to see symbols being used repeatedly, interactively and generatively, during a meaningful ongoing activity" (p. 14). Advocates of this approach believe that the use of a naturalized setting to teach functional communication may produce more generalization than standard behavioral techniques because it makes the treatment situation more like situations in everyday life (Hart & Risley, 1975; Koegel, O'Dell, & Koegel, 1987).

Beukelman and Mirenda (1992) submitted that much of the dysfunctional communication behaviors demonstrated by AAC users is the result of failed opportunities for meaningful learning. Opportunities to practice meaningful communication within the natural context are critical to the generalization of learned skills. There is a growing body of literature that supports the notion that one-to-one mass trial training approaches have significant limitations in achieving reasonable generalization (Goossens, Crain, & Elder, 1992; Mirenda & Calculator, 1993; Reichle & Keogh, 1985; Rogers-Warren & Warren, 1980). Given the *gestalt* learning styles of individuals with autism and their apparent inflexible adherence to sameness or routines, it is not surprising that issues related to generalization are of paramount importance with any AAC intervention.

Naturalistic Language Training. A number of authors have demonstrated the need to use naturalized interventions that promote effective training and the generalization of learned communication skills (Beukelman & Mirenda, 1992; Koegel et al., 1987; Mirenda & Donnellan, 1986; Rydell & Mirenda, 1991; Schuler & Prizant, 1987; Warren & Kaiser, 1986; Watson, Lord, Schaeffer, & Schopler, 1989; Wetherby, 1989). To develop useful communication, it is important to work with the behaviors that are initiated by the individual with autism. This is the context from which many dysfunctional forms of communication can be transformed into more appropriate means of expression (Wetherby, 1989).

The natural language teaching paradigm (Koegel et al., 1987) and the TEACCH (Treatment and Education of Autistic and related Communication handicapped CHildren) communication curriculum (Watson, 1985; Watson et al., 1989) are two examples of intervention programs that have successfully maintained a structured behavioral approach while using child-directed principles. These child-directed principles were summarized by Beukelman and Mirenda (1992) as: "a) providing contingent, functionally related reinforcement for children's communicative attempts; b) taking turns and allowing children to choose tasks; c) varying tasks to prevent frustration or boredom; d) sharing control of interactions; and e) teaching during naturally occurring, functional activities using relevant contextual cues" (p. 280).

Koegel et al. (1987) looked at two important paradigms of treatment: traditional analog and natural language teaching. The traditional analog method of treatment represented a type of intervention that is typically teacher-directed using isolated, mass stimulus-response training procedures that target specific language skills. The natural language teaching method identified several basic parameters of normal language interactions. These language parameters were pursued within child-directed activities typical of a child's naturalized learning environments. The results of the study showed that the training of language communication for children with autism who are nonverbal can be effectively addressed when the conditions of learning are child directed and more naturalistic. This study further demonstrated that the traditional analog treatments typically used with children with autism were substantially less effective in teaching basic language communication. The research conducted by Koegel et al. (1987) has helped facilitate an important step forward in presenting evidence that intervention techniques that use natural language teaching strategies should be considered for children with autism.

The TEACCH program is a comprehensive intervention program that focuses on the treatment of communication, socialization, and independence. These three areas are simultaneously integrated throughout the activities of the child's day. The TEACCH program does not view communication as a separate skill-based deficit, but as a pervasive disability that crosses cognitive, affective, and social domains. These components require communication interventions to be systematically incorporated into all aspects of the child's educational program. The TEACCH instructional model uses child-directed principles while maintaining structured teaching methods.

Most children who enter the TEACCH program are nonverbal and are unable to use any conventional means of communication to express their basic wants and needs. Treatment begins by placing priorities on helping young children with autism to develop a means of effective communication while encouraging the possible development of a verbal system of communication. Augmentative communication systems are regularly used to support the child's immediate and ongoing communication needs throughout the day in various environments. In keeping with child-directed principles, communication training is focused on developing the child's emerging communication skills by engineering the classroom environment for frequent opportunities for communication.

One of the core goals of the TEACCH program is the training of functional communication. This is initiated by conducting an inventory of the child's communication demands across various program contexts (e.g., play time, circle time, work time, snack time). This inventory is then used to identify those situations that can be engineered for communication. It is here that the child's emerging communication skills are shaped into more conventional forms of expression using AAC setups as warranted. Much effort is given to developing the conditions from which natural consequences can be used to reinforce the communicative attempts offered by the child.

The TEACCH program and others like it recognize the importance of creating an instructional plan for integrating the child's AAC system into the structure and routines of the day. Picture symbol systems are frequently used to provide a visual representation of the child's daily schedule. This picture schedule system is often attached to a velcro base to allow for the direct manipulation of pictured items to be moved from an active space (*We are doing _____ today*) to an inactive one (*We did _____ today*). Various picture symbol systems can be an effective way to provide the child with augmented input concerning the sequence of events. This type of setup can also provide for the structure that is commonly necessary for children with autism. The picture schedule is sometimes the child's first meaningful exposure to a graphic symbol system. The experiences associated with the sequence of a schedule can often be shaped into other variations of AAC use.

Another example of AAC integration into the TEACCH program can be seen during work sessions. A work session might be designed to train a specific task such as following one-step gross motor directions (e.g., "touch your head" or "touch your nose"). Following simple gross motor directions by themselves might at first seem to provide little functional opportunity for communication; however, as many young children with autism have significant difficulty comprehending spoken language, the use of pictured symbols to augment simple directions can provide a needed visual cue for comprehension. A facilitator might choose to wear a communication vest that displays various picture symbols appropriate for the task. Using Aided Language Stimulation techniques, the facilitator touches the symbol(s) that represent the directions as he or she speaks. The child is initially cued by the picture symbol to complete the direction. As the child correctly learns to follow these simple one-step directions, he or she can then be taught to respond to a simple question: "What did you do?" It is here that the child can be encouraged to touch the corresponding picture symbols describing his or her movements. Work sessions use behavioral training methods. Yet through the use of AAC, isolated skills can be generalized into turn-taking interactions.

Koegel et al. (1987) and Watson et al. (1989) have done much to advance child-directed principles. This includes the perspective that children with autism need to learn communication skills in the natural environments in which they are most likely to communicate. Practitioners are increasingly pressed to identify effective interventions that can promote functional communication skills within naturalized settings while maintaining behavioral and child-directed principles. The TEACCH model and the natural language teaching paradigm research provide two good examples of how communication training can be integrated into the ongoing curricula of a program.

Engineering Opportunities for Communication

Most individuals with autism who use AAC experience significant difficulties in the spontaneous use of their communication systems (Halle, 1987; Light, 1988; Mirenda & Schuler, 1988). Numerous factors may contribute to these problems. An analysis of the individual's environment can often reveal limited opportunities for meaningful communication. Many AAC users find themselves in situations where the opportunity to communicate is frequently interrupted by others who attempt to anticipate their every want and need (Halle, Baer, & Spradlin, 1981). These conditions rarely produce the positive social behaviors that can lead to effective communication (Goossens, Crain, & Elder, 1992).

The failure to communicate is not so much the result of limited ability, but failed conditions. When children who use AAC do use their systems, it is often in the respondent role, yielding minimal responses (Calculator & Dollaghan, 1982; Light, Collier, & Parnes, 1985). Often the interactions between a facilitator using natural speech and the child using AAC are dominated by the facilitator, thus producing very little spontaneous communication from the AAC user (Light, Dattilo, English, & Gutierrez, 1992). Children with severe expressive communication disabilities must learn early on to use multimodal AAC methods to manipulate their environments, otherwise, communication will remain seriously impeded (Light, 1988).

Research continues to demonstrate the range of communicative functions produced by AAC users to be significantly restricted due to flawed or short-sighted training. As previously discussed in this chapter, AAC users with autism are frequently taught the symbols (vocabular-ies) of their communication system by using discrete trial training methods. This training is often conducted in an isolated stimulus-response manner, which has been shown to be less effective in promoting generalization than those strategies that employ more naturalized methods (Bristol, 1985; Koegel et al., 1987). Discrete trial language training frequently results in the lack of initiation and in dependency on cues (Prizant & Schuler, 1987). Mirenda and Calculator (1993) stressed the importance of including in classroom communication programs specific procedures by which teachers and others can increase the number of opportunities that students have to interact with a wide range of people in the school, home, and community.

Milieu Training Strategies for AAC Skills

In recent years there has been increased interest in more "naturalistic" approaches to training functional AAC skills. Milieu teaching strategies represent some of those attempts at facilitating language communication using incidental teaching techniques. As reported by Beukelman and Mirenda (1992), the term *milieu teaching* was first introduced to describe a number of systematic natural context interventions by Hart and Rogers-Warren (1978). Milieu strategies were initially applied to children who were language delayed and culturally disadvantaged; however, subsequent studies have successfully demonstrated the use of milieu strategies to teach requesting to persons with autism or severe disabilities (Halle, Baer, & Spradlin, 1981; Halle, Marshall, & Spradlin, 1979; Haring, Neetz, Lovinger, Peck, & Semmel, 1987; Oliver & Halle, 1982; Peck, 1985). Three strategies in particular, *incidental teaching* (Warren & Kaiser, 1986), the *mand-model technique* (Halle, 1982), and a *time delay procedure* (Halle et al., 1979, 1981) have been successfully used to improve functional communication skills.

Milieu teaching strategies require that facilitators learn to identify situations and engineer opportunities for communication. Setup strategies include (a) giving individuals opportunities to make choices, (b) blocking access to a desired item, (c) giving the individual items that are out of context (e.g., providing a pencil instead of a spoon during snack time), or (d) placing a desired item out of reach. All these strategies are meant to elicit spontaneous use of the individual's AAC system. For an outline of milieu teaching strategies as a means of providing communication opportunities, the reader is referred to Beukelman and Mirenda (1992).

Mand-Model Technique. The mand-model technique can be used to teach basic requesting skills to AAC users who do not use their system(s) to make choices. One of the easiest places to engineer opportunities for communication is during a snack activity. A snack activity can be set up to elicit multiple opportunities for making requests for food items. In preparation for this activity, the facilitator arranges an array of desirable snack food items out of the reach of the AAC user. The child's AAC device is developed with appropriate symbols and vocabularies for the selected snack food items. The facilitator has complete control over the food items, which are out of the child's reach. It is likely that the child will use various nonsymbolic forms of communication (e.g., reaching, eye contact, vocalizations) to indicate his or her desire for food items. At this moment the facilitator initiates communication by asking the child, "What do you want?" If the child does not respond by using the AAC system, the facilitator then models the desired AAC behavior (i.e., pointing to the symbol on the AAC system that corresponds to the desired food item) and pauses for a response. If the child still does not use the AAC system to request the snack food item, the facilitator pro-

vides a second model and a physical prompt if necessary to assist imitation. For example, "You tell me what you want" + model + physical prompt. The child is then reinforced with verbal praise and the requested snack food item.

Incidental Teaching. Incidental teaching strategies are used to promote initiation and to develop more sophisticated forms of communication. As with all milieu teaching strategies, it is important to create a variety of communication opportunities in natural contexts wherever possible. The multiple situations that the facilitator engineers for communication are designed to elicit the use of a child's AAC system. For example, the facilitator can place highly desirable items out of reach, "forget" to give a child a spoon when getting ready to eat pudding, give the child a cup when he or she is expecting a fork, or pretend not to understand what the child has said when he or she uses unconventional nonsymbolic forms of communication (e.g., vocalizations, gestures, eye contact).

Incidental teaching strategies involve imaginative strategies to improve the functional communication skills of AAC users. There is nothing boring or routine about using incidental teaching strategies. There are virtually no limitations on how creative a facilitator can be in arranging the conditions for effective use of AAC systems. For example, an elementary school-age child arrives at his classroom and routinely places his book bag in the designated cubby. The student's milk money is located in the front pocket of his bookbag. Without the child's knowledge, the facilitator moves the milk money to the side pocket of the book bag. Later that morning, students are directed to get their money to purchase a milk ticket. As this child attempts to retrieve his money, he soon realizes that it is not in the front pocket of his book bag. At this point, the student has a realistic need to use his AAC system to request help. Another example might be to place several books in the child's cubby that will block his ability to put his book bag away. Once again, this creates an opportunity for the child to use his AAC system to problem-solve a new situation. These type of foils, designed to promote communication skills in real-life situations, can be engineered throughout the student's day with a great deal of creativity.

It is not uncommon for children with autism to develop the necessary language for independent communication, yet fail to use it for functional communication. The failure of children with autism to achieve effective AAC skills is often the result of having developed an overreliance on multiple cues and prompts to communicate. The consistent yet varied use of incidental teaching strategies can help individuals with autism use their AAC skills to express themselves without the dependency on direct prompts or cues.

There are four levels of prompts that can be used and faded over time to promote independent AAC use (Hart & Risley, 1975). The first is a natural prompt. The natural prompt can take the form of a question ("What do you want?") or give direct attention to the child (e.g., closer proximity). If a child does not demonstrate the desired communication behavior using a natural prompt, then a minimum prompt is used to elicit the target AAC behavior. A minimum prompt is an unspecified verbal direction from the facilitator, such as "Tell me what you want." If the minimum prompt does not produce the desired communication behavior, then the facilitator should use a medium prompt. A medium prompt is a request for a partial imitation. The facilitator might say "Tell me what you want. You want (*item*)," while pointing to the symbol on the AAC user's system to signal a response. If the medium prompt fails to elicit an appropriate response then a maximum prompt should be used. A maximum prompt is when the facilitator asks "What do you want? Tell me (*item*)" while modeling the target behavior on the child's AAC system. A maximum prompt should be used as a last resort.

Remember that many children with autism who use AAC systems have developed an overdependency on direct prompts and cues from their communication partners. This prompt dependency may be one contributing reason why some children have difficulty becoming independent AAC users. The use of a maximum prompt should only be used when the other less-invasive prompts have been tried with unsuccessful results. Once a prompt results in the child responding correctly, reinforce the AAC behavior verbally and give the desired item to the child.

Time Delay Procedure. The time delay procedure is most often used to encourage the initiation of communication skills and to break the dependency of the AAC user to wait for a facilitator's verbal prompt or cue. Most of the time when a child does not use a prescribed communication system, it is because he or she has chosen a nonsymbolic form of communication over the use of the AAC system. These nonsymbolic forms of communication are recognized to be an important part of any child's communication repertoire; however, used by themselves, they are often not adequate to meet functional communication demands.

Many children with autism become overly dependent upon their communication partners to anticipate their every want and need. These children are less likely to initiate effective communication on their own. It is because of this overreliance on others that less sophisticated forms of communication are used over more effective ones. Given this situation, the child with autism may not learn to initiate communication using any AAC system unless there is a substantial change in the communication expectations.

The time delay procedure is one teaching strategy that can make a significant contribution to the way therapists teach the initiation of learned AAC skills. As with all milieu teaching strategies, the time delay procedure requires that the facilitator identify and engineer various communication opportunities for the AAC user in his or her immediate environment. This procedure starts by closely watching the child's behavior to see if he or she indicates wanting something in the environment. Very often, the child will demonstrate his or her desire for something by looking at or approaching a desired item. When this type of behavior is observed, the facilitator then approaches the child within 3 feet without saying anything. It is here that the facilitator makes his or his presence known to the child through the use of body language (e.g., eye contact, shrugging the shoulders, or clearing the throat). Once the presence of the facilitator is known to the child, the facilitator pauses for 15 seconds for the child to initiate the desired communication behavior (e.g., verbalizing a request for the item or using a picture communication symbol to request the item). The facilitator provides the desired item to the child when the desired communication behavior has occurred. If the child does not respond after the pause, the facilitator can provide a visual prompt by pointing toward the item that the child wants. Sometimes the facilitator may find it useful to use exaggerated facial expressions and body language as if to say "I don't know what you want." The last resort is to model the desired communication behavior or use incidental teaching prompts.

It is important to remember that the desired item should only be provided when the target communication behavior has been demonstrated by the child. Using these strategies, the consistent use of time delay procedures can transform dysfunctional communication patterns into effective AAC skills that are self-initiated by the child with autism.

The generalization of AAC skills to children with autism has always presented a significant challenge. The milieu teaching strategies of incidental teaching, mand-model, and time delay procedures are all used in a similar fashion, but are applied to different situations. This provides facilitators with a great deal of flexibility in responding to a wide range of student learning needs (Halle, 1982). The use of milieu teaching strategies helps create conditions for effective AAC learning and use. The primary reasons for using these milieu strategies have come from two sources: (a) the growing body of evidence that users of AAC systems are not learning functional communication skills that are interactive and generative (Bristol, 1985; Light et al., 1992; Goossens et al., 1992); and (b) the more traditional, one-to-one massed trial training approaches are limited in achieving reasonable generalization of communication skills (Costello, 1983; Harris, 1975; Prizant & Schuler, 1987; Reichle & Keogh, 1985; Warren & Rogers-Warren, 1980). Milieu teaching strategies give practitioners the tools to address idiosyncratic learning behaviors specific to autism in the natural environment. It should be the goal of every communication program to teach communication skills in real situations in which communication is likely to take place. The use of milieu teaching strategies is one approach that can support communication training programs for students with autism.

CONCLUSION

Children with severe speech and language disabilities, developmental apraxia of speech, and pervasive developmental disabilities including autism have been shown to benefit from the use of AAC technologies. School systems today are beginning to recognize some of the tangible benefits of providing augmentative and assistive technology services to these individuals. Giving children who are nonverbal or limited speakers the means to communicate has done much toward achieving desirable educational outcomes. These children should be considered candidates for intervention with AAC strategies that promote both receptive and expressive language skills.

There is little doubt that early AAC intervention is a critical step in creating the right conditions for building a strong foundation for communication. AAC interventions require practitioners and parents to participate in a well-planned and coordinated instructional intervention that promotes multimodal communication in all settings. Whether a child has speech or the potential for speech, the use of multimodal communication strategies is warranted. No single communication system is right for all situations. The combined use of various forms of nonsymbolic and symbolic communication is necessary as a child learns to maneuver multiple environments. AAC training must include strategies that teach functional communication skills in situations where children are most likely to communicate. A comprehensive approach to AAC intervention begins with a shared commitment from caregivers and educators to engineer and manage AAC systems for meaningful communication. Without this commitment, children with developmental disabilities will continue to demonstrate dysfunctional communication void of independence and initiation. The goal of an AAC intervention program is to assist individuals with severe communication disorders to become more communicatively competent while increasing their opportunities to interact with a wide range of people in school, at home, and in the community.

REFERENCES

American Psychiatric Association. (1994). *Diagnostic and statistical manual of mental disorders* (4th ed.). Washington, DC: Author.

American Speech-Language-Hearing Association. (1991). Report: Augmentative and alternative communication. *Asha, 33*(5), 9–2.

Bebko, J. M. (1990). Echolalia, mitigation, and autism: Indicators from child characteristics for the use of sign language and other augmentative language systems. *Sign Language Studies, 66*, 61–78.

Berkowitz, S. (1990). A comparison of two methods of prompting in training discrimination of communication book pictures by autistic students. *Journal of Autism and Developmental Disorders, 20*(2), 255–262.

Beukelman, D., & Garrett, K. (1988). Augmentative and alternative communication for adults with acquired severe communication disorders. *Augmentative and Alternative Communication, 4*, 104–121.

Beukelman, D., & Mirenda, P. (1992). *Augmentative and alternative communication: Management of severe communication disorders in children and adults.* Baltimore, MD: Paul H. Brookes Publishing.

Biklen, D. (1990). Communication unbound: Autism and praxis. *Harvard Educational Review, 3*, 291–314.

Blackstone, S. (1989). Individuals with developmental apraxia of speech. *Augmentative Communication News, 2*(2), 1–7.

Blackstone, S. W., & Painter, M. (1985). Speech problems in multihandicapped children. In J. Darby (Ed.), *Speech and language evaluation in neurology: Childhood disorders* (pp. 219-242). Orlando, FL: Grune & Stratton.

Bondy, A. S., & Frost, L. A. (1993). Mands across the water: A report on the application of the picture-exchange communication system in Peru. *The Behavior Analyst, 16*, 123–128.

Bristol, M. M. (1985). Designing programs for young developmentally disabled children: A family systems approach to autism. *Remedial and Special Education, 6*(4) 46–53.

Brown, L., Nietupski, J., & Hamre-Nietupski, S. (1976). The criterion of ultimate functioning and public school services for severely handicapped students. In M. A. Thomas (Ed.), *Hey, don't forget about me: Education's investment in the severely, profoundly, and multiply handicapped* (pp. 2–15). Reston, VA: Council for Exceptional Children.

Bryson, S. E., Clark, B. S., & Smith, I. M. (1988). First report on a Canadian epidemiological study of autistic syndromes. *Journal of Child Psychology and Psychiatry, 29,* 433–445.

Burd, L., Fisher, W., Knowlton, D., & Kerbeshian, J. (1987). Hyperlexia, a marker for improvement in children with pervasive developmental disorders? *Journal of the American Academy of Child and Adolescent Psychiatry, 26*(3), 407–412.

Burd, L., & Kerbeshian, J. (1983). A North Dakota prevalence study of schizophrenia presenting in childhood. *Journal of the American Academy of Child and Adolescent Psychiatry, 26,* 347–350.

Cafiero, J. (1995). *Teaching parents of children with autism picture communication symbols as a natural language to decrease levels of family stress.* Unpublished doctoral dissertation, University of Toledo, OH.

Calculator, S., & Dollaghan, C. (1982). The use of communication boards in a residential setting: An evaluation. *Journal of Speech and Hearing Disorders, 47,* 281–287.

Carr, E. G., (1989). Functional equivalence of autistic leading and communicative pointing: Analysis and treatment. *Journal of Autism and Developmental Disorders, 19*(4), 561–578.

Colby, K., & Smith, D. (1971). Computers in the treatment of nonspeaking autistic children. In J. H. Masserman (Ed.), *Current psychiatric therapies* (pp. 1–17). New York: Grune & Stratton.

Costello, J. M. (1983). Generalization across settings: Language intervention with children. In J. Miller, D. E. Yoder, & R. L. Schiefelbusch (Eds.), *Contemporary issues in language intervention* (pp. 275–297). Rockville, MD: American Speech-Language-Hearing Association.

Crary, M. (1993). *Developmental motor speech disorders.* San Diego: Singular Publishing Group.

Culp, D. (1989). Developmental apraxia and augmentative or alternative communication: A case example. *Augmentative and Alternative Communication, 5*(1), 27–34.

Culp, D., & Carlisle, M. (1988). *Partners in augmentative communication training.* Tucson, AZ: Communication Skill Builders.

Cumley, G., & Jones, R. (1992). Persons with primary speech, language, and motor impairments. In R. Beukelman & P. Mirenda (Eds.), *Augmentative and alternative communication: Management of severe communication disorders in children and adults* (pp. 229–251). Baltimore, MD: Paul H. Brookes.

Denckla, M. B. (1986). Editorial: New diagnostic criteria for autism and related behavioral disorders: Guidelines for research protocols. *Journal of the American Academy of Child Psychiatry, 25,* 221–224.

Fay, W. H., & Schuler, A. L., (1980). *Emerging language in autistic children.* Baltimore: University Park Press.

Ferguson, D. (1994). Is communication really the point? Some thoughts on interventions and membership. *Mental Retardation, 32,* 7–18.

Ferry, P., Hall, S., & Hicks, J. (1975). 'Dilapidated' speech: Developmental verbal dyspraxia. *Developmental Medicine and Child Neurology, 17,* 749–756.

Fish, B., Shapiro, T., & Campbell, M. (1966). Long-term prognosis and the response of schizophrenic children to drug therapy: A controlled study of trifluoperazine. *American Journal of Psychiatry, 123,* 32–39.

Frost, R. E. (1984). Computers and the autistic child. In D. Peterson (Ed.), *Intelligent schoolhouse* (pp. 246–250). Reston, VA: Prentice-Hall.

Gerber, S., & Kraat, A. (1992). Use of a developmental model of language acquisition: Applications to children using AAC systems. *Augmentative and Alternative Communication, 8*(1), 19–32.

Gillberg, C. (1989). The role of the endogenous opioids in autism and possible relationships to clinical features. In L. Wing (Ed.), *Aspects of autism: Biological research* (pp. 31–37). London: Gaskell, The National Autistic Society.

Gillberg, C. (1990). Autism and pervasive developmental disorder. *Journal of Child Psychology and Psychiatry, 31*(1), 99–119.

Goldberg, T. (1987). On hermetic reading abilities. *Journal of Autism and Developmental Disorders, 17,* 29–44.

Goldstein, H. (1991). Significant progress in child language intervention: An 11 year retrospective. *Research in Developmental Disabilities, 12*(4), 401–424.

Goossens, C. (1989). Aided communication intervention before assessment: A case study of a child with cerebral palsy. *Augmentative and Alternative Communication, 5*(1), 14–26.

Goossens, C., Crain, S., & Elder, P. (1992). *Engineering the preschool environment for interactive, symbolic communication*. Birmingham, AL: Southeast Augmentative Communication Conference.

Gorenflo, C., & Gorenflo, D. (1991). The effects of information and augmentative communication technique on attitudes toward nonspeaking individuals. *Journal of Speech and Hearing Research 34,* 19–26.

Hall, P. (1992). At the center of controversy: Developmental apraxia. *American Journal of Speech-Language Pathology, 1*(3), 23–25.

Hall, P., Jordan, L., & Robin, D. (1993). *Developmental apraxia of speech: Theory and clinical practice*. Austin, TX: Pro-Ed.

Halle, J. (1987). Teaching language in the natural environment: An analysis of spontaneity. *The Journal of the Association for Persons with Severe Handicaps, 12,* 28–37.

Halle, J. W. (1982). Teaching functional language to the handicapped: Integrative model of natural environment teaching techniques. *The Journal of the Association for Persons with Severe Handicaps, 7,* 29–37.

Halle, J. W., Baer, D., & Spradlin, J. (1981). Teachers' generalized use of delay as a stimulus control procedure to increase language use by handicapped children. *Journal of Applied Behavior Analysis, 14,* 389–409.

Halle, J. W., Marshall, A., & Spradlin, J. (1979). Time delay: A technique to increase language use and facilitate generalization in retarded children. *Journal of Applied Behavior Analysis, 12,* 431–439.

Haring, T., Neetz, J., Lovinger, L., Peck, C., & Semmel, M. (1987). Effects of four modified incidental teaching procedures to create opportunities for communication. *Journal of the Association for Persons with Severe Handicaps, 12,* 218–226.

Harris, S. L. (1975). Teaching language to nonverbal children with emphasis on problems of generalization. *Psychological Bulletin, 82,* 565–580.

Hart, B., & Risley, T. R. (1975). Incidental teaching of language in the preschool. *Journal of Applied Behavior Analysis, 8,* 411–420.

Hart, B., & Rogers-Warren, A. (1978). Milieu teaching approaches. In R. Scheifelbusch (Ed.), *Language intervention strategies*. Baltimore: University Park Press.

Hayden, D. (1994). Differential diagnosis of motor speech dysfunction in children. *Clinics in Communication Disorders, 4*(2), 119–141.

Hayden, D., & Square, P. (1994). Motor speech treatment hierarchy: A systems approach. *Clinics in Communication Disorders, 4*(3), 162–174.

Hedbring, C. (1985). Computers and autistic learners: An evolving technology. *Australian Journal of Human Communication Disorders, 13,* 169–188.

Helfrich-Miller, K. (1994). A clinical perspective: Melodic intonation therapy for developmental apraxia. *Clinics in Communication Disorders, 4*(3), 175–182.

Hodge, D. (1994). Assessment of children with developmental apraxia of speech: A rationale. *Clinics in Communication Disorders, 4*(2), 91–101.

Hodge, D., & Hancock, H. (1994). Assessment of children with developmental apraxia of speech: A procedure. *Clinics in Communication Disorders, 4*(2), 102–118.

Hoyson, F., Jamieson, B., & Strain, P. (1984). Individualized group instruction of normally developing and autistic-like children: The LEAP curriculum model. *Journal of the Division for Early Childhood, 8,* 157–172.

Kangas, K., & Lloyd, L. (1988). Early cognitive skills as prerequisites to augmentative and alternative communication use: What are we waiting for? *Augmentative and Alternative Communication, 4,* 211–221.

Kanner, L. (1943). Autistic disturbances of affective contact. *Nervous Child, 2,* 217–250.

Kiernan, C. (1983). The use of nonvocal communication techniques with autistic individuals. *Journal of Child Psychology and Psychiatry, 24,* 339–375.

Klick, S. (1994). Adapted cueing technique: Facilitating sequential phoneme production. *Clinics in Communication Disorders, 4*(3), 183–189.

Koegel, R. L., & Rincover, A. (1977). Research on the difference between generalization and maintenance in extra-therapy responding. *Journal of Applied Behavior Analysis, 10*(1), 1–12.

Koegel, R., O'Dell, M., & Koegel, L. (1987). A natural language teaching paradigm for nonverbal autistic children. *Journal of Autism and Developmental Disorders, 2*(17), 187–199.

Kravitz, E., & Littman, D. (1990). A communication system for a nonspeaking person with hearing and cognitive impairments. *Augmentative and Alternative Communication, 6*(2), 100.

Kumin, L. (1994). Understanding motor planning skills and problems. *Communicating Together, 2,* 1–4.

Light, J., (1988). Interaction involving individuals using augmentative and alternative communication systems: State of the art and future directions. *Augmentative and Alternative Communication, 4,* 66–82.

Light, J., Collier, B., & Parnes, P. (1985). Communicative interaction between young nonspeaking physically disabled children and their primary caregivers: Part I: Discourse patterns. *Augmentative and Alternative Communication, 1,* 74–83.

Light, J., Dattilo, J., English, J., & Gutierrez, L. (1992). Instructing facilitators to support the communication of people who use augmentative communication systems. *Journal of Speech and Hearing Research, 35*(4), 865–875.

Lovaas, O. I. (1987). Behavioral treatment and normal educational and intellectual functioning in young autistic children. *Journal of Consulting and Clinical Psychology, 55,* 3–9.

Marquardt, T., Dunn, C., & Davis, B. (1985). Apraxia of speech in children. In J. Darby (Ed.), *Speech and language evaluation in neurology: Childhood disorders* (pp. 113–132). New York: Grune & Stratton.

Marquardt, T., & Sussman, H. (1991). Developmental apraxia of speech: Theory and practice. In D. Vogel & M. Cannito (Eds.), *Treating disordered speech motor control* (pp. 341–390). Austin, TX: Pro-Ed.

McGregor, G., Young, J., Gerak, J., Thomas, B., & Vogelsberg, R. T. (1992). Increasing functional use of an assistive communication device by a student with severe disabilities. *Augmentative and Alternative Communication, 8,* 243–249.

Mirenda, P., & Calculator, S. (1993). Enhancing curricular designs. In L. Kupper (Ed.), *The national symposium on effective communication for children and youth with severe disabilities,* (pp. 253–280). McLean, VA: Topic Papers, Readers Guide and videotape.

Mirenda, P., & Donnellan, A. (1986). Effects of adult interaction style on conversational behavior in students with severe communication problems. *Language, Speech, and Hearing Services in Schools, 17,* 126–141.

Mirenda, P., & Mathy-Laikko, P. (1989). Augmentative and alternative communication applications for persons with severe congenital communication disorders: An introduction. *Augmentative and Alternative Communication, 5*(1), 3–13.

Mirenda, P., & Schuler, A. (1988). Augmenting communication for persons with autism: Issues and strategies. *Topics in Language Disorders, 9,* 24–43.

National Joint Committee for the Communicative Needs of Persons with Severe Disabilities. (1992). Guidelines for meeting the communication needs of persons with severe disabilities. *Asha, 34*(Suppl. 7), 1–8.

Nelson, N. W. (1992). Performance is the prize: Language competence and performance among AAC users. *Augmentative and Alternative Communication, 8,* 3–18.

Oliver, C. B., & Halle, J. W. (1982). Language training in the everyday environment: Teaching functional sign use to a retarded child. *Journal of the Association for the Severely Handicapped, 8,* 50–62.

Paluszny, M. J. (1979). *Autism: A practical guide for parents and professionals.* Syracuse, NY: Syracuse University Press.

Pannbacker, M. (1988). Management strategies for developmental apraxia of speech: A review of literature. *Journal of Communication Disorders, 21*(5), 363–371.

Panyan, M. (1984). Computer technology for autistic students. *Journal of Autism and Developmental Disorders, 14,* 375–382.

Peck, C. A. (1985). Increasing opportunities for social control by children with autism and severe handicaps: Effects on learner behavior and perceived classroom climate. *Journal of the Association for Persons with Severe Handicaps, 10,* 183–193.

Pennington, B. F., Rogers, S., & Welsh, M. (1987). Word recognition and comprehension skills in hyperlexic children. *Brain and Language, 32,* 76–96.

Peterson, S. L., Bondy, A. S., Vincent, V., & Finnegan, C. S. (1995). Effects of altering communicative input for students with autism and no speech: Two case studies. *Augmentative and Alternative Communication, 11,* 93–100.

Prizant, B. M. (1982). Gestalt language and gestalt processing in autism. *Topics in Language Disorders, 3,* 16–23.

Prizant, B. (1983). Language and communicative behavior in autism: Toward an understanding of the "whole" of it. *Journal of Speech and Hearing Disorders, 46,* 241–249.

Prizant, B. (1987). Communicative intent: A framework for understanding social-communicative behavior in autism. *Journal of the American Academy of Child and Adolescent Psychiatry, 26*(4), 472–479.

Prizant, B., & Schuler, A. (1987). Facilitating communication: Theoretical foundations. In D. J. Cohen & A. M. Donnellan (Eds.), *Handbook of autism and pervasive developmental disorders* (pp. 289–300). New York: John Wiley & Sons.

Prizant, B., & Wetherby, A. M. (1988). Providing services to children with autism (ages 0 to 2 years) and their families. *Topics in Language Disorders, 9*(1), 1–23.

Reichle, J., & Karlan, G. (1985). The selection of an augmentative system of communication intervention: A critique of decision rules. *Journal of the Association for Persons with Severe Handicaps. 11,* 68–73.

Reichle, J., & Keogh, W. J. (1985). Communication intervention: A selective review of what, when and how to teach. In S. F. Warren & A. K. Rogers-Warren (Eds.), *Teaching functional language* (pp. 25–59). Austin, TX: Pro-Ed.

Ricks, D., & Wing, L. (1976). Language, communication, and the use of symbols. In L. Wing (Ed.), *Early strategies for learners with severe disabilities* (pp. 93–134). Baltimore: Paul H. Brookes.

Rimland, B. (1964). *Infantile autism.* New York: Appleton-Century-Crofts.

Rimland, B., & Fein, D. (1988). Special talents of autistic savants. In L. K. Obler & D. Fein (Eds.), *The exceptional brain* (pp. 474–492). New York: Guilford Press.

Ritvo, E. R., & Freeman, B. J. (1978). National Society for Autistic Children: Definition of the syndrome of autism and childhood schizophrenia, *8,* 162-167.

Robin, D. (1992). Developmental apraxia of speech: Just another motor problem. *American Journal of Speech-Language Pathology, 1*(3), 19–22.

Rogers-Warren, A., & Warren, S. (1980). Mands for verbalization: Facilitating the display of newly-taught language. *Behavior Modification, 4,* 361–382.

Romski, M. A., & Sevcik, R. (1988). Augmentative and alternative communication systems: Considerations for individuals with severe intellectual disabilities. *Augmentative and Alternative Communication, 2,* 83–93.

Romski, M., & Sevcik, R. (1992). Augmented language development in children with severe mental retardation. In S. Warren & J. Reichle (Eds.), *Causes and effects in communication and language intervention* (pp. 113–130). Baltimore: Paul H. Brookes.

Romski, M. A., & Sevcik, R. (1993). Language comprehension: Considerations for augmentative and alternative communication. *Augmentative and Alternative Communication, 9,* 281–285.

Rosenbek, J., & Wertz, R. (1972). A review of fifty cases of developmental apraxia of speech. *Language, Speech and Hearing Services in Schools, 3*(1), 23–33.

Rutter, M. (1978). Diagnosis and definition of childhood autism. *Journal of Autism and Childhood Schizophrenia, 8,* 136–161.

Rydell, P., & Mirenda, P. (1991). The effects of two levels of linguistic constraints on echolalia and generative language production in children with autism. *Journal of Autism and Developmental Disorders, 21,* 131–157.

Schuler, A., & Prizant, B. (1987). Facilitating communication: Pre-language approaches, In D. Cohen & A. Donnellan (Eds.), *Handbook of autism and pervasive developmental disorders* (pp. 301–315). New York: John Wiley & Sons.

Shriberg, L. (1994). Developmental phonological disorders: Moving toward the 21st century—forwards, backwards, or endlessly sideways? *American Journal of Speech-Language Pathology, 3*(3), 26–28.

Siegel-Causey, E., & Guess, D. (1989). *Enhancing nonsymbolic communication interactions among learners with severe disabilities.* Baltimore: Paul H. Brookes.

Silberberg, N., & Silberberg, M. (1967). Hyperlexia-specific word recognition skills in young children. *Exceptional Child, 34,* 41–42.

Silverman, F. (1995). *Communication for the speechless*. (3rd ed.). Boston: Allyn & Bacon.

Simeonnson, R. J., Olley, J. G., & Rosenthal, S. L. (1987). Early intervention for children with autism. In M. J. Guralnick & F. C. Bennett (Eds.), *The effectiveness of early intervention for at-risk and handicapped children* (pp. 275–296). Orlando, FL: Academic Press.

Square, P. (1994). Treatment approaches for developmental apraxia of speech. *Clinics in Communication Disorders, 4*(3), 151–161.

Sternberg, M. (1994). *The American Sign Language Dictionary on CD-ROM*. HarperCollins Interactive.

Stokes, T. F., & Baer, D. M. (1977). An implicit technology of generalization. *Journal of Applied Behavior Analysis, 10*(2) 349–367.

Strode, R., & Chamberlain, C. (1993). *Easy does it for apraxia and motor planning*. East Moline, IL: LinguiSystems, Inc.

Strode, R., & Chamberlain, C. (1994). *Easy Does It for Apraxia: Preschool*. East Moline, IL: LinguiSystems, Inc.

Tager-Flusberg, H. (1981). On the nature of linguistic functioning in early infantile autism. *Journal of Autism and Developmental Disorders, 11*, 45–56.

Treffert, D. A. (1988). The idiot savant: A review of the syndrome. *American Journal of Psychiatry, 145*, 563–571.

Volkmar, F. R., Cohen, D. J., (1988). Neurobiologic aspects of autism. *The New England Journal of Medicine, 21*(318) 1390–1391.

Warren, S., & Kaiser, A. (1986). Incidental language teaching: A critical review. *Journal of Speech and Hearing Disorders, 51*, 291–298.

Warren, S. F., & Rogers-Warren, A. K. (1980). Current perspectives in language remediation. *Education and Treatment of Children, 5*, 133–153.

Watson, L. (1985). The TEACCH communication curriculum. In E. Schopler & G. Mesibov (Eds.), *Communication problems in autism,* (pp. 187—206). New York: Plenum.

Watson, L., Lord, C., Schaeffer, B., & Schopler, E. (1989). *Teaching spontaneous communication to autistic and developmentally handicapped children*. New York: Irvington.

Wetherby, A. (1985). Speech and language disorders in children: An overview. In J. Darby (Ed.), *Speech and language evaluation in neurology: Childhood disorders* (pp. 3–32). Orlando, FL: Grune & Stratton.

Wetherby, A. (1989). Language intervention for autistic children: A look at where we have come in the past 25 years. *Journal of Speech-Language Pathology and Audiology, 13*(4), 15–28.

Wetherby, A., & Prizant, B. (1990). *Communication and Symbolic Behavior Scales* (CSBS). Tucson, AZ: Communication Skill Builders.

Zahner, G., & Pauls, L. D. (1987). Epidemiological surveys on infantile autism. In D. J. Cohen & M. A. Donnellan (Eds.), *Handbook of autism and pervasive developmental disorders* (pp. 199–207). New York: John Wiley.

Brooke's AAC Story: Developmental Apraxia of Speech

Sharon L. Glennen

When Brooke was 20 months old, she said her first word. Her mother, Patricia, was concerned because Brooke was not speaking as early as her older brother, but the pediatrician told her not to worry about it. By the age of 30 months, it was obvious that Brooke's speech development was not progressing normally. Brooke would try to talk, but her family could not understand her. Brooke grew frustrated at her inability to communicate and threw frequent temper tantrums when she couldn't make herself understood. Patricia discussed her concerns again with the pediatrician, who suggested a hearing test. Patricia arranged for an audiology evaluation at the local hearing and speech agency. The audiologist found that Brooke had normal hearing, and recommended a speech and language evaluation.

At the age of 2 years, 9 months, Brooke was seen for her first speech and language evaluation. The speech-language pathologist found that her receptive language abilities were within normal limits for her chronological age. However, her expressive speech and phonological development were extremely delayed. Brooke attempted to communicate using phrases but her speech was less than 10% intelligible. An extensive speech analysis found that she frequently deleted initial, medial,

and final consonants of words. The only consonant that was ever used consistently in words was /g/. She also used the semivowels and glides /w, j, h/. Her vowels were often distorted. An oral motor evaluation found that Brooke had difficulty imitating simple oral motor movements in nonspeech and speech activities but had normal oral motor skills when feeding. The speech-language pathologist diagnosed Brooke with a severe developmental apraxia of speech with an accompanying expressive language delay. Brooke was referred to the infant and toddlers program in her area to begin receiving home-based speech and language services. She was also enrolled in twice weekly therapy sessions at the speech and hearing agency.

Expressive Language Development Through AAC

Brooke's speech-language pathologist discussed therapy options with Patricia. Brooke was becoming increasingly frustrated at her inability to communicate and needed a way to develop expressive communication skills until her speech abilities improved. The speech-language pathologist suggested using sign language. Patricia was very concerned that if Brooke learned sign language, she would never learn to talk and would have to attend a school for children with hearing impairments. Patricia also worried that Brooke's grandparents and extended family would not be able to understand her signs.

Several sessions were spent discussing Patricia's concerns. During each session she would begin to see the need for an augmentative method of communication, then go home to discuss the issues with her husband and family. Each week, she would return to the next session with even more questions. The speech-language pathologist finally asked that both parents come together to the next session to discuss augmentative communication issues. During this session it was stressed that sign language would only be used to augment Brooke's existing speech abilities. It was pointed out to the family that Brooke was already supplementing her speech with naturally occurring gestures such as pointing, head nods, facial expressions, and a few idiosyncratic gestures that the family had developed. Speech therapy goals would also simultaneously focus on improving Brooke's oral motor abilities and speech. To assist with the decision-making process, the family was put in contact with the parent of an older child with developmental apraxia of speech who learned to communicate through sign language at an early age but was now talking. Patricia later said that discussing the issues with another parent who had been through the experience was helpful. Two months into the speech-language therapy process, Brooke's family decided that sign language could be used to augment her expressive language.

Brooke quickly learned functional single signs to express common wants and needs. *Eat, drink, apple, more, all-done, mommy, daddy, baby, sleep, open*, and *car* were rapidly learned within a few sessions. Once Patricia saw the effect of sign language on Brooke's communication abilities, she jumped into the AAC process

whole-heartedly. She enrolled in a sign language course at the local community college and began modeling sign phrases to Brooke across all daily activities. Brooke began to imitate the models and quickly learned to combine signs together into two and three word phrases. By the age of 3 years, 3 months, Brooke had a sign language vocabulary of over 100 words that she was using effectively at home. Once sign language skills were established, Brooke was prompted to simultaneously combine her existing speech with signs.

Brooke's speech-language pathologist also implemented a more traditional speech therapy program. Because of her young age, progress was slow. Brooke learned to imitate simple oral motor movements. She was able to smile and stick out her tongue on command. Sound imitation skills were still extremely limited. Brooke could put her lips together to produce an /m/ sound and an approximation of /b/. The therapist tried to have Brooke generalize these sounds to words without any success. A few new sounds began to appear in Brooke's spontaneous speech. She inconsistently produced /n/ and /d/ as consonant substitutions in the final position of words. Her intonation patterns also sounded more sentence-like. However, these changes did not significantly enhance her intelligibility because her message length was also simultaneously increasing. The few words that she could say in a single word context lost their intelligibility when embedded into a sentence. Brooke was still less than 10% intelligible.

AAC in Preschool

During the spring of Brooke's third year, the speech-language pathologist from the infant and toddler program began to discuss preschool options with the family. The local school district had a preschool classroom for children with severe communication impairments. The teacher and classroom aide used sign language and several children in the class relied on signs as their primary method of communication. Patricia made a trip to the school to observe the class before making a final decision. She liked the teacher and program but was concerned that most of the preschoolers did not understand language as well as Brooke. She was worried that Brooke would be bored in the class and wouldn't learn preschool skills that would be needed for kindergarten. Several service delivery options were discussed with the family. Patricia finally decided that Brooke would enroll in the communication preschool program three days each week, receiving her speech and language services as part of the classroom program.

Patricia still wanted Brooke to have an opportunity to interact with preschoolers from the neighborhood. She went to observe the preschool program at their neighborhood recreation center. The director of the center and the teacher were excited about the possibility of Brooke attending their program. However, they were concerned that they wouldn't be able to communicate with her because they didn't know sign language. Patricia decided to enroll Brooke in the neighborhood program two mornings each week. She would attend preschool with Brooke to act as her interpreter and to facilitate communication.

Brooke began preschool that fall when she was 3 years, 10 months old. Her sign language vocabulary had grown considerably. She was consistently signing three and four word sentences while simultaneously speaking. Over the summer, the original classroom teacher for the communication preschool classroom had been transferred. The new teacher knew some sign language, but could not understand all of Brooke's signs. Because her sign language knowledge was limited, the teacher had difficulty consistently modeling new signs and sentences to Brooke. The normal

frustrations of transitioning into a classroom were amplified for Brooke because of her inability to be understood by others.

Brooke was less frustrated in the neighborhood preschool program because her mother was present to interpret her signs. However, Brooke's reliance on her mother made it difficult for her to engage in interactions with classroom peers. Brooke tended to play with her mother, and did not seek attention from the teacher or other children. If Patricia invited other children into the play activity, Brooke would interact with them. Patricia would try to move away from the activity so Brooke could directly interact with the other children. As soon as Brooke noticed, she would leave the activity and go stand beside her mother.

The speech-language pathologist assigned to the preschool for children with communication disorders immediately noticed that Brooke's sign language vocabulary was beyond the teacher's signing abilities. She also noticed that the new teacher was not using picture-based methods of communication with any of the classroom children. She began meeting with the teacher to discuss using picture communication boards. Rather than overwhelming the teacher, it was decided to integrate a single picture communication board into one of the existing classroom language activities.

The next week, the speech-language pathologist conducted a cooking activity with the teacher and provided the children with a simple picture communication board to make requests for objects and actions. After several class sessions of modeling board use through communication activities, Brooke's teacher decided to make picture communication boards for other classroom activities. Resources related to engineering preschool classrooms with multiple activity-based picture communication displays were shared with the teacher, who began a collaborative process of developing communication boards.

As picture communication boards began appearing in the preschool class, Brooke's communication frustration decreased. Brooke continued to rely on her speech and signs as a primary method of communication, but if she wasn't understood, she could walk to a picture display and point to a picture to establish her communication topic. Once the topic was established, her teacher could usually figure out what Brooke wanted through a combination of speech, signs, and lots of yes/no questions. In October, Brooke's mother Patricia came to school for a Halloween party. Brooke's teacher had made a special picture communication board to use with the class for a face painting activity at the party. Patricia immediately realized that if Brooke had similar picture communication boards to use at her other preschool, she could independently interact with teachers and classroom peers. Patricia scheduled a meeting with the speech-language pathologist to discuss using picture communication boards at home and in the other preschool program. They decided to develop a picture communication book with activity-based pages for Brooke.

Brooke's mom never did anything halfway. Once she decided to create a picture communication system for Brooke, she immediately copied symbol materials from the school and developed vocabulary pages. Within 3 weeks, Brooke was using a picture communication book at home and at school. Initial attempts to create communication pages were not always thought out systematically. Symbol arrangements were often inconsistent and pictures were added to pages randomly. For example, the *teacher* picture symbol was in the upper right corner of some pages and along the left column of others. When the *snack-time* page filled up, additional food items were placed on the *coloring* page that came next. The speech-language pathologist worked with Brooke's

mother to systematically organize the communication book.

As Brooke's ability to use the picture communication book improved, her mother was able to reduce her role as a communication facilitator at the neighborhood preschool. Patricia would bring Brooke to school and stay for the first 30 minutes, then she would leave the room for the rest of the morning. Over several months, Brooke began to realize that the teachers and peers in her neighborhood preschool did not understand most of her signs. At that school, she used her speech, picture communication book, and a few signs that she knew her teachers understood. At home, Brooke relied completely on signs and speech. The picture communication book was only used if her mother prompted her to get it. In the communication preschool, Brooke relied on her speech and signs, but would supplement both modalities by frequently pointing to pictures in her book. By the end of the school year, Brooke had turned into a multimodal communicator who was aware of which modality was needed for different communication situations.

The Transition to High Tech AAC

Brooke's speech and language program at school remained focused on teaching sign language and picture communication skills throughout preschool. Her sign vocabulary increased and she was able to sequence signs together into sentences to communicate messages. Picture communication was used with those who did not understand her signs. Brooke also made moderate progress at improving her speech. She could imitate a wider range of speech sounds in the initial and final position of single syllables (/m, b, w, y, d, l, n, g/ and /ng/) but could not easily generalize the sounds to spontaneous words. She could produce voiceless sounds /p, f, t, k/ in isolation, but was unable to make the sounds in a syllable context. Her vowel approximations were improving but vowel productions were still distorted.

Near the end of 2 years of preschool, Brooke's speech could be understood over 50% of the time by her immediate family if the context of her communication was known. She achieved this intelligibility by reverting back to shorter two and three word phrases, and by slowing down her rate of speech. Brooke had also learned to produce a limited core of single words with intelligible phonemic approximations. These words were functional vocabulary that had been practiced over and over again. Although her word productions were not normal, most strangers could understand them in context.

Brooke was now ready for kindergarten. Although she continued to have a significant communication disorder, her family, school, and therapists felt that she should enroll in an inclusive kindergarten program at her neighborhood school. Many of the children from her community preschool program would be enrolling in the neighborhood kindergarten, which would provide her with peer support. The speech-language pathologist felt strongly that Brooke should begin using a voice output high tech AAC system in kindergarten. She felt that the larger class size, the teacher's inexperience with children who were nonspeaking, the teacher's lack of sign language skills, and Brooke's need to independently interact with other children warranted the need for a device that could talk. Brooke was referred to the AAC team within her county's school district for an evaluation.

The county's AAC team evaluated Brooke by reviewing information gathered by the school team. When Brooke was originally evaluated at the age of 2, her receptive language skills were normal for her age. However, standardized tests for 2-year-olds are primarily based on parent interviews, comprehension of single word vocabulary, and comprehension of simple commands. Now that Brooke was older and could be evaluated more thoroughly, her receptive language abilities showed significant scatter. Although many of her skills were within normal ranges for her age, there were several specific receptive skills such as understanding simple analogies, or following complex directions, that were difficult for her. These abilities needed to be taken into consideration in making the decision to use a complex high tech AAC system.

Brooke was observed by the school's AAC team interacting in her classroom program. They then met with Brooke's family and school team to discuss her communication needs and potential high tech AAC options. Brooke's language abilities dictated that she needed a device that organized and retrieved messages using picture symbols. The AAC system would need to provide her with enough vocabulary to function in a regular kindergarten classroom. She also needed a system that would let her begin to explore forming words through writing. Because Brooke was walking, the device needed to be portable so that it could be carried throughout the classroom.

After considering several different devices, the team decided that either a Dynavox 2C, or DeltaTalker would meet Brooke's AAC needs. Brooke was briefly evaluated by the AAC team to determine if she had the language skills necessary to use both devices. The Dynavox 2C has a touch screen that allows the user to select between multiple picture communication displays using a master menu. Because the Dynavox 2C could be set up similar to her existing picture communication book, Brooke quickly transitioned to it and within a few minutes was using it to communicate in a play activity. The DeltaTalker was programmed with Unity software. The DeltaTalker has a single fixed page of symbols that are sequenced together to create words. Light cues are provided to locate symbols for a given sequence. This device functioned very differently from Brooke's existing picture-based system. Brooke initially had difficulty remembering the symbol sequences. However, after 30 minutes of training, she was able to remember up to 10 two-symbol sequences to make simple requests in a play activity.

Trying to make a decision between the DeltaTalker and Dynavox 2C was like comparing apples and oranges. Although both systems were appropriate for her, they functioned very differently from one another. It was decided to let Brooke try each device for a 1-month trial before making any final decisions. Because the Dynavox 2C was immediately available, she tried that device first. Several of her existing picture communication book pages were programmed into the device. Brooke easily learned to use the device to communicate in specific play activities. The only disadvantage was that Brooke's communication was limited to what was previously programmed into the system by school staff. There were times when she wanted to communicate about other topics that weren't available in the system.

Brooke then had an opportunity to try the DeltaTalker with Unity software. The DeltaTalker was initially difficult for Brooke. The subtle receptive language difficulties that were found during her recent evaluation translated into difficulty remembering the symbol sequences. The speech-language pathologist worked with Brooke on the symbol sequences, teaching her specific vocabulary for functional activities, and rule-based vocabulary that used similar symbol sequences. By the end of the month, Brooke had learned 36 words and could combine some of them together into two-word phrases. Once Brooke caught onto the concept of rules for sequencing, she was able to learn new words within a rule-class relatively quickly.

Brooke's AAC team gathered together to discuss their final recommendations. Patricia had attended many of Brooke's therapy sessions during the trial AAC device loan period. She had an opportunity to see Brooke's progress with both devices. During the loan period, she had contacted local vendors for the products to get more information. She also contacted parents of other children who were using both devices. When the team came together, she was still confused about which device to choose. She had heard pros and cons about both systems, and was reluctant to select one device over the other. The speech-language pathologist helped Patricia make the final decision. Although Brooke had the potential to use both devices successfully, the transition into kindergarten and an inclusive environment was going to be difficult, especially in light of Brooke's newly discovered receptive language disabilities. It was felt that Brooke needed a device that would give her immediate success with a minimum of training. Because the Dynavox 2C could be set up identically to Brooke's existing picture communication book, the transition to a new communication system would be less difficult. The team discussed this option at length, and finally agreed to obtain a Dynavox 2C for Brooke to use in kindergarten.

To Kindergarten and Beyond

Brooke began kindergarten with her new Dynavox 2C. Patricia took responsibility for programming the device, and began by programming in all of the pages from Brooke's existing picture communication book. She then arranged to meet with Brooke's teacher and speech-language pathologist on a weekly basis to develop vocabulary for new pages. The speech-language pathologist was thrilled to be working with a parent who liked programming

AAC devices and encouraged her to volunteer at the school to program other AAC devices. Although Brooke's Dynavox 2C allowed her to communicate with her teacher and class peers, she often communicated using signs and gestures. Her teacher and speech-language pathologist decided to incorporate a classroom-based sign language training program for all of the kindergarten children. During morning circle time, the teacher introduced one or two new signs to all of the children. The sign vocabulary was related to the weekly teaching theme and students were encouraged to use the signs during classroom activities. This inclusive teaching method served two functions. It taught Brooke new sign vocabulary related to her classroom lessons, and it made the other students aware that Brooke's signs and gestures were communicative.

Throughout her kindergarten year, Brooke made steady progress using the Dynavox 2C and sign language in the school setting. She also continued with private speech therapy sessions focused on improving her speech. Her improvements in this modality came in small increments, but in time, speech became her primary method of communicating at home. In spite of this progress, Brooke's speech was still difficult for others to understand. Patricia realized that Brooke would need to use augmentative methods of communication for several years to come. Until Brooke's speech improved, AAC provided her with a means to communicate and participate in her school and community.

Key Points to Remember

• Children with severe developmental apraxia of speech need exposure to augmentative methods of communication at an early age. AAC can be used to strengthen underlying expressive language and communicative abilities while waiting for speech abilities to improve.

• Parents of children with apraxia of speech often have difficulty making the decision to use augmentative methods of communication. They often receive conflicting information from different professionals regarding treatment options. Discussing the issues with other parents is often helpful. Parents should be referred to support groups or introduced to other interested parents to help them work through the decision-making process.

• Young children need to be exposed to all potential modalities of communication. Speech, sign language, and picture-graphic methods of communication should be included in the child's therapy and classroom program. Teaching all three modalities ensures that the child will have the ability to communicate in the home, school, and community.

• Children with developmental apraxia of speech need intensive therapy services. Implementing augmentative methods of communication is a time-consuming process for professionals and families. In addition, these children need intensive therapy services to improve their oral-motor and speech abilities. Professionals need to create service delivery methods that can provide all of these intervention services.

• Most children with developmental apraxia of speech eventually rely on speech as their primary method of communication. Augmentative methods are naturally retired as spoken language abilities improve. When speech becomes the primary method of communication the child should still be monitored to determine if there are specific communicative environments that require AAC. It is important for the child to learn when to switch from speech to augmentative methods of communication, and which augmentative method to choose in a given situation.

Life Stories

Sam's AAC Story:
Autism and AAC

Sharon L. Glennen

Rachel knew that Sam was very different from her other children. Sam didn't speak, didn't seem to understand anything that was said to him, and enjoyed sitting on the floor spinning the wheels of his cars for hours on end. When Sam was 18 months old, his pediatrician suspected that he was severely retarded and referred the family to the infants and toddlers program in their area. Sam was evaluated and qualified for early intervention services with a diagnosis of severe communication delay. Rachel began attending a parent-child group sponsored by the infants and toddlers program to learn how to facilitate his language development. At those meetings, she realized that Sam did not act like the other children with communication delays. Most of them could understand some speech, whereas Sam acted as if he were deaf. Sam had strange behaviors that the other children didn't have. He flicked his fingers at the ceiling lights, spun objects over and over again, lined up blocks in neat rows, and screamed and held his ears when other children in the group cried.

Rachel brought Sam to a special autism program when he was 3 years old. She had already decided that Sam was autistic, based on information she absorbed from professionals the infants and toddlers program, and through reading articles and books. Professionals from the autism program simply confirmed the diagnosis that she had already made on her own. Sam's initial evaluations indicated that he was good at nonverbal visual skills. He could line up blocks in order from smallest to largest, match blocks onto pattern grids, and string beads into patterns.

Sam's receptive and expressive language abilities were severely impaired. The only spoken words that he responded to consistently were his name, *no* and *mommy*. Otherwise, he needed gesture cues to respond to simple commands such as *give it to me* or *sit down*. He vocalized using high pitched giggles when happy, and screamed when upset. When he wanted something, he simply went and got it himself. He sometimes used his mother to get him things that were out of his reach. For example, he would grab her by the hand and lead her to the refrigerator to get food, or to the back door to go outside. It was noted that he understood object and situation cues in his environment. Rachel reported that, if she put on her coat, Sam would go stand by the back door. If she started serving dinner onto plates, Sam would go sit at the table. Rachel noticed that Sam enjoyed looking at pictures in books. He would sit still for long periods of time staring at pictures before turning each page. She noted that he preferred looking at pictures of people's faces, and liked to look through her women's magazines to see the cosmetic ads because the faces were extra large on the page.

Shortly after Sam was seen in the autism program, he was evaluated by Bess, the AAC specialist in the infants and toddlers program. The communicative and perseverative behaviors that were noted in previous evaluations were certainly present during the first AAC evaluation. Initial attempts to explore Sam's ability to communicate using either pictures or sign language were unsuccessful. Bess discussed various AAC options and decided to implement a communication program consisting of both signs and picture symbols as an exploratory intervention. Because Sam would be entering a preschool program in 6 months, the goal of his AAC intervention program was to determine which AAC methods worked best. That information would then be used to create an AAC intervention plan for his preschool classroom.

AAC Assessment
Through Intervention

Rachel was taught four signs to use with Sam throughout his day at home. These were *more, all done, eat,* and *open.* She was shown how to model each sign within naturally occurring activities. Bess taught her how to create natural language training activities that would require him to produce the signs frequently. For example, instead of giving Sam his entire snack at once, Rachel was instructed to give him small pieces to prompt him to ask for more. Rachel was shown how to provide hand over hand guidance to assist Sam in imitating the signs. Sam quickly learned to imitate the signs, however he rarely initiated using any of the signs spontaneously.

A picture communication board was developed with photographs of four favorite play objects. Rachel was shown how to model pointing to the pictures during play activities, and how to physically guide Sam to point to the pictures to request them. Sam quickly learned that if he touched the board, he got an object that he wanted. However, he rarely looked at the pictures when pointing. He would glance at the real toy, then randomly slap his hand repeatedly on the picture board. Bess, his AAC specialist, noted that there was no incentive for Sam to discriminate which photograph he was touching since he was equally motivated to select all four items.

After several weeks without progress, Bess decided to use a modified version of the Picture Exchange Communication System (PECS) (Bondy & Frost, 1993). PECS was used to get Sam to make better discriminative choices between the pictures, and to understand that the pictures were communicative. She decided to separate the four photographs onto individual index cards, with each one mounted on different background colors. The cards were spread far enough apart so that Sam would have to make a deliberate choice between them. He was taught to pick up a card then hand it to his mother to get a play toy. Bess also replaced one of the four photographs with a photo of an object that wasn't motivating. Sam would need to begin to make choices between the four photographs to ensure that he requested an object that he really wanted.

Sam quickly adapted to the PECS format of making requests through the photographs. After several sessions, it was noted that he never selected the photograph related to the nonmotivating item. He also selected his favorite object more than 80% of the time. Bess noted that Sam rarely looked at the photographs before picking them up and giving them to his mother. She suspected that Sam had memorized the location of the favorite object card and was selecting it based on that information. She decided that Rachel should begin to vary the location and ordering of the photo cards from session to session. This would prompt Sam to look at the photos before making a choice. Initially, Sam had great difficulty when the photo cards were moved. He kept going back to the familiar location for his favorite object symbol card. When Rachel would give him the object he asked for (which was not the object he wanted), he would push it away. Rachel then physically guided Sam to the location of the preferred item. In time, Sam would habituate to the new location and consistently ask for the motivating object.

It took several weeks of consistent training, but gradually Sam began to visually scan through the photographs before selecting the symbol for his favorite object. Once Sam was able to ask for his favorite objects consistently, Bess began to systematically move the pictures closer together during training sessions until they were arranged into a simple communication board format. Sam was still selecting pictures and handing them to his mother to receive favorite objects. Bess decided to transition Sam back to simply pointing to the pictures. The four photographs were arranged on a communication board. Sam was given physical guidance to touch the pictures to receive his choice. Across several sessions Sam began to touch, then point to, the picture that he wanted to request.

Three months after the AAC program was implemented, it was obvious that Sam had learned to discriminate between the four photo choices to request preferred objects. He frequently pointed to his favorite object, and occasionally would point to one of the other preferred choices. Sam never pointed to the photo of the toy object that he didn't like. Throughout this 3-month period, Rachel consistently modeled the four signs that were selected for training. However, Sam rarely attended

to the sign models. When he did attend, he would sometimes imitate the sign with an approximation of the movement. Based upon his progress, Bess decided to expand the AAC picture communication training program and to reduce sign training down to a single sign that Sam could learn to produce by rote. Because he already pushed away objects that he didn't want, it was decided to focus on transferring the pushing movement into an *all done* gesture.

Bess then created a new photo communication board consisting of four food choices. Three of the choices were preferred snacks, and one of the choices was a snack that Sam always pushed away after smelling. Rachel was taught to implement the snack board at home. Because Sam was appropriately pointing to photographs on his toy board, it was hoped that he would transition quickly to the new communication pictures; however, success did not happen overnight. Sam initially didn't visually scan the pictures on the board. Additional visual cues were added and the pictures were spread further apart. The pictures were also placed directly in front of each food item. When Sam reached for the food, he was redirected back to the corresponding picture. Across 2 months of daily sessions, Sam gradually began making appropriate choices using the snack photographs.

Sam's symbolic AAC breakthrough came one day when he wanted a food item that wasn't on his communication board. After looking at the four food choice symbols, he led Rachel by the hand to a food coupons flyer that he had leafed through earlier in the day. He flipped through the pages until he found a photo of his favorite cereal and pointed to it. Although Rachel was ecstatic about Sam's spontaneous generalization to a new picture, Sam did not repeat the behavior again for several weeks. He gradually began to infrequently point to new photos in magazines, on signs, or in books to make requests.

Sam's progress at learning to produce by rote the *all done* sign was slow. Initially, Rachel tried to get him to use it across a variety of situations and contexts. Sam began to spontaneously produce the sign, but would use it indiscriminately whenever he was involved in a communicative exchange. He didn't appear to comprehend the meaning of the sign, nor when to use it appropriately. Bess then recommended modeling the sign in a single highly specific situation that could be repeated frequently. The *all done* sign was only modeled during manipulative play activities (i.e., coloring, clay, or form puzzles) that took place when he was sitting in his chair at his small table. After 2 minutes of play, Bess would model the *all done* sign and motion for Sam to get up from the chair. Play activities were gradually lengthened before Bess would model the sign and let Sam leave the table. Sam was prompted to imitate the sign before being excused. Bess then began to introduce activities that she knew would not be as motivating for him. Sam was allowed to imitate the *all done* sign and leave the table within a minute. After several weeks of daily sessions, Sam learned that the *all done* sign could be used to get up from the table. His mother was instructed to let him leave the table whenever the sign was produced spontaneously, even if he had just sat down. In time, Sam began discriminating when to make the sign at the table. When favorite activities were occurring, he would sit for several minutes before signing *all done*. Activities he didn't like resulted in an immediate request to leave. Although Sam could produce the sign independently at the table, he did not generalize it to any other contexts.

It was finally time to transition Sam into a preschool environment. Bess and Rachel worked with his new classroom team to develop an AAC intervention plan. Based upon his progress with signs and picture symbols at home, it was decided to continue using both methods in the classroom. However, picture symbols would be his primary method of communication. Because Sam had difficulty generalizing his communication skills to different symbols or situations, Bess worked with classroom staff to develop communication situations and a set of photo symbols that were similar to what he had already learned. It was decided to begin the school year working with the eight photo symbols that he had learned at home. Rachel provided the class with the toy objects from home that corresponded to his communication board. Once Sam learned to generalize his old set of photographs to new classroom situations, new symbols would be added to match classroom activities. The *all done* sign would be modeled during table activities in the classroom, with the goal of generalizing the sign to new activities once Sam became comfortable with the classroom routine.

Key Points to Remember

- Many children with autism have difficulty generalizing communication skills across multiple situations. They often have better initial success when communication skills are worked on in specific discrete contexts that occur frequently.
- Sam's preschool AAC program was developed to teach communication in specific situations, then gradually generalize to new situations. Initially, he was only exposed to familiar symbols in familiar routines. The school team then systematically introduced him to new symbols the context of familiar routines, and used familiar symbols within the context of new routines.
- Cause-effect communication occurs when a child understands that touching or doing something with a symbol gets the child what he or she wants. This level of

communication is relatively easy to train and does not require the ability to discriminate between symbols.

- Many children with autism have difficulty learning to make discriminations between symbol choices. When a child does not "know" a symbol, AAC training can be used to teach the symbol's concrete meaning through expressive language tasks. If a child is consistently rewarded with a particular item every time he or she touches a particular symbol choice, the child gradually learns to associate the symbol with the object.
- Many children with autism or severe mental retardation have difficulty learning to make visual discriminations between picture symbols. Multiple visual, tactile, locative, or auditory cues are often needed to assist with this process. Examples include mounting symbols onto separate cards with different background colors, keeping symbols in a specific locations that don't vary, or using voice output AAC systems to provide auditory feedback. These cues provide the child with additional information to make discriminations between choices. Once the child is able to use the cues to make appropriate choices, the cues can be gradually faded until the child is making discriminations with the picture symbol itself.
- Some children are never able to discriminate between picture symbols without additional cues. For these children, the cue itself becomes a symbol that represents the desired object or action. For example, one child with autism could successfully discriminate between four different symbols as long as they were always positioned in the same location on the communication board. When the symbols were moved, he lost the ability to discriminate between them. The location on the board was the "symbol" for the child.

Chapter 12

AAC AND INDIVIDUALS WITH SEVERE TO PROFOUND DISABILITIES

Stephen N. Calculator

Just as AAC is a relatively new field, the concept of providing instruction to individuals with severe to profound disabilities and expecting these individuals to be active participants in their communities continues to evolve. There remain vestiges of practices driven by beliefs that these individuals are best served in custodial programs where basic needs can be anticipated and responded to by others. For example, individuals may be "placed" in self-contained classrooms that purport to meet their special needs. This author questions how special these needs are, upon considering the rationale for placing a dozen or more other students in the same classroom, and exposing all to the same generic curriculum.

Rather than a formal curriculum, life skills such as toothbrushing, toileting, dressing, and survival skills may be taught. Much attention is paid to preskills such as prevocation, prewriting, and prereading (or, to be stylish, preliteracy). Eventually, these individuals find their way to a network of adult services that rarely build on, much less inquire about, the various "skills" that were addressed

through these individuals' first 18 to 21 years of life.

MOVING AWAY FROM CUSTODIAL CARE

Deviations from a custodial track began to arise in the 1960s, as training programs began to explore methods of integrating people with severe and profound disabilities into their communities (Blatt & Kaplan, 1966). Initially, only those who were "ready" were afforded the opportunity to participate in sheltered workshops and similar self-contained programs. Their peers remained in special programs where they were allegedly readied to join sheltered workshops at some future time.

In the early 1970s, normalization (a forerunner to the concept of least restrictive environment) was introduced by Wolfensberger (1972). It suddenly became popular to promote practices that prepared individuals for community life in group homes and similar residential and work environments.

Meanwhile, in the educational sphere, the passage of P.L. 94-142 heralded an era in which all handicapped children were entitled to a free and appropriate public education in the least restrictive environment (Education for All Handicapped Children Act, 1975). The first educational programs were driven by developmental theories that posited the need for children to acquire prerequisite skills along a developmental continuum. In many cases, learning these skills constituted the student's entire curriculum. Where a student was not viewed as "ready" for communication instruction, skills that were felt to be precursors to such training were addressed. For example, students received intensive instruction in vocal and motor imitation, object permanence, means-end, causality, and so forth. Vestiges of these practices remain prevalent today as professionals continue to buy computer software and design programs that target these skills.

On to Functional Skills

Moving to the late 1970s and early 1980s, a philosophic shift occurred in service provision to children and adults with severe and profound handicaps. The focus now became functional skills, defined as activities that would need to be performed by others if individuals failed to learn to perform the skills themselves (Brown et al., 1979; Brown, Nietupski, & Hamre-Nietupski, 1976). The shift to functional programming ushered in a new era characterized by the following practices (Jorgensen & Calculator, 1994):

1. Teach functional skills.
2. Teach skills in the environments in which they are ultimately expected to be performed (i.e., community-based instruction).
3. Use age-appropriate materials and tasks.
4. Provide systematic opportunities for integration with students without disabilities.

5. Promote participation in community activities.

As the 1980s came to a close, checklists of "best practices" emerged. Once again there was a primary emphasis on functional skills (Baine & Sobsey, 1983; Meyer, 1987; Thousand, 1987). Additional themes that emerged at this time included:

6. Age-appropriate placement in public schools.
7. Integrated delivery of educational and related services.
8. Systematic data-based instruction.
9. Home-school partnerships.
10. Team collaboration.

Changes in Communication Programming

Communication and AAC practices over this time period mirrored these broader directions in education and general practice. For example, the 1980s ushered in recommendations that communication programs should (a) be integrated into education, home life, and other aspects of daily living rather than constituting a separate program entity; (b) target functional skills that would enable individuals to participate more actively in community living; and (c) teach skills in natural environments (Yoder & Calculator, 1981).

INTEGRATION TO INCLUSION

As the 1980s came to a close, greater efforts were invested to integrate individuals with severe and profound disabilities into their communities. The concept of integration soon evolved to a perspective that valued "inclusion." Agencies that once strived to provide systematic opportunities for individuals to occasionally leave their special settings and participate in typical environments now examined ways of restructuring and even merging what were once two independent entities: regular education and special services (Forest, 1989; Gartner & Lipsky, 1987; O'Brien & Forest; 1989; Sizer, 1992; Strully & Strully, 1985; Thousand & Villa, 1992; West, 1990).

Once again, the progression to inclusive practices spawned changes in communication and AAC services as well. Calculator (1994a) recommended viewing AAC as a support for interaction and inclusion, as opposed to a discrete area of the curriculum. Mirenda and Calculator (1993) suggested that AAC instruction for school-aged children with severe and profound disabilities should:

- Be carried out in regular classrooms and other natural environments.
- Be structured to promote natural interactions between students both with and without disabilities.
- Be carried out by a variety of individuals including instructors, classmates, family members, and others, rather than being within the exclusive realm of the speech-language pathologist.

GOALS OF AAC INSTRUCTION

The inclusion perspective forces us to examine the effectiveness of AAC programs very differently than past methods dictated. For example, programs that were, or continue to be, driven by a developmental perspective may cite positive outcomes such as (a) Tom's average length of message has progressed from 1.3 to 1.8 symbols; (b) Sarah's communication display has primarily been changed from photographs and pictures to line drawings; (c) the average latency of Tim's response in activating a switch to operate a battery-operated toy has diminished by 30 seconds.

Practitioners who operate from an inclusion perspective question whether any of these changes are necessarily associated with positive AAC outcomes relative to an individual's presence in their community. They point out that it is no longer enough to consider an outcome important just because it represents a statistically significant change in performance relative to baseline functioning. Changes are examined with respect to their significance to individuals' lives, or, social validity (Baer, Wolf, & Risley, 1987; Brown & Lehr, 1993; Kazdin, 1977). Practitioners are encouraged to solicit opinions from teachers, parents, and others about the value of a student's change in communication performance.

Positive outcomes of AAC may be measured in a variety of ways (Calculator, 1994a). Table 12–1 lists some of these outcome-based measures. AAC outcomes can be determined by noting positive changes in the attitudes of teachers, classmates, co-workers, and others toward the individual. Impressions can be gathered informally, through interview, or more formally through the use of different sociometric scales. Other measures involve documenting the increased frequency of natural, spontaneous interactions initiated toward the individual by persons either disabled or nondisabled. Particularly significant are interactions with individuals who are not paid to do so, such as co-workers, friends, and other peers. Professionals can also measure increases in the amount of time an individual spends in inclusive settings and changes in active participation in those settings. Changes in the frequency of opportunities for communication, increases in the range of inclusive settings that provide interaction opportunities, and increases in the number of available communication partners can also be documented as positive outcomes.

Another measurement of communication outcomes is to document increased use of positive social behaviors, often in-

Table 12–1. Positive outcome goals for AAC instruction.

- Positive changes in attitudes of communication partners.
- Increased spontaneous interactions with partners.
- Increased opportunities for communication.
- Increases in the variety of communication partners.
- Increased time spent in inclusive settings.
- Increased range of inclusive settings available for communication.
- Active participation within inclusive settings.
- Increased use of positive social behaviors with decreases in challenging behaviors.
- Increased opportunities for decision making.
- Indications of enhanced status and acceptance by others.
- Reductions in the number of unsuccessful communicative interactions.
- Improvements in the availability and accessibility of AAC.
- Increases in the number of partners taking responsibility for management of AAC.
- Changes in listener responsiveness to unaided and aided communication.
- Increases in listener encouragement to use AAC to assist with communication breakdowns.

Source: From: "Communicative Intervention as a Means to Successful Inclusion," by S. Calculator, 1994, in S. Calculator and C. Jorgensen (Eds.), *Including Students with Severe Disabilities in Schools: Fostering Communication, Interaction and Participation* (pp. 188-190), San Diego, CA: Singular Publishing Group, Inc. Copyright 1994 by Singular Publishing Group. Adapted with permission.

corporating AAC methods, with concomitant decreases in challenging behaviors such as crying, tantrums, self-injury, and aggression. After identifying the functions challenging behaviors serve for individuals, such as obtaining desired objects, gaining attention, and escaping from unpleasant activities, AAC methods can be introduced as replacements for these behaviors (Donnellan, Mirenda, Mesaros, & Fassbender, 1984; Reichle & Johnston, 1993). As Durand (1993) pointed out, it is essential that the form of communication taught match the functions of the challenging behavior and evoke the same consequences as the challenging behavior. The replacement behavior should potentially be more efficient and equally effective as the behavior being replaced. It should se-cure the desired response for the individual and require no greater effort than the challenging behavior it is replacing.

Another positive communication outcome is the ability of individuals who are nonspeaking to have greater choice, control, and responsibility for events and decisions affecting them. This might include making decisions regarding how they dress, where and with whom they play, what classes they take, what jobs they take, with whom they work, who serves as their aide or personal care assistant, and so forth. With more responsibility for decision making, changes in the perceptions and actions of communication partners are often noted. Indications that partners view an individual who is nonspeaking with enhanced status and accept the individual more readily are measurements of positive communicative and social change. Reports of diminished frequency of episodes associated with unsuccessful communicative interactions is a measure of change from the perspective of both the listener and individual who is nonspeaking.

Finally, evidence that partners are increasingly accepting of an individual's AAC system is a positive outcome that can be measured by noting changes in the availability and accessibility of AAC technology; the range of individuals who assume responsibility for assisting and managing AAC equipment; active encouragement from listeners to use AAC methods to manage communication breakdowns; and a listener's responsiveness to messages involving aided and unaided AAC.

Having introduced a perspective for identifying and addressing the AAC needs of individuals with severe and profound disabilities, we now delve into additional issues germane to this population. The author begins by defining the population and pointing out special AAC concerns and considerations that arise when supporting this population. Next, assessment and intervention strategies are presented, with a focus on informal procedures that can be implemented in various natural environments.

DESCRIPTION OF THE POPULATION

The principle of inclusion has been embraced nationally, however its actual implementation has proved elusive to many. It has been suggested that students with severe disabilities remain the most segregated group in American public schools (Danielson & Bellamy, 1989; McDonnell & Hardman, 1989).

Calculator (1994b) pointed out that educators and others risk experiencing an "inclusion delusion" (p. xxv) when they lack the resources or the willingness, or

both, to implement principles consistent with this model. McLean (1993) expressed this by commenting that, at the current time, our deeds do not match the promise of our laws or our language. He pointed out that philosophies and values are useful in setting targets for individuals, but provide little information about how to achieve these ends.

The extent to which individuals with severe to profound disabilities can be successfully included in society depends heavily on the ability of others to identify and then respond to their individualized needs for special modifications and adaptations to otherwise natural settings and contexts. Gold (1980) suggested that the height of individuals' functioning is not determined biologically but instead by the type and magnitude of supports society is willing to allocate to assist them.

The population of children and adults with severe disabilities comprises individuals whose needs and abilities are constantly changing. The nature and extent of their needs for communication intervention are determined largely by the resources that are available to them, and the effectiveness with which these resources are meted out.

AAC supports that are consistent with inclusive practices will be discussed later in this chapter. First, we define this population a bit more specifically.

The National Joint Committee for Meeting the Communicative Needs of Persons with Severe Disabilities (1992) suggested that the term *severe disabilities* refers to a heterogeneous group of individuals that includes those with severe to profound mental retardation, autism, and other disorders that result in severe sociocommunicative and cognitive communicative impairments. The population may also include persons with physical disabilities, dual sensory impairments, and individuals previously identified as multiply handicapped. It is thus a population whose diagnostic label provides minimal information about individual needs, learning styles, and competencies. These can only be determined through comprehensive, longitudinal assessments as described later in this chapter.

AAC CONCERNS AND ISSUES RELATED TO PERSONS WITH SEVERE TO PROFOUND DISABILITIES

Material in this section should be consistent with principles discussed elsewhere in this book, with some special twists. General principles will be noted here, with additional discussion to follow in the subsequent assessment and intervention section of this chapter.

AAC Candidacy Criteria

There is one circumstance that would preclude the introduction of AAC to individuals with severe to profound disabilities: the fact that their immediate and projected communicative needs are being adequately met with their present methods of communication. This is not a simple determination, nor one that should be made until all necessary information is compiled and discussed by the team.

AAC needs cannot be determined by a single individual, whether that is a parent, employer, teacher, sibling, or other. Part of the assessment process should consist of interviews and supplementary observations of the individual communicating with different partners. A perceived lack of need for AAC may result from a situation in which an individual's communication needs are being anticipated or unwittingly circumvented. Given this situation, it may be concluded that the existing system of communication is satisfactory. The social context may need to be changed by introducing new friends and acquaintances as

communication partners, increasing a partner's communication expectations, and providing more opportunities for individuals to make choices and decisions. As communication opportunities and experiences change, the inadequacy of an individual's present methods of communication may be revealed and candidacy for AAC may be revisited. Chapter 5 provides additional information on the needs assessment process.

In summary, candidacy determination should be a dynamic and longitudinal process. The communicative needs of an individual change with different partners and in different settings. Similarly, new experiences, interests, work opportunities, living arrangements, and future goals may be a basis for re-examining an individual's candidacy for AAC.

Zero Exclusion Policy

Every child or adult referred for an AAC assessment is a potential candidate for AAC. As discussed in Chapters 3, 4, and 6, AAC entails a broad range of output and input modes, symbol systems, accessing strategies, and so forth, each of which presupposes certain cognitive, physical, and social-emotional skills. The critical point remains that the field now presents a sufficient range of options to be a source of benefit for any individual whose current communication needs are not met sufficiently. Despite these views, candidacy criteria for AAC intervention still exists. On some occasions, a physical disability is viewed as so severe that an access mode cannot be identified. On others, limited cognitive abilities exclude individuals from consideration for AAC intervention. It is the author's contention that such restrictions on candidacy do not reflect AAC user incompetencies but instead reflect limited resources, inadequate knowledge, and attitudinal and policy barriers that are fabricated and perpetuated by society.

Cognitive Prerequisites and Discrepancy Formulas. There is a growing body of literature that questions the relevance of cognitive abilities, particularly those that have previously been cited as prerequisites to communicative functioning, such as object permanence, causality, imitation, and means-end behavior (Casby, 1992; Cole, Dale, & Mills, 1990; Kangas & Lloyd, 1988; Miller, Chapman, & Bedrosian, 1977). These authors have questioned the rationale for teaching these skills directly, prior to in-troducing communication training.

It has been the author's experience that communication instruction can provide an excellent medium for concurrently addressing these cognitive abilities. For example, a child may demonstrate a lack of understanding of means-ends behavior, indicated by a failure to seek out adults to satisfy basic wants and needs. This limitation could be addressed within a communication framework in several ways:

- Encouraging potential partners to present more opportunities and reasons for the child to communicate.
- Increasing others' responsiveness to the child's communication attempts, making certain that their behaviors are contingent on the behavior of the child. Here it is critical that listeners be aware of the communicative function of each message produced by the child.
- Modeling and prompting communicative behaviors that are within the child's immediate or prospective grasp.

Casby (1992) reported that 31 of 50 states in the United States continue to use cognitive prerequisites, discrepancy formulas, or both to determine students' eligibility for communication instruction. When employing discrepancy formulas, service eligibility is determined on the basis of significant gaps between an individual's language and intellectual ability. For example, students may not be eligible for services unless their overall language skills fall a minimum of 1.5 standard deviations below the mean for their mental age. Where gaps do not exist, or are not of sufficient magnitude, instruction is deemed to be unwarranted. Cutoff scores vary from state to state, with some locations going so far as to specify the particular tests used to make these determinations. These practices persist despite cautionary advice from the American Speech-Language-Hearing Association (Committee on Language Learning Disorders, 1989).

Speech-language pathologists should assume leadership in changing outdated policies that deny services to individuals on the basis of erroneous assumptions. Certainly this would be a battle that parents and advocates would support, either through pressure to enact new legislation or acts of litigation.

MULTIPLE MODES OF COMMUNICATION

AAC as a Misnomer?

Just as all individuals with severe to profound disabilities are assumed to be capable of benefiting from AAC intervention, all individuals are assumed to be communicating prior to considering AAC options. It is the quality of their existing methods of communication that prompts deliberations about AAC. Candidates for AAC are not viewed as individuals who lack a present means of communication. Instead, their need for AAC arises because their existing communication methods lack effectiveness in meeting present or projected communication needs.

The introduction of AAC usually complements and augments an individual's existing means of communication. On some occasions, most notably those in which individuals rely on challenging behaviors to convey communicative functions, alternative methods of communication may be introduced. However, these individuals also typically possess other preexisting communicative behaviors that remain an effective means by which they can continue to communicate with some partners, in some situations, following the introduction of AAC. Additional AAC options can then be offered to enhance their success in communicating with the same and other partners in different situations.

Because the acronym AAC connotes augmentative and alternative communication, some practitioners may provide services that suggest they view candidates as falling into two different groups: those in need of supplementing, as opposed to those needing to replace, existing methods of communication. As already indicated, all individuals should be expected to possess some effective means of communication that should be integrated into the use of new AAC methods. Still, there are situations that suggest the need for alternate forms of communication, some of which have already been discussed.

Situations Calling for Alternative Means of Communication

As discussed earlier, an alternative communicative behavior may be considered when the present method of expression involves the use of challenging behaviors. Other conditions that have been cited (Calculator, 1994c; Reichle, Feeley, & Johnston, 1993) as reasons to teach alternative communicative behaviors to replace existing communication include the following:

1. The behavior is socially unacceptable (e.g., throwing a plate on the floor to indicate one is finished eating and would like to leave the table).
2. The behavior involves the controlled use of an undesired reflex (e.g., using an asymmetric tonic neck reflex to extend one's arm toward a desired object).
3. The behavior is tiring for the student (e.g., picture pointing requires tremendous effort, leaving the individual exhausted after a brief interaction).
4. The behavior is so idiosyncratic that even familiar listeners find it ambiguous, and are unable to respond contingently.
5. The behavior is potentially harmful to the individual and/or others (e.g., self-abuse and aggression).
6. The behavior is relatively inefficient and ineffective, placing undue stress on the message sender and receiver.

Modes for All Occasions

AAC efforts should include identifying effective methods of communication in different contexts and then promoting an individual's use of these methods across all settings and contexts. When a particular method of communication is ineffective, the individual should have access to other modes. Ideally and over time the cue for using a particular augmentative or alternative communication mode should be internalized. Upon realizing that a certain AAC method results in an unfavorable consequence, the individual should spontaneously resort to another AAC method from his or her repertoire. This is preferable to external prompting and cajoling by a clinician, teacher, or peer to use their AAC system. Ideally, individuals relying on AAC must recognize when to use their aided systems to avoid communication breakdowns, and when to shift to and away from these systems to repair conversational breakdowns.

ROLE OF THE ENVIRONMENT

The environment plays a particularly significant role in AAC activities with this population; this is discussed in greater detail in the next section dealing with assessment. In the course of providing AAC consultations, the author has been confronted with a particularly troublesome situation on many occasions. It was frequently noted that the settings themselves did not support or value communication. Opportunities for individuals to communicate were rare. Instead, staff anticipated an individual's wants and needs, rarely moved close enough to provide opportunities for using a communication system, and rarely made AAC systems accessible to individuals. When individuals attempted to communicate, their messages were typically ignored and/or they were redirected to another activity chosen by the staff.

Such situations require AAC interventions aimed at potential partners and policymakers, with minimal initial attention paid directly to the prospective AAC user. Unless and until an environment that supports communication is established, efforts to develop AAC skills will be unsupported and quickly extinguished, either wittingly or unwittingly. Rather than investing resources on systems and instruction, AAC specialists and others need to collaborate to effect changes in the environments in which individuals participate. Such efforts may extend to recommending changes of educational placement, staffing, employment, and residence.

The author has been involved in several situations in which AAC assessments were suddenly terminated, and staff notified that, under the circumstances, a communication assessment for an individual was premature. These included cases in which a child was being encouraged to use a communication board with partners who were unable to see or understand the symbols, a man who was hit by several of his peers when he attempted to engage them in interaction, and a young girl in a self-contained classroom in which the levels of noise and chaos precluded interaction.

Rather than proceed with the assessment as planned, time was spent with staff discussing factors that contributed to and detracted from a positive social environment. A plan was developed in each case and individual responsibilities assigned to progress toward creating environments that were more supportive of communication. Staff were encouraged to monitor changes in each individual's communicative behavior as they altered the environment. This dynamic assessment process served as the prelude to later assessments of the individuals and their respective environments.

SELF-DETERMINATION

Individuals with severe to profound disabilities have often been described as passive. The term underfunctioning is also used frequently to describe a commonly observed pattern in which these individuals rely on others to anticipate and meet their needs, rather than acting on their own behalf, despite evidence of their ability to do so. The likelihood that such behaviors are biologically determined is minimal. Instead, individuals may adopt these styles of behavior in response to participating in instructional, residential, and employment contexts that fail to promote or reward their attempts at decision making.

Self-determination implies that these individuals operate as consumers, making their own decisions and choices rather than agreeing to options preselected by well-meaning professionals and others. Individuals are encouraged to assume roles as change agents for themselves. Table 12–2 provides examples of AAC activities designed to promote self-determination. Although examples are presented separately for children and adults, there is certainly overlap in implementing these activities across the life span.

Table 12–2. Examples of AAC activities that promote self-determination in children and adults with severe to profound disabilities.

Children

1. Assigning chores and responsibilities that benefit them personally, as well as others (e.g., their classmates).
2. Shopping for their own clothing.
3. Identifying children with whom they would like to establish friendships.
4. Inviting other children to their homes.
5. Participating in active planning processes.
6. Selecting elective classes.
7. Negotiating their way into an ongoing group activity.
8. Instructing others how to use their AAC system.
9. Protesting when a decision is made for them without first soliciting their input.

Adults

1. Determining who is and is not able to visit them at home.
2. Determining who lives with them.
3. Actively participating in the process of interviewing a prospective personal care assistant or aide.
4. Developing a weekly menu.
5. Decorating their own room.
6. Scheduling their own medical and other personal appointments.
7. Indicating job preferences.
8. Indicating the types of physical and emotional support from others that they do and do not find helpful.

Self-Determination for Children

One method of self-determination for children is to assign chores or responsibilities that benefit the individual personally. These assignments can also benefit peers or other partners in the communication environment. For example, each day Tommy is asked to match photographs of his teacher and paraprofessionals to jobs with which he requires their adult assistance. Sarah is offered a choice of a sponge or a washcloth, and is then assisted in cleaning her work area.

Shopping for clothing can also provide self-determination for nonspeaking individuals. For example, colored pictures of Looney Tunes characters are placed on Megan's communication board. Each time she indicates one of the pictures, larger glossy prints of that character are presented and a brief cartoon is viewed. A classmate records the picture that Megan points to most frequently. At the end of the day, Megan brings a note home to her parents indicating that if they are thinking about buying a new tee shirt, Megan has a preference for the Tasmanian Devil.

Individuals can also indicate which persons they would like to have as friends. For example, Reggie is encouraged to use his AAC device to indicate to his aide the student he would like to be positioned next to during circle time. Tiffany is encouraged to use her communication book to indicate that she is unhappy with her present location, and her wish to be positioned elsewhere in the classroom. This can be expanded to inviting friends for a home visit. Todd is encouraged to approach several classmates and then activate a prerecorded invitation to a party at his home. Todd's mother has already contacted the respective students' families to inform them about the party.

Individuals who are nonspeaking can also participate in active planning processes. Items necessary for William and two other classmates to complete a task are purposely not provided by the teacher. The classmates are encouraged to use William's communication board to correct this situation. Following their modeling, William also requests the necessary materials. Planning and decision making can also extend to selecting elective classes. Jessie meets with the high school guidance counselor and indicates that she would prefer to participate in the horticulture class, rather than food preparation. In advance of this meeting, Jesse visited each setting and staff observed her relative interest in activities in each class.

Children can also learn to negotiate their way into ongoing group activities. Terry is encouraged to approach a small group of children, one of whom has been recruited as a confederate, and ask to join their game of kickball. Learning to protest when a decision is made for them without first soliciting their input is also an important step in acquiring self-determination. Sandra's aide is asked to interrupt activities that Sandra is obviously enjoying two times each day. Initially, a classmate is recruited to physically prompt Sandra to point to a message asking that she be allowed to continue what she was doing. The aide then complies with Sandra's request.

Self-determination can also be developed by teaching children to instruct others in how to use their AAC system. Molly is taught to begin each interaction with a greeting, and then to call her listener's attention

to a brief set of directions on her wheelchair tray explaining how she communicates.

Self-Determination for Adults

Adults can also learn to make decisions and determine outcomes for themselves. Determining who is and is not able to visit them at their home is one method of increasing self-determination. For example, Helen's staff is reminded to always notify her in advance of visitors. Once they arrive, visitors are informed that they must ask Helen's permission to go to her room; otherwise they are expected to remain in the common area of the group home. Adults can also play a role in determining who lives with them. Staff meet to talk about the types of people Ann appears to be drawn to versus those she tends to avoid. Qualities of prospective roommates are listed in order to use this information as a basis for identifying a support person to live with Ann in an apartment.

Adults should be allowed to actively participate in the process of interviewing a prospective personal care assistant or aide. A series of questions are prerecorded on Sheila's communication device prior to a prospective candidate arriving at her home. Messages that give information about Sheila's interests, experiences, and needs are also available. Within the home setting, the process of developing a weekly menu or decorating a room can be implemented. For example, pictures corresponding to different food choices are presented two at a time, and Sam indicates his choices. He then affixes the pictures to a weekly calendar to create a menu. Five possible bedspreads are presented to Marie, two at a time, and Marie reaches for her preference.

Within community interactions, adults can schedule their own medical and other personal appointments. For example, three people will be coming to Tom's house on Tuesday. He is given the opportunity to indicate the order of their visits. Adults can also indicate job preferences. Susan arrives at work each day and is provided with a communication board arranged with job tasks. She is asked to select what work she would like to complete that day. Self-determination also involves indicating the types of physical and emotional support from others that adults do and do not find helpful. Paul is encouraged to be more explicit when he asks for assistance from others.

NATURAL SUPPORTS

Jorgensen (1992) argued that if the long-term goal for an individual with severe to profound disabilities is to eventually live and work in inclusive, typical settings, then instructional approaches should draw upon resources available to individuals who are nondisabled. In the case of a student with severe disabilities, the primary or sole source of support may be a personal aide. All others defer to this delegated expert to manage the student's needs during the school day. This contrasts markedly from typical students who are often able to obtain support and assistance from their peers.

An approach using natural supports might take the form of the school speech-language pathologist consulting with the regular education teacher and others about how to communicate effectively with the individual. Other professionals might collaborate with the classroom teacher to identify equipment needs, alternative or adapted curricula, and instructional methods, such as cooperative learning, that would foster the child's participation at school. Classmates would be instructed how to program the AAC system, with the individual's permission.

In identifying natural supports, it has been suggested that the process begin by delineating resources that are readily available in a particular setting. Depend-

ing on the nature of the situation, one might then progress up a hierarchy from least to progressively more intrusive supports (Jorgensen, 1992). Applying this model, support might first be sought from classmates or co-workers, progress to teachers and employers, and, under extreme circumstances, involve other professional staff. Supports from professionals such as speech-language pathologists are generally offered in the form of consultation to others who are in direct contact with the individuals.

AAC ASSESSMENT AND INTERVENTION STRATEGIES FOR INDIVIDUALS WITH SEVERE TO PROFOUND DISABILITIES

Teaming

In light of the diversity and magnitude of their needs, individuals with severe to profound disabilities require comprehensive, integrated programs supported by professionals and others representing multiple disciplines. Where the competence necessary to address a particular concern is unavailable in the core team, professionals should refer clients and their families to the appropriate sources. Ultimately, all information gleaned can be shared and then acted on by the team. It should not be forgotten that the most significant members of the team are the client and his or her family or support staff. Input and ongoing feedback must be solicited from these individuals throughout the assessment and intervention process if we are to provide services that will stand the test of social validation.

The remainder of this section will focus on the role of the professional in the assessment and intervention process. The reader is referred to Chapter 2 for more information regarding teaming and service delivery.

Getting to Know the Student

The assessment process should begin with systematic efforts to become familiar with the individual— past, present, and future. Individuals with severe to profound disabilities often receive disjointed services that vary with the whims and personal priorities of different service providers who are transients in their lives.

Several procedures have been introduced recently to help team members learn about individuals, their instructional priorities, and their long-term goals. Three of these procedures, M.A.P.S., Personal Futures Planning, and C.O.A.C.H. are described next. Material presented here applies to assessment and intervention as these are continuous, intertwined processes.

M.A.P.S.

The McGill Action Planning System, or M.A.P.S. (Vandercook, York, & Forest, 1989), entails a process by which an individual and his or her support personnel, family, and friends identify supports and procedures for including the individual in school and other settings. The process begins by having participants answer the question, "Who is this person?" Strengths, likes, and dislikes are identified. This information is later supplemented with the results of formal evaluations. However, at this stage of the process discussion is informal and special terminology is avoided.

Next, the educational, medical, and family history of the individual is reviewed. Participants discuss where the individual came from, critical experiences in the person's life, and the relevance of this information to future planning.

The M.A.P.S. process then involves a discussion pertaining to the dreams of this individual, parents, care providers, and others. Discussions can provide an invaluable source of long-range goals that cross

traditional disciplinary boundaries, such as the desire to live independently, to find a paying job, to make friends, and to acquire certain skills and hobbies, among other goals.

Next, the group discusses the individual's nightmare, or, what may happen if the dream does not come true. Frequent themes that arise at this stage include fears that the individual will be institutionalized, have no friends, be neglected, and have no say in events imposed on him.

Special abilities possessed by the individual are then discussed, again relative to fostering increased participation and inclusion in the community and elsewhere. Supports that would facilitate this process are also identified, first in terms of immediate needs and then relative to the individual's long-term dreams. Specific roles and responsibilities are delegated to different team members in order to effect the desired outcomes.

Based on the M.A.P.S. process and supplementary interviewing and observation, the team might assume responsibilities such as:

1. Linking up the child with a "Big Brother" or "Big Sister" to assist in expanding the array of places and activities experienced by the child. These become contexts and settings for AAC intervention, in that they provide changing environments that afford opportunities for communication. The speech-language pathologist can provide consultation to the volunteer regarding communication and methods of promoting self-determination through communication.

2. Making certain that vocabulary stored on the communication aid is up to date, and affords opportunities for the individual to share information that is relevant in different settings.

3. Structuring opportunities for the individual to make choices, indicate preferences, and provide input to group decisions.

4. Collaborating with the classroom teacher and others in identifying curriculum and other modifications that are necessary to foster participation and inclusion of the individual. For example, this might include developing overlays for the communication board that are subject-specific for the different classes and routines the individual participates in from one day to the next.

5. Collaborating with the classroom teacher and others to identify adaptive equipment that will foster inclusion and participation opportunities.

6. Encouraging the individual to assume responsibility for maintaining the AAC device in good working order (e.g., by letting others know when there is a problem and, to the extent they are able to do so, describing the nature of the problem).

7. Modeling appropriate methods of interacting with the individual, and encouraging/praising others for doing so. Ideally, this would occur in classrooms and other natural settings.

8. Fostering friendships and relationships. For one student at a local high school, this took the form of professionals operating in a matchmaking capacity. A young man was assisted in inviting a sophomore to his junior prom. Photographs taken at the prom served as topic setters and the substance of conversations for several weeks following this event!

Personal Futures Planning (Mount, 1987; Mount & Zwernik, 1988)

Like M.A.P.S., Personal Futures Planning begins with discussions of the individual's past, progresses to descriptions of present abilities, interests, and activities, and culminates with individuals and their families expressing their goals or dreams for the individual. Whereas the M.A.P.S. process generally consists of one or two meetings and follow-up, Personal Futures Planning involves a more protracted process. A support network is formed and expanded over time as new participants are added to the process. Roles of participants in helping to support the individual are delineated, along with activities to achieve goals that are short- and long-term priorities for the individual. Progress is reviewed over time.

Choosing Options and Accommodations for Children (C.O.A.C.H.)

Unlike the preceding processes, C.O.A.C.H. is a family-centered procedure that serves as a prescriptive tool in developing a student's Individualized Education Plan (IEP) (Giangreco, Cloninger, & Iverson, 1993). Family members and others are interviewed to identify present educational needs and long-term visions for the student. A document similar to an I.E.P. is developed as broad, discipline-free goals are refined in the form of short-term objectives for the school year. Persons are identified to implement different phases of the program and, perhaps what is most unique about the process, program content is defined in the form of a personalized curriculum that can be implemented in regular classrooms and other settings.

The Program Development Process

Jorgensen (1994) described a series of steps that can be used to get to know students and to begin the program development process. These procedures, summarized in Table 12–3, incorporate principles from the three processes described.

Step One. At Step One of the program development process, the individual's prior experiences with AAC are discussed. The team reviews prior roles and responsibilities of the individual, family members, and other sources of support in AAC instruction and use. The relative effectiveness with which the individual and others use different AAC systems is reviewed, and ra-

Table 12–3. An individualized inclusion oriented program development process.

Step 1. Describe the individual's abilities and needs by using M.A.P.S., Personal Futures Planning, the C.O.A.C.H., or a similar device. Supplement with interviews and observations of the individual, peers, and others.

Step 2. Identify barriers to inclusion and develop plans and timelines to address those barriers.

Step 3. Develop a process for facilitating friendships and natural supports.

Step 4. Choose priority learning goals for the year.

Step 5. Specify how the individual will participate in different settings and revise needs for support in each setting.

Step 6. Develop short-term objectives based on observation of the student's current skills, discrepancy analysis, formal testing, and other means.

Step 7. Develop teaching and curriculum modifications based on the individual's learning style and others interaction styles. Revise regularly, depending on changing needs and opportunities.

Step 8. Evaluate the quality of inclusion and effectiveness of instruction in helping the individual to achieve priority learning outcomes. The role of the AAC system in promoting versus unwittingly impeding inclusion and full participation should be reviewed systematically and longitudinally.

Source: From "Developing Individualized Inclusive Educational Programs," by C. Jorgensen, (1994), in S. Calculator and C. Jorgensen (Eds.), *Including Students with Severe Disabilities in Schools: Fostering Communication, Interaction, and Participation* (p. 36), San Diego, CA: Singular Publishing Group, Inc. Copyright 1994 by Singular Publishing Group. Adapted with permission.

tionales for moving from one system to another are discussed. The team identifies current communication abilities and challenges facing the individual.

Step Two. Barriers to inclusion are identified, and plans to address those barriers are developed in Step Two. Several barriers that are specific to AAC commonly arise. Frequently there is an inappropriate number of support staff. On some occasions there may be an insufficient number of staff members. However, the more common scenario involves ample or even excessive numbers of staff members available, with inefficient use of these resources. The author has visited classrooms in which natural supports are supplemented by two or more aides who are assigned to individual children. The aides are not viewed as classroom supports, but instead are limited in their responsibilities to serving specific students. Although they are physically present, they may be of little help in meeting the broader needs of the classroom teacher. Other programs have determined that it is both necessary and preferable to employ fewer staff, rely more on natural supports, and consider all resources as available to *all* students.

Another barrier is the need for inservice training of staff, family members, friends, and others at school, home, and the worksite regarding effective interaction strategies. This can also be negatively impacted by a lack of opportunities, reasons, and places for the individual to communicate. In addition, there may be a limited number of people with whom the individual has the opportunity and desire to communicate. The need to identify funding sources for the possible purchase of AAC devices and other adaptive equipment is also an often identified barrier to inclusion.

Step Three. In Step Three of the program development process, means of facilitating friendships and natural supports are developed. AAC efforts might include discussions about how to engineer environments to promote increased interactions between the individual and peers who are nondisabled. Activities that are enjoyable to the individual and projected to be more likely to foster participation by peers are introduced.

For example, at one time Jason was taken to the back of his classroom several times each day to work on a computer. He had his software in a box next to the software that was available to the rest of his classmates. Over time, his cause-effect programs were replaced by a TV monitor on which he and his peers earned time to play Super Nintendo together. Classmates spontaneously problem-solved ways of getting Jason involved with the games, using his switch. For example, they might relegate a single function to Jason, such as keeping the character moving on the screen, while they took care of jumping, shooting, and other types of mayhem associated with this particular game.

Jorgensen (1994) presented a variety of methods for promoting friendships in inclusive settings. Most critical to point out here is the fact that, unlike natural relationships, friendships with individuals with severe to profound disabilities often do not occur without outside intervention. Parents often cite the development of friendships as a top priority for their children. AAC can serve a major role in fostering peer friendships and interactions.

Recently, two 7-year-old children were observed collaborating on the coloring of a dinosaur picture. The child without a disability systematically presented choices of crayons and monitored her friend's eye gaze. She also provided hand-over-hand support during coloring. Each child reinforced one another's actions throughout the process. These actions occurred following teacher modeling and subsequent reinforcement of the classmate's positive interactions with the student.

Step Four. In Step Four, the team prioritizes general annual goals for the student. Ideally, goals are discipline-free in that they cut across many of the traditional do-

mains: academic, motor, social, communication, self-care, and so forth. Examples may include increasing the amount of time spent in an inclusive classroom, having a student eat at the same table as his or her classmates who are not disabled, spending leisure time with friends, finding a job, expanding the number and range of interests or hobbies, visiting more places in the community, participating in a community recreation program, and volunteering time to a local service program.

Each of these goals could require a need for communication intervention. Irrespective of whether the individual was in the community, classroom, or work setting the quality of interactions would depend heavily on the ability to initiate, maintain, and respond to conversational exchanges. An AAC specialist would be instrumental in collaborating with others to develop a functional means of communication that fosters participation in each setting.

For example, when a student goes to lunch he or she should have a means of sharing novel information with peers. It is not enough to communicate messages such as *eat, drink, more,* and *all done.* Nor is it enough to be able to label 50 possible food items. These are not skills that foster interactions with other students. Vocabulary that enables the student to comment on what others are eating, trade snacks with peers, or engage in small talk is more likely to promote inclusion in the cafeteria. Possible topics of interest to the student might also be of interest to partners.

Step Five. The team specifies how the individual will participate in different settings and examines the need for support in each setting. Here the role of AAC in fostering participation is described. Equipment needs and other supports necessary in each setting are cited.

An adult named Ron who used a Macaw to interact with his customers on his newspaper route was observed. Routines were scripted to enable this gentleman to interact with his customers. He also exchanged greetings and small talk about the weather, the plight of the Boston Red Sox, and the foibles of well-known politicians, even though it was questionable whether or not he himself understood the messages he was conveying. Staff felt that Ron's lack of understanding was irrelevant, and supported their argument by pointing out changes in his demeanor following the introduction of the communication program.

In the case of Tony, the team talked about ways of involving him during silent reading. A strategy was worked out that involved recruiting different classmates to read to Tony. The classmate would pause after each page and wait for Tony to touch the page to indicate his desire to continue the story. When Tony did not respond on his own, the classmate was taught to prompt and cue him as necessary. Classmates were also encouraged to stop the story and talk about pictures in which Tony showed an interest by looking at, smiling, and touching the pictures.

Step Six. Short-term objectives, still largely discipline-free, are developed in this step. Examples of short-term objectives that foster participation include:

- Sharing novel information with classmates during "show and tell."
- Activating a device to participate in the morning Pledge of Allegiance.
- Activating a Big Mack that signals classmates it is time to move on to the next activity.
- Ordering a meal in the cafeteria.
- Selecting a partner to assist on the playground.
- Choosing and purchasing items to decorate a room.
- Notifying a supervisor when a new task is not understood.

Step Seven. This step involves the development of teaching and curriculum modifications based on the individual's learning style and others' interaction styles. These are revised regularly, depending on changing needs and opportunities. Modifications might involve:

- Incorporating symbols, including those contained on the student's AAC communication display, into group classroom lessons.
- Having the teacher model the use of an AAC system for a student's classmates.
- Teaching an employer to simplify his or her verbal input so that it is more understandable to an employee.
- Having an aide present questions in ways that provide increased opportunities for choice making.

Step Eight. Finally, in Step Eight the team evaluates the quality of inclusion and overall effectiveness of instruction in helping the individual to achieve the targeted outcomes. The role of the AAC system in promoting versus unwittingly impeding inclusion and full participation should be reviewed systematically and longitudinally. Methods of assessing outcomes of AAC were discussed earlier in this chapter.

The eight step process emphasizes the need for team members to explore individuals' personal backgrounds and experiences, to describe their abilities and needs, to identify their dreams and barriers to achieving these aspirations, and then to develop a systematic plan to assist these individuals in meeting their goals. The primary focus remains consistent throughout the process: fostering participation and inclusion. Discussions arising in connection with this process can form a foundation for identifying the role of AAC relative to an expanding venue of social and vocational options for individuals with severe disabilities.

The remainder of this section on assessment strategies augments general principles noted in Chapter 5's discussion of AAC evaluation strategies. As will be seen, assessment of individuals with severe to profound disabilities is a dynamic process that extends beyond the individual to consider listeners and settings in which interactions arise. Current communication skills and needs are identified relative to present and projected environmental demands. As new skills are introduced, their impact relative to fostering participation and interaction are evaluated and modified continuously.

Identification of Communication Skills

The process of getting to know the individual includes a thorough description of past and present communication skills. For individuals with severe to profound disabilities, levels of phonologic, syntactic, semantic, and pragmatic ability are viewed in the broader context of interaction and functional skills. Within this framework, the team's primary concern is with the effectiveness of communication across partners and settings, as opposed to the particulars of message transmission. Some examples of assessment concerns in each language dimension, expressively and receptively, are depicted in Table 12–4.

The evaluation of present levels of communicative function is supplemented with other sources of information seen as critical to program development. These include examinations of symbol knowledge, aptitude and interest in unaided methods of communication, and the degree to which individuals are able to meet communication demands that arise naturally in different settings. The latter is examined through the use of discrepancy analyses and similar procedures.

Symbol Knowledge

Mirenda and Locke (1989) identified the following hierarchy of increasing difficulty

for symbolizing common objects: actual objects, color photographs, black and white photographs, miniature objects, black and white line drawings, Pictographs, Blissymbols, and written words. The authors found that individuals varied greatly in their understanding of different symbol sets, and recommended that this determination be made on a client-by-client basis.

Assessments of symbol knowledge are often made using matching tasks. For example, the individual may be presented with two or more objects and a symbol that represents one of these objects. The presentation of the symbol cues the individual to act on the corresponding object in some way. This author often prefers to evaluate symbol knowledge by more functional means. Symbols can be presented to an individual, perhaps on an existing communication display, with no prior training. Based on background information about the individual, situations are set up in which individual is expected to be intrinsically motivated to point to or otherwise select particular symbols. Pointing to the symbols earns natural consequences. If spontaneous pointing does not occur, uses of the symbol are modeled and additional opportunities for use are presented. The evaluator notes the individual's initial responses without training, and the length of time or number of trials that are necessary before the individual uses the symbol without prompting. Finally, retention and generalization of symbols is examined as subsequent opportunities for use are presented on successive days and weeks. A variety of symbol sets can be explored in this manner.

Mirenda and Santogrossi (1985) described a prompt-free strategy similar to that suggested here, by which a young child with moderate to severe mental retardation was taught to use a picture communication board. Their procedure involved functional reinforcement of spontaneous picture touching, in a series of graduated

Table 12–4. Examples of assessment concerns across language dimensions.

Phonology

1. Degree of intelligibility (with and without existing AAC systems) to different listeners in different situations.

2. Extent to which AAC may enhance intelligibility.

3. Degree to which speech/vocalizations contribute to message success and the extent to which vocal behavior can be shaped, following possible introduction of AAC, to further enhance intelligibility.

Syntax

1. Relationship between length of message and intelligibility.

2. Range of syntactic-semantic relations conveyed and understood.

3. Word preferences relative to grammatical constituencies (e.g., nouns, verbs, adjectives, adverbs).

4. Understanding of semantic compaction, abbreviated spelling, and other message acceleration techniques that require activating the keys of a communication aid in a particular order.

Semantics

1. Vocabulary needs.

2. Understanding of basic and abstract concepts.

3. Ability to store and retrieve vocabulary items, depending on how they are symbolized and organized. Understanding of superordinate categories and themes for more effective and efficient use of Minspeak, topic-specific communication boards, and other applications.

Pragmatics

1. Availability and choice of conversational partners.

2. Frequency and relative success of initiated messages

3. Characteristics of partners with whom interactions are most common, and most often successful.

4. Range of communicative functions, with different conversational partners.

5. Modes (conventional and nonconventional forms of communication, challenging behaviors, aided and unaided methods) by which communicative functions are conveyed.

6. Ability to communicate in 1:1, small, and large group situations.

7. Turn-taking skills in conversations.

---

steps. Interestingly, none of these steps involved verbal cueing. A verbal prompt-free strategy has also been proposed for individuals with more severe disabilities (Mirenda & Dattilo, 1987).

The assessment of symbol sets often results in findings that individuals may benefit most from communication displays that include a variety of symbols. These modes are then used in conjunction with unaided modes of communication. The subject of unaided communication is discussed briefly here.

Aptitude and Interest in Unaided Communication

The assessment should also include a description of present unaided methods of communicating (e.g., vocal, gestural, pantomime, sign), and the relative effectiveness of each with different partners in different situations. Individuals with profound disabilities will likely use natural gestures and some idiosyncratic gestures. The primary issue here is the usefulness of these behaviors with familiar and, more importantly, unfamiliar listeners. An ambiguous gesture is of no greater value than an unintelligible word.

Individuals with severe disabilities can be expected to be capable of developing large repertoires of unaided signs and gestures. Limitations are related to the cognitive and motor requirements (hand shape, location on body, type of movement) of the signs themselves, and interactions among these various components (Doherty, 1985; Dunn, 1982; McEwen & Lloyd, 1990). No less important, however, is the degree to which this communication mode is modeled, reinforced, and responded to by others in the immediate environment.

Decisions about the viability of unaided communication require input from physical and occupational therapists. These professionals can provide information about an individual's positioning needs, hand and finger dexterity, range of motion, ability to produce different hand shapes, and so forth.

Discrepancy Analyses

The literature contains many specific examples of discrepancy analyses conducted on individuals with severe to profound disabilities (Beukelman & Mirenda, 1992; Calculator, 1994c; Calculator & Jorgensen, 1991; Cipani, 1989). These procedures have several features in common. All require the examiner to assess the individual's communication skills relative to those that appear to be necessary in order to fully participate in corresponding events and activities. In some cases, necessary and desired skills are identified by observing other individuals who are participating successfully in the same setting. The individual's abilities are then examined relative to this reference group, and discrepancies are noted. Subsequent intervention then targets these limitations.

In some cases, this means teaching the missing skills. For example, a student who is rarely successful in having his or her messages responded to might be taught to be certain to get the listener's attention prior to conveying the rest of the message.

On other occasions, introducing alternative means of acquiring desired outcomes may be warranted. An adult who is unable to leave a dining table on his or her own may be taught to push the food tray to the middle of the table to indicate that he or she is finished eating and wants assistance leaving the table. A third outcome of a discrepancy analysis might be to introduce different modifications to tasks, changing others' expectations of the individual in a particular context, and so forth.

Discrepancy analyses also frequently examine opportunities for communication in particular settings. Where opportunities exist and individuals are not taking advantage of them, AAC interventions may be considered.

Calculator and Jorgensen (1991) described a procedure for doing a discrepancy analysis on-line. Their Functional Analysis of Opportunities to Participate in Regular School Activities can be applied to children or adults in different settings.

Using this procedure, the examiner notes actions of the individual relative to those engaged in by others. This permits later analyses of the extent to which the individual is an active participant in daily routines. Notations are made regarding the environment, such as the physical arrangement of furniture and adaptive equipment, materials available to the individual and others. Sources of support (aides, regular and special education teachers, peers, and others) are also identified during the on-line observations.

Material recorded in the Functional Analysis of Opportunities to Participate in Regular School Activities (Calculator & Jorgensen, 1991) is then reviewed with other team members. The team recommends ways of fostering the individual's participation in activities occurring in the classroom and other settings through changes in support, curriculum, and other modifications. Finally, short-term objectives that reinforce long-term goals for the individual are identified and embedded into these activities.

The assessment practices described in this chapter are intended to explore the extent to which individuals are able to communicate functionally in different settings and under different circumstances. Assessment and intervention are continuous, interrelated processes. The most significant assessment information for individuals with severe disabilities is often derived by examining their responsiveness to AAC instruction. Factors that influence their rate of learning, amount of learning, and variability in applying learned skills all serve as a basis for modifying AAC programs and continuing to assess the benefits of instruction.

Continuity is a basic principle of AAC instruction for children and adults with severe to profound disabilities. Other principles are summarized in Table 12–5.

AAC INTERVENTION FOR INDIVIDUALS WITH SEVERE TO PROFOUND DISABILITIES

The principles cited in Table 12–5 share a broader theme of viewing AAC intervention relative to fostering inclusion, participation, and interaction. Changes in communication without concomitant changes in these domains are not viewed positively. Several of these principles were discussed earlier and thus will not be addressed at this time. Others are explained in greater detail here.

Continuity of Instruction

AAC interventions should be carried out throughout the day, rather than being addressed in a static block of time. The speech-language pathologist collaborates with other team members to identify situations throughout the day that lend themselves to addressing each individual's pri-

Table 12–5. Basic principles in providing AAC interventions to children and adults with severe to profound disabilities.

1. Maintain continuity of instruction.
2. Use a variety of natural settings to promote the acquisition and generalization of AAC skills.
3. Recruit a variety of partners or natural supports to promote the acquisition and generalization of AAC skills.
4. Embed AAC instruction into ongoing activities.
5. Emphasize the acquisition and generalization of functional skills.
6. Collaborate with home, school, workplace, and elsewhere to identify, prioritize, and address instructional priorities.
7. View all individuals, and prospective partners, as potential candidates for AAC instruction. Employ a zero-exclusion policy relative to eligibility decisions.
8. Teach AAC skills that individuals are likely to acquire in a reasonable period of time (ease of acquisition).
9. Foster communication/interaction as opposed to the isolated use of any one particular mode of communication. View AAC as a tool rather than a prop for interaction. Encourage multiple modes of communication to meet multiple communication needs with different listeners in different situations.
10. Develop environments that promote opportunities for interaction and participation.
11. Foster self-determination.
12. Maintain and model high expectations.

ority goals. Previously noted procedures such as discrepancy analyses and the Functional Analysis of Opportunities to Participate in Regular School Activities are useful here.

Rather than a professional taking an adult aside to work on "greetings" in an isolated one-to-one context, experiences are offered by different individuals (with monitoring by the speech-language pathologist and others) throughout the day to reinforce the acquisition and generalization of this skill. Several examples of AAC implementation using this principle are given.

Mr. Sutherland is a young man who, with support from an aide, picks up recyclable goods from local merchants in the community each morning. The merchants have learned to approach William as he arrives, and then pause in expectation of a greeting from him. When necessary, they cue/prompt this behavior through an expectant gaze and hand gesture and, under rare circumstances, look to William's aide to assist him in this regard.

Ms. Phillips is employed as a messenger for several local businesses. On occasion, her customers are asked by Ms. Phillips' assistant to intentionally provide inadequate information or directions to her. For example, they may mumble their message. The aide reports back to the speech-language pathologist how Ms. Phillips responded in these situations. Ms. Phillip's goal is to be aware of when these situations occur and then to use her communication display or any other means to request clarification.

Tom, a fourth grader, is encouraged to offer positive comments to classmates. His communication aid has been programmed with phrases such as, "that's awesome," and, "wow, I really like that." He is cued by his aide to use these expressions when approached by classmates holding their work in art class. Classmates activate the same messages as they refer to his work. Although it is unclear whether

or not Tom himself understands the content of these messages, they serve as appropriate means of greeting and stimulating conversations with classmates.

Sources of Discontinuity

Recently another connotation was offered relative to continuity of AAC instruction. Smith-Lewis (1994) examined changes over time in AAC system development for individuals. She categorized each AAC system change as being either continuous or discontinuous. Continuous changes reflected appropriate progressions in complexity from one aided device or symbol system to another.

Smith-Lewis's (1994) expert panel cited numerous sources of discontinuity of aided systems and symbol sets upon reviewing the AAC programs of a group of school-aged learners. These included: (a) protracted periods of trial-and-error assessment with new devices and symbol sets; (b) professionals' personal biases and preferences for one system or another; (c) inconsistent involvement of parents in their children's AAC programs; (d) emergence of new technology, and (e) lack of guidelines concerning how to change from one system to another over time.

Other insights about program discontinuity can be gleaned from reports by AAC users (Huer & Lloyd, 1990; Smith-Lewis & Ford, 1987). Individuals have expressed frustration with professionals who make decisions for them without soliciting their input. They also express concerns about the competency of AAC professionals in making program decisions, and others' lack of appropriate expectations for them.

Employ a Variety of Natural Settings

Within the context of an individual's daily settings, AAC needs are identified relative to opportunities for interactions that arise. The ability of the individual to use AAC to respond to routine and novel situations across various settings should also be a focus of intervention. Similarly, AAC outcomes are evaluated relative to changes in an individual's level of participation in these settings.

Recruit a Variety of Partners or Natural Supports

The goal is to enhance AAC skills with an infinite number of current and prospective communication partners. This requires providing AAC methods and training strategies that lead to efficient, unambiguous modes of communication. It also implies the need for ongoing training of staff, family members, and others regarding nuances in how different individuals communicate, and their respective roles in fostering effective interactions.

Collaborate with Others to Identify Priorities

Calculator and Jorgensen (1992) described a program, with accompanying timelines, for providing technical assistance to schools in support of inclusive AAC and related practices. Their program included steps by which teams (a) identify their need for training and technical assistance; (b) get to know students and their families; and (c) develop and then implement plans for inclusion.

More recently, Wisniewski and Alper (1994) detailed the following five phases:

1. Develop networks within the community, following an assessment of attitudes toward inclusion.
2. Assess school and community resources. Determine how best to arrange resources, in terms of service delivery options, to optimize benefits to students.
3. Review strategies for inclusion such as grouping of students, peer tutors and

other natural supports, computer-assisted instruction and other assistive technologies, community-based training sites, and visits by staff to model/demonstration project sites.
4. Install strategies that lead to inclusion.
5. Develop a system of feedback and renewal.

Wisniewski and Alper evaluated the success of inclusion relative to increased independence in functional skills, increased participation and use of generic/public facilities and services, and increased input and choice regarding individuals' daily activities and overall lifestyle.

Embed AAC Instruction into Ongoing Activities

Calculator and Jorgensen (1991) provided numerous examples of AAC objectives that are integrated into daily educational practices. Generalizing this discussion to the adult population, objectives such as the following might arise:

In response to hearing his name, Mr. Schultz will establish eye contact with his prospective conversational partner. Partners will neither initiate nor maintain interactions in the absence of inappropriate eye contact.

Upon returning to work each Monday, Ms. Jackson will inform co-workers of two interesting things she did over the weekend. These will appear as prerecorded AAC system messages, accompanied by souvenirs of activities and events in which she participated. For example, the program to a play she attended, a ticket stub, a store coupon, and other props can be used to prompt interactions at work.

Teach AAC Skills That Are Quickly and Easily Acquired

Individuals who are nonspeaking with significant cognitive deficits constitute a population whose lack of effective communication skills places them at great risk of being isolated from their home communities. As important as it is to plan for tomorrow, these individuals have urgent needs for communication that must be addressed now.

Professionals might begin with simple solutions to AAC needs, relying initially on low cost and quickly fabricated devices and programs. The assessment process itself should pilot immediate intervention ideas, and provide support to staff and family on immediate implementation.

As an example, while observing Mr. Thompson at a local Burger King, his personal care assistant provided little opportunity for him to direct the meal that was fed to him. During the assessment, it was determined that Mr. Thompson was responsive to instruction that encouraged him to look and reach for foods (hamburger, french fries, shake) with which he then needed his assistant's help. He also shifted his eye gaze and averted his head in response to being offered foods that he did not want. These behaviors were incorporated into this setting, and were later augmented using a picture communication system to order his meal and to request that his assistant help him dispose of his trash at the end of the meal.

Maintain and Model High Expectations

Perhaps more important than any other consideration is the need to promote and maintain high expectations for all individuals with severe to profound disabilities. Among this population are individuals who presently live in their own apartments and homes, attend colleges and universities, are employed competitively, have broad networks of friends and other relationships, are married with children of their own, and so forth. Other individuals who were once regarded as highly aggressive and "noncommunicative" have re-

vealed their personalities and enjoyment of relationships with others after gaining access to AAC.

Certainly, the achievements of these individuals can be credited in part to the types of supports that have been available to them and the extent to which they have learned to advocate for themselves. AAC will continue to be germane to both of these pursuits, to the extent that professionals and others can overcome personal and social barriers that prevent them from seeing "the vision" in its full potential.

SUMMARY

This chapter began with a discussion of the evolution toward inclusive practices for children and adults with severe disabilities. AAC and other services were framed within the broader context of their impact on fostering active participation in schools and communities. Where individuals are physically present in settings, yet are not provided with the services they need to be actively involved, the benefits of inclusion may be questioned. Inclusion must continue to imply not only presence, but also meaningful involvement.

Assessment practices described in this chapter operate under a basic assumption that all individuals are potential candidates for AAC instruction. Needs for instruction are highly individualized and change not only across but also within specific settings, depending on factors such as communication demands, opportunities for communication, and communication partners. The AAC assessment process is dynamic, with examiners continuously evaluating the effectiveness of interventions relative to levels of inclusion and participation.

As discussed, some situations such as the use of challenging behaviors to convey communicative functions, call for developing alternative modes of communication. However, it is more likely that the assessment process will result in various options for augmenting communication skills already established in an individual's repertoire.

Practices reviewed in this chapter expand the focus of concern beyond individuals with severe disabilities to also consider their current and prospective conversational partners, and the settings in which interactions occur. If individuals are to have maximal input into events affecting them, and to exercise maximal control over their lives or self-determination, they must interact in settings in which they are valued. Their conversational partners must maintain high expectations of them and afford them sufficient opportunities for interaction and participation. These outcomes are enhanced by recruiting and fostering natural supports as necessary.

An assessment process was described in which teams begin by devoting significant effort to getting to know individuals, identifying their skills, determining long range priorities, identifying possible obstacles, and developing a plan to meet their goals. Examples of AAC activities that corresponded with each step of this process were discussed. The chapter concluded with a set of principles on which to base AAC intervention.

As was indicated earlier, this is a population that is at great risk of being segregated from the rest of society. To the extent that AAC and other services can prevent or reverse such an outcome, the value of such interventions cannot be disputed.

REFERENCES

Baer, D., Wolf, M., & Risley, T. (1987). Some still-current dimensions of applied behavior analysis. *Journal of Applied Behavior Analysis, 20*, 313–327.

Baine, D., & Sobsey, R. (1983). Implementing transdisciplinary services for severely handicapped persons. *Special Education in Canada, 58*(1), 13–14.

Blatt, B., & Kaplan, F. (1966). *Christmas in purgatory.* Boston: Allyn and Bacon.

Beukelman, D., & Mirenda, P. (1992). *Augmentative and alternative communication: Management of severe communication disorders in children and adults.* Baltimore: Paul H. Brookes.

Brown, F., & Lehr, D. (1993, Summer). Making activities meaningful for students with severe multiple disabilities. *Teaching Exceptional Children,* 12–16.

Brown, L., Branston, M. B., Hamre-Nietupski, S., Pumpian, I., Certo, N., & Gruenwald, L. (1979). A strategy for developing chronological age-appropriate and functional curricular content for severely handicapped adolescents and young adults. *Journal of Special Education, 13*, 81–90.

Brown, L., Nietupski, J., & Hamre-Nietupski, S. (1976). The criterion of ultimate functioning in public school services for severely handicapped students. In M. A. Thomas (Ed.), *Hey! Don't forget about me: Education's investment in the severely, profoundly and mulitply handicapped* (pp. 2–15). Reston, VA: Council for Exceptional Children.

Calculator, S. (1994a). Communicative intervention as a means to successful inclusion. In S. Calculator & C. Jorgensen (Eds.), *Including students with severe disabilities in schools: Fostering communication, interaction and participation* (pp. 183–214). San Diego, CA: Singular Publishing Group, Inc.

Calculator, S. (1994b). Designing and implementing communicative assessments in inclusive settings. In S. Calculator & C. Jorgensen (Eds.), *Including students with severe disabilities in schools: Fostering communication, interaction and participation* (pp. xiii–xxviii). San Diego, CA: Singular Publishing Group, Inc.

Calculator, S. (1994c). Communicative intervention as a means to successful inclusion. In S. Calculator & C. Jorgensen (Eds.), *Including students with severe disabilities in schools: Fostering communication, interaction and participation,* (pp. 113–181). San Diego, CA: Singular Publishing Group, Inc.

Calculator, S., & Jorgensen, C. (1991). Integrating AAC instruction into regular education settings: Expounding on best practices. *Augmentative and Alternative Communication, 7,* 204–214.

Calculator, S., & Jorgensen, C. (1992). A technical assistance model for promoting integrated communication supports and services for students with severe disabilities. *Seminars in Speech and Language, 13*(2), 99–110.

Casby, M. (1992). The cognitive hypothesis and its influence on speech-language services in schools. *Language, Speech, and Hearing Services in Schools, 23,* 198–202.

Cipani, E. (1989). Providing language consultation in the natural context: A model for delivery of services. *Mental Retardation, 27,* 317–324.

Cole, K., Dale, P., & Mills, P. (1990). Defining language delay in young children by cognitive referencing: Are we saying more than we know? *Journal of Applied Psycholinguistics, 11,* 291–302.

Committee on Language Learning Disabilities. (1989). Issues in determining eligibility for language learning. *Asha, 31,* 113–118.

Danielson, L., & Bellamy, G. (1989). State variation in placement of children with handicaps in segregated environments. *Exceptional Children, 55,* 448–455.

Doherty, J. (1985). The effects of signs characteristics on sign acquisition and retention: An integrative review of the literature. *Augmentative and Alternative Communication, 1,* 108–121.

Donnellan, A., Mirenda, P., Mesaros, R., & Fassbender, L. (1984). Analyzing the communicative functions of aberrant behavior. *Journal of the Association for Persons with Severe Handicaps, 9,* 201–212.

Dunn, M. (1982). *Pre-sign language motor skills.* Tucson, AZ: Communication Skills Builders.

Durand, M. (1993). Functional communication training for challenging behaviors. *Clinics in Communication Disorders, 3*(2), 59–70.

Education for All Handicapped Children Act. (1975). P.L. 94-142.

Forest, M. (1989). *It's about relationships.* Toronto: Frontier College Press.

Gartner, A., & Lipsky, D. (1987). Beyond special education: Toward a quality system for all students. *Harvard Educational Review, 57,* 367–395.

Giangreco, M., Cloninger, C., & Iverson, V. (1993). *Choosing options and accommodations for children (C.O.A.C.H.): A guide to planning inclusive education.* Baltimore: Paul H. Brookes.

Gold, M. (1980). *Try another way training manual.* Champaign, IL: Research Press.

Huer, M., & Lloyd, L. (1990). AAC users' perspectives on augmentative and alternative communication. *Augmentative and Alternative Communication, 6*(4), 242–249.

Jorgensen, C. (1992). Natural supports in inclusive schools: Curricular and teaching strategies. In J. Nisbet (Ed.), *Natural supports in school, at work, and in the community for people with severe disabilities* (pp. 179–215). Baltimore, MD: Paul H. Brookes.

Jorgensen, C. (1994). Developing individualized inclusive educational programs. In S. Calculator & C. Jorgensen (Eds.), *Including students with severe disabilities in schools: Fostering communication, interaction and participation* (pp. 27–74). San Diego, CA: Singular Publishing Group, Inc.

Jorgensen, C., & Calculator, S. (1994). The evolution of best practices in educating students with severe disabilities. In S. Calculator & C. Jorgensen (Eds.), *Including students with severe disabilities in schools: Fostering communication, interaction and participation* (pp. 1–25). San Diego, CA: Singular Publishing Group, Inc.

Kangas, K., & Lloyd, L. (1988). Early cognitive skills as prerequisites to augmentative and alternative communication use: What are we waiting for? *Augmentative and Alternative Communication, 4,* 211–221.

Kazdin, A. (1977). Assessing the clinical or implied importance of behavior change through social validation. *Behavior Modification, 1,* 427–451.

McDonnell, A., & Hardman, M. (1989). The desegregation of America's special schools: Strategies for change. *Journal of the Association for Persons with Severe Handicaps, 14,* 68–74.

McEwen, I., & Lloyd, L. (1990). Some considerations about the motor requirements of manual signs. *Augmentative and Alternative Communication, 6,* 207–216.

McLean, J. (1993). Assuring best practices in communication for children and youth with severe disabilities. *Clinics in Communication Disorders, 3,* 1–6.

Meyer, L. (1897). *Program quality indicators (PQI): A checklist of most promising practices in educational programs for students with se-*

vere disabilities. Syracuse, NY: Division of Special Education and Rehabilitiation, Syracuse University.

Miller, J., Chapman, R., & Bedrosian, J. (1977). *Defining developmentally disabled subjects for research: The relationship between etiology, cognitive development, and language and communicative performance.* Paper presented at the Second Annual Boston University Conference on Language Development, Boston, MA.

Mirenda, P., & Calculator, S. (1993). Enhancing curricula design. *Clinics in Communication Disorders, 3,* 43–58.

Mirenda, P., & Dattilo, J. (1987). Instructional techniques in alternative communication for students with severe intellectual handicaps. *Augmentative and Alternative Communication, 3,* 143–152.

Mirenda, P., & Locke, P. (1989). A comparison of symbol transparency in nonspeaking persons with intellectual disabilities. *Journal of Speech and Hearing Disorders, 54*(2), 131–140.

Mirenda, P., & Santogrossi, J. (1985). A prompt-free strategy to teach pictorial communication system use. *Augmentative and Alternative Communication, 1,* 143–150.

Mount, B. (1987). *Personal futures planning: Finding directions for change.* Ann Arbor: University of Michigan Dissertation Information Service.

Mount, B., & Zwernik, K. (1988). *It's never too early, it's never too late.* St. Paul, MN: Metropolitan Council. (Publication No. 421-88-109)

National Joint Committee for Meeting the Communicative Needs of Persons with Severe Disabilities. (1992). Guidelines for meeting the communication needs of persons with severe disabilities. *Asha, 34* (3, Suppl. 7), 1–8.

O'Brien, J., & Forest, M. (1989). *Action for inclusion.* Toronto, Ontario: Centre for Integrated Education, Frontier College.

Reichle, J., Feeley, K., & Johnston, S. (1993). Communication intervention for persons with severe and profound disabilities. *Clinics in Communication Disorders, 3,* 7–30.

Reichle, J., & Johnston, S. (1993). Replacing challenging behavior: The role of communication intervention. *Topics in Language Disorders, 13*(3), 61–76.

Sizer, T. (1992). *Horace's school: Redesigning the American high school.* Boston: Houghton Mifflin Co.

Smith-Lewis, M. (1994). Discontinuity in the development of aided augmentative and alternative communication systems. *Augmentative and Alternative Communication, 10,* 14-26.

Smith-Lewis, M., & Ford, A. (1987). A user's perspective on augmentative communication. *Augmentative and Alternative Communication, 3*(1), 12–17.

Strully, J., & Strully, C. (1985). Friendship and our children. *Journal of the Association for Persons with Severe Handicaps, 10,* 224–227.

Thousand, J. (1987). *Best practice guidelines for students with intensive educational needs.* Burlington: University of Vermont Center for Developmental Disabilities.

Thousand, J., & Villa, R. (1992). *Restructuring for caring and effective education.* Baltimore: Paul H. Brookes.

Vandercook, T., York, J., & Forest, M. (1989). The McGill action planning system (M.A.P.S.): A strategy for building the vision. *Journal of the Association for Persons with Severe Handicaps, 14,* 205–215.

West, F. (1990). Educational collaboration in the restructuring of schools. *Journal of Educational and Psychological Consultation, 1*(1), 23–40.

Wisniewski, L., & Alper, S. (1994). Including students with severe disabilities in general education settings: Guidelines for change. *Remedial and Special Education, 15* (1) 4–13.

Wolfensberger, W. (1972). *The principle of normalisation in human services.* Toronto: National Institute on Mental Retardation.

Yoder, D., & Calculator, S. (1981). Some perspectives on intervention strategies for persons with developmental disorders. *Journal of Autism and Developmental Disorders, 11,* 107–123.

Matthew's AAC Story: Breaking Through

Elizabeth Delsandro with Sharon L. Glennen

Matthew was born with more than his fair share of complications. He was diagnosed shortly after birth as having atypical Treacher-Collins syndrome. Matthew had a cleft palate and malformations of the outer and middle ear which are common features of this syndrome. He also had severe mental retardation, a moderate to severe hearing loss, and chronic reactive airway disease which resulted in a tracheostomy and feeding gastrostomy tube. His mother initially tried to take care of him but he had frequent medical complications during his early months. During one of his early hospital stays, he was abandoned and left a ward of the state. Matthew lived in a pediatric long-term care hospital during the first 5 years of his life. Although the nurses cared about him, they were severely understaffed to meet the needs of an extremely active toddler. Matthew spent many hours confined in his hospital crib or a playpen with a safety cover to prevent him from crawling out. Although he was given toys and attention, this lack of stimulation did little to develop early communication skills and set Matthew on a developmental course that was difficult to change.

When Matthew was 3, he began to attend a special preschool program for children with multiple disabilities. At preschool, he was given an opportunity to play and explore his environment. Matthew was now walking and spent much of his time excitedly running around being chased by his teachers. Because he was nonverbal and hearing impaired, his teachers and school speech-language pathologist began a program to teach him sign language. Several of the children in his classroom were also learning signs. Matthew's teachers worked hard to provide consistent models across all class activities. The school also began a program to get him to wear his hearing aids on a consistent basis. This was extremely difficult given his activity level. His tolerance for the hearing aids ranged from immediately pulling them out, to pulling them out and throwing them while running away from his teachers.

Sign language was a difficult modality for Matthew to learn. He was an extremely active child with a limited attention span. Because his hearing loss was profound, his teachers relied on visual cues to get his attention. Once they got his attention to look at their sign models, he would quickly glance, then shift his attention toward the next visually stimulating object. Matthew also had gross and fine motor delays that prevented him from easily imitating sign models. At the end of his first year of preschool, Matthew had learned how to use a reaching gesture to indicate his desire for a particular object or person; however, he had not demonstrated comprehension nor production of any true signs.

During this period, Matthew continued to live at the hospital facility. Each morning a special van took him to the preschool program. Every afternoon he returned to the hospital. The signs that were used in the school environment were never modeled or used by nursing staff at the hospital. Matthew's high activity level and hearing loss made him a difficult child to monitor in a hospital environment. Given hospital staffing patterns, it was difficult to provide him with consistent attention or communication models. Rotating staff meant that he did not bond emotionally or communicatively with any caregivers. Although he was constantly supervised, changes in caregivers made it difficult for Matthew to learn a reliable and efficient means of communication. As he continued to grow, he still spent much of his time in beds or special play areas designed so that he could not crawl out. He began to engage in perseverative stimulatory behaviors such as twirling strings, staring at the lights, flapping his hands, and showing high interest in round objects such as balls.

When Matthew was 4, he returned to his preschool program. Despite his lack of progress during the previous year, his teacher and speech-language pathologist continued with their program to teach him sign language. Because of lack of progress during the previous year, Matthew's speech and language services were dropped to a consultative level. The speech-language pathologist met with his teacher once each month to review Matthew's progress and make recommendations for continued language goals. Even though he was one year older, Matthew's activity level and attention span had not improved. If anything, he was more difficult to manage because

he was bigger and significantly stronger. He also acquired the coordination and strength to get into cupboards, containers, and other items in the class that were previously too difficult. Because of his behavior, Matthew was assigned a one-to-one aide to stay by his side in the preschool program. The aide was able to model signs to Matthew more frequently. She also provided hand-over-hand physical guidance to assist him in producing signs. His teachers hoped that the additional assistance would help him acquire a few functional signs. However, by the end of Matthew's second year of preschool, he could not comprehend or produce any signs.

Imagine being a child without the ability to understand or communicate expressively to others. Without an effective means of communication, Matthew had to resort to the only communication methods he knew. Over the years, he learned that if he cried or tantrumed, someone would eventually pay attention to him. If he tantrumed hard and banged his head, someone would run over to make him stop. If he hit himself while tantruming, he could get immediate attention. If he hit or kicked others, attention was also quickly given. Although Matthew was severely mentally retarded, he was able to learn the cause effect communicative relationship between his behaviors and gaining adult attention.

By the time Matthew was 5, his only way to communicate effectively was through maladaptive behaviors. He screamed, cried, hit, kicked, banged his head, and bit himself. His only positive communication skill was the reach gesture that he learned at the age of 3. During his kindergarten year, his behavior deteriorated to the point where he was becoming a danger to himself and others. He couldn't be trusted to sit next to any other children in the class. His one-to-one aide spent most of the day holding him in her lap to prevent him from hitting himself. At the hospital, he was watched constantly to prevent him from banging his head on the side of the crib. A helmet was tried, but he quickly learned to take it off. As Matthew grew, controlling his behaviors became increasingly difficult for his teachers and hospital staff. His behavior was so uncontrollable that he was in danger of losing placement in his school program.

OPENING THE DOOR

During the spring of his kindergarten year, Matthew was referred to a hospital program for children with severe maladaptive behaviors. Outpatient behavior programs were initially tried for a few months without any changes or improvement in his behavior. It was decided to admit him to the inpatient hospital unit designed to address severe behaviors. This unit was staffed by psychologists, educators, and speech-language pathologists trained to systematically work with children with severe maladaptive behaviors. It was immediately apparent to everyone who worked with Matthew that his lack of appropriate communication skills had led to many of his maladaptive behaviors.

Matthew's initial behavior therapy program had several goals. The primary goal was to provide him with socially appropriate methods of gaining attention from others, making requests, and asking to leave or end a situation (known as asking for an escape). The expectation was for a decrease in his maladaptive behaviors as his functional communication skills improved. Another goal was to find an appropriate home and school program that could meet his needs after discharge. Everyone agreed that returning to his previous long-term care hospital program might cause a relapse in his maladaptive behaviors.

Matthew's behaviors, hearing loss, and lack of communication skills meant that he initially could not be evaluated using standard assessment methods. After reviewing Matthew's communicative history, it was apparent that sign language training had not been effective. With that knowledge as a starting point, Matthew's initial assessment consisted of observing his existing play and communicative abilities in naturally occurring situations. As we got to know Matthew we realized that, despite his inability to communicate, he was able to learn. He could be shown how to play with a new toy and was able to imitate those play behaviors. He smiled appropriately when staff accidentally dropped things on the floor. He enjoyed being swung around by staff and would reach out over and over again to request another turn. We decided to begin using an object-based augmentative communication system to teach Matthew to request favorite toys or activities. Small objects representing three favorite activities were selected for the initial stages of training. With hand-over-hand guidance, Matthew was taught to touch one of the objects to request the activity. Within two training sessions, he began to spontaneously touch the objects. He would even walk across the room to the objects to make a request.

Following Matthew's initial success, an additional object representing a nonpreferred activity was added to the communication array. Matthew selected this object once, immediately rejected it by pushing it away, and never selected it again. Across several therapy sessions, we began moving the objects around on the board to determine if he could make a symbolic discrimination and find the objects representing his favorite activities. Time after time, he was able to consistently request his favorite toy. Within 1 week, it was decided to progress to a picture symbol communication system.

Matthew's initial picture communication system consisted of four large colored picture symbols matching the objects that were previously used. Matthew initially swatted randomly at the picture communication board with both hands. After several sessions, it was decided to reduce the system to a single picture that could be paired with an object. The object was placed into a clear container that he could not open. The picture symbol was velcroed to the outside of the container. Matthew was given hand-over-hand guidance to pull the picture off the container to request the object. This behavior was then modified to simply touching the picture. Once he was able to touch a single picture to make a request, a second container was added so that he could begin to make choices. Within 2 weeks, he was touching pictures to make requests between four different containers. The pictures were then placed on the table in front of each container. Gradually the pictures were moved farther away from the containers until Matthew was making choices by touching the pictures with the containers hidden out of sight. We worked with behavior unit staff to begin using the pictures to make play choices across Matthew's program. As his ability to appropriately communicate increased, staff began to see a decrease in his maladaptive behaviors.

Once Matthew began using the four choice picture communication board across his day, his communication options needed to be increased. Additional pictures were added to the original board so that Matthew could request from even more favorite activities. The pictures were gradually reduced to a 1-inch size and Matthew was taught to point to them with his index finger. Matthew began to spontaneously look for his board when he had something to communicate. He also began to lead staff by the hand to the location where his board was kept.

Matthew's play skills were also improving. When he was initially admitted, most of his play consisted of repetitive perseverative actions with favorite objects. His communication choices were requests for strings, balls, and bubbles, all of which he played with perseveratively. We began to introduce him to simple imaginative play activities: feeding a baby doll, pushing a car into a garage, stirring play foods in a pot, and walking Fisher-Price people and animals around a play farm. Matthew began to imitate these play behaviors, then began to spontaneously request these play activities. Appropriate play behaviors were modeled and gradually expanded. For example, Matthew was shown that the Fisher-Price animals could eat food and drinks, and could be placed into cars for rides.

As Matthew's imaginative play behaviors developed, his communicative choices were simultaneously expanded through the use of activity-based communication boards with abstract symbol concepts. His favorite activity was blowing bubbles. A board with symbols representing people, objects, and actions related to the bubble activity was created. Initially, Matthew did not understand the purpose of the additional symbols. He kept pointing over and over again to the picture of *bubbles* to request them. A small penlight was used to highlight other symbol choices such as *wand, open lid, blow,* and *pop*. Matthew was given hand-over-hand guidance to point to the other choices. Through consistent modeling, he began to spontaneously select some of the other symbols. Across several weeks of twice daily therapy, Matthew learned to use multiple activity-based communication boards that each had 8 to 10 picture symbols. Because the introduction of multiple boards can be confusing, symbols that were used across all of the boards were consistently located in the same place and highlighted with colored markers. Five of the boards were eventually placed into a communication book. Matthew learned to look through the communication book to find the activity he wanted. When he finished an activity, he would indicate he was done by turning to a new page.

Picture communication boards provided Matthew with the means to express his wants and needs. However, because of his hearing loss, he lacked the ability to understand others. We began to reintroduce sign language in conjunction with the communication boards. Picture symbols representing *me, you, more, stop, all done, yes,* and *no* were added to the activity-based communication boards. During play activities an aide would point to the symbols with a pen light while the speech-language pathologist produced the signs. Over time, Matthew began to comprehend the meaning of *more, all done,* and *stop.* Although he did not produce any of the signs himself, staff could sign to him to communicate. Learning the meaning of *stop* was an important step in controlling his behavior. Like most young children, he didn't always stop when asked, but it at least gave his behavior therapists a tool to communicate what they wanted him to do. *All done* was an equally important sign. Matthew learned that when the *all done* sign was produced he could leave an activity. With continued hand-over-hand modeling, Matthew learned to produce the *all done* sign following a model. This gave him a way to "escape" out of activities without resorting to maladaptive behaviors.

Despite Matthew's rapidly expanding communication abilities, his behavior problems did not miraculously disappear overnight. Matthew's maladaptive communication skills were deeply ingrained. Although he experienced success with his communication boards, he still resorted to tantrums, hitting, and head banging if his demands were not immediately met. In addition, Matthew was still extremely active. His attention span for any play activity was less than 2 minutes. His energy and lack of focus meant that he quickly ran through his favorite repertoire of activities. As soon as he grew bored, he would begin to look for new things to occupy himself. He was constantly climbing furniture, opening and dumping drawers, running through unlocked doors, and other exploits that exhausted the staff. The process of replacing maladaptive behaviors with more appropriate communication and play skills was a long slow battle.

Complicating the process was the difficulty of finding an appropriate home placement. Everyone involved was concerned that if Matthew went back to his previous hospital program his behaviors would immediately revert. He was placed on a waiting list of children needing specialized foster care. His stay in the behavior program was extended for several weeks because of the lack of an appropriate placement. This extension in his hospital stay provided us with an opportunity to expand his communication abilities even more. Matthew's speech-language pathologist decided to introduce a voice output AAC system. Even though Matthew would not be able to hear what the system was saying, voice output would give him a better way to get the attention of others. An AlphaTalker augmentative communication system was introduced on loan. The AlphaTalker has a 32 symbol display. It was easy to convert the activity-based communication boards that Matthew was already using to the format required by the system. This device was also chosen because of the red LED lights displayed with each symbol. As keys are selected, the lights blink. This provided Matthew with a visual cue that he had pressed hard enough to make a selection. During individual speech and language sessions, Matthew learned to use the AlphaTalker to communicate his needs to others. The decision was made to pursue funding for Matthew's own AlphaTalker system.

ENTERING THE COMMUNITY

Four months after Matthew was admitted to the inpatient behavior program, a specialized foster care placement was found. Matthew's new foster family began attending training sessions at the hospital to learn to manage his behavior. As part of the training process, they were shown how to implement his activity-based communication boards. Matthew had progressed to using eight different boards appropriately. A visit was made to his new home to determine new picture symbol vocabulary that would be appropriate in the home environment. Before Matthew's discharge, several new activity-based boards were created for his use at home. Several sessions were spent training Matthew's foster mother how to model vocabulary using the boards, and how to integrate sign language with the picture system.

Matthew's foster family lived in the same school district that he formerly attended. It was decided that he would return back to the same school but in a different classroom. His new class was composed of 10 children with severe multiple disabilities and behavior problems. Initially, the teachers and staff who previously knew him were skeptical of using picture communication boards. However, a videotape of him using the boards was shown to them for training purposes. We assisted school staff in creating several additional activity-based communication boards for his use at school. Matthew's IEP was revised to provide him with 60 minutes of classroom-based speech and language services each week.

Matthew was then discharged from the inpatient behavior program. He was actively followed by his behavior therapists and speech-language pathologist on an outpatient basis. Three months after Matthew's discharge, funding for his AlphaTalker was approved. The device was ordered and implemented right away. All of his existing communication boards had been made using the AlphaTalker overlay format. These low technology picture boards then became the picture overlays for his high tech system. The transition to the AlphaTalker was easier for Matthew than it was for his new family and school. Matthew's foster mother and school initially had difficulty implementing the AlphaTalker on a consistent basis because of difficulty learning to change pages in the system and a lack of appropriate vocabulary choices. His foster mother began to bring Matthew in for weekly speech therapy visits at the hospital. The goal of each visit was to develop vocabulary for one new activity-based communication board, to make the picture display during the session using BoardMaker software, and to program the vocabulary into the AlphaTalker. Matthew and his foster mother would then engage in related play activities with the speech-language pathologist who demonstrated how to teach him to use the system.

An activity-based picture communication board was developed for Matthew to request play activities with his foster brothers and sisters. Matthew enjoyed requesting attention from his siblings using the device. The siblings enjoyed the voice output and readily pushed the pictures to communicate with Matthew. Matthew and his siblings began taking turns requesting play activities using the AlphaTalker. This incident made Matthew's foster mother aware of the interactive power of a voice output AAC system. After that occurrence, she began to make sure that Matthew always had access to his AlphaTalker system.

NEW COMMUNICATION BARRIERS

Matthew's school was not as successful at implementing the AlphaTalker. Despite initial attempts to train school staff to program the device, and monthly follow-up consultations, it became apparent that additional activity-based communication boards were not being developed by Matthew's teachers or speech-language pathologist. After several months, Matthew's teacher admitted that the device was rarely used in class. In fact, his teacher had independently decided that sign language should be his primary method of communication. Because sign language was written into his IEP (along with use of picture-based methods of communication), his foster mother had never been notified of the change. Matthew's teacher noted that he was beginning to make progress in learning to comprehend and produce signs. He could independently sign a few functional requests (*all done, more, eat,* and *drink*). However, his ability to communicate using the picture communication boards was significantly better than his signing.

Several meetings were held between Matthew's school, family, and hospital staff. It was agreed that Matthew needed exposure to multiple modalities of communication, including the AlphaTalker simple communication boards, and sign language. School staff disagreed on who was responsible for developing picture communication displays and vocabulary. The school speech-language pathologist argued that she was only at the school 8 hours per week, and did not have the time to observe his class, interview the teacher, develop vocabulary, make picture communication displays, and program the AlphaTalker. His teacher argued that she was already overworked with 10 children in her class. She felt uncomfortable programming the device and changing activity pages. She was also worried about the school's liability if other children in the classroom broke the device.

We offered to develop classroom vocabulary displays and to program the AlphaTalker. However, when we observed his classroom, it was immediately apparent that class activities were designed for children at lower levels of functioning. Matthew was capable of communicating

higher level activity-based concepts, but the classroom routine did not require any of these skills. His teacher did not want to change her classroom activities as they were appropriate for most of the children in the class. It was decided to seek a transfer into a more appropriate classroom program that could meet Matthew's communication needs. After several additional meetings, it was agreed that he would transfer into a classroom for children with severe communication impairments at the beginning of the next school year.

BREAKING THROUGH

Matthew was 7 when he began attending his new school. Staff at the school were experienced at teaching all modalities of communication. In fact, there were already four other children in the class using voice output AAC systems. Picture communication displays were arranged in the classroom environment for all of the children to use. The school speech-language pathologist provided all of her services within the context of the classroom. She worked with the teacher to develop picture communication displays for commonly occurring classroom activities. She also trained Matthew's one-to-one aide to program the AlphaTalker. Managing vocabulary evolved into a collaborative effort. The teacher and speech-language pathologist would plan vocabulary pages, the aide would make the picture displays using BoardMaker, and the aide would program messages into the AlphaTalker.

Matthew blossomed during his seventh year. He continued to use picture-based methods of communication. By the end of the school year, he was beginning to rotely sequence picture symbols together to create messages (i.e., *I want + crayons,* and *I want + paper*). In addition, his ability to comprehend and produce signs significantly improved. He consistently accompanied his use of pictures with signs and gestures. Staff estimated that he was able to independently sign 20 different messages. As his ability to communicate improved, his maladaptive behaviors gradually disappeared. This did not mean that he was an easy child. Although he was no longer hitting, kicking, tantruming, or biting, he still had an extremely short attention span and lots of energy. Staff still spent lots of time chasing him from one activity to another. In addition, he had no sense of danger and continued to climb on furniture, run out unlocked doors, and dump or knock over boxes and containers. His foster mother began to refer to him as her "little tornado," which definitely characterized him.

Matthew's AAC journey is now almost 2 years old. AAC has provided him with the means to connect with other people in his world. It has given him a voice to make himself and his needs heard. Without that voice, he resorted to extreme behaviors to gain attention. Through AAC, he has learned how to appropriately communicate and interact with others and his personality is beginning to emerge. Matthew is finally breaking through to communication.

KEY POINTS TO REMEMBER

- Many individuals with severe maladaptive behaviors learn to communicate through hitting, kicking, biting, tantruming, and head banging, among other behaviors. Professionals need to determine the communicative function served by the behavior, and to replace the behavior with socially appropriate communication skills. This one-for-one conversion is easy in theory, but difficult to implement. It often takes months, if not years, to exchange one communicative behavior for another. What is easier is to try to avoid teaching the maladaptive communication behaviors in the first place.

- Matthew's first school program exposed him to sign language and speech, but ignored picture-based communication methods. Consequently, Matthew lost valuable learning time. Early intervention strategies for children with multiple disabilities need to include all potential communication methods. Over time, the preferred communication modality will emerge and less successful methods can be faded.

- Children with multiple disabilities cannot be evaluated easily using standardized assessment methods. Matthew's evaluation consisted of therapeutic observations over a long period of time. Through the gradual implementation of AAC strategies, a better picture of Matthew's true communication potential emerged.

- When AAC modalities are used, comprehension does not always precede expression. Matthew learned to use pictures while making expressive functional requests. Initially, he was probably only responding to the location of the symbol, its color, or some other visual cue related to the picture. Through expressive modeling and cause-effect pairings, he gradually learned the underlying meaning of each symbol. As he continued to expressively use symbols, he was able to generalize the symbol to new activity-based communication boards. This generalization indicated that he was able to identify the symbol and understand its communicative function.

- For children, voice output AAC devices are important in developing peer interactions. Simple picture communication boards or sign languages are effective for communicating with adults, but do not provide opportunities to independently communicate with peers.

- The process of developing and implementing picture-based communication strategies is time consuming. Many families and school staff have difficulty finding time to complete the process. Breaking the process down into small structured steps is often helpful. Matthew's foster mother was asked to help plan one new picture display each week. His weekly speech therapy sessions were used to complete the process. This provided her with the structure she needed to complete multiple picture communication displays.

Chapter 13

AAC AND ADULTS WITH ACQUIRED DISABILITIES

Patricia Pyatak Fletcher

Neurogenic communication disorders occur in adult populations as the result of a variety of diseases or conditions. Although some individuals retain their speech, language, and cognitive functioning in the presence of these disorders, others exhibit significant difficulty in effectively communicating with their families, friends, colleagues, and co-workers. Many individuals with acquired neurological disorders have severe communication impairments and benefit from using augmentative and alternative communication (AAC) strategies. This chapter explores the development of an interdisciplinary AAC evaluation and treatment team within the adult rehabilitation environment. It includes the incorporation of training activities within functional contexts as a means of facilitating a user's highest level of communicative functioning. The importance of extensive user and family education is also described, including how the completion of education and counseling regarding AAC issues facilitates device selection and may ultimately make the difference between consumer satisfaction and system abandonment. Finally, AAC device

maintenance and carryover techniques are reviewed.

DESCRIPTION OF THE POPULATION

Within the adult population, there are numerous diseases and conditions that may result in an acquired loss of communication abilities. Such conditions include traumatic brain injuries, cerebrovascular accidents, spinal cord injuries, various oncological conditions, and neurodegenerative diseases such as amyotrophic lateral sclerosis, multiple sclerosis, and progressive supranuclear palsy. According to the American Speech-Language-Hearing Association, nearly 2 million Americans are nonspeaking (ASHA, 1991). Adults with acquired communication disorders who are nonspeaking or have limited speaking ability are often good candidates for AAC systems. AAC can be defined as all forms of communication that enhance or supplement speech and writing skills (National Institute on Disability and Rehabilitation Research [NIDRR], 1992). LaPlante (1992) reported that 56% of speech technology device users in the United States were over the age of 65. People 24 years and under comprised only 23.5% of the sample. The high incidence of adult users may reflect the greater prevalence of people with impairments who can benefit from AAC intervention in the adult population.

People with acquired communication deficits can be organized into two groups: those whose conditions result in communication or physical conditions that remain relatively unchanged postonset or improve over time; and those that are characterized by a steady or erratic decline in communication or physical status over time. Table 13–1 illustrates this dichotomy. Information about population groups is explored further in this chapter.

Static or Improving Neurological Conditions

Neurological conditions such as traumatic brain injury, stroke, spinal cord injury, and various oncological conditions do not typically result in progressive loss of functioning. A person's level of communication with these conditions may remain static or may improve over time. The use of AAC strategies can serve to improve the user's communicative effectiveness, given a prerequisite degree of cognitive and communicative functioning.

Traumatic Brain Injury

A traumatic brain injury (TBI) occurs when trauma to the brain results in physical, cognitive-linguistic, emotional, and vocational changes (National Head Injury Foundation [NHIF], 1985). Over 2 million TBIs occur per year with 500,000 of these cases requiring hospitalization (National Institutes of Health [NIH], 1994). In a study examining the prevalence of traumatic brain injury as a cause of nonspeaking conditions among a sample of individuals who were nonspeaking, DeRuyter and Lafontaine (1987) found that, of 200 people who were seen at the Nonoral Center at the Rancho Los Amigos Medical Center in Downey, California, 31.5% were individuals with TBI. Primary causes of TBI in the adult population are motor vehicle accidents, automobile-pedestrian accidents, falls, gunshot wounds, work-related accidents, sports injuries, and assaults. Males are two times more likely to sustain a TBI than females (Ylvisaker, 1985).

Although people who sustain traumatic brain injuries may experience deficits in speech production, cognitive-communication, perception, and motor skills, these deficits do not generally progress in severity once diagnosed. Research by Thompsen (1983) reported that in the brain injury population, the status of those who

Table 13–1. Static and progressive neurological conditions.

Neurological conditions that are static or improving

Traumatic Brain Injury (TBI)

Cerebrovascular Accident (CVA)

Spinal Cord Injury (SCI)

Oncologic Conditions

Neurological conditions that are progressive

Amyotrophic Lateral Sclerosis (ALS)

Multiple Sclerosis (MS)

Progressive Supranuclear Palsy (PSP)

presented with dysarthria changed little up to 13 years postinjury. AAC efforts are directed at identifying the earliest point in the person's recovery in which they may benefit from AAC intervention as a component of a multimodal communication system. Low tech (i.e., a communication board) or high tech AAC systems are continuously modified and adjusted as the individual's skills improve and as his or her communication needs change. Modifications of technology are necessary throughout the client's recovery, beginning in the early stages.

The early stage of recovery from TBI is marked by the client's ability to consistently demonstrate purposeful responses in the environment and the inconsistent ability to follow commands (Ylvisaker, 1985). At this stage of recovery, the individual may be considered a candidate for use of very simple AAC systems, including the training of a yes/no signal and use of a single switch connected to a nurse's call button or electric appliance to request attention.

At the middle phase of recovery, the individual exhibits confusion yet improved consistency in the ability to attend to environmental stimuli and follow commands. The individual can be trained in the use of communication boards or in electronic devices with simple picture overlays of limited complexity (e.g., four pictures of four familiar functional objects). In the late stage of recovery from TBI, performance is marked by generally appropriate behavior with limitations in self-monitoring, sustained attention, memory, and reasoning/problem solving. AAC systems that can be investigated at this point in recovery include dedicated high tech or nondedicated multipurpose systems that can be useful within numerous contexts such as vocational and recreational situations (Cohen & DeRuyter, 1982).

Cerebrovascular Accident

Cerebrovascular accident (CVA), commonly known as stroke, is the leading cause of disability in the United States today. Approximately 2.5 million survive the stroke and require rehabilitation services (Foley & Pizer, 1990). A CVA is an injury to the nervous system that occurs when an adequate supply of oxygen and nutrients fails to reach portions of the brain due to thrombus, embolism, or hemorrhage. The majority of strokes occur between the ages of 70–80. Risk factors include gender and race. Statistics show that men are more likely to have a stroke and African Americans are 60% more likely than Caucasians to have a stroke (Caplan, Dyken, & Easton, 1994). Approximately 20% of all stroke patients experience aphasia, with 20–30% of these individuals exhibiting severe communication deficits for at least a portion of their recovery (Collins, 1986).

Survivors of CVA may have difficulties achieving an AAC system-user match, because of their possible deficits in reading, auditory comprehension, sequencing, and organization. Despite largely intact cognitive abilities, existing language deficits may result in the person's inability to use the communication system of his or her choice and may cause a person to be dissatisfied or frustrated with the use of simple AAC systems. For example, the speech-language pathologist may find that a person's low literacy level precludes him or her from using a system with written messages that are selected from a menu of printed words, or messages that are accessed through letter codes. Indeed, the language deficits of many persons with aphasia make it extremely difficult for them to operate linguistically based AAC systems (Hux, Beukelman, & Garrett, 1994). Further, clients who have difficulty in comprehending pictorial stimuli or in recalling a symbol's semantic meaning may become frustrated when interacting with many commercially available AAC systems. It is frequently the client's and evaluating clinician's challenge to secure a system that achieves a balance between the individual's communicative needs and existing communication deficits.

Spinal Cord Injury

A spinal cord injury (SCI) occurs when there is an "abrupt nonprogressive disruption of the spinal cord" (Ozer, 1988, p. 6). The incidence of persons who sustain permanent spinal cord injuries annually is estimated to be in the range of 7,600–10,000 people (National Spinal Cord Injury Statistical Center, 1994). The person most frequently prone to a spinal cord injury is male (4:1), injured in a motor vehicle, diving, or sports-related injury, or injured by a knife or gunshot wound (Ozer, 1988). Young, Burns, Bowen, and McCutchen (1982) found that the median age of people sustaining spinal cord injuries was 25 with almost half not yet high school graduates.

The SCI lesion may be complete, causing total loss of sensation and voluntary muscle control below the level of damage, or incomplete, resulting in a partial loss of functioning. In the SCI population, cognitive-communicative skills are intact unless there is a preexisting condition (e.g., mental retardation), or if other conditions occur at the time of the spinal cord injury (e.g., SCI combined with TBI). Beukelman and Yorkston reported that in persons with SCI, "the physical impairment alone is typically responsible for speaking and writing disorders" (Beukelman & Yorkston, 1989, p. 47).

According to Vanderheiden and Smith (1989), individuals with spinal cord injuries benefit greatly from the use of three primary AAC and other assistive technology strategies: strategies for writing, computer access, and environmental control. To enhance writing abilities, persons with cervical level 3–5 injuries (C3–C5) benefit from communication techniques that incorporate adaptive equipment including universal cuffs (adaptive hand-held equipment that enables the consumer to hold various items without functional fine motor ability) and wrist-stabilizing splints. Computer access can be maximized through the use of typing aids and keyguards (Kirby, 1989). These pieces of equipment not only facilitate system access but can also enhance motor access accuracy and speed (Bay, 1991). In a C6–C7 injury, although the person is typically independent in the use of typewriters, computers, and in turning pages of a book, the person may require AAC intervention during extended conversational exchanges (e.g., meetings at work, lectures) due to decreased respiratory support or vocal volume. Chapter 3 provides more information regarding specific AAC systems and devices.

Oncological Conditions

Head and neck cancers are among the oncological conditions that may result in a need for AAC intervention. Cancer of the larynx (including vocal folds), tongue, and mandible are frequently diagnosed in the elderly with associated risk factors of smoking or chewing tobacco and alcohol consumption (Sonies, 1987). Deficits in speech and swallowing may result from resectioning malignant tissues and radiation treatment. Other oncologic conditions include brain tumors, with resultant deficits similar to those noted in stroke. That is, given the site of the primary or metastatic tumor, the person may present with neurogenic speech, language, cognitive-communicative, or swallowing difficulties.

The needs of the AAC user with oncological conditions may change throughout the course of the disease and treatment phase. Electrolarynges are among the AAC systems that have been found to be appropriate for individuals with oncological conditions. These devices are available in both neck placement and intraoral varieties (see Chapter 16 for more information). Some individuals may prefer to use simple AAC systems such as a notebook or a "magic slate" containing frequently used utterances. AAC systems that enable the person to type messages or to select words or symbols with prestored messages have also been found to be useful.

Neurological Conditions That Are Progressive

Neurodegenerative diseases, marked by a progressive decline in functioning, can prove to be extremely challenging for clinicians considering AAC intervention. The progressive and unstable nature of these diseases requires ongoing adjustment in therapeutic management, including prescription of assistive technology and incorporation of this technology into the person's daily routines. AAC technology that provides flexibility in selection techniques, vocabulary, and cognitive-communicative demands is critical for individuals with neurodegenerative diseases.

Amyotrophic Lateral Sclerosis (ALS)

ALS, a disease affecting both the upper and lower motor neurons, results in a flaccid-spastic paralysis that ultimately affects all muscular functions (Darley, Aronson, & Brown, 1975). The disease does not affect cognition. The decrement in motor skills, including lingual, labial, buccal, palatal, laryngeal, and respiratory musculature strength and functioning, results in dysarthria, dysphagia, and ultimately, aphonia.

In the early stages of ALS, the individual may have reduced speech intelligibility due to dysarthria of mixed flaccid-spastic type (Darley et al., 1975) with hypernasality and dysphonia seen in conjunction with prosodic impairments (Sonies, 1987). AAC efforts may be directed toward education about various communication options, including communication boards, dedicated systems with speech output, and sophisticated computer-based AAC systems. Peo-

ple with early-stage ALS who demonstrate reduced speech audibility or intelligibility may benefit from speech amplification systems or simple AAC systems that use notebooks containing frequently used utterances or blank pages for writing messages.

As the disease progresses and the existing speech deficits increase in severity, end-stage communication skills are characterized by effortful verbal output due to severe respiratory and speech muscular impairments. In a study by Saunders, Walsh, and Smith (1981) involving 100 hospice patients in late stage ALS, 28% of the people were anarthric, 47% demonstrated dysarthria severe enough to produce speech with decreased speech intelligibility, and only 25% spoke with functional speech intelligibility at the time of their death. Swallowing skills are also severely impaired at end stages, with the individual's nutritional needs typically being met via parenteral tube feedings. Furthermore, deterioration in other areas of motor function occurs with the progression of the disease. Whereas the client may have accessed early-stage AAC systems via direct selection, many users by the late stage of ALS frequently use scanning AAC devices via single or double switches for system access. A system that provides flexibility in motor selection technique as the disease progresses ultimately decreases the amount of training time required for the user while accommodating changes in physical status.

Multiple Sclerosis

Multiple sclerosis (MS), is caused by the progressive demyelination of the central nervous system (Erickson, Lie, & Wineinger, 1989). Deficits associated with MS include dysarthria with difficulties in controlling vocal volume, pitch, and prosody (Sonies, 1987). Deficits in cognition may include decreased attention, orientation, memory, nonverbal learning, problem solving, and reasoning (Staples & Lincoln, 1979). Communication systems that provide the person with a variety of selection techniques and features enable the individual to effectively utilize the communication system throughout the progression of the disease.

AAC systems that provide ample communication flexibility and require moderate amounts of consumer training (e.g., complex AAC software packages, use of Minspeak) may initially be selected by the evaluating team as best meeting the consumer's needs. However, it is critical to select an AAC system that can be simplified over time without replacing the entire package. A device that initially compensates for the person's reduced vocal volume and mildly impaired fine motor skills through use of a keyguard may be completely inaccessible as the disease progresses to the middle and late stages. The decrement in cognitive-communicative skills frequently seen in late stage MS supports the use of AAC systems that provide flexibility in vocabulary, simplicity in operation, ease of maintenance, and can be accessed via a variety of motor selection techniques.

Progressive Supranuclear Palsy

Progressive supranuclear palsy (PSP), or Steele-Richardson-Olzewski syndrome, may include clinical characteristics of dysarthria, aphonia, and oral/pharyngeal dysphagia (Sonies, 1987). Dementia and lability may also be present in PSP (Jankovic, 1984). PSP progresses rapidly during a 2–3 year period, resulting in significant difficulties in communication due to oral-motor system deficits and severe head and neck rigidity. Communication systems that are useful with clients with PSP include communication boards with written or pictorial stimuli and dedicated AAC systems with speech output.

ASSESSMENT STRATEGIES

Interdisciplinary Evaluation Process

Given the multi-faceted profile of disabilities in adults with acquired communication deficits, there are numerous advantages to an interdisciplinary team approach for assessment purposes. Support for this claim was made at the AAC intervention consensus validation conference 1992 where it was argued that an interdisciplinary team approach was highly effective in the management of consumers with AAC needs. Table 13–2 illustrates sample interdisciplinary evaluation roles, including recommended primary and supportive clinical services. This process is supported by ASHA's *Preferred Practice Patterns* regarding AAC (1992).

Within the adult rehabilitation setting, selection of team members and clinical roles within the AAC evaluation process is dependent upon the client's diagnosis and communication needs. Patients with a diagnosis of ALS frequently have an evaluation team comprising a speech-language pathologist, an occupational therapist, a physical therapist, a rehabilitation engineer, and a social worker. The individual frequently has a physiatrist or neurologist who provides consultative services throughout the evaluation process. In contrast, the "team" for persons with head and neck oncological conditions may comprise only a speech-language pathologist and a physician for consultation services. These clients frequently do not require occupational or physical therapy services as they typically do not have other motor impairments, nor are they in need of rehabilitation engineering as customized equipment is usually not warranted. People with oncologic conditions may already be participating in supportive psychological services provid-

Table 13–2. Interdisciplinary evaluation team in the adult rehabilitation setting.

Core AAC Team Members

- **Speech-Language Pathologist**

Reading Comprehension	Oral Motor/Speech	Environmental AAC Needs
Auditory Comprehension	Expressive Language	Vocabulary Selection
Social Skills	Sequencing	Device Recommendations
Problem Solving	Memory	Encoding System
		Device Training

- **Occupational Therapist**

Fine Motor Abilities	Hand Functioning	Switch Access
Muscle Tone	Visual Motor Skills	AAC Selection Technique
Positioning	Visual Perceptual Skills	Environmental Accommodations
Coordination		Equipment Adaptations

- **Rehabilitation Engineer**

Equipment Design	Equipment Adaptations	Equipment Integration
Mounting Equipment	Equipment Fabrication	

Supportive AAC Team Members

- **Physical Therapy**

Lower Extremity	Range of Motion	Seating
Gait Training	Balance	Positioning
Muscle Tone		

- **Physiatrist**

Diagnosis of Medical Status	Recommend Equipment Needs

- **Nurse**

Ongoing Medical Care	Communication Needs	AAC Implementation

- **Social Worker**

Client and Family Liason	Funding Liason	Client and Family Counseling

- **Vocational Rehabilitation Counselor**

Vocational Counseling	Work Site Evaluation	Work Site Accommodations
Employer Counseling	Employer Education	Job Training

- **Neuropsychologist**

Neuropsychologic Assessment	Client and Family Counseling

ed by a social worker or psychologist and may need to be referred for these services only if they have not been secured prior to the AAC evaluation process.

Composition of the AAC evaluation team is also dependent upon the vocational needs of the consumer. Clients with acquired communication deficits who wish to return to work may have an evaluation team compring not only a speech-language pathologist, occupational therapist, physical therapist, rehabilitation engineer, neuropsychologist, and social worker, but also a vocational rehabilitation counselor. This team member supplements team efforts by generating vocationally based goals and assisting other team members in gearing their goals toward vocational needs.

Team members and their respective roles may be determined by other factors, including the expertise of various team members or the limitations inherent to the facility where AAC services are provided. In some facilities, occupational therapy or rehabilitation engineering services, for example, may not be available. In the case where needed clinical services are not readily available, consultative services may be obtained to provide comprehensive services or the individual may ultimately need to be referred to a facility that can provide comprehensive AAC evaluation and treatment services (Trefler, 1987). For more information on teaming and service delivery issues, please refer to Chapter 2.

Preliminary Data Collection

AAC Interview Assessment

Use of an initial interview assessment is useful in gathering client and family information for evaluation purposes. A questionnaire developed at the National Rehabilitation Hospital (NRH) has been found to be a highly effective means to gather information while efficiently identifying the consumer's needs. NRH's questionnaire covers information in areas from "Reason for Referral" through physical and communication skills (Goldsmith, O'Donnell, Carin, Schein, & Harrison, 1988). Incorporation of rating scales is useful in determining the consumer's and family's priority of needs. An example of this rating scale is presented in Figure 13–1.

It is critical to obtain information regarding the consumer's medical status, as this may ultimately affect the patient's outcome. Information obtained can guide the interdisciplinary team in AAC device selection and equipment purchase as well as in determining prognosis and treatment techniques. Medically related questions in

a comprehensive questionnaire should include questions regarding diagnosis, etiology, and medical management. Questions such as, "What is your medical diagnosis?" "Date of onset/injury?" "Are you currently taking any prescribed medications?" "Have you recently had any medical or surgical procedures?" and "Are any medical or surgical procedures planned in the near future?" assist therapists in determining evaluation processes. Questions targeting physical factors such as trunk control, mobility, and upper extremity use will also enable the therapists to plan evaluation measures that take into consideration concomitant medical diagnoses (e.g., scoliosis) and wheelchair use (e.g., time spent in the wheelchair each day, type of wheelchair).

Preevaluation questions related to perception and memory are recommended to determine the consumer's visual-perceptual and cognitive abilities. Information regarding the person's ability to visually track pictorial and orthographic stimuli can direct the evaluator to the appropriate size and color of presented symbols. If the person responds affirmatively to a question such as "Do you confuse similar written words?" (e.g., "cat" for "hat"), the evaluation team should investigate the individual's visual-perceptual status for reading purposes. Ultimately, the team may need to opt for use of enlarged pictorial stimuli rather than written words for communication system purposes.

In addition to questions targeting medical and physical status, a thorough questionnaire should also include questions related to communication. Questionnaire items should be posed in a variety of formats to enable the consumer or family member to respond to questions in a comprehensive manner. Sample communication questions are also included in Figure 13–1.

Lastly questions designed to tap the consumer's vocational and community needs and goals should be included in a comprehensive questionnaire. Recommend-

AAC Preliminary Needs Interview

Patient Name: _____   Date: _____

Rank order the following communication environments for which an AAC system would be used (1 = very important; 2 = somewhat important; 3 = not important).

1 2 3 At Home	1 2 3 In the Community
1 2 3 At School	1 2 3 Social Contexts (Parties, etc.)
1 2 3 At Work	1 2 3 Telephone

Are you able to make sounds using your voice?   Yes   No
Can you say words?   Yes   No
Can you indicate yes and no consistently?   Yes   No
Can you use facial expressions to communicate?   Yes   No
Can you use body language to communicate?   Yes   No

How do you reliably communicate the following:

Comm Need	Method	Comm Need	Method
Pain		Happiness	
Frustration		Refusal	
Hunger		Fatigue	
Discomfort		Boredom	
Toileting		Other	

If your listener doesn't understand you, what is your reaction (i.e., do you repeat yourself, become angry, rephrase what was said, or give up)?

How often do other persons not understand you?

Do some persons have more difficulty understanding you than others (i.e., family versus strangers)?

Figure 13–1. AAC preliminary needs interview. (From *AAC Questionnaire*, by T. Goldsmith, K. O'Donnell, S. Carin, R. Schein, & A. Harrison, 1988, Unpublished paper. Washington, DC: National Rehabilitation Hospital. Reprinted with permission.)

ed items should address the types of jobs held, skills used, dates employed, years of education, as well as activities completed in the home and community settings and length of time the respondent engaged in these activities.

Information gathered from interviews with the consumer and caregiver also assists the evaluator in developing and refining an assessment protocol. For example, a consumer may report that following surgery for removal of a portion of the larynx, he or she has no difficulties in auditory and reading comprehension, writing, memory, or problem-solving skills, and would like to identify a communication system with speech output. Assessment measures would typically be developed that involve informal assessment of communication needs and education regarding the various communication systems available.

Training of a Reliable Yes/No Response for Evaluation Purposes

People who use AAC technology are often unable to verbally respond to traditional assessment measures. In order to circumvent this disability, the examiner needs to determine the person's most reliable manner of response to test questions. Assessment strategies should include the identification of a motor response that is, according to Kirby (1989, p. 187), "speedy, accurate, and nonfatiguing." To do this, the evaluator needs to determine if there are two distinguishable movements exhibited by the client. In a study by Bay (1991), therapeutic positioning with support for the trunk and extremities and control of abnormal movements (e.g., primitive reflexes) facilitated the individual's ability to use movements for communication purposes. Once these reliable movements are identified, the evaluator is able to train one movement to mean "yes" and one to signal "no." If only one movement is identi-

fied, yes and no can be signaled by one movement meaning "yes" and two repetitions of the movement meaning "no". Preserved voluntary movements used to communicate "no" may also spontaneously emerge (e.g., a person emerging from coma due to a severe traumatic brain injury indicating "no" by pushing things away with his or her upper extremity). It is therefore recommended that evaluation and training of motor movements be completed within contextually based environments to obtain responses that have increased frequency of use and possess a higher degree of naturalness for the user. Behaviors and motor responses for yes/no communication are illustrated in Table 13–3. Once a reliable yes/no response is attained, administration of various formal and informal assessment tools can be completed.

FORMAL ASSESSMENT MEASURES

In assessing the cognitive-communicative skills of individuals who are nonspeaking, it is not uncommon to adapt or modify standardized assessment measures. Numerous assessment tools have been published that are routinely administered to individuals who have sustained a TBI or CVA. These assessments target individuals who have sustained neurological injury, yet had intact functional speech, language, and cognitive-communicative abilities prior to the injury. Many of these assessment measures can be used to extrapolate information for AAC purposes, including determination of the client's communication diagnosis and generation of treatment goals. Information obtained during the preliminary interview assessment will help the team to determine the components of the evaluation process by focusing on specific skill areas.

Assessment tools can be modified so that test stimuli are presented in either a

Table 13–3. Behaviors and motor responses for yes/no communication.

1. eye gaze/movements
2. finger movements
3. eye blinks
4. squeezing/opening hand
5. facial movements/expressions
6. gestural body movements

yes/no or multiple choice format (see Chapter 5 for more information). The evaluator should be cautious in test interpretation, as changing the stimuli presentation format inherently changes the validity of the tool; however, valuable diagnostic information may nonetheless be yielded. A list of these "traditional" measures and suggestions for their "nontraditional" use within AAC evaluations includes the tests that follow.

Reading Comprehension

Reading Comprehension Battery For Aphasia

The *Reading Comprehension Battery for Aphasia* ([RCBA]: LaPointe & Horner, 1984) has many subtests that can be adapted to evaluate reading abilities in the adult population with acquired disabilities. Recommended subtests include: I. Word-Visual; II. Word-Auditory; III. Word-Semantic; IV. Functional Reading; VI. Sentence-Picture; and VII. Paragraph-Picture.

The initial three subtests of the RCBA include presentations of three single words with one pictorial stimulus. The client is instructed to point to the word that matches the picture. Increased difficulty is introduced at the "Functional Reading" subtest level, as the person is required to read various sentence-level stimuli within a functional framework (e.g., a medication label, a weather report) and in-

structed to point to the picture or position within a narrative that is described in the presented sentence.

Administration of these RCBA subtests can provide information regarding the consumer's literacy level as well as identify the level at which the person experiences difficulty in interpreting orthographic information. Such information is helpful in determining the person's ability to receptively identify printed symbols on a communication board or system overlay. It also directs the evaluator in generating realistic goals for treatment, including the use of single words or phrases on the overlay and helps in determining the ideal length of stored messages. If an individual cannot respond accurately to sentence-length stimuli, single words or simple phrases should be stored in the client's message inventory.

Despite this measure's reported limitations as valid indicator of reading ability (Nicholas, MacLennan, & Brookshire, 1986), the RCBA can provide the clinician with valuable AAC diagnostic information. The test presents pictorial and orthographic stimuli that are frequently familiar to the consumer and are presented in a format that does not visually overload the user.

Boston Diagnostic Aphasia Examination

The *Boston Diagnostic Aphasia Examination* ([BDAE]; Goodglass & Kaplan, 1983) also has sections that can yield corroborative evidence regarding functional reading status.

Symbol Discrimination. The person is presented with various single letters printed in one style, and instructed to point to the same letter, written in a different style, from an array of five letters. Observations made during test administration can be helpful in determining what type of print size and style the therapist and family members should use on the consumer's communication system. If the person exhibits difficulty in interpreting written script during test administration, it is not recommended that script be incorporated into the communication system.

Word Recognition. The client is instructed to point to the word that is spoken by the examiner from a horizontally arranged list of five words. Four other lines of stimuli (each with five words per line) are visually presented while addressing the targeted line. This subtest not only provides information related to the individual's single word reading, but also subjective information regarding the degree to which visually loaded stimuli can be presented while maintaining accurate reading skills. This information can be helpful in fabrication of AAC systems that maximize communication options without visually overloading the user.

Word-Picture Matching. This subtest provides information regarding the consumer's ability to match picture stimuli with written orthographic stimuli. Information extrapolated from this subtest may include the person's ability to match symbols with pictures and whether pictures or words are more readily identified by the individual.

Reading Sentences and Paragraphs. This subtest requires the consumer to respond to 10 stimuli of increasing complexity and length, progressing up to paragraph-level stimuli. In addition to providing information regarding the person's reading skill status, this subtest may also provide subjective information about the individual's

speed of reading, attention, cognitive endurance, and vigilance. This information assists the clinician in determining device selection, use of orthography within the user's communication system, and vocabulary selection.

If the client reports adequate reading skills for functional materials (magazines, work-related briefs), use of assessment tools that assess complex reading skills (i.e., The Nelson-Denny Reading Test; Brown, Bennett, & Hanna, 1981) may also be used. Conversely, if less complex assessment items are needed due to greater reading impairment, various subtests from the Western Aphasia Battery (Kertesz, 1982) such as Reading Commands and Reading Comprehension of Sentences are suggested.

Auditory Comprehension

The following evaluation procedures can be used to assess the unique auditory comprehension deficits that often accompany acquired neurological conditions.

Boston Diagnostic Aphasia Examination
([BDAE]; Goodglass & Kaplan, 1983)

Word Discrimination. Although the items targeted in this subtest may not be considered uniformly relevant to all user's communication needs or environment (e.g., *cylinder, dripping*), the subtest taps comprehension of a large variety of semantic categories, including objects, letters, forms, actions, colors and numbers.

A nonstandard administration style of this subtest (that is, administration of only a limited number of items to obtain a preliminary impression of auditory word discrimination skills) is recommended as this assessment tool is easily administered and requires limited client training to complete. Many of the test items may not be relevant to the consumer's communication needs. Follow-up testing can be adapted with the use of words identified by the consumer or family members or other advocates as being relevant for their daily communication needs.

Body-Part Identification. Selected items from this subtest are frequently used with patients who present with adult-onset communication disorders. Items such as *shoulder, knee, chest, neck,* and *thigh* are often seen in adult communication systems because of the need to express concerns regarding pain in these areas and changing medical concerns. It is recommended that the clinician use the list of body-part targets in the subtest as a guide to be presented in a multiple choice format. For example, the evaluator can point to three different sites on the person and ask at each site, "Is this your leg?" The person can use their yes/no response system to answer each question, yielding a measure of the individual's ability to identify body parts. Test items should be repeated to determine response reliability.

Additional tools that can be utilized to assess an individual's auditory comprehension skills include the Complex Ideational Material subtest of the BDAE (Goodglass & Kaplan, 1983), the *Revised Token Test* (McNeil & Prescott, 1978), the Oral Directions subtest of the *Detroit Tests of Learning Aptitude-2* (Hammill, 1985) and an informal yes/no battery that includes yes/no questions related to personal, environmental, and factual questions.

Speech Intelligibility

A modified version of the *Computerized Assessment of Intelligibility of Dysarthric Speakers* ([CAIDS]; Yorkston, Beukelman, & Traynor, 1984) can be administered to assess an adult's speech intelligibility status. This tool provides a percentage of speech intelligibility and can yield information regarding the level of reliance a user may have on verbal output in con-

junction with assistive technology. A modified administration of this tool can be completed (e.g., presentation of a portion of the test items) if the individual demonstrates fatigue during administration of the entire tool. It should be noted that although this assessment measure is useful in determining the user's level of speech intelligibility, it does not assess skill level within functional contexts. This assessment tool should be used in conjunction with an informal assessment of speech intelligibility within meaningful contexts as identified by the user or user's family. Assessment should include the determination of speech intelligibility for spontaneously produced words and utterances as well as for utterances produced within imitative contexts. More information on this topic is available in Chapter 5.

Expressive Language

By the nature of the individual's disability as well as the fact that many formal assessment measures do not adequately assess the client's skill level within functional contexts, many clients needing AAC intervention frequently require informal assessment procedures to determine their level of expressive language functioning. Assessment measures completed within functional contexts such as in the community, workplace, or home enable the clinician to assess the client's actual communication functioning as well as needs within these familiar contexts. If the person has functionally unintelligible speech production, it is difficult for the evaluator to assess the individual's expressive language performance. If residual speech output exists, recording and analysis of the individual's spontaneous conversation may be helpful in informally assessing the individual's vocabulary, syntax, level of concreteness or abstraction, and organizational skills. Video- or audio-taping an evaluation enables the clinician to transcribe off-line the person's expressive language interactions and to determine skill status.

In addition to verbal communication, assessment procedures should address the individual's existing gestural and written expression skills. In many cases, these nonverbal communication modalities serve to supplement the client's use of verbal communication. It is helpful to determine the individual's ability to gesture common feelings such as cold, sick, angry, tired, pain, happiness, hunger. It is also helpful to assess the client's ability to gesture common objects such as bed or pillow, wheelchair, medication, car, and hospital as a means to communicate an utterance such as "I need my medication."

Assessment should initially involve observation of the client within a familiar context to determine his or her ability to communicate functional messages through the use of gestures. If no gestures are observed, or the client is unsuccessful in effectively communicating meaningful information using gestures, the clinician should provide a model of the targeted gesture without using the intended object to determine if the client can imitate the gesture. If needed, increased structure can be provided by modeling the gesture with the appropriate object (i.e., actually pointing to or holding a pillow) and then requesting the patient to imitate the gesture. Refer to Rao (1994) for a review of gestural assessment and treatment strategies in persons with severe aphasia.

Functional assessment of expressive language skills should also include evaluation of the client's written expression. Assessment should include the person's ability to write his or her name, address, phone number, and basic needs and feelings. Findings should include the length of the written utterance along with accuracy and legibility of the written message.

Memory/Sequencing

The Rivermead Behavioural Memory Test

The *Rivermead Behavioural Memory Test* ([RBMT]; Wilson, Cockburn, & Baddeley, 1985) was designed to investigate everyday memory abilities of adults between the ages of 16 and 69. Test items include the recall of an appointment, picture recognition, prose recall, face recognition, immediate and delayed recall of a route, taking and delivering a message, recall of orientation items, and recall to request a hidden belonging. Although this test does not directly assess the skills needed for AAC system use, the clinician is frequently able to observe the presence or absence of requisite skills during test administration, including the ability to visually recognize and sequence pictorial stimuli. Subjective data regarding the consumer's level of attention and problem solving can also be obtained.

INFORMAL ASSESSMENT MEASURES

Informal administration of various tasks within the areas of receptive and expressive language, cognition, and pragmatics can provide pivotal information for a comprehensive evaluation. In some cases, formal measures cannot be administered and the evaluator must rely on informal findings to generate the cognitive-linguistic diagnosis, prognosis, and treatment goals. For individuals with severe deficits such as those in the early stage of recovery from TBI or those with severe aphasia, the assessment protocol is typically composed of informal measures addressing auditory and reading comprehension status, existing verbal expression/speech production skills, and cognitive-communication level. Table 13–4 illustrates various informal measures that can be administered during a comprehensive AAC evaluation. Based upon the client's diagnosis, existing deficits, and communication needs the evaluator can select items from this informal assessment battery.

AAC TRAINING STRATEGIES

Application of AAC technology involves numerous clinical skills, as the clinician assists the user in mastering a way to access the communication system as well as how to incorporate the system into functional contexts. AAC implementation also involves the training of family members and friends in facilitating communication interactions with the user in specific contexts. In the adult population, the evaluation process continues throughout training, with ongoing adjustments made to the system as a person's communication status improves (as in TBI) or regresses (as in ALS). Indeed, evaluation and training of a

Table 13–4. Informal AAC assessment measures.

• Attention	Informal observations
	Divided attention tasks
	Tracking colors, shapes, numbers
• Auditory Comprehension	Reliable responses to yes/no questions
	Ability to follow 1, 2, and 3 step commands
• Receptive Vocabulary	Identification of well known objects
	Identification of photographs
	Identification of colored drawings
	Identification of black and white line drawings
• Memory	Recall of time, place, self
	Recall of objects and pictures
• Sequencing	Sequencing pictures to represent a routine activity
	Sequencing pictures to represent a 2-3 word message
• Reading	Matching pictures to words and sentences
• Spelling	Matching letters
	Identification of named letters
	Selecting letters to complete spelling words
• Pragmatics	Ability to initiate communication
	Eye contact
	Use of gestures
• Speech	Intelligibility of single words
	Intelligibility of phrases, sentences, conversation
	Stimulability for pacing or overarticulation strategies

system in this adult population is different from all other populations being trained in AAC device use as most of these adults come to the communication arena with functional preexisting communication skills. An adult's actual participation in functional contexts with an AAC device reveals the merging of premorbid speech, language, cognition, and pragmatic language skills with existing deficits.

It is extremely helpful to train not only the user but all individuals frequently involved in the user's AAC environment (e.g., family, caregiver, clinicians). Research by McNaughton and Light (1989) found that the incorporation of a communication partner in the training process can be critical to the success of an AAC system. Training all persons involved in the AAC process serves to reinforce system use in a variety of contexts and interactive manners (Nelson, Leonard, Fisher, Esquenzai, & Hicks, 1989). The training process should include mastery of a selection technique, beginning with the attainment of a consistent and reliable body movement, single switch, eye gaze, or direct selection technique. Training for vocabulary and symbol selection should also be completed.

Selection Technique

Consistent/Reliable Body Movement

The mastery of a consistent motor response is fundamental to selection technique training. Initial training involves the identification of a reliable movement and then the development of activities that reinforce the client's consistent and reliable use of this movement. The clinician needs to chart the ability to turn the head to auditory stimuli, to focus eyes on the clinician, to look up and down, to blink the eyes, to move individual fingers and groups of fingers and to move lower extremities (e.g., tapping the foot). Use of tracking sheets, including those developed by Ladtkow

and Culp (1992) can be helpful in the consistent documentation of the client's motor responses.

It is important to note that, in the adult population, the user may employ a variety of access methods as his or her medical status changes. In the case of an individual with a neurodegenerative disease such as multiple sclerosis, the user may initially use direct selection. As his or her physical status declines, the user may be considered a candidate for use of a joystick, and with further physical decline, may need to use a single switch for row-column scanning. Conversely, a user who has sustained a traumatic brain injury or cerebrovascular accident may initially use a single switch due to pervasive motor deficits but then progress to direct selection as his or her motor deficits resolve. The next section will review options for accessing AAC systems. These include single switch methods, eye gaze, and direct selection. Chapter 7 provides more information on motor access evaluation and training methods.

Cause-Effect Single Switch Use

Simple AAC systems can be fabricated that incorporate the training of a body part movement through a cause-effect paradigm. Such AAC systems can include the use of single switches hooked up to assistive technology appliances. An example of this type of system used in a hospital setting includes the use of a single switch hooked up to a nurse's call button. A large-surfaced single switch interfaced with an environmental control unit (ECU) permits an individual to turn on and off lights, fans, and other appliances. Such assistive technology systems are very reinforcing as cause-and-effect is immediately attained. Once consistent single switch use is attained, training efforts can be directed at switch operation for scanning purposes.

When the individual can reliably activate the ECU in a cause-effect manner, training can progress to where the client activates the switch within a specified period of time. Training tasks should address the person's ability to accurately and quickly activate a switch, as these are requisite skills for functional AAC communication system use.

Scanning Training

Tasks can next be designed that train circular scanning via various low tech AAC devices such as the commercially available Versascan, which has a clock hand pointer that rotates around a dial. The client is encouraged to activate the switch at specific locations on the dial, beginning initially with a single location and progressing to 2–3 locations. Increased task difficulty can be introduced by progressing from pictures to printed word stimuli. In this manner, the client can begin training in consistent use of a switch in a circular scanning format.

Given successful training of simple scanning skills, training activities can next address the client's ability to use scanning to access simple AAC systems containing multiple symbols. Various scanning techniques should be attempted to determine the scanning method that the client can use with the greatest consistency and accuracy. Modification in the selection technique variables, such as step scanning, direction of scan (e.g., circular, linear), speed of scan, and delay at each location should be assessed so that training can be completed using the most efficient mode of scanning.

For users with memory impairments, it is helpful to include a visual cue (i.e., picture or written menu) of sentences and symbols either on the user's laptray or on the AAC system to enhance recall of symbol sequences during training sessions. Technology that employs symbol prediction or predictive scanning is useful in enhancing recall of sequences as well as access speed, as only those sequences programmed into the device are able to be selected. The user can be trained to utilize a trial-and-error method in order to recall sequences. Alternatively, a problem-solving based strategy may be employed, with the user scanning possible sequence items and identifying the most plausible symbols. This reasoning strategy is most effective in users with functional problem-solving and reasoning abilities but inconsistent symbol sequence recall ability.

Eye Gaze Training

In those individuals whose disabilities preclude them from reliably moving most parts of their body (e.g., ALS, brainstem stroke), eye gaze is a direct selection option for an alternative selection technique. Eye gaze training initially involves improving the person's ability to direct his or her gaze in a given direction for a designated amount of time. Direction and style of eye gaze training should be driven by the person's visual preference or physical status. A person may demonstrate a preference to look to the right, may have difficulty disassociating eye movements from head movements, or may exhibit an oculomotor deficit that requires looking only to the right and left, and not up or down. In all training sessions, tasks should be designed that address the person's accuracy and consistency in eye gaze for communication system use.

Training activities should include stimuli that are readily seen, including adequate size and color contrast. Tasks should begin with the client maintaining eye gaze on a stimulus for a designated period of time. Tasks that use picture stimuli are useful with individuals who present with decreased attention or who require stimuli with a high degree of familiarity and concreteness. AAC systems with single words can be presented to clients at their functional literacy level.

Once consistent and reliable responses to a single picture or word are attained, task difficulty can be upgraded whereby two to five items are presented (typically mounted on a clear plastic board) and the individual shifts his or her gaze from one choice to the other, as directed by the therapist.

Presentation of additional symbols can be introduced once the individual can reliably identify a small set of stimuli (less than 5 items). The client is asked to select a named picture (e.g., "Show me the wheelchair") with tasks progressing in difficulty as accurate responses are noted (i.e., using contextual cues, "Show me the item that helps you get around in your house").

Stimuli can be arranged in various formats, including alphabetical groupings of letters (see Figure 13–2). The user looks at a group of letters that contains the target, then looks at the listener. The listener in turn verbally scans through the letters, looking for a prearranged signal by the user that signals the intended letter. This process is repeated until the word is completed. Chapters 3 and 4 present additional information on developing eye gaze systems.

Another format or technique designed to access stimuli involves an Eye Link technique. This technique uses stimuli (either orthographic or pictorial) that are arranged evenly across a clear plastic mounting surface and held vertically in front of the user. The user fixes his or her gaze on the targeted symbol and the partner moves the board until eye contact is made with the user. The listener says the target name and the user confirms it with a prearranged signal.

Direct Selection Training

Direct selection is one of the easier selection techniques to train as it is usually the most natural mode of access. Eye gaze is a form of direct selection. However, eye gaze techniques do not involve physical contact with the AAC system. Direct selection methods involve pointing to an item on the AAC device using a body part (as in typing with a finger, depressing a key via a mouth stick, or activating a LCD via a lightpointer). This selection technique is generally more efficient than scanning techniques.

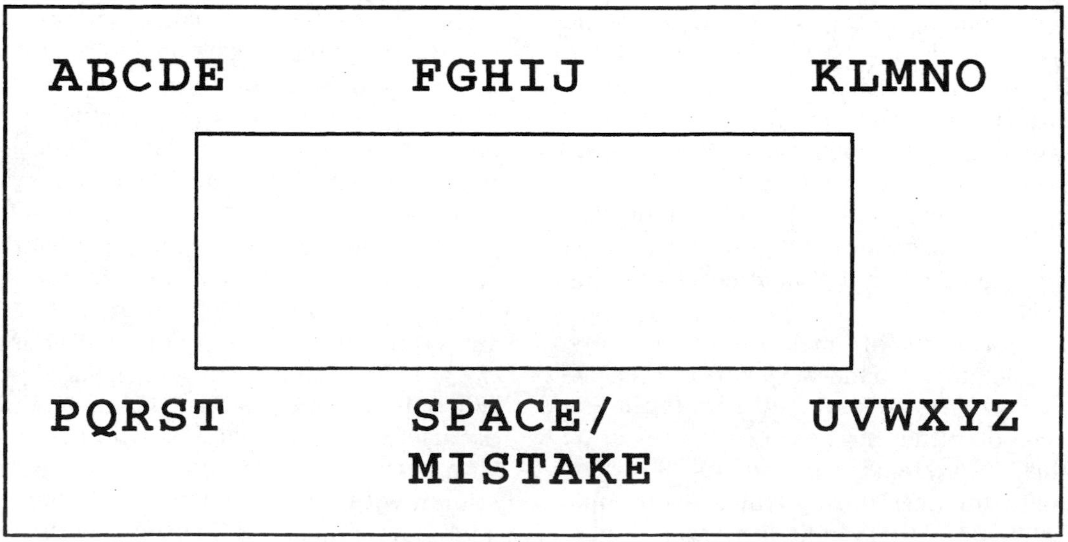

ABCDE	FGHIJ	KLMNO
PQRST	SPACE/ MISTAKE	UVWXYZ

Figure 13–2. Eye gaze communication board combined with listener-assisted scanning.

Direct selection can be paired with various pieces of assistive technology to fabricate an accessible communication system. Use of a QWERTY keyboard layout can be utilized with people who have previous keyboard experience. For non-QWERTY users, an alphabetically arranged keyboard/overlay or alphabet board can be used if letter selection is completed at a faster rate in this manner.

Numerous modifications to direct selection may enhance access speed and accuracy. Such modifications take into consideration the user's fine motor, visual motor, and visual perceptual abilities. Modifications might include the use of keyguards, enlarged keyboards, miniature keyboards, light pointers, chin sticks, mouth sticks, and hand-held pointers. Chapter 3 contains detailed information on specific device modifications.

In training for direct selection of symbols, it is helpful to use a hierarchy that systematically increases the level of task difficulty. A sample task hierarchy would be:

1. Present a limited number of symbols on a flat surface positioned for accurate client access (i.e., on the laptray or on a clear piece of plastic positioned vertically in front of the patient). It is recommended that stimuli are not permanently positioned on the display so that they can be repositioned as needed.
2. Instruct the user to select a target given a direct cue (e.g., "Show me the TV"). Be sure that the user can physically access all stimuli to determine that some are not positioned in areas that are out of functional range of movement or in areas that are affected by a hemispatial neglect.
3. Instruct the user to identify a stimulus given a contextual cue (e.g., "Point to what you would use if you wanted a drink"; the user identifies "cup").

4. Facilitate carryover of AAC communication system use by employing the system in a variety of contexts including the client's room, cafeteria, therapy area, community outings. Progressively fade cues within functional contexts to facilitate the user's ability to initiate communication within all contexts 90% of the time.

Vocabulary Selection

Selection of vocabulary is a critical step in the implementation of AAC technology, as the vocabulary that is chosen ultimately effects the user's level of communicative effectiveness. In order to provide the user with the maximum amount of semantic and syntactic flexibility, vocabulary groups should be selected to truly reflect the user's needs. Vocabulary groups can be collected through numerous processes. Categorical listing of semantic targets by the user, family, and clinical staff, team generation of targets through an unstructured listing approach, and use of a vocabulary checklist can be highly effective in yielding appropriate vocabulary lists. Regardless of the approach, it is critical that the adult user be directly involved in the selection process. It is not uncommon for caregivers to report their own vocabulary preferences and syntactic patterns, without adequately considering how the AAC user would produce the same utterance.

Another consideration in selecting vocabulary is the vocabulary size. Users who present with cognitive-communicative and language deficits frequently benefit from vocabulary lists that do not exceed their recall and organizational abilities. Beukelman, Yorkston, Poblete, and Naranjo (1984) found that a vocabulary of 500 words was adequate to cover 80% of what their adult AAC users communicated over a 14-day period. Further, any approach utilized by a clinical team for vocabulary selection should be sensitive to the cognitive-linguistic impairments of the user. Vocabulary lists for users who present with such deficits should contain words that are highly familiar and concrete. Concrete and familiar vocabulary facilitates improved recall and sequencing of the corpus of available words. Although larger word lists can provide the user with increased semantic flexibility, the clinical team needs to balance the number of words used with the user's cognitive abilities. In some cases, a list that is limited in number but readily accessed by the user due to its high level of familiarity facilitates a greater degree of communicative competence. Holland (1975) found that a small vocabulary corpus is beneficial to users who had language disorders. Chapter 4 provides more information on vocabulary and symbol selection methods.

Categorical Listing

The use of categorically organized lists can be useful in the generation of vocabulary. This approach is readily adopted by many clinicians within a treatment environment, as categorization tasks that facilitate the development of vocabulary lists reinforce existing treatment goals. Categorization tasks for improvement in memory or word-finding, for example, can reinforce and ultimately enhance performance within tasks that address the development of a vocabulary list. Categories for vocabulary organization include: people, feelings, needs, actions, body parts, places, objects, and social phrases.

It is advantageous to use the entire interdisciplinary team, as well as the user and family members, to generate vocabulary targets. A team approach can yield a large variety of semantic targets that are functional, relevant to daily needs, and assist the user in managing his or her medical, social, and personal needs. Illustration of this categorical generation of vocabulary for a user with a severe TBI is illustrated in Table 13–5.

Vocabulary should reflect the user's daily interaction environments. Samples should be obtained from varied settings including the hospital, home, social contexts, school, and work. The findings of Morrow, Mirenda, Beukelman, and Yorkston (1993)

Table 13–5. Categorical vocabulary for a client with TBI.

People	Feelings	Needs	Body Parts	Miscellaneous
Husband	Happy	Comb Hair	Arm	Hello
Sister	Sad	Take Shower	Leg	Goodbye
Brother	Tired	Lie Down	Stomach	How Are You?
Daughter	Excited	Get Dressed	Head	I Love You
Son	Angry	Need Glasses	Back	Thank You
Friend	Fine	Turn on Radio	Shoulder	
	Cold	Turn on TV	Chest	
	Hot	Need Medicine	Throat	
	Hungry	Brush Teeth		
	Dirty	Reposition		
	Pain			
	Sick			

supported the use of an ecological inventory in attaining a relevant vocabulary corpus. It is also extremely time efficient to employ the assistance of the user and the user's caregivers in maintaining diaries of prospective vocabulary words. The clinician should encourage the user and caretaker to maintain lists of words that would be verbally communicated if the user did not have communication difficulties. Examples of context-specific vocabulary are illustrated in Table 13–6.

Table 13–6. Context specific vocabulary lists.

Hospital Context				
People	**Needs**	**Actions**	**Leisure**	**Feelings**
Family	Call Button	Suction Me	Book	Mad
Doctor	Urinal	Reposition Me	Cards	Upset
Nurse	Medication	Turn Me	Radio	Afraid
Chaplain	Bedpan	Bed Up/Down	TV	Cold
SLP	Glasses	Transfer Me	Paper	Hot
OT	Hearing Aid	Clean	Magazine	Pain
PT	Dentures	Come	Video	Confused
Social Worker	Food	Sit		Understand
	Razor	Eat		Worry
	Brush	Drink		Sick

Home Context				
People	**Needs**	**Actions**	**Leisure**	**Feelings**
Mom	Breakfast	Help	Book	Frustrated
Dad	Lunch	Feed	TV	Confused
Sister	Dinner	Drink	Video	Bored
Brother	Snack	Go	Magazine	Embarrased
Spouse	Bed	Get/Want	Nintendo	Hungry
Children	Bathroom	Don't	Outside	Lonely
Medicine	Open	CD Player	Thirsty	

Social Community Context			
People	**Places**	**Actions**	**Phrases**
Friend	Movie	Watch	I don't understand
Neighbor	Park	Play	Glad to meet you
Stranger	Pool	Swim	I don't know
Minister	Church	Sit	I'm fine
Clerk	Store	Buy	Please
Driver	Bus	Ride	Excuse me

(continued)

Table 13–6. *(continued)*

| | Work Context | | |
People	Objects	Actions	Phrases
Boss	Desk	Sit	Would you move this?
Colleague	Computer	Work	I need more time.
Supervisor	Copier machine	Copy	How does this work?
Friend	Paper	Write	What is the answer?
Secretary	File Drawer	Find	Where is it?
Receptionist	Chair	Discuss	I'll have it finished soon.

Unstructured Listing Approach

This approach employs the use of a blank piece of paper where team members (e.g., professionals, the family, and the user) write all of the words that they feel are necessary for the user's daily experiences and should be included in the AAC system. This open-ended strategy requires the team to generate a comprehensive vocabulary corpus purely from memory, thus placing a high degree of cognitive demand on all those involved. Within the adult population, this approach is frequently effective with individuals who exhibit anticipatory insight and functional cognitive-communication. This client group may already have a list of words or utterances that they want to communicate in order to enhance their personal and medical interactions.

This listing approach, however, may be less effective with individuals who exhibit cognitive-communicative impairments or reduced psychosocial adjustment to existing deficits. Clinical experience in the rehabilitation hospital setting reflects the user's and frequently the family members' difficulty in accommodating communication difficulties with AAC interventions. Further, this approach places a high level of responsibility on the user and caregiver to independently generate the vocabulary corpus. This approach inherently requires divergent reasoning, word finding, and organizational and pragmatic language skills, which are commonly the areas impaired in populations with acquired communication deficits. Users with these deficits who attempt to employ this strategy frequently generate vocabulary lists that omit critical words and subsequently do not adequately communicate their needs.

Vocabulary Checklists

In this approach, the user and caregiver are presented with word lists and instructed to check off words that they feel should be included in the user's vocabulary list. Words are included on the list based on the clinician's assessment of the user's needs for medical and personal purposes. Various predetermined word lists can be utilized, including a vocabulary checklist developed by Berger (1967) or Baker, Higgins, Costello, and Stump (1986). Lists can also be used that are computer-generated based on programs containing words rank-ordered by frequency (i.e., AAC Vocabulary Manager, see Appendix A). This approach provides the person with the highest degree of structure as compared to the other methods because the words are already generated and simply need to be checked off. However, this approach limits word choices. Further, although the words on the list are high frequency words in the English language, they may not be needed on a daily basis by the user. Findings by Yorkston, Honsinger, Dowden, and Marriner (1989) suggested that vocabulary checklists are efficient tools when used as a supplement to other vocabulary generation strategies as they provide access to a large variety of semantic items. Similar findings were reported by Yorkston, Dowden, Honsinger, and Marriner (1988), who recommended that client-specific words be obtained through various methods (i.e., categorical listing) and then used to supplement vocabulary items that are obtained through the use of vocabulary checklists.

Symbol Selection

After developing the system's vocabulary, if the user requires a picture cue with the vocabulary word, therapy tasks should address the generation of a group of pictures that reflect the vocabulary items. Pictures that possess a high degree of color contrast and are easily seen by the user are especially effective with people who have impaired visual-perceptual abilities. Many elderly adults have declining visual skills and require enlarged symbols. Photographs are recommended because they are highly familiar to the user and may provide increased user motivation. In some cases, simple black and white line drawings or white drawings on a highly contrasting background (e.g., black) can be utilized for easy identification. Chapter 4 reviews existing commercially available symbol sets.

When users have existing premorbid literacy abilities, consideration should be given to communication displays that combine written words with picture symbols. Some users may reject the use of picture symbols and request communication displays that consist of only written words. Bilingual adult users can retain portions of each language and may need words incorporated into the display across both languages. The individual's visual skills should be taken into consideration, and if necessary, enlarged text should be used.

Once an appropriate type of contrast is identified, picture or written word symbols should be arranged in a format that facilitates accurate and efficient access. For users with recall or organizational impairments, symbols can be categorically arranged with each category presented in a different background color. In this format, the need to scan the entire system layout can be reduced if the user is unable to recall the picture's location. The user need only recall the target symbol's category and the color of the category and then visually scan that category for the particular symbol. Use of a categorical listing format can decrease random visual scanning of the system and subsequently increase access speed. In some cases, positioning of favorite photographs within the user's neglected visual field may facilitate and maintain greater attention to this area.

Symbols can also be arranged in a format that is easiest for the user to physically reach. For example, if the user is selecting items with a mouth stick, positioning the targets of greatest user frequency at midline is beneficial, as this is the location most readily accessed. Stimuli of lesser frequency can be positioned on the perimeter of these targets. In contrast to this midline organization, users who access targets via use of a mobile arm support can benefit from an arrangement that positions stimuli on the lateral border of the communication device that is on the same side as the mobile arm support. For a user with a mobile arm support, symbols should be positioned in locations that are accessible within the user's range of motion. Chapter 7 reviews motor access issues.

AAC DEVICE SELECTION

There are multiple variables involved in determining an AAC system that is best suited for the user. The ultimate system should not only meet the user's communication needs within specific contexts but also maximize his or her existing speech, language, cognitive-communicative, and motor skills to facilitate functional communicative competence (August & Weiss, 1992). Selection should be driven by the client's needs, including the communication environment and the type of message to be produced (length of message, printed or spoken). System selection should not be driven by the center's AAC system inventory (August & Weiss, 1992). A summary of variables that should be considered when determining a technology-user match is outlined in Figure 13–3.

When working with adults with acquired communication disabilities the concept of "the simpler the better" should be considered in the AAC device selection process. Consider using simple systems such as communication boards or concrete easy to use dedicated devices rather than complicated high tech AAC systems. Many individuals with acquired disabilities have never been introduced to computers or even typewriters in their lifetime. Further, simple AAC systems are more cost effective and easily purchased by individuals who may have exhausted their insurance coverage or have fixed or limited incomes.

It is also important that the recommended AAC system be portable and lightweight. Many times persons with acquired

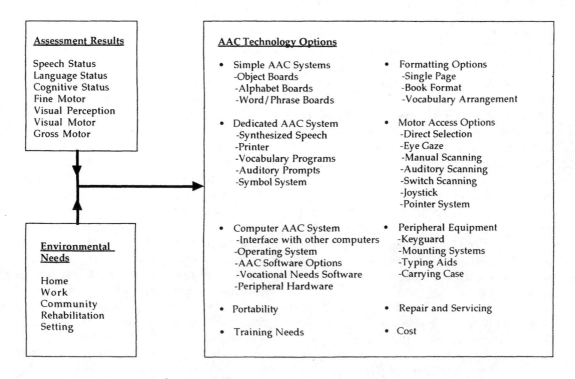

Figure 13–3. Considerations in AAC system selection.

disabilities prioritize these factors as more important than system flexibility or capability. Users frequently report the desire to use an AAC system that can be easily concealed, or carried independently when using a cane.

When electronic voice output AAC systems are recommended, the ergonomics of the device should be considered. Will the user be able to turn the volume control knob independently, can he or she read the display screen, or understand the speech output of the system? It is not uncommon for adult users to state a preference for digitized speech over synthesized speech. Digitized speech is usually preferred as it is more familiar and can be the voice of a loved one or family member.

Many adult users are well-informed buyers who want to play an integral role is the selection of their communication system. Some adults will tell the evaluation team what system they want, what features are needed, and what vocabulary they need upon initial arrival to an evaluation session. It is not uncommon for an AAC system that is recommended by an evaluation team to be declined by a consumer. A particular system may be clinically appropriate, but the consumer judges the system to be ineffective in meeting their communication and personal needs. The system selection process should therefore include the following components: presentation of all evaluation results to the consumer and advocate; description and demonstration of AAC options that were judged to meet the consumer's needs; cursory description and demonstration of equipment that was not judged to meet consumer's communication needs, including a rationale for elimination; field testing of appropriate AAC options; and a follow-up question and answer session where the consumer and advocate can ask questions relating to AAC communication system use.

It is critical to incorporate the users requests and preferences with features that are clinically appropriate and necessary in system selection in order to attain an optimum technology match. In the end, the AAC system chosen by the adult user may not be the same system selected by the evaluation team. An informed consumer or advocate who has had a role in selecting an AAC system following a comprehensive evaluation process will be more likely to use the AAC system effectively and less likely to abandon the device. The user will feel a greater sense of involvement in the device selection process and increased commitment to system use (Smith-Lewis & Ford, 1987).

ABANDONMENT

Individuals requiring assistive technology who receive an AAC evaluation and then purchase an AAC system often follow a pattern of adoption and abandonment. Information gathered by Batavia and Hammer (1990) revealed that when an individual is using AAC technology the following pattern occurs: the client obtains an assistive device; uses the device and finds that it does not meet his or her needs; either continues to use the device although dissatisfied until it is no longer usable, or abandons the device; and sometimes chooses another AAC device.

The consequences of abandonment are significant to both the AAC user and society at large. Abandoning a communication device may not only result in decreased independence, but perhaps extensive financial loss to both the consumer and involved caregivers. Abandonment also means inefficient use of third party payers, financial resources, resulting in reduced funding for additional assistive technology equipment in the future.

According to Batavia, Dillard and Phillips (1990), several factors appear to be related to system abandonment. These factors include inadequate product performance;

lack of improvement in the user's functional performance; difficulty in operating the device; and high cost and limited availability of service and repair. Furthermore, Batavia et al. (1990) stated that although a device may meet one of the user's needs, it may simultaneously compromise other needs. The user may feel that the system does not enhance his or her existing communication skills or functional performance and subsequently abandon the device.

Anecdotal evidence of this was found with an individual who purchased a dedicated communication system following an AAC clinical evaluation. The person accessed the communication device via direct selection with a light pointer mounted on his head. The client was functional in his use of the device in non-interactional contexts (e.g., while using his personal computer); however, the consumer reported poor performance in interactions with listeners, as the device communicated his messages at the expense of eye contact, proxemics, and gesture. Support for this frustration in communication due to decreased integration of pragmatic features was reported by Beukelman (1989). Indeed, the user stated that his pragmatic language skills were physically "blocked" by the communication system. The user eventually opted for a simple communication board requiring listener-directed scanning that maintained communication competence without compromising pragmatic language interactions. The dedicated light-pointer AAC system was abandoned for communication purposes.

Phillips and Zhao (1993) maintained that abandonment can be reduced by comprehensively training all clinical professionals who prescribe assistive technology equipment in their respective areas of expertise and by thoroughly educating consumers about the equipment that they will be using.

The use of rental options for AAC equipment should be considered as a way to decrease device abandonment for adult users. Although rental involves a financial outlay, this amount is typically much lower than actual equipment purchase. Renting helps to defray financial responsibilities as many companies offer low-cost rental options for AAC equipment. Equipment rental provides users who have changing skills with the flexibility of renting different AAC systems as needed. Renting also accomodates individuals who may be able to purchase devices but are ambivalent regarding the system's appropriateness or their consistent use of the equipment in the home setting. Equipment rental affords the ability to use AAC equipment on a trial basis without the fear of purchasing equipment that may be abandoned later.

The incorporation of a Consumer Satisfaction Measure (CSM) can serve as an additional tool to prevent AAC system abandonment. Consumer satisfaction surveys, such as the CSM published by the American Speech-Language-Hearing Association (1989) give the service provider information regarding the user's satisfaction with the evaluation and treatment process. This tool, or one that is tailored specifically for AAC needs, could enlighten service providers regarding aspects of the AAC process with which the consumer was (dis)satisfied. Research by Rao, Goldsmith, Wilkerson, and Hildebrant (1992, p. 35) that looked at four various CSMs found "considerable similarity and overlaps" in quality dimensions identified as valuable in assessing consumer satisfaction. Items that were consistently included on the CSMs included questions regarding technical quality, courtesy of personnel, access, convenience and cost of services, and continuity of care. The inclusion of a CSM, coupled with service-provider training and consumer education, may serve to decrease the occurrence of AAC system abandonment and heighten consumer satisfaction.

MAINTENANCE

Maintenance of a communication system is critical for achieving effective AAC communication skills. The selection of a communication device is only a preliminary step in obtaining communicative competence (Trefler, 1987). A pivotal step in facilitating functional AAC system use is the training of all those involved (user, family, friends, caregiver, clinicians) in the maintenance of the communication system. The following guidelines may be helpful in assuring optimal AAC communication system operation: (1) Identify a person to maintain device, (2) Ensure that the user and caregiver thoroughly understand the communication device's owners manual and the operation guidelines, (3) Determine that the user and caregiver know how to contact the vendor for resolution of system failures or operation errors, (4) Ensure that the user and involved partners participate in training sessions that include instruction in system operation and maintenance procedures, (5) Develop a back-up system to be used in the event of primary system failure (e.g., a simple communication board or communication book).

As stated in the maintenance guidelines, all users should be trained in the operation of the communication device, including programming. Although some programming is not critical for effective system use (e.g., changing the voice on a multiple voice speech synthesizer system), simple programming processes are important for the user to master, either independently or by directing someone else to complete the process. Priority programming processes include message storage and editing. Users with compromised memory and organizational skills can be systematically trained to complete the steps in system programming through the use of a cueing hierarchy where cues are faded as the user demonstrates functional completion of individual process steps. Mas-

tery is attained when independent completion of the process is demonstrated within functional contexts.

It is recommended that the user's communicative partner complete training sessions so as to be independent in system programming as well as comfortable in facilitating the user's programming skill. This dual training of user and partner assures that the system can be programmed at any time, even if the user is unable to independently perform the task. It also provides a vehicle for additional skill training and carryover as the partner is able to practice programming exercises with the user outside of the clinical setting. Mastery of programming can be achieved by the partner either through completion of vendor-provided training courses or through participation in therapy sessions where the treating clinician provides the user and partner with sequential training of the programming process.

CARRYOVER OF AAC TECHNIQUES

As a user leaves the supportive clinical setting and returns home or to a nursing facility, his or her communication needs may change. The contexts in which the user may need to communicate may not be as supportive or conducive to AAC use as the clinical setting. A number of techniques can be incorporated to facilitate increased communicative effectiveness within the nonclinical setting. Most of these techniques require training listeners in the target environment. However, users who are cognitively able can be trained to proactively facilitate good listener skills. Specific techniques that can enhance AAC carryover into the natural environment include the following:

- Communicate with the user in a variety of contexts, including the user's home, neighborhood, work, or school.

- Always provide an environment where communication can occur. For example, always have the user's communication board available and appropriately positioned.
- Facilitate communication by not asking too many yes/no questions. Instead, present questions that require a specific answer.
- Provide the client with plenty of time in which to respond.
- Model and reinforce the user's communication technique whenever possible.
- Use repair strategies. When breakdowns occur, request that the user begin the message again; encourage the client to pause after the listener repeats the letter or word so as to assure confirmation of the target; encourage the user to paraphrase utterances rather than rotely repeating previously misunderstood utterances.
- Reinforce all attempts at communication, including the initiation of communication and use of communication techniques.

Pragmatics Training

Learning to effectively use the AAC system to communicate a variety of information in the natural environment is another important component of training. Present the user with tasks that facilitate requesting information, providing information, questioning, stating opinions and feelings, and commenting in group contexts. These tasks provide the client with interactional opportunities with a variety of communicative partners. Tasks should employ frequent turn-taking by the communicative partner rather than one-sided response-format interactions, where the listener poses questions and the user responds.

It is helpful to include an utterance in all communication systems that explains why the individual needs the communication system and how the device is used. Explanation utterances assist a person who has never seen an AAC device in becoming more comfortable with the user

and assists the listener in interacting with the user. Various explanation utterances can include: *I use this device to communicate because I've had an accident and have a difficult time talking; Please look at the letters on my machine, I want to spell something for you; Please be patient with me I have had a stroke and use this computer to help me speak.*

SUMMARY

It is the goal of professionals working with users of assistive technology to facilitate use of an AAC communication system in functional communication contexts. For some users, this may mean independent use of the communication system in the home setting for daily living skill purposes, whereas for others it may be independent system use in the work environment. Through participation in an interdisciplinary evaluation and training process the consumer maximizes his or her opportunity to attain the highest level of communicative competence possible. Becoming an AAC user is a lengthy and complex process for adults with acquired communication disorders, yet is often critical for enhancing communicative independence. The heterogeneous nature of this population requires the ongoing adjustment of evaluation and training procedures to meet the ultimate goal of communicative competence within a variety of functional contexts. Although the communicative disorders that are seen within this population may vary, treating clinicians may find greater clinical success by incorporating the following recommendations.

- Be flexible within the evaluation process, including the selection of an interdisciplinary team. Team members should possess expertise in the evaluation and management of clients with acquired communication disorders who require the use of AAC systems. Demonstrate flexibility when developing and administering an assessment protocol comprising a variety of informal and formal measures.

- Provide training services within functional contexts. The consumer must be surrounded by a supportive clinical team in which all clinicians possess a working knowledge of the AAC communication system and develop training objectives that complement other clinical areas. Training should be provided to those people who interact with the consumer on a daily basis, including the individual's family, caregivers, co-workers, and friends.
- Provide extensive consumer and family education and counseling throughout the entire AAC process to enhance client adjustment to the newly acquired communication system and to incorporate its use into daily routines. Education completed during this AAC process can make the difference between consumer satisfaction and system abandonment.

REFERENCES

American Speech-Language-Hearing Association. (1989). *ASHA consumer satisfaction measure*. Rockville, MD: ASHA.

American Speech-Language-Hearing Association. (1991). Report: Augmentative and alternative communication. *ASHA, 33*(Suppl. 5), 9–12.

American Speech-Language-Hearing Association. (1992). *Preferred practice patterns*. Rockville, MD: ASHA.

August S., & Weiss, P. (1992). A human factors approach to adapted access device prescription and customization. *Journal of Rehabilitation Research and Development, 29*(4), 64–77.

Baker, B., Higgins, J., Costello, J., & Stump, R. (1986). *Systematic approaches to vocabulary selection for communication aid users*. Short course presented at the annual convention of the American Speech-Language-Hearing Association annual convention, Detroit, MI.

Batavia, A., Dillard, D., & Phillips, B. (1990). How to avoid technology abandonment. In H. Murphy (Ed.), *Proceedings of the Fifth Annual Conference, Technology and Persons with Disabilities* (pp. 55–64). Los Angeles, Office of Disabled Student Services, California State University, Northridge.

Batavia, A., & Hammer, G. (1990). Toward a consumer-based criteria for the evaluation of assistive devices. *Journal of Rehabilitation Research and Development, 27*(4), 425–436.

Bay, J. (1991). Positioning for head control to access an augmentative communication machine. *The American Journal of Occupational Therapy, 45*(6), 544–549.

Berger, K. (1967). The most common words used in conversation. *Journal of Communication Disorders, 1*, 201–214.

Beukelman, D. (1989). There are some things you just can't say with your right hand. *Augmentative and Alternative Communication, 5*(4), 257–258.

Beukelman, D., & Yorkston, K. (1989). Augmentative and alternative communication application for persons with severe acquired communication disorders: An introduction. *Augmentative and Alternative Communication, 5*(1), 47.

Beukelman, D., Yorkston, K., Poblete, M., & Naranjo, C. (1984). Frequency of word occurrence in communication samples produced by adult communication aid users. *Journal of Speech and Hearing Disorders, 49*, 360–367.

Brown, J., Bennett, J., & Hanna, G. (1981). *The Nelson-Denny Reading Test*. Chicago: The Riverside Publishing Company.

Caplan, L. R., Dyken, M., & Easton, J. (1994). *Family guide to stroke treatment, recovery, and prevention* (p. 47). New York: American Heart Association, Times Books.

Cohen, C., & DeRuyter, F. (1982). Technology for the communicatively impaired: A perspective for future clinicians. *Journal of the National Student Speech Language Hearing Association, 10*, 67–76.

Collins, M. (1986). *Diagnosis and treatment of global aphasia*. San Diego: College-Hill Press.

Darley, F., Aronson, A., & Brown, J. (1975). Motor speech disorders. Philadelphia: W. B. Saunders.

DeRuyter, F., & Lafontaine, L. (1987). The nonspeaking brain-injured: A clinical and demographic database report. *Augmentative and Alternative Communication, 3*(1), 18–25.

Erickson, R., Lie, M., & Wineinger, M. (1989). Rehabilitation in multiple sclerosis. *Mayo Clinic Proceedings, 64,* 818–828.

Foley, C., & Pizer, H. F. (1990). *The stroke fact book.* Golden Valley: Courage Press.

Goldsmith, T., O'Donnell, K., Carin, S., Schein, R., & Harrison, A. (1988). *AAC questionnaire.* Unpublished paper, Washington, DC: National Rehabilitation Hospital.

Goodglass, H., & Kaplan, E. (1983). *Boston Diagnostic Aphasia Examination.* Philadelphia: Lea & Febiger.

Hammill, D. (1985). *Detroit Tests of Learning Aptitude-2.* Austin: Pro-Ed.

Holland, A. (1975). Language therapy for children: Some thoughts on context and content. *Journal of Speech and Hearing Disorders, 40,* 514–523.

Hux, K., Beukelman, D., & Garrett, K. (1994). Augmentative and alternative communication for persons with aphasia. In R. Chapey (Ed.), *Language intervention strategies in adult aphasia.* Baltimore: Williams & Wilkens.

Jankovic, J. (1984). Progressive supranuclear palsy: Clinical and pharmacologic update. *Neurologic Clinics, 2,* 473–486.

Kertesz, A. (1982). *Western Aphasia Battery.* New York: Grune & Stratton.

Kirby, N. (1989). The individual with high quadriplegia. *Nursing Clinics of North America, 24*(1), 179–191.

Ladtkow, M., & Culp, D. (1992). Locked-in syndrome and augmentative communication. In K. Yorkston (Ed.), *Augmentative communication in the medical setting.* Tucson: Communication Skill Builders.

LaPlante, M. P. (1992). Assistive technology devices and home accessibility features: Prevalence, payment, need, and trends. *Advance Data, Centers for Disease Control/National Center for Health Statistics, 217.*

LaPointe, L., & Horner, J. (1984). *Reading Comprehension Battery for Aphasia.* Tigard, OR: C. C. Publications, Inc.

McNaughton D., & Light, J. (1989). Teaching facilitators to support the communication skills of an adult with severe cognitive disabilities: A case study. *Augmentative and Alternative Communication, 5*(1), 35–41.

McNeil, M. R., & Prescott, T. E. (1978). *Revised Token Test.* Baltimore: University Park Press.

Morrow, D., Mirenda, P., Beukelman, D., & Yorkston, K. (1993). Vocabulary selection for augmentative communication systems: A comparison of three techniques. *American Journal of Speech-Language Pathology, 1,* 19–30.

National Head Injury Foundation (NHIF). (1985). *An educator's manual: What educators need to know about students with traumatic brain injury.* Framingham, MA: NHIF.

National Institute on Disability and Rehabilitation Research (NIDRR). (1992). *Augmentative and alternative communication intervention, Consensus validation conference position statement.* Washington, DC: NIDRR.

National Institutes of Health, National Institute of Neurological Disorders and Stroke. (1994). *Interagency head injury task force reports.* Bethesda, MD: NIH.

National Spinal Cord Injury Statistical Center. (1994). *Spinal cord injury facts and figures at a glance.* Birmingham, AL: The University of Alabama.

Nelson, V., Leonard, J., Fisher, S., Esquenazi, A., & Hicks, J. (1989). Prosthetics, orthotics, and assistive devices. 2. Specialized seating and assistive devices. *Archives of Physical Medicine and Rehabilitation, 70,* 202–205.

Nicholas, L., MacLennan, D., & Brookshire, R. (1986). Validity of multiple sentence reading comprehension tests for aphasic adults. *Journal of Speech and Hearing Disorders, 51,* 82–87.

Ozer, M. (1988). *The management of persons with spinal cord injury.* New York: Demos Publications.

Phillips, B., & Zhao, H. (1993). Predictors of assistive technology abandonment. *Assistive Technology, 5,* 36–45.

Rao, P. (1994). Use of Amer-Ind Code by persons with aphasia. In R. Chapey (Ed.), *Language intervention strategies in adult aphasia* (3rd ed., pp. 358–367). Baltimore: Williams & Wilkens.

Rao, P., Goldsmith, T., Wilkerson, D., & Hildebrandt, L. (1992). How to keep your customer satisfied: Consumer satisfaction survey. *Hearsay, Journal of the Ohio Speech and Hearing Association, 7*(1), 35.

Saunders, C., Walsh, T., & Smith, M. (1981). Hospice care in the motor neuron diseases. In C.

Saunders & J. Teller (Eds.), *Hospice: The living idea* (pp. 12–15). London: Edward Arnold Publishers.

Smith-Lewis, M., & Ford, A. (1987). A user's perspective on augmentative communication. *Augmentative and Alternative Communication, 3*(1), 12–17.

Sonies, B. (1987). Oral-motor problems. In H. Mueller & V. Geoffrey (Eds.), *Communication disorders in aging assessment and management*. Washington, DC: Gallaudet University Press.

Staples, D., & Lincoln, N. (1979). Intellectual impairment in multiple sclerosis and its relation to functional abilities. *Rheumatology Rehabilitation, 18*, 153–160.

Thompsen, V. (1983). Standardized methods of assessing and predicting outcome. In M. Rosenthal, E. Griffith, M. Bond, & J. Miller (Eds.), *Rehabilitation of the head injured adult* (pp. 256–289). Philadelphia: W. B. Saunders.

Trefler, E. (1987). Technology applications in occupational therapy. *The American Journal of Occupational Therapy, 41*, 697–700.

Vanderheiden, G., & Smith, R. (1989). Application of communication technologies to an adult with a high spinal cord injury. *Augmentative and Alternative Communication, 5*(1), 62–66.

Wilson, B., Cockburn, J., & Baddeley, A. (1985). *The Rivermead Behavioural Memory Test*. Titchfield, Fareham, Hant: Thames Valley Test Company.

Ylvisaker, M. (1985). *Head injury rehabilitation*. San Diego: College-Hill Press, Inc.

Yorkston, K., Beukelman, D., & Traynor, C. (1984). *Computerized Assessment of Intelligibility of Dysarthric Speech*. Tigard, OR: C. C. Publications, Inc.

Yorkston, K., Dowden, P., Honsinger, M., & Marriner, N. (1988). A comparison of standard and user vocabulary lists. *Augmentative and Alternative Communication, 4*, 189–210.

Yorkston, K., Honsinger, M., Dowden, P., & Marriner, N. (1989). Vocabulary selection: A case report. *Augmentative and Alternative Communication, 5*, 101–107.

Young, J. S., Burns, P. E., Bowen, A. M., & McCutchen, R. (1982). *Spinal cord injury statistics: Experience of the regional spinal cord injury systems*. Phoenix: Good Samaritan Medical Center.

Life Stories

Steve's AAC Story:
Traumatic Brain Injury and AAC

Patricia Pyatak Fletcher

teve began his AAC journey when he was 27 years old. Like many young male adults, he was speeding down a rural highway when an accident happened. A passenger in his car was able to walk away from the accident, but Steve wasn't so lucky. When initially admitted to the emergency room, he had a Glasgow Coma Scale rating of 11. He opened his eyes when his name was called, and reacted to touch stimuli. Vocalizations consisted of moans. The hospital's initial evaluations found a number of physical and neurological traumas. A cat scan (CT scan) of his face indicated bilateral Leforte II fractures and temporomandibular dislocation. A CT scan of his head was negative for intracerebral hemorrhage but showed frontal scalp edema. Steve's injuries included bilateral thoracic level 3 and 4 laminar fractures and a right transverse process fracture at thoracic level 5. A left lower extremity crush injury was also sustained which resulted in a left above-the-knee amputation. Finally, it was determined that heterotopic ossification was present in Steve's right elbow joint.

Steve spent the first 8 weeks following his accident in the acute care hospital. He was intubated for 4 days, then received a tracheostomy. He spent 5 weeks on a res-

pirator, unable to communicate except to blink his eyes on command. He was gradually weaned from the respirator but continued to breathe through the tracheostomy. Eight weeks after the accident, he was discharged to an adult rehabilitation hospital. Throughout his stay in the acute care hospital, Steve had not been provided with any means of communication. His AAC journey finally began when he entered the rehabilitation hospital.

AAC Evaluation

Steve had significant communication difficulties when he was first admitted to the rehabilitation hospital. He could not communicate verbally, nor was he able to use gestures, writing, or pointing to make his needs known. These communicative deficits prevented him from effectively interacting with his family and medical staff and from providing input regarding his medical status, medical decisions, or level of pain. The initial AAC goal was to evaluate Steve's potential to communicate basic functional and medical needs to others in the hospital environment. In order to address this goal, various cognitive and communicative evaluation procedures needed to be given. The first portion of the assessment consisted of developing a reliable method of responding to test questions. It was noted that Steve had difficulty consistently following one-step commands. Two-step commands were impossible for him to complete. He was instructed to answer yes/no questions using a smile-look up/frown-look down method. Steve had difficulty remembering the system and could not consistently answer simple questions regarding his age, name, and other personal information. He was then shown two index cards with the words yes and no written in large print. Using these cards he was able to answer simple yes/no questions using eye gaze responses with better consistency. Even then, Steve's inability to remain alert impacted his ability to respond to test questions.

Steve was evaluated using the yes/no responding procedures and other eye gaze methods to determine the extent of his cognitive and language deficits. Testing consisted of both informal and formal measures of arousal/alerting, attention, orientation, discrimination, categorization, sequencing, and memory. Areas targeted in the communication evaluation included auditory comprehension, reading comprehension, oral-motor skills, expressive language, and written expression. Steve's evaluation revealed severe cognitive and communicative deficits with severely impaired auditory comprehension. He also had severe impairments in the areas of working memory and reasoning flexibility.

An expressive communication evaluation found that Steve was unable to vocalize secondary to an unplugged tracheostomy tube. He had a severe oral and pharyngeal dysphagia and was fed through a G-tube. These oral motor difficulties carried over to speech motor skills, resulting in severe dysarthria. When sitting upright, he could grossly move his left hand and arm to point to test stimuli. When lying in bed, he could only use eye gaze. Otherwise, he had no means of communication.

In addition to his communication difficulties, Steve also required intensive rehabilitation in other areas. He was unable to independently complete any functional daily living skills. He could only tolerate sitting upright in a wheelchair for 2 hours at a time. He was incontinent for both bowel and bladder control. In order to make sufficient progress to be discharged from the hospital, Steve's communication goals would need to be tied to his overall rehabilitation program.

AAC Treatment Goals

Steve's rehabilitation team met to develop interdisciplinary team goals. Communication goals were designed to increase his ability to initiate communication, and to improve his ability to effectively interact about his basic medical needs to hospital staff and family using an AAC system. Specific interdisciplinary AAC treatment goals were focused on immediate communication needs in the rehabilitation environment. These included:

- The ability to independently and accurately use an AAC device while maintaining appropriate positioning seated in his wheelchair,
- The ability to alert nursing staff via a call button or through activation of an AAC device to communicate his need to use the toilet or urinal,
- The ability to use an AAC system to express his comfort level to hospital staff and family (i.e., too hot, in pain),
- The ability to use the AAC system to request something to eat,
- The ability to use an AAC system to indicate his wish to transfer into and out of bed,
- The ability to reliably answer simple yes/no questions regarding basic needs using eye gaze methods.

AAC Implementation Strategies

The first stage of Steve's treatment program focused on setting up a voice output AAC system that could be used to communicate basic medical and functional needs to the hospital staff. A voice output AAC device was necessary so Steve could independently initiate communication without staff intervention or monitoring. Steve was seen for an assessment with the occupational therapist and speech-language pathologist to determine the best method of motorically accessing a device. Because Steve was only tolerating his wheelchair for short periods of time, the motor access method would need to work for him in the wheelchair and while lying semi-upright in bed. Steve initially tried using a Zygo Macaw AAC system set up with a 32-location display matrix with 1-inch symbols. He had good range of motion with his left hand to reach symbols across the entire display, however his fine motor abilities prevented him from accurately targeting individual symbols accurately.

Row-column scanning using the Macaw's 32-location display was considered. Steve was easily able to access a Jelly Bean switch on command with his left hand. However, he had difficulty using the Macaw when it was set up for scanning. He could not consistently press the switch at the right times, and had difficulty remembering the two-step row-column selection process. In addition, the speed of scanning was slow, which significantly impacted on his ability to communicate. By the time the device scanned to a particular symbol, Steve often forgot the question he was answering.

Direct selection options were reviewed again. The Macaw was reconfigured with an 8-location display matrix. Steve had no difficulty motorically accessing the large 2-inch symbols on this display. The Macaw was positioned next to Steve's left arm when he was lying in bed and in front of him on a laptray when he was seated in his wheelchair. Because Steve had significant cognitive and language impairments, it was decided to initially limit his communication options to a single picture display. A simple picture symbol display for basic medical needs was developed using large colored pictures. Steve's overlay included the following functional vocabulary: *bathroom, drink, eat, urinal, hot, pain, wheelchair,* and *bed.*

The speech-language pathologist initially focused on simultaneously training Steve to use the Macaw while also teaching family and staff to implement use of the device. Training was provided to interdisciplinary team members, including occupational and physical therapy, nurses, physicians, and social workers. Training of staff in conjunction with family members was used to enhance carryover across different rehabilitation settings.

Steve's progress with the Macaw was slow. Because he was in immense pain much of the time, he had difficulty focusing on therapy goals. His significant physical and medical impairments meant that he spent much of his time in bed feeling too ill for intensive therapy sessions. He also had difficulty tolerating his wheelchair. When lying in bed, he was monitored closely, and did not come into contact with many individuals. This severely limited his need to communicate interactively and independently to others. He rarely initiated using the Macaw during this time. Instead, staff relied on yes/no questions that could be answered through eye gaze using written word cards as symbols.

After 3 months of rehabilitation, Steve's pain gradually lessened, and his ability to tolerate sitting in the wheelchair increased. He was seen more frequently for speech and language services to increase his use of the Macaw. Steve's ability to consistently identify each of the eight symbols improved. He gradually began independently selecting some of the symbols to request basic needs. There were many times when he would perseveratively request the same item over and over again. For example, the physiatrist had orders for him to sit in his wheelchair for up to 3 hours before being placed back into bed. Steve would begin to communicate Put me in bed shortly after being placed in the chair. Hospital staff would inform him of the current time and let him know when he could get back into bed. However, within a few minutes Steve would press the symbol again. Steady improvements in short-term memory and auditory comprehension gradually lessened his need to make these perseverative requests. However, by the time of discharge, the problem had still not completely disappeared.

After 5 months of rehabilitation, Steve was finally medically ready for discharge. He was able to use the Macaw to independently request assistance using the bathroom, to get attention from others, to request ice chips, and to indicate that he was in pain. Use of the Macaw was an essential component of achieving other rehabilitation goals, including bowel and bladder continence. With the Macaw he was able to request assistance to go to the bathroom and gained full control of these functions by the time of discharge.

Ongoing AAC Needs

Steve was discharged home to his family and encouraged to initiate outpatient rehabilitation services. During his inpatient stay, funding for a Macaw had been obtained so that Steve could continue using the device at home. Steve's case was transferred to a home-based speech language pathologist who could assist the family to implement the Macaw in the home and community. Vocabulary specific to these environments would need to be developed and Steve would need ongoing functional communication training to learn to use the Macaw independently and effectively at home.

Key Points To Remember

- During the early stages of rehabilitation following a traumatic brain injury many individuals are too sick, too disoriented, or in too much pain to learn to use complex AAC systems. AAC solutions need to be kept simple both motorically and cognitively.
- Many times low technology simple solutions are more effective than high technology solutions during the early stages of rehabilitation. Steve was able to respond much better using yes/no eye gaze cards when he was initially admitted to the rehabilitation hospital. As he recovered, his ability to use the Macaw improved and he was finally able to achieve independent communication.
- Perseverative communicative behaviors are common for individuals with frontal lobe brain injuries who are nonspeaking. The memory deficits associated with frontal lobe injuries result in an inability to remember recent communication events, and a tendency to repeat messages. Individuals who are able to speak will repeat their verbal questions over and over again, individuals using AAC devices will continuously press the same messages repeatedly.
- Within a rehabilitation environment, AAC needs have to be linked to the communicative skills necessary to achieve other rehabilitation goals. Steve might not have achieved the goal of bowel and bladder control if he did not have a method of independently requesting bathroom help from the nursing staff.
- Discharge planning is an important part of AAC treatment. The home-based speech-language pathologist will need to assist Steve and his family in expanding his communication options to the home and community environment.

Life Stories

Mike's AAC Story: Multiple Sclerosis and AAC

Patricia Pyatak Fletcher

When Mike was 23 years old, he was diagnosed with multiple sclerosis (MS). Prior to the diagnosis, he had felt numb tingling sensations in his fingers and arms. He sometimes dropped little things and seemed to fatigue easier. After the diagnosis, Mike continued on with his life and initially made few concessions to the disease. He was able to complete 2 years of college with minimal assistance. After a few years Mike began having frequent relapses. After each relapse, he would lose physical function. By the time Mike was 30, he resided in a nursing home and was dependent for all daily living tasks. Mike spent much of his day seated in front of the television in a reclining wheelchair, or watching television from his bed.

When Mike was initially admitted to the nursing home, he was still able to communicate using single words and phrases. Nursing staff members were able to understand him if the context of his messages was known. However, as Mike's MS progressed, nursing home staff members were no longer able to understand his speech. Mike was referred for an AAC evaluation because he was increasingly unable to communicate his needs due to severe speech and motor deficits. Severe motor deficits made it impossible for him to gesture or write, though he was able to use a gross gesture for pointing. He could nod his head yes or no, but when fatigued, these movements were difficult for him to initiate. He had a severe dysarthria which significantly decreased his intelligibility. He was unable to intelligibly communicate with his family or with nursing home staff.

AAC Assessment

When Mike was first seen for AAC services, staff at the nursing home were unclear about his auditory comprehension abilities, his memory, and cognitive skills. The first stage of AAC assessment would be to determine his speech, language, and cognitive-communicative status. This information would then be used to develop an appropriate AAC system. Mike's motor and communicative impairments made it difficult to admister formal evaluation tools. Informal evaluation methods were used to obtain the assessment information. Mike fatigued easily during the evaluation. He needed frequent breaks after 15 to 20 minutes of testing. The assessment took place over several visits to his nursing home.

Mike was able to respond to yes/no questions by using a head nod with accompanying vocalizations. This modality was used to evaluate his auditory comprehension, memory, general orientation, and other cognitive skills. Informal assessment found that Mike was able to correctly respond to personal questions with 90% accuracy, environmental questions with 80% accuracy and factual questions with 50% accuracy. He was oriented to people and places within his environment, but not to the date as assessed via yes/no questions. Informal assessment of his ability to follow directions revealed a 75% accuracy level for familiar one-step commands (i.e., "close your eyes"). He had difficulty responding to two-step commands, even when directions were repeated.

Most individuals with advanced stages of MS have significant visual perceptual deficits which cause difficulty discriminating between test stimuli and consequently, AAC symbols. Mike definitely fit this pattern. The *Boston Diagnostic Aphasia Examination* (BDAE) Word Discrimination subtest was discontinued due to Mike's difficulty in discriminating items on test stimuli. He was then evaluated informally to determine if he had the ability to identify picture symbols. Eye gaze methods of responding were used for this portion of the assessment. He was able to reliably identify photographs of commonly used objects that were familiar in his environment (i.e., bed, glasses, chair). Identification of photographs of objects that were not common to his environment were identified less than 25% of the time.

The *Reading Comprehension Battery for Aphasia* Word-Visual and Word-Auditory subtests were also discontinued due to Mike's visual-perceptual deficits; modified assessment revealed reliable comprehension of familiar written single words (e.g., bed, shoe) yet unreliable responses for tasks targeting comprehension of less frequent, single words (e.g., vacation). Mike

was unable to read any familiar items at the phrase and sentence level.

Due to Mike's significant communication deficits, The *Rivermead Behavioural Memory Test* could not be completed. Informal assessment of his ability to recall functional information through yes/no questions (i.e., "Did you have lunch yet?") and to problem-solve a simple situation (i.e., "Should we stop now and go to occupational therapy?") indicated a moderate cognitive-communicative deficit, characterized by slow processing speed, decreased immediate and working memory, and decreased abilities in the areas of problem solving and reasoning.

Mike's verbal speech consisted of vocalizations that were sometimes used to gain attention, and to accompany gestures and head nods. He also was able to produce single words, but these were subjectively judged to be less than 20% intelligible, even when contextual cues were present. Oral motor assessment revealed severely impaired lingual, labial, and palatal active range of motion with resultant severe dysarthria. His nonverbal communication abilities were characterized by head nods, gross pointing, and eye movements.

Mike's pragmatic communication abilities were directly impacted by his motor and expressive communicative disabilities. His interactions were characterized by inconsistent eye contact, an inability to control body proxemics or to generate gestures, and an inability to initiate communication topics or maintain an ongoing topic of conversation. He was generally alert and aware of his environment and frequently initiated interactions with the nursing and clinical staff via body movements or verbal approximations.

Based on findings from the informal assessment measures, the following diagnosis was made.

- Mike had severe receptive and expressive language deficits. He was able to respond to simple yes/no questions, to receptively identify familiar photographs, and to follow one-step directions. He had no functional ability to read, write, or verbally express himself.

- Mike had moderate cognitive-communication deficits. He was able to attend to structured tasks for 15–20 minutes, and to recall simple and familiar sequences within his environment. He had difficulty responding appropriately to cognitive or communicative information outside the context of his immediate setting.

- Mike had severe dysarthria due to severely impaired lingual, labial, and palatal strength; limited oral motor range of motion; and little functional intelligible speech.

AAC Implementation Strategies

Mike's cognitive and communication abilities were then combined with his motor abilities to develop an AAC system that would meet his needs in the nursing home setting. Because Mike had difficulty responding to complex auditory information and had significant memory deficits, it was decided that he would need an AAC system that could be accessed through direct selection. Although single-switch scanning AAC systems would be less physically fatiguing, Mike would have difficulty maintaining his attention on the system throughout the scanning process. In addition, the process of teaching him to select symbols appropriately on a scanning system would be difficult given his memory and visual constraints.

Mike was able to use his right hand to make large swiping gestures. However, he did not have the accuracy of movement to use his arm or hand for direct selection AAC systems. These gestures were also extremely fatiguing. In contrast, Mike was very accurate when using eye gaze to look at objects, persons, and photographs.

Through additional informal testing it was determined that he could reliably use eye gaze to make selections between 12 familiar photographs that were 2 inches in size. The symbols needed to be placed far apart with 2 inches of blank spacing between symbols due to his visual perceptual deficits.

After conferring with nursing staff and family about his communication needs, photographs were taken of persons and objects that were essential communication topics. The photos were arranged and laminated together into a clear lightweight communication board. A simple frame for the communication board was constructed for his wheelchair tray using PVC pipe. The communication board was attached to the frame with velcro. When Mike was in bed, the communication board could be removed from the PVC frame and held in place by nursing staff.

Eye gaze AAC systems are powerful communication tools. However, it is impossible to initiate communication with an eye gaze system unless the user is able to get the attention of a listener. Mike needed to call the nursing staff so that he could communicate his needs with the eye gaze system. A large Big Red switch was mounted onto the right side of his wheelchair tray. The switch was attached to a chime that alerted staff that Mike wanted their attention. The same switch and chime were also mounted onto the right side of Mike's bed railing using velcro so that he could call the nurses from his bed.

The next implementation step was to teach the nursing home staff how to use the communication system. They were trained to place the eye gaze board and switch onto his wheelchair tray. The nurses were then shown how to read Mike's eye gaze, and how to prompt him to respond if he seemed confused. They were also shown how to mount the switch by his bedside and hold the eye gaze board to communicate when he was in bed. Following two training sessions with nursing staff, Mike was able to use the communication system at a functional level within the structured nursing home setting. Staff reported that they were setting up the system on a daily basis and using it regularly to communicate with Mike.

Ongoing AAC Needs

The initial AAC evaluation and implementation stages were only the beginning of Mike's AAC journey. He required consultative monitoring by the speech-language pathologist to make sure that his AAC system continued to be effective. The degenerative nature of MS meant that Mike's communicative, motor, visual-perceptual, and cognitive status would change over time. Mike's AAC system would need to be decreased in complexity as these changes occurred. Nursing home staff were instructed to monitor Mike's accuracy in system use, as well as any changes in his cognitive-communicative and physical status. The other concern was ongoing staff turnover at the nursing home. The speech-language pathologist saw Mike for consultative AAC services every 2 months to monitor use of the system and to provide ongoing training for new staff.

Key Points To Remember

- The assessment of visual perceptual abilities is important in any AAC evaluation. This is especially true for individuals with degenerative conditions because changes in sensory abilities frequently accompany declines in motor and cognitive abilities.
- Many adults with severe motor impairments will need to be evaluated using informal assessment methods. Fatigue and motor abilities need to be considered when determining the best method of assessment.
- When low tech methods of communication are implemented, the ability to successfully initiate interactions needs to be considered. Individuals confined to wheelchairs or beds who are non-speaking cannot walk up to a listener to initiate communication. Call signals, chimes, or voice output AAC devices need to be implemented as part of the overall AAC system.
- Individuals with degenerative conditions need to have their AAC systems monitored on a regular basis. Regular monitoring ensures that the AAC system will change as their physical, communicative, perceptual, and cognitive abilities change.

Section 3

AAC IN
SPECIFIC ENVIRONMENTS

Chapter 14

AAC IN THE FAMILY AND HOME

Dianne H. Angelo

Providing assistive devices to children with severe speaking and writing disabilities creates numerous opportunities and challenges not only for the user but for the family as well. The clinical practice of augmentative and alternative communication (AAC) has focused traditionally on meeting the needs of children and adults who AAC systems to compensate for severe expressive communication disorders. As professionals, we are committed to helping these individuals achieve their fullest potential and have greater control over their lives through technology. Most everyone would agree that assistive technology can affect significant changes in the lives of individuals with disabilities. Through assistive technology, the ability to participate more fully and contribute more meaningfully in home, school, work, and community settings can be realized.

The impact of technology on the lives of users has been documented and can be found in professional books and journals (e.g., *Augmentative and Alternative Communication, The Exceptional Parent*), affiliated publications (e.g., *Augmentative Communication News, Alternatively Speaking, Communication Outlook, Communicating Together*), and newsletters or magazines of commercial AAC device manufacturers (e.g., *Echo On, The Key*). The trials and tribulations of communicating through assistive devices are most often described in personal narratives and third-person accounts that humanize the AAC experience (e.g., Brown, 1954; Nolan, 1987). From this documentation, the impact of AAC systems on the lives of users can be discerned.

Professionals in the field are developing an appreciation for the user's perspective on augmentative and alternative communication. In reviewing the literature, Huer and Lloyd (1990) summarized the perspectives of users and found that several predominant themes emerged and tended to recur. AAC users' personal insights regarding attitudes toward professionals, availability of communication partners, benefits and limitations of aided techniques, intervention priorities, and personal reactions and experiences were cited frequently. From their own perspectives, users have offered advice to professionals and have proposed recommendations for change in assessment and intervention practices.

What was and continues to be most important about consumer information is that it does influence the practices and approaches of professionals in AAC. For example, users have repeatedly expressed their dissatisfaction with professionals who disregard the perspectives of the user or family and dominate the decision-making process (Huer & Lloyd, 1990; Smith-Lewis & Ford, 1987). Today, users and family members are regarded as essential members of interdisciplinary teams. Contemporary best practices now enlist users and their families to participate with professionals in decision making and goal setting. The reality is that families are more likely to assume "ownership" of interventions when goals and decisions are formulated with their input and agreement (Beukelman & Mirenda, 1992). Their participation can foster family satisfaction and promote positive regard for professionals (Crais, 1991).

A concern that emerges from the literature is that AAC users believe there is a need for greater consideration of both users and family members in AAC decision making. Although family members participate on teams and are involved in assessment and intervention, professionals have only a limited understanding of how the family affects AAC outcomes or how AAC devices and services affect the family. Immediate family members have been described by users as the most significant communication partners in their lives (Huer & Lloyd, 1990). In personal accounts provided primarily by adult users, successful outcomes were almost always attributed in some way to the support and commitment of family members over time. In predicting intervention outcomes, family acceptance of AAC systems has been found to be an important variable (Silver-

man, 1989; Van Dyck, Allaire, & Gressard, 1990). Clearly, families are important, and because they can significantly affect outcomes, it is necessary to address family issues in AAC.

AAC FAMILIES AND MULTICULTURAL ISSUES

To date, our understanding of AAC families is limited and taken primarily from a literature base that reflects the mainstream culture. Unfortunately, it lacks attention to cultural, ethnic, social, or linguistic considerations. As a profession, we are now studying relevant issues in AAC from a cultural perspective (e.g., aided and unaided symbol selection, interaction styles and patterns, cognitive styles). This is an exciting time to increase our knowledge of all AAC families in a rapidly changing American society.

In the United States, contemporary society is becoming more culturally diverse, a demographic trend that is expected to continue into the next century. In 1990, almost 28% of American people were persons of color, and it is estimated that this number will increase to one third of the nation by the year 2010 and one half of the population by 2050 (Taylor, 1994). Based on the U.S. 1990 census, (Statistical Abstract of the United States, 1990), the rate of growth for Asian-American, Hispanic, African-American, and American Indian populations has far exceeded that of Caucasians due to unexpected immigration trends (Battle, 1993). The result of these changing demographics is a society that is significantly more culturally and linguistically diverse than ever before.

Individuals with severe expressive communication disorders are found in every culture. This being the case, professionals are challenged to better understand the families whom they serve by adopting innovative approaches and practices in assessing and treating communication disorders among multicultural populations. How a family accepts and values services for a family member with a disability can vary widely across and within cultures (Battle, 1993; Blackstone, 1993). The beliefs and values held by culturally and linguistically diverse families regarding communication styles, disabilities, technology, education and rehabilitation services, health and health care will influence the delivery of services to these populations (Cheng, 1993; Harris, 1993; Kayser, 1993; Terrell & Terrell, 1993). In addition, the extent to which a family adapts to a new or different culture and becomes "acculturated" may also affect service delivery (Buzolich, 1994).

In AAC, cultural diversity is becoming an important consideration in assessment, prescription, and intervention. Sophisticated technology is increasingly available to help those with severe expressive communication disorders achieve communicative competence. However, access to AAC services and devices may be difficult for members of cultural minorities, particularly if the family does not speak the dominant language (Blackstone, 1993).

When recommending interventions that include technology and technology services, many cultural issues must be considered. For example, Taylor (1994) suggested that consumer satisfaction with technology and technology-based interventions may have a cultural component. Family attitudes toward technology may determine the extent to which a family is accepting of technology or specifies the conditions under which technology is used. In addition, communication behavior, including that which is technology-based, is culturally determined (Taylor, 1994). For any particular group, what defines communication behavior or constitutes a communication disorder is a reflection of cultural values, norms, perceptions,

attitudes, and history which may differ considerably from traditional views of Caucasian, middle-class Americans (Battle, 1993; Harris, 1994; Soto, 1994).

Clearly, we need to conduct research investigations to study relevant issues in AAC from a cultural perspective. The addition of this essential information to the literature will extend our understanding beyond that of the mainstream culture to all families and improve service delivery to them. Increasing our knowledge base will result in professional philosophies and approaches in AAC that are both culturally sensitive and family centered.

PARENTS AND COMMUNICATIVE COMPETENCE

For most children, and across cultures, the family is the essential context for language learning and communication development (Anderson & Battle, 1993). Family members, and particularly parents or adult caregivers, are the primary communication partners for their children. They encourage the child's communicative competence within the expectations of the family (Anderson & Battle, 1993). Family members promote opportunities for social interaction, create needs to communicate, provide appropriate communication and language models, and respond contingently to the child's communication efforts (Donahue-Kilburg, 1992).

Acquiring communicative competence has been described as a process in which the child "acquires readable behaviors that can be interpreted as communicative bids" (Dunst & Lowe, 1986, p. 12). Early successful communication exchanges are necessary for developing the child's social communicative competence. However, for many parents of children with disabilities who are users or potential users of AAC systems, being the child's communication partner can be a challenging and frustrating experience. Because disabilities often mask communication behaviors, the child's attempts to interact may go unrecognized. Parents may have difficulty in reading and interpreting their child's behaviors as attempts to communicate because these behaviors can be subtle or unconventional. By failing to respond contingently to the child's attempts, opportunities for social interactions are lost.

Parents or adult caregivers provide the essential social experiences and practice opportunities for developing the child's social and communication competence. As a result, it seems that the roles of family members and the impact of augmentative and alternative communication on the entire family should be carefully explored. To understand the significance of the family in AAC, several questions will be discussed. First, are families involved in AAC assessment and intervention? Second, how are families involved and to what extent is their level of involvement? Third, are there barriers to family involvement? Fourth, in what ways can families and professionals work together to ensure successful outcomes for their children? And finally, what is the impact of AAC on families?

PARENTAL ROLES IN AAC

Parent Involvement and Roles in AAC

A review of the literature in AAC suggests that professionals certainly recognize the importance of working with families. Clinical experience suggests that the success of our interventions is highly dependent on the family's involvement and shared commitment to the goals of intervention. This section will highlight family involvement with particular emphasis on par-

ents' roles. This is not intended in any way to minimize the role of other family members (e.g., siblings, grandparents). It is recognized that, in some cultures, these roles may be assumed by or shared with other adult caregivers (Blackstone, 1993). However, because parents are often the primary caregivers, this discussion will focus on their contributions as reported in the literature.

Parent involvement can be described in terms of the roles and responsibilities that are related to assessment and intervention. Clearly, these change over time as family priorities shift and user needs arise. One area of parent involvement that is reported in the literature is vocabulary selection. Parents are often asked to generate vocabularies and messages for their children that reflect their communication needs at home or in the community. Parents play a particularly important role in generating vocabularies for their preliterate and nonliterate children. This has led several investigators to conclude that parents are necessary contributors in the vocabulary selection process for AAC users (Carlson, 1981; Fried-Oken & More, 1992; Light, Beesley, & Collier, 1988; Yorkston, Dowden, Honsinger, Marriner, & Smith, 1988; Yorkston, Fried-Oken, & Beukelman, 1988). Chapter 4 provides more information on the vocabulary selection process.

Parent involvement is probably best documented in the area of communication training (Beukelman, 1991; Culp & Carlisle, 1988; Cumley & Beukelman, 1992; Light et al., 1988). Professionals often work with families to carry out interventions designed to develop the functional communication competence of the user. AAC parents are trained to teach and practice skills at home that promote their child's operational, linguistic, strategic, and social competencies. Learning to use the child's assistive device is a necessary first step that leads to integrating the AAC system in the home and community. A sampling of tasks that parents are involved with includes selecting and compiling symbols and symbol sets, creating symbol displays, programming messages, operating and maintaining the assistive device, and modifying the physical environment to accommodate the technology (Table 14–1).

Other areas of parent involvement include promoting literacy learning (Koppenhaver, Evans, & Yoder, 1991) and developing the child's knowledge base (Beukelman & Mirenda, 1992). Ensuring educational opportunities and supporting the AAC child in achieving educational goals is usually a priority among parents. Parents also serve as advocates, transition coordinators, and liaisons among service providers and service agencies as needed. According to Berry (1987), family members often play an essential role in the transfer of information about technology, interaction styles, and other components of the child's augmentative communication program throughout the child's educational career.

Barriers to Parent Involvement

Clearly, parents assume many different responsibilities in AAC assessment and intervention. Their contributions are important and deserving of recognition. However, if we look carefully at how parents are involved in AAC, it appears that true partnerships with professionals are the exception rather than the rule. This may be particularly true for culturally diverse groups, especially when cultural and linguistic factors that influence family involvement are not taken into account. Traditional service models have often dictated a limited and passive role for family members in spite of attempts to involve them. Much of our effort has been aimed at directing parents to carry out interventions at home as prescribed by "experts." Within traditional service models that tend to be diagnostic and prescriptive in nature, services are based on goals, objectives, and preferences that are most likely derived from the professional's own cultural perspective. This situation, however, is not unique to the field of AAC. Most developmental, educational, and health care delivery systems have addressed families only through involvement in educational or training programs (Campbell & Leifield, 1993).

A problem with this orientation is that parents and family members may lose their enthusiasm and commitment over time. Professionals may not recognize that

Table 14-1. Common areas of parent involvement.

Vocabulary/Message Selection

Symbol Selection

Language and Communication Training

Literacy Training

Technology Programming

Technology Problem-Solving

Educational Tutoring

Advocacy

Transitioning

Coordinating Services

the demands placed on families can be overwhelming. Using and maintaining assistive devices requires additional time, energy, resources, and supports. Integrating assistive devices in the home will most likely increase roles and responsibilities of individual family members. These are in addition to their many other caregiving obligations as parents and family members. It should not be surprising then that, as the novelty of assistive technology fades, parent involvement may also decline. The magic and anticipation that accompanies the arrival of an assistive device can be neutralized by the reality of making assistive devices "fit" within demanding daily routines and schedules.

Ongoing demands related to assistive devices may discourage families and diminish their involvement over time. It is not uncommon for professionals to learn that parents and family members fail to follow through with prescribed interventions at home. Comments such as "we never use the device at home" or "I don't know how to program the device" are heard. For children, school is reported to be the predominant setting for using an assistive device (Culp, 1987). Carryover to other settings is considerably less. In several studies, parents as informants indicated limited device use by their children at home and in the community (Allaire, Gressard, Blackman, & Hostler, 1991; Culp, 1987; Culp, Ambrosi, Berniger, & Mitchell, 1986). Abandonment of assistive devices in the home has also been reported (Blackstone, 1992; Culp, 1987).

Our clinical experience suggests that parent involvement may be necessary but not sufficient for achieving successful outcomes in AAC. How to maintain family involvement over time is an important issue. Getting parents involved initially and keeping them involved throughout intervention has been a constant challenge for professionals in the field of communication disorders (Crais, 1991). The consider-able investment that parents and family members must make in order to use and maintain assistive devices in the home requires that professionals work together with families in ways that promote family satisfaction. Because family satisfaction with AAC systems may have a cultural component, it is important that cultural issues that influence family involvement with any service delivery system be carefully considered. It is no longer enough that parents simply satisfy the needs of the experts in carrying out interventions at home.

Overcoming Barriers

One way to counter problems associated with lack of parent involvement is by promoting family-professional collaboration. Lack of involvement may be a symptom of family-professional relationships in which experts dictate all aspects of service delivery. Limited device use and rejection of assistive devices in the home may simply be another symptom. Collectively, these serve as a "wake-up call" for professionals to be more sensitive and responsive to the expressed needs, priorities, and preferences of all families. This message also reinforces the concerns expressed by users to be more considerate of family members.

It is possible that families perceive their needs differently from professionals who determine intervention goals and plans for them. This is especially true for families from culturally diverse backgrounds. Most professionals specializing in AAC are members of the mainstream culture (Blackstone, 1993). Many families may not attach the same value to certain aspects of intervention deemed most important by professionals. For example, a family may reject use of an assistive device at home because members can effectively read and interpret the child's unaided communication techniques. Family needs for social closeness or intimacy with their child may conflict with needs of professionals to provide practice opportunities with assistive devices in the home. Failure to follow through may be misinterpreted by professionals as a lack of commitment on the part of family members.

Within collaborative relationships, families enjoy equal partnerships with professionals in all aspects of decision making, goal setting, and intervention planning. Opportunities for identifying and prioritizing family needs for services and expected outcomes allow families to determine the extent of their involvement in assessment and intervention. This is in sharp contrast to traditional practices in AAC. Professionals need to offer help that is in response to family identified needs and congruent with the family's appraisal of their needs (Campbell & Leifield, 1993). "While the need for and availability of support will vary over time, the family's perception that an appropriate amount of support is being given, relative to the degree of need, is what counts" (Blackstone, 1993, p. 2). With culturally diverse groups, differing perceptions may result in absenteeism, tardiness, and termination of services (Nellum-Davis, 1993).

In summary, professionals recognize and value families in AAC assessment and intervention. Knowing how to work with AAC families, and especially those of culturally and linguistically diverse backgrounds, in ways that promote and sustain family involvement may require a whole new set of philosophies, attitudes, values, and practices on the part of both professionals and family members. Limited use and rejection of assistive devices in the home strongly suggest that there is a need to evaluate critically our working relationships with AAC families. Fortunately, we can draw from contemporary family support movements and apply the philosophies and best practices of family-centered services to the field of AAC.

FROM PARENT INVOLVEMENT TO FAMILY-CENTERED SERVICES

Within the discipline of communication disorders, there is a growing interest in family-centered interventions and services (Andrews & Andrews, 1990; Crais, 1991; Donahue-Kilburg, 1992). "Parent involvement" is gradually being replaced with terminology reflecting the significance of the family and the impact of the family system on the child with a communication disorder.

Previously, the importance of the family, and parents or adult caregivers in particular, was discussed with regard to the child's emerging communicative competence. Within the broader context of contemporary service delivery, families are considered to be the constant throughout the child's life whereas service systems and service providers within those systems may be involved only episodically (Campbell & Leifield, 1993; Crais, 1991). It is likely that AAC families may interact with scores of professionals and have numerous associations with health, social service, and education agencies over their lifetimes. This places families in a prime position to foster and support the child's development, regardless of the child's age or disability, across the life span.

What is a family? There is no one, universally agreed upon definition of *family* in today's society. In fact, a definition of *family* is different for families from different cultures (Anderson & Battle, 1993). As American society becomes more culturally rich and diverse, traditional notions of the family are being replaced by changing family configurations. In addition to the nuclear family (i.e., mother, father, and children), there are also growing numbers of single-parent, blended, and extended or multigenerational families. Because it is difficult to agree upon a single characterization, contemporary commentators propose an expanded definition of family.

Hartman (1981, p. 8) described family as "two or more individuals who define themselves as a family and who, over time, assume those obligations to one another that are generally considered an essential component of family systems." This definition suggests that a family functions as a system. This perspective takes into account the "mutual influencing factors which surround individuals and families and recognizes that changes in any part of the 'system' can affect the entire system" (Crais, 1991, p. 4). The family is viewed as a social unit embedded within other extended social units and networks which are interdependent (Dunst, Trivette & Deal, 1988). This has led family specialists to advocate for an ecological or systems-based perspective in working with families (Andrews & Andrews, 1990; Bronfenbrenner, 1979; Donahue-Kilburg, 1992; Dunst, Trivette, & Deal, 1988).

In family-centered services, priorities and choices of the family drive the delivery of services. Because the needs of each child and family differ, services are individualized to meet those unique needs. Several models for working with families were described by Dunst, Johanson, Trivette, and Hamby (1991) and fall along a continuum of family-centered services (see Figure 14–1). At one end of the continuum is the *professional-centered model*, in which professionals determine a family's needs from their own "expert" perspective. In a *family-allied model*, professionals identify a family's needs and enlist family members to carry out interventions deemed necessary for the benefit of the family. A family-focused model differs from the previous models in that family members and professionals together determine a family's needs. Families are encouraged, however, to rely primarily on professional services and networks to meet their needs. At the other end of the continuum is a *family-centered* model. Similar to the family-focused model, families and professionals together identify family needs that guide all aspects of service delivery. However, this model aims to strengthen a family's own capacity to meet their individual family-identified needs. In AAC, the professional-centered and the family-allied models were used almost exclusively in the past. Family-focused and family-centered models have only emerged in recent years.

Although it is not within the scope of this chapter to elaborate in detail on family-centered practices and services, there are several excellent resources on the topic (Andrews & Andrews, 1990; Campbell & Leifield, 1993; Crais, 1991; Dunst, Trivette, & Deal, 1988; Winton, 1992; Zipper, Weil, & Rounds, 1991). Family specialists in early intervention, early childhood education, and health care have defined characteristics of family-centered services that reflect contemporary philosophies and best practices in working with families. These include

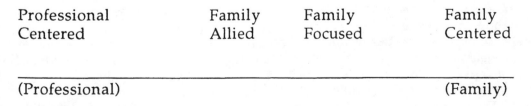

Professional Centered	Family Allied	Family Focused	Family Centered

(Professional)   (Family)

Figure 14–1. A continuum of models for working with families. Compiled from: From C. J. Dunst, C. Johanson, C. M. Trivette, and D. Hamby, 1991. "Family oriented early intervention policies and practices: Family-centered or not?" *Exceptional Children, 58,* 116-126.

practices that are family-focused, ecologically based, needs-based, individualized, and culturally sensitive (Crais, 1991; Winton, 1992). Families should experience coordinated service delivery, collaborative partnerships between families and professionals, and normalized services that integrate both the child and family within the community (Campbell & Leifield, 1993). In addition, family-centered services should strive to empower families to feel competent in meeting the needs of their own family (Campbell & Leifield, 1993; Crais, 1991; Winton, 1992)

McBride, Brotherson, Joanning, Whiddon, and Demmitt (1993) summarized the major assumptions of family-centered services that provide a framework for practice. The first major assumption is that the family is the focus of services. This represents a significant departure from more traditional models in that the family, not the child, is the focus of intervention and service delivery. Recognizing the family as the unit of intervention acknowledges the importance of the family system that is composed of interdependent members (Dunst, Trivette, & Deal, 1988). The second major assumption is that families have the right to decide what is important for themselves and their children. Supporting and respecting family decision making is essential. Empowering families to make decisions fosters their sense of control and provides a basis for partnerships in parent-professional relationships (Dunst, 1985). The third major assumption is the importance of providing services to families in order to strengthen family functioning. Family-centered services are intended to provide services that strengthen the family's ability to meet their needs and those of their child (McBride et al., 1993). By strengthening and supporting the family unit and not just the child, the chance of making a significant positive impact upon all family members is enhanced considerably (Dunst, Trivette, & Deal, 1988).

Support for family-centered services in AAC can be found in federal legislation. In 1986, P.L. 99-457 was passed by Congress and became known as the 1986 Amendments to the Education of the Handicapped Act (EHA). Part H of the Act created and established a philosophical basis for a family-centered approach in early intervention (Bender & Baglin, 1992). It mandated services for infants and toddlers identified with developmental delays from birth to age 3, or those who were "at risk" for developmental delay, and their families. In 1991, the law was strengthened through reauthorization. P.L. 101-476 changed the name of the law to the Individuals with Disabilities Education Act (IDEA).

IDEA created major challenges and opportunities for the development and delivery of family-centered early intervention services to infants and toddlers with disabilities and their families. Part H of IDEA, with its strong emphasis on the family, provided the strongest legislative direction to date for family-centered services (Zipper, Weil, & Rounds, 1991). In 1991, Part H was reauthorized by Congress and P.L. 102-119 became known as the Individuals with Disabilities Education Act Amendments of 1991. Additional early intervention services, such as assistive technology devices and services, were included.

Because assistive technology devices and services are included, there is a strong incentive for adopting family-centered philosophies and practices in the field of AAC. Family-centered services are already mandated for infants and toddlers in early intervention programs. There is also growing support for extending this family focus to 3- through 5-year-old eligible children (Rose & Smith, 1994).

At the present time, there is no mandate for family-oriented services to school-aged children. However, professionals within educational systems are required to provide assistive technology services to promote educational opportunities for these students. Use of augmentative communication devices and strategies must be linked directly with educational goals on the Individualized Education Plan (IEP). Unfortunately, different missions and mandates of organizations may make it difficult for professionals to have a family focus in their provision of services to students using assistive technology. It may be possible, however, to move toward a more family-oriented focus through the IEP goals. For example, IEP goals can address the child's communication needs across various environments including home and community. Communication boards and devices can be designed to bridge communication needs between home and school. The family can be included in the planning and decision-making process regarding vocabulary selection, overlay design, and strategies for use.

It seems reasonable, however, that the family-centered focus that families experience while their children are very young should continue to guide service delivery across the life span of the child. One best practice of family-centered services that may serve to support and extend the family-centered focus beyond early intervention is that of cultural sensitivity. Professionals are required not only to be sensitive to the cultural diversity of families, but also to be proactive in providing culturally competent services (Campbell & Leifield, 1993). Cultural competence refers to the ability to honor the cultural diversity of families in the provision of services (Roberts, 1990). It requires professionals to recognize and respect the racial, ethnic, cultural, and socioeconomic diversity of families (Campbell & Leifield, 1993). With the changing demographics of American society, a service delivery system that is sensitive to these differences and offers services that are consistent with family values, traditions, norms, and beliefs may have the greatest appeal to all AAC families across the life span and may yield the

most successful outcomes for individuals using technology.

NEEDS OF AAC FAMILIES

Within family-centered models, services are provided within the context of the family system (Donahue-Kilburg, 1992). Assessment of a family's perceived needs determines the scope of services and translates into goals for intervention. Bailey (1991) defined family needs as the family's expressed concerns and priorities of all family members that guide all aspects of service delivery. As stated previously, a defining characteristic of family-centered services is a need-based approach.

Needs assessment is important to AAC professionals in determining goals for family-centered interventions. It is an initial step that can lead to identification of family strengths. When needs are identified from a family perspective, professionals can assist families in accessing information and mobilizing resources and supports that meet their unique needs. Instead of focusing on limitations or constraints, there is an emphasis on developing or strengthening a family's unique capacity to meet their own needs (McBride et al., 1993). The goal is to help families to become competent, rather than dependent upon professionals, in ways that support and strengthen the family (Dunst, Trivette, & Deal, 1988). In family-centered practices, a needs-based approach allows the family and professionals to work together in identifying and obtaining services from the perspective of a family's priorities.

In an effort to better understand AAC families, Angelo, Jones, and Kokoska (1995) conducted a survey to identify the needs, priorities, and preferences of parents with young children using assistive devices and technology services. Using the Assistive Device Technology Needs Scale (Angelo &

Jones, 1991) this study identified the top five priority needs related to assistive devices and technology services of mothers and fathers. The results of the study must be interpreted with caution because of the limited population sample. For the most part, the families who responded to the survey consisted of educated, Caucasian, middle-class, two-parent households. Obviously, the responses of the mothers and fathers who participated in the survey are unlikely to be representative of all parents with young children using technology. Further research is needed to understand the diverse needs and concerns of AAC families of varied racial, ethnic, cultural, and socioeconomic backgrounds.

As seen in Tables 14–2 and 14–3, the study identified priority needs for mothers and fathers. For fathers, the need for increasing knowledge of assistive devices ranked first. This finding supports related studies in which fathers of young children with disabilities expressed their greatest needs for informational supports (Bailey & Simeonsson, 1988; Cooper & Allred, 1992; Linder & Chitwood, 1984). Cooper and Allred (1992) contend that fathers want to be more informed and also want to share the "liaison" role between professionals and families traditionally assumed by mothers. Brotherson and Goldstein

(1992) found that mothers want more opportunities for fathers to be involved with programs and services. For mothers, the need for knowledge about assistive devices ranked third. Again, the mothers in this study were similar to other mothers of children with disabilities as reported by Cooper and Allred (1992) and Bailey and Simeonsson (1988) in their need for information. Obviously, both parents have strong needs for being well-informed and knowledgeable about technology. According to Glicksman (1989), the need for information is also linked to the need to share information which has put parents in leadership roles in organizing parent-initiated networks including *Closing the Gap* and the *National Special Education Alliance*.

Given the rapid pace of technological advancements, professionals should plan and promote opportunities for learning about assistive devices. Opportunities for increasing knowledge may include hands-on equipment training sessions, lab tours, vendor demonstrations, technology workshops, and conferences. In addition to providing these informational supports, creative family-centered scheduling (e.g., weekends or evenings) should be explored to accommodate the demanding schedules of both parents and ensure that both parents' needs are being met. Assist-

Table 14–2. Ranking of mothers' priority needs for assistive devices and services.

First:	Integrating assistive devices in the community.
Second:	Developing community awareness and supports for assistive device users.
Third (tied):	Increasing own knowledge of assistive devices.
Third (tied):	Getting computer access for her child.
Fourth:	Planning for her child's future communication needs.
Fifth (tied):	Finding advocacy groups for parents of children using assistive devices.
Fifth (tied):	Finding trained professionals to work with her child.

Source: "A family perspective on augmentative and alternative communication: Families of young children," by D. Angelo, S. Jones, and S. Kokoska, 1995. *Augmentative and Alternative Communication, 11*, 193–201. Reprinted with permisison.

Table 14–3. Ranking of fathers' priority needs for assistive devices and services.

First:	Increasing own knowledge of assistive devices.
Second:	Planning for his child's future communication needs.
Third:	Finding volunteers to work with his child.
Fourth:	Getting funding for an assistive device or services.
Fifth (tied):	Integrating assistive devices in the home.
Fifth (tied):	Knowing how to teach his child to use an assistive device.

Source: "A family perspective on augmentative and alternative communication: Families of young children." by D. Angelo, S. Jones, and S. Kokoska, 1995. *Augmentative and Alternative Communication, 11*, 193-201. Reprinted with permisison.

ing with or coordinating transportation arrangements (e.g., carpools) may also improve access, particularly for families in areas with limited local resources. In addition, professionals may consider strategies to provide on-site child care during scheduled events (e.g., enlisting community volunteers, university students) to further free parents to benefit from learning opportunities.

Planning for future communication needs, which includes assistive device options and services, was among the top priorities of both fathers (second) and mothers (fourth). Like the Cooper and Allred study (1992), families expressed strong needs for information about future child services. Professionals and service agencies need to recognize the importance of planning for the future. Linking families to parent support groups, advocacy groups, professional organizations, volunteer services, and social service agencies is an important step for identifying and accessing resources and meeting both present and future needs. Several support groups, parent organizations, and empowerment initiatives (e.g., *Hear Our Voices,* Broehl, 1990) have emerged over the years to help families. Related to future planning, it is also necessary for professionals to coordinate our service delivery systems to minimize the demands on families to do this

(Brotherson & Goldstein, 1992). Focusing on transitions across all life phases and developing transition plans and strategies should be a primary goal of professionals so that no child "slips between the cracks."

Related to the need for increasing knowledge about assistive devices is the need for knowing how to teach the child to use an assistive device, and integrating assistive devices at home. Similar to the Cooper and Allred study (1992) which found that fathers needed information about how to teach their children, these two needs were tied and ranked fifth highest among priorities for fathers. Unlike the mothers in the Cooper and Allred study, mothers did not rank these particular needs as top priorities. Instead, mothers expressed greater needs for integrating assistive devices in the community (first) and developing community awareness and supports for assistive device users (second). A similar finding was reported by Culp (1987) in that families identified training of the general public as an important concern. The introduction of assistive devices often requires both parents to assume new or expanded roles and responsibilities within the family. Margalit (1990) contends that "each parent takes on the most personally relevant and appropriate role, regardless of traditional distinctions"

(1990, p. 83) when technology becomes part of the home and family.

The need for finding trained professionals and the need for finding advocacy groups were both ranked as fifth priority for the mothers. Both are linked to needs for informational supports that were addressed earlier. Glicksman (1989) contended that parents who are proactive learn to access specialized information and become knowledgeable about various disciplines whose specialty has an impact on their child. In addition, these parents "know which needs of our children are served by different disciplines; what the professional organizations are that lead these disciplines; and who the principle investigators and practitioners are." (Glicksman, 1989, p. 15). Fathers also expressed a need for volunteers to work with their children (third). Memberships in organized groups and networks may assist families in addressing issues that pertain to service delivery, personal advocacy, public policy reform, and funding issues (Broehl, 1990).

For fathers, the need to get funding for an assistive device or services was ranked among the top priorities (fourth). Because few insurance policies provide for AAC devices and services, the burden of expense may rest with the family and is often prohibitive. Lack of information about sources of funding for technology and technology services is frequently reported by families (RESNA, 1989). Professionals need to work closely with families to explore funding through insurance, educational, or vocational sources, or to find creative ways to finance technology, such as volunteer and religious organizations, when other options cannot be accessed (Parette, Hofmann, & VanBiervliet, 1994). Chapter 9 provides more information on funding resources.

Mothers also expressed a strong need for getting computer access for their children (third). For many users, a computer is the key to educational and social inclusion as well as future competitive or supported employment. In a study by Margalit (1990) of parents of children with disabilities using computers, a large proportion of mothers indicated their belief that a computer would significantly assist their children in dealing with their learning difficulties. It was suggested that the introduction of computers in the family has the potential to empower parents by introducing new challenges into their existing roles (Margalit, 1990).

Needs expressed by families in this study suggested that mothers and fathers do indeed have parent preferences for goals and services related to assistive technology. Because parents may have differing needs, it is important to assess both mothers and fathers in two-parent households. Having only one "spokesperson" may unintentionally limit goals and services available to the family. In addition, parents' needs and priorities may differ from those of the professionals working with them. Differing values assigned to various aspects of intervention can create dissension between parents and professionals. Families of children with disabilities often report that professionals do not listen or respond to the needs of individual families (Turnbull & Turnbull, 1985). It is important that professionals be willing to respect family needs, priorities, and preferences. By collaborating with families, identifying and obtaining services according to their priorities is possible (Crais, 1991).

It is important to reemphasize that the needs expressed by Caucasian, middle class, two-parent families cannot be generalized to all AAC families. Identification of needs of culturally diverse families must take into account the traditions, norms, values, and beliefs of the family. A family's perception of a disability and the child's communicative competence, value of an AAC device, and acceptance of the professional community will undoubtedly influence their needs for technology and technology services.

Determining needs of culturally diverse families in AAC may require different approaches. A common practice in early intervention and health care has been to use checklists or questionnaires to determine a family's strengths, needs, and resources. A problem with this approach is that these instruments are developed by professionals of the mainstream culture with little consideration for multicultural or multilingual issues. Another concern is that families of cultural minorities may not be responsive to questionnaire formats. One alternative is the use of an ethnographic approach to research which appears to offer a more viable means of identifying family needs. Research methods include formal and informal interviews with members of the family and observations in the home to determine meaningful needs from a cultural perspective. An ethnographic approach to research is likely to "contribute substantial information to our attempts to define communicative competence, the efficacy of intervention strategies, delivery and use of technology, and partner training" for our culturally diverse AAC populations (Blackstone, 1993, p. 6).

THE IMPACT OF AAC ON THE FAMILY

Developing an understanding of family issues and perspectives in AAC assessment and intervention is an important goal for professionals. Although the impact of technology on the user is documented, what is less clear and certainly less frequently reported is the impact of AAC systems on the family. The most obvious impact on families is that AAC offers a way to communicate and reduces the demand on family members to anticipate or interpret the child's communication. In one study, parents and family members indicated

that AAC allowed the primary caregiver to leave the user in the care of others as a result of using the AAC system (Culp, 1987).

The introduction of AAC systems in the family can be very stressful. "Without special awareness of families and their needs while adapting to a child with an impairment or disability, it is easy for professionals, even with the best of intentions, to increase the stress that family members feel" (Donahue-Kilburg, 1992, p. 81). As professionals begin to address the needs and priorities of family members, the impact of assistive devices and technology services on families becomes more apparent. To date, little information is available regarding the impact of AAC systems on family members. There is, however, related research that suggests that a variety of stressors are associated with a child's need for and use of assistive technology (Parette, 1994).

Identifying sources of stress in families with children with disabilities has been a focus of research activity over the past decade. The issue of stress in AAC families, however, has only recently been investigated. According to Berry (1987), "family stress may be exacerbated when the child's ability to communicate is severely impaired" (p. 90). Like other families, AAC families are confronted with the emotional and stressful challenges of adapting and adjusting to the ongoing, day-to-day demands of family life. Unlike other families, these family members must also accommodate assistive technology devices and equipment, technology services, assistive technology specialists, and agencies within their already demanding and complicated social and professional networks. The potential impact on family tasks, roles, and responsibilities should be considered early in the assessment process. Because acceptance of technology may be culturally influenced, this becomes particularly relevant for cultural and linguistic minorities. It seems reasonable that assessment should include identification of factors related to parental stress as well as the resources and supports that families use to help buffer the effects of these stressors (Margalit, 1990).

Jones, Angelo and Kokoska (1994) reported sources of parenting stress among parents with children using assistive devices. In this study, parents were surveyed and responded to the *Parenting Stress Index* (Abidin, 1986). This instrument was used to evaluate parent stressors arising from either child- or parent-related sources. Both mothers and fathers indicated that the top three child-related parenting stressors included acceptance, demandingness, and adaptability of the child. With regard to parent-related parenting stressors, results revealed differences for fathers and mothers. The three highest scores for parent-related stressors for mothers were relationships with their spouse, health, and social isolation. Fathers identified attachment to the child, social isolation, sense of competency, and parent health as the parental characteristics associated with the greatest level of stress. Results indicated that only a small percentage of mothers and fathers were experiencing other stressful life events such as unemployment or illness in the family. However, 39.7% of the mothers and 36.6% of the fathers had total stress scores indicating extremely high stress levels and the need for assistance.

There are many potential sources of stress for mothers and fathers of children using assistive devices. Stress can result from the demands of parent involvement described earlier. Finding the time and energy to assume new roles and responsibilities can be overwhelming. In addition to being caregivers, parents also become teachers, therapists, consultants, technology programmers and problem-solvers, transporters, transition coordinators, program evaluators, and advocates. These additional caregiving responsibilities can compromise parent health and well-being. In addition, financial resources and marital relations may be affected.

Other sources of stress arise from changes in family routines. Parents are frequently asked to integrate the AAC system in daily activities. The inclusion of AAC systems within daily routines can complicate or extend routines as parents attempt to learn and use the assistive device at home. Physical modifications in home and community environments needed to accommodate the AAC system may also produce stress in families. Many parents who rely on unaided communication techniques at home may find it cumbersome, if not unnecessary, to use an aided assistive device in daily activities. Parents may abandon the AAC system if it is not easily assimilated into family routines or if parents are uncomfortable with their ability to use the system with their child.

Restrictions of activities can also be stressful to parents. Transitioning from one activity or setting can be difficult as parents attempt to integrate the use of their child's technology into daily activities and in various family and neighborhood settings. Such transitions require not only the physical transport of the technology but may require modifications or re-programming of the device to reflect vocabulary needs of a specific setting or activity. Not only does this require specific skills and knowledge on the part of the parents but it demands additional time and energy. These added demands may discourage parents from engaging in activities. Restrictions of activities can also lead to social isolation for parents and families.

Obviously, not all parents experience stress stemming from these sources. It is not simply the number of stressors that affect parents and family functioning but the coping strategies, resources, and supports that families use to ameliorate the effects of stress. Coping is an ongoing process whereby family members attempt to master, tolerate, or reduce the demands that are straining their resources (Lazarus & Folkman, 1984). Parents and family members cope in a variety of ways depending on the child's disability and needs, as well as the family's needs, resources, and supports (Zipper, Weil, & Rounds, 1991). Although AAC families report stressors in their lives, the benefits derived from assisting their child to develop competence, increase self-esteem, and gain independence can be rewarding and fulfilling. As professionals, we need to assist families in identifying and mobilizing resources and supports that will help them cope with stress and minimize any negative impact of assistive devices on the family.

FUTURE DIRECTIONS IN AAC

Developing collaborative relationships between families and professionals requires innovative policies and practices. It also requires changes in the ways in which all services and supports have been traditionally provided for children with disabilities and their families. In AAC, it is suggested that professionals move toward family-centered philosophies, practices, and attitudes of what is referred to as contemporary family support movements. The goals of family support programs and services are to "enable and empower people by enhancing and promoting individual and family capabilities that support and strengthen family functioning" (Dunst, Trivette, Starnes, Hamby, & Gordon, 1993, p. 4).

It is reasonable to assume that family-centered services will require professionals to gain different skills and attitudes. Knowledge of cultural and linguistic issues in AAC is essential to understand the families of our changing society and to provide culturally competent and culturally sensitive services to these populations. Professionals will need to focus on offering services that are consistent with the expec-

tations of the family by recognizing and honoring the cultural, racial, ethnic, and socioeconomic diversity of all families.

It is also important that professionals develop necessary competencies for working with families across the life span. Clearly, we need to gain a better understanding of individual AAC families. Because working with families is an important responsibility, additional training may be needed to be competent in this area. Many AAC professionals have not had specific training in working with families and need to acquire skills in areas such as partnership building, consensus building, interviewing, counseling, consultation, collaboration, goal setting, and decision making (Beukelman & Mirenda, 1992; Donahue-Kilburg, 1992).

Further investigation is needed to increase our understanding of parent and family issues in AAC and measure the impact of AAC on all families. Professionals in the field must be willing to make a commitment to multicultural issues in AAC as reflected in our research, professional education, and clinical practice. An ethnographic approach to research and clinical practice will undoubtedly improve the quality of services provided to families of multicultural populations in the future.

REFERENCES

Abidin, R. R. (1986). *Parenting Stress Index: Manual* (2nd ed.). Charlottesville, VA: Pediatric Psychology Press.

Allaire, J. H., Gressard, R. P., Blackman, J. A., & Hostler, S. L. (1991). Children with severe speech impairments: Caregiver survey of AAC use. *Augmentative and Alternative Communication, 7*(4), 248–255.

Anderson, N. B., & Battle, D. E. (1993). Cultural diversity in the development of language. In D. E. Battle (Ed.), *Communication disorders in multicultural populations* (pp. 158–185). Boston: Andover Medical Publishers.

Andrews, J. R., & Andrews, M. A. (1990). *Family based treatment in communicative disorders: A systemic approach.* Sandwich, Il: Janelle Publications, Inc.

Angelo, D. H., & Jones, S. D. (1991). *Assistive device technology needs scale.* Unpublished manuscript, Bloomsburg University, Bloomsburg, PA.

Angelo, D., Jones, S., & Kokoska, S. (1995). Family perspective on augmentative and alternative communication: Families of young children. *Augmentative and Alternative Communication, 11,* 193–201.

Bailey, D. B. (1991). Issues and perspectives on family assessment. *Infants and Young Children, 4*(1), 26–43.

Bailey, D. B., & Simeonsson, R. J. (1988). Assessing needs of families with handicapped infants. *Journal of Special Education, 22,* 117–127.

Battle, D. E. (Ed.). (1993). *Communication disorders in multicultural populations.* Boston: Andover Medical Publishers.

Bender, M., & Baglin, C. A. (1992). *Infants and toddlers: A resource guide for practitioners.* San Diego: Singular Publishing Group.

Berry, J. O. (1987). Strategies for involving parents in programs for young children using augmentative and alternative communication. *Augmentative and Alternative Communication, 3*(2), 90–93.

Beukelman, D. R. (1991). Magic and cost of communicative competence. *Augmentative and Alternative Communication, 7*(1), 2–10.

Beukelman, D. R., & Mirenda, P. (1992). *Augmentative and alternative communication: Management of severe communication disorders in children and adults.* Baltimore: Paul H. Brookes Publishing Co.

Blackstone, S. W. (1992). Abandonment of assistive technology: What consumers know and professionals need to find out. *Augmentative Communication News, 5*(3), 2.

Blackstone, S. W. (1993). For consumers: Culture in the community. *Augmentative Communication News. 6*(2), 1–10.

Broehl, D. (1990). Hear our voices—An empowerment initiative. *Communication Outlook, 12*(2), 12-13.

Bronfenbrenner, U. (1979). *The ecology of human development: Experiments by nature and design.* Cambridge: Harvard University Press.

Brotherson, M. J., & Goldstein, B. (1992). Time as a resource and constraint for parents of young children with disabilities: Implication for early intervention services. *Topics in Early Childhood Special Education, 12*(4), 508–527.

Brown, C. (1954). *My left foot.* London, England: Secker & Warbug.

Buzolich, M. J. (1994). *Multicultural issues in augmentative and alternative communication.* Miniseminar presented by Buzolich, M. J., Harris, O., Lloyd, L. L., Soto, G., & Taylor, O. L. at the American Speech-Language-Hearing Association Annual Convention, New Orleans, LA.

Campbell, P., & Leifield, L. (1993). *A model for statewide faculty training.* Philadelphia: Northeastern Early Intervention Faculty Training Institute.

Carlson, F. (1981). A format for selecting vocabulary for the nonspeaking child. *Language, Speech and Hearing Services in Schools, 12,* 140–145.

Cheng, L. L. (1993). Asian-American cultures. In D. E. Battle (Ed.), *Communication disorders in multicultural populations.* Boston: Andover Medical Publishers.

Cooper, C. S., & Allred, K. W. (1992). A comparison of mothers' versus fathers' needs for support in caring for a young child with special needs. *Infant-Toddler Intervention: The Transdisciplinary Journal, 2*(3), 205–221.

Crais, E. R. (1991). *A practical guide to embedding family-centered content into existing speech-language pathology coursework.* Chapel Hill, NC: Carolina Institute for Research on Infant Personnel Preparation. Frank Porter Graham Child Development Center.

Culp, D. M. (1987). Outcome measurement: The impact of communication augmentation. *Seminars in Speech and Language, 9*(2), 169–184.

Culp, D. M., Ambrosi, D. M., Berniger, T. M., & Mitchell, J. O. (1986). Augmentative communication aid use—A follow-up study. *Augmentative and Alternative Communication, 2*(1), 19–24.

Culp, D. M., & Carlisle, M. (1988). *Partners in augmentative communication training.* Tucson, AZ: Communication Skill Builders, Inc.

Cumley, G. D., & Beukelman, D. R. (1992). Roles and responsibilities of facilitators in augmentative and alternative communication. *Seminars in Speech and Language, 13*(2), 111–119.

Davis, P. B., & May, J. E. (1991). Involving fathers in early intervention and family support programs: Issues and strategies. *Children's Health Care, 20*(2), 87–92.

Donahue-Kilburg, G. (1992). *Family-centered early intervention for communication disorders: Prevention and treatment.* Gaithersburg, MD: Aspen Publishers, Inc.

Dunst, C. J. (1985). Rethinking early intervention. *Analysis and Intervention in Developmental Disabilities, 5,* 165–201.

Dunst, C. J., & Lowe, L. W. (1986). From reflex to symbol: Describing, explaining, and fostering communicative competence. *Augmentative and Alternative Communication, 2*(1), 11–18.

Dunst, C. J., Johanson, C., Trivette, C. M., & Hamby, D. (1991). Family-oriented early intervention policies and practices. Family-centered or not? *Exceptional Children, 58,* 115–126.

Dunst, C. J., Trivette, C. M., & Deal, A. G. (1988). *Enabling and empowering families: Principles and guidelines for practice.* Cambridge, MA: Brookline Books.

Dunst, C., Trivette, C., Starnes, A., Hamby, D., & Gorden, N. (1993). *Building and evaluating family support initiatives: A national study of programs for persons with developmental disabilities.* Baltimore, MD: Paul H. Brookes Publishing Co.

Fried-Oken, M., & More, L. (1992). An initial vocabulary for nonspeaking preschool children based on developmental and environmental language sources. *Augmentative and Alternative Communication, 8*(1), 41–56.

Glicksman, H. (1989). AAC: A parent's perspective. *Communication Outlook, 10*(3), 14–15.

Harris, G. A. (1993) American Indian cultures: A lesson in diversity. In D. E. Battle (Ed.), *Communication Disorders in multicultural populations.* Boston: Andover Medical Publishers.

Harris, O. (1994). *Multicultural issues in augmentative and alternative communication.* Miniseminar presented by Buzolich, M., Harris, O., Lloyd, L., Soto, G., & Taylor, O. L. at the American Speech-Language-Hearing Convention, New Orleans, LA.

Hartman, A. (1981). The family: A central focus for practice. *Social Work,* (1), 7–13.

Huer, M. B., & Lloyd, L. L. (1990). AAC users' perspectives on augmentative and alternative communication. *AAC Augmentative and Alternative Communication, 6*(4), 242–249.

Jones, S. D., Angelo, D. H., & Kokoska, S. M. (1994). *Stressors and needs: Families with children using augmentative and alternative communication technology.* Unpublished manuscript.

Kayser, H. (1993). Hispanic cultures. In D. E. Battle (Ed.), *Communication disorders in multicultural populations.* Boston: Andover Medical Publishers.

Koppenhaver, D. A., Evans, D. A., & Yoder, D. E. (1991). Childhood reading and writing experiences of literate adults with severe speech and motor impairments. *Augmentative and Alternative Communication, 7*(1), 20–33.

Lazarus, R. S., & Folkman, S. (1984). *Stress, appraisal and coping.* New York: Springer.

Light, J., Beesley, M., & Collier, B. (1988). Transition through multiple augmentative and alternative communication systems: A three-year case study of a head injured adolescent. *Augmentative and Alternative Communication, 4*(1), 2–14.

Linder, T. W., & Chitwood, D. G. (1984). The needs of fathers of young handicapped children. *Journal of the Division for Early Childhood, 8*(2), 133–139.

Margalit, M. (1990). *Effective technology integration for disabled children: The family perspective.* New York: Springer-Verlag.

McBride, S. L., Brotherson, M. J., Joanning, H., Whiddon, D., & Demmitt, A. (1993). Implementation of family-centered services: Perceptions of families and professionals. *Journal of Early Intervention, 17*(4), 414–430.

Nellum-Davis, P. (1993). Clinical practice issues. In D. E. Battle (Ed.), *Communication disorders in multicultural populations.* Boston: Andover Medical Publishers.

Nolan, C. (1987). *Under the eye of the clock: The life story of Christopher Nolan.* New York: Dell.

Parette, H. P. (1994). Assessing the influence of augmentative and alternative communication devices on families of young children with disabilities. *Perceptual and Motor Skills, 78,* 1361–1362.

Parette, H. P., Hofmann, A., & VanBiervliet, A. (1994). The professional's role in obtaining funding for assistive technology for infants and toddlers with disabilities. *Teaching Exceptional Children,* 22–28.

RESNA. (1989). *Technology related assistance for individuals with disabilities. Summaries of successful grant applications awarded under P.L. 100–407.* Washington, DC: RESNA Press.

Roberts, R. N. (1990). *Developing competent programs for families of children with special needs?* (2nd ed.). Washington, DC: Georgetown University Child Development Center.

Rose, D., & Smith, B. J. (1994). Providing public education services to preschoolers with disabilities in community-based programs: Who's responsible for what? *Young Children, 49*(6), 64–68.

Silverman, F. H. (1989). *Communication for the speechless.* (2nd ed.). Englewood Cliffs, NJ: Prentice-Hall.

Smith-Lewis, M. R., & Ford, A. (1987). A user's perspective on augmentative communication. *Augmentative and Alternative Communication, 3*(1), 12–17.

Soto, G. (1994). *Multicultural issues in augmentative and alternative communication.* Miniseminar presented by Buzolich, M., Harris, O., Lloyd, L., Soto, G., & Taylor, O. L. at the American Speech-Language-Hearing Association Annual Convention, New Orleans, LA.

Statistical abstract of the United States. 1990. (110th ed.). Washington, DC: U.S. Department of Commerce. Bureau of Census.

Terrell, S. L., & Terrell, F. (1993). African-American cultures. In D. E. Battle (Ed.), *Communication disorders in multicultural populations.* Boston: Andover Medical Publishers.

Taylor, O. L. (1994). *Multicultural issues in augmentative and alternative communication.* Miniseminar presented by Buzolich, M., Harris, O., Lloyd, L., Soto, G., & Taylor, O. L. at the American Speech-Language-Hearing Association Annual Convention, New Orleans, LA.

Turnbull, A. P., & Turnbull, H. R. (1985). *Parents speak out.* Columbus, OH: Charles E. Merrill.

Van Dyck, M. C., Allaire, J. H., & Gressard, R. (1990). AAC decision-making. *Communication Outlook, 11*(4), 12-14.

Winton, P. J. (1992). *Working with families in early intervention: An interdisciplinary preservice curriculum* (2nd ed.). Chapel Hill, NC: Frank Porter Graham Child Development Center, University of North Carolina.

Yorkston, K. M., Dowden, P. A., Honsinger, M. J., Marriner, N., & Smith, K. (1988). A comparison of standard and user vocabulary lists. *Augmentative and Alternative Communication, 4*(4), 189-210.

Yorkston, K. M., Fried-Oken, M., & Beukelman, D. R. (1988). Single word vocabulary needs: Studies from various nonspeaking populations. *Augmentative and Alternative Communication, 4*(3), 149.

Zipper, I. N., Weil, M., & Rounds, K. (1991). *Service coordination for early intervention: Parents and professionals.* Chapel Hill, NC: Carolina Institute for Research on Infant Personnel Preparation, Frank Porter Graham Child Development Center, University of North Carolina.

Life Stories

Alexander's Story:
A Parent's Perspective

Denise DeCoste

The following life story is derived from a parent interview with Ann regarding her son Alexander's history with AAC. It speaks to the highs and lows of AAC and the many issues that are pressed on parents, perhaps before they are really prepared for them. Ann's comments are written in italics.

I remember when he had no way to express himself; no way to even say yes or no. He had no way to communicate his preferences, no way to control his relationships with others, no way to express his interests or convey even the germ of an idea. All he could do was look with his eyes.

Alexander appeared to be developing normally until he was about 4 months old. Beginning at that time, he had repeated illnesses, including parasitic infections at 7 and 15 months of age. By 8 months there was a clear loss of developmental skill and he was eventually diagnosed with spastic quadriparesis with significant underlying low tone.

The augmentative communication and assistive technology team became acquainted with Alexander and his family when he entered the public schools at age 6. He initially appeared quite passive. He had very poor head control and he demonstrated little volitional movement. He

would occasionally smile or laugh, otherwise his face and body were very still. It was impossible to know what was inside this child, what he was thinking and feeling. Because he had little active movement outside of his eyes, the prospect of finding a method of motor access that this child could use to operate a communication device was slim. In fact, it took years.

Alexander learned a continuum of ways to express himself, moving from eye gaze gradually to the use of voice output. The AAC team began by teaching him the basic elements of how to look at a person and use his eyes to communicate. They found ways for him to indicate yes or no. This is not something that happens by accident. A child has to be taught these things.

It was clear to the AAC team that communication would begin with eye gaze strategies. Much effort went into teaching Alexander the process of communication using his eyes. Gradually, Alexander learned the procedures: look at the communication partner, look at the desired object, and then look back at his partner. Parallel training was also initiated on single switch use. A variety of movements and control sites were explored during the first year in school without much initial success: gross shoulder movement, thumb movement, and head movement were paired with different types of single switches. Single switch computer activities and circular scanning using the Versascan were introduced. Consistent movements that could be paired with a yes or no response were also explored.

Parents of children who are nonspeaking have to be very patient. It is so difficult to see the big picture when you're just starting out. It's hard to see how the pieces fit together and where it all leads you.

The difficulty for the school team was that few of the AAC strategies, except for eye gaze, could be depended upon for purposes of communication with any degree of confidence. Was this due to motor problems, or cognitive issues, or was it a motivational problem? We still had more questions than answers. The problem for the family was that new methods were constantly being introduced, with no definitive reasons why chosen methods were not effective for Alexander. The parents and the team felt sure that this child wanted to communicate; the big question was "How?"

Over the next four years, eye gaze continued to be Alexander's most reliable method of communication and eye gaze strategies were upgraded to include letter-color encoding strategies. Improving head control to operate a switch for automatic scanning in linear and row column patterns continued to be emphasized. Over the course of 4 long years, Alexander moved from a Scan Wolf to a Light Talker, but progress with scanning accuracy sufficient for communication was slow. During this time, other AAC strategies were evaluated to determine whether direct selection methods of access were as yet a possibility. Head pointers, light pointers, and upper extremity controlled scanning were all tried without success. Although eye gaze continued to be the most reliable, it was always adult initiated and did not give

Alexander control over his communication with others.

You have to find some way not to become overwhelmed. There were so many strategies being tried with Alexander and progress was slow. At the beginning, when we were relying on an eye gaze board we tried to keep up with all the picture symbols and keep pace with his vocabulary needs. At times, it seemed totally unmanageable.

In the first 5 years, many methods were tried, and many devices were introduced. Each time this occurred, the family was presented with new information to sort through and new techniques to learn. Of course all of this occurred against a backdrop of a wide variety of complicated home and school issues (e.g., surgeries, homework issues, literacy learning issues, inclusion logistics); AAC was by no means the only issue of concern to the family and school team.

Communication from school to home took place via phone calls, occasional meetings, and a daily message book. Each year at the annual review meetings, the school team presented Alexander's current strengths and weaknesses, while the family struggled to make sense of it all. All hoped that next year would bring greater gains in all areas, with the common belief that active, accurate, and independent communication was still Alexander's biggest personal and education need.

It is important for parents to be thoughtful as to how all these communication devices fit into your family, and yet be open to other possibilities. For example, at one point we tried to use a voice output device at dinner time. It just didn't work for our family and created some disappointment overall. It can be hard to find the right balance.

Most families find it difficult to incorporate communication technology into their daily routines at home. At the point at which a child with physical disabilities seems ready to use an electronic voice output device, most families have already established successful low tech strategies for day-to-day communication. Staff are often so eager to enlist a family in the use of a voice output device that they don't stop to realize that this can be an additional stress on the family, requiring more time and energy than the family has on reserve. For staff, communication across many environments is a high priority. Parents often understand this, but cannot make it happen so easily. What seems easy at school may not be so easy at home. School objectives may not match home priorities.

As another example of this, the school team was interested in exploring power mobility for Alexander. The family indicated that they were not ready to incorporate a power wheelchair into their family life; it would require a new van with a wheelchair lift, as well as home accommodations. However, they eventually agreed to a set trial period with an electric wheelchair at school. Alexander was only somewhat successful during the trial period and a much longer trial period would have been needed to sort out the best method for Alexander to operate his wheelchair. Alexander seemed only marginally interested, the family dealt with another assistive technology strategy that did not materialize, and staff were disappointed that power mobility did not empower Alexander toward greater independence.

Alexander's progress was incremental. When I look back, it's hard to believe all that he's accomplished, and yet we still have such a long way to go. But you have to take the long view on all of the issues that pertain to you child.

At age 11, Alexander was introduced to a dynamic screen voice output device called the System 2000. By this point, his head control was much improved and his ability to stay visually focused on a task was better. Automatic row column scanning was still slow, but more accurate. Decisions regarding the type of head switch, the position of the switch, and the switch mount had reached consensus. When Alexander turned 13, his family made a big leap to purchase a DynaVox with DynaWrite for him. This was a monumental decision for this family; by this point they were understandably skeptical of the promise of technology. Use of such a device demands collaboration and cooperation from many individuals, both at home and school, to keep it operational and to make it meaningful.

For us, the AAC team has been a guide through a complicated maze. They have helped us along the "communication pathway," instructing us on AAC strategies and counseling us on which devices were best for our child.

Alexander is currently doing well with the DynaVox, which is used principally for schoolwork and homework. The auditory scan features combined with the visual scan features and the ability to limit items on a page without limiting overall vocabulary have been beneficial for Alexander. Increasing scanning speed, writing using DynaWrite with word prediction, and better use of the DynaVox to communicate socially and interactively with his peers is still a high priority. As his mother relayed, Alexander still has a long way to go. He will be transitioning to a middle school next year and by its nature, this forces the family and the school team to explore meaningful and realistic goals for the years to come. Members of the AAC team will be there to make the transition with Alexander. It is the AAC team's objective to make this transition with the family as true partners. Not as experts directing the parents, not dominating the decision-making process, but with a shared sense of ownership of the goals and objectives for Alexander and a healthy respect for the family's expressed needs and priorities.

As I look back over the years, the most significant door that opened for Alexander is communication and the ability to actively participate in the world around him. It moved him from being a passive observer to an active participant who was much more engaged in his surroundings. Over time, Alexander's sense of humor has emerged. We've gotten to know who he is through the use of his different communication systems.

KEY POINTS TO REMEMBER

- Instructing and training parents is a critical part of the AAC intervention process, but they do not represent the full spectrum of parent-school involvement. Parents also need to be included in the ongoing formulation and decision-making aspects of AAC assessment.
- The AAC assessment process is ongoing. It can take years to find the right combination of strategies — some will be immediately successful and others will not. Professionals need to help parents understand the trial and error aspects of AAC assessment, and that unsuccessful strategies are not a sign of failure, but a process of working toward what works best.
- Parental feelings of being overwhelmed are not uncommon. Different families have different "carrying capacities." Professionals need to be sensitive to this and provide support.
- Avoid overstating the promise of technology. Technology is only a tool. Degrees of success are influenced by many variables (e.g., general health and development, maturity, physical ability, staff and home commitment, the presence of environmental barriers); some can be controlled and others cannot.
- Parents need to be given opportunities to express their own needs and priorities. Parents have a right to choose which AAC strategies they will use at home. School priorities and home priorities often differ. Professionals need to respect these differences.
- AAC strategies recommended for use at home should fit into home routines without causing undue stress to the family. Professionals need to be cognizant of a family's time and energy demands.
- A variety of communication routes should be available between home and school. Regularly scheduled two-way communications keep everybody involved. Communication with families should be honest, but gentle.
- Children with multiple disabilities and complex issues need to be followed proactively on a long-term basis. Even when final "solutions" are reached and plateaus occur, the team needs to be there for the family during times of transition, such as the move to a new school or during the transition to work.
- Effective AAC takes time to develop, but it is well worth the combined efforts of the family and the AAC team.

Chapter 15

AAC IN THE
EDUCATIONAL SETTING

Sylvia Gray

A s awareness and acceptance of the field of augmentative and alternative communication (AAC) has increased, the need for public schools to provide AAC for students with severe communication disabilities has become more evident. Speech-language pathologists, educators, parents, and other professionals are becoming more informed regarding students who might benefit from AAC and the legislation that ensures the right to a "free, appropriate, public education" for students with disabilities. For many students with severe communication disabilities, the provision of AAC will be a necessary component of a "free, appropriate, public education." This chapter examines the provision of AAC services to students in public schools. Aspects of providing these services in the public schools which are addressed in this chapter include a description of the public school environment; models of AAC service delivery in a variety of school systems; assessment issues specific to schools; "best practice" implementation strategies for students; and age-specific intervention strategies.

DESCRIPTION OF THE EDUCATIONAL ENVIRONMENT

The Public School Environment

Public schools are primarily the responsibility of state and local governments. The state education agency has the primary responsibility for developing state regulations such as establishing attendance rules, determining teacher qualifications, and, in some instances, establishing curriculum standards. It is also the responsibility of the state education agency to ensure that the local education agencies are in compliance with state and federal guidelines. Within these guidelines, implementation of state and federal laws is left to the discretion of local school boards and local school district administration. Local education agencies or school districts are given some flexibility in how the district fulfills state and federal mandates and in determining curriculum.

Public schools are primarily funded by local tax dollars. Funding may also be supplemented by state and federal funds. Federal funds are provided to assist local education agencies in implementing federal programs that are mandated. Schools may receive federal money for bilingual programs, vocational programs, special education programs, and other programs such as Headstart.

Although a school district receives federal funds in order to provide special education, there is not a separate federal fund allocated specifically for the provision of AAC devices and services. Funding for AAC services and devices must be allotted from the district's overall special education budget. For example, a district might set aside a portion of the budget in order to purchase, lease, or repair AAC equipment. Special education funds may be used to purchase AAC devices that are necessary in order to implement a student's Individualized Education Plan (IEP); provide staff development for an AAC team; or, if needed, contract with an independent consultant or evaluation center to assist in providing AAC assessment. School districts may also choose to pursue other funding sources for AAC devices and services such as health insurance, grants, or charities. Chapter 9 addresses AAC funding sources in depth.

General Education and Special Education

Traditionally, schools have been organized based on student outcomes. Schools are expected to teach students basic skills such as reading, writing, math, and problem solving. Schools are expected to prepare the student for college, employment, and other life activities. There is a significant portion of the student population that experiences difficulty with academic progress and is not successful within the general education curriculum. In an effort to ensure equality of education for all students and to increase academic success,

the federal government has initiated remedial programs for students who are disadvantaged (Title I), students who have second-language backgrounds, and students with disabilities (special education). The result of this has been the creation of separate educational programs within a system. Students with disabilities are provided services through a special education program. Recently, there has been a move to reduce or eliminate separate programs and to create a unified curriculum (Gartner & Lipsky, 1987; McLaughlin & Warren, 1992; Wang, Reynolds, & Walberg, 1994).

The general education environment consists of educators who are trained in teacher preparation programs which focus on content areas (such as reading, math, science, music) and instructional methodologies designed for students who are typically developing. General education teachers are responsible for ensuring that students in the general education classroom master the curriculum objectives that have been identified by state or local guidelines. Teachers in the general education environment are often responsible for a large number of students. If a student experiences difficulty in meeting the demands of the general education curriculum, the general education teacher refers that student to programs that are designed to assist students with special needs.

The special education environment consists of educators who are trained in specialized instructional strategies for specific disability groups, such as learning disability, mental retardation, or serious emotional disturbance. The special education teacher is responsible for ensuring that students in special education master the objectives of the Individualized Education Plan (IEP). The content of the instructional program for special education is determined by the IEP committee, not by state or local guidelines. Typically, special education teachers are only responsible for students who are identified as special education students. There usually are fewer students in a special education classroom. The special education environment also consists of related services such as physical therapy, occupational therapy, or speech therapy which are designed to assist a student in benefiting from the special education program.

Least Restrictive Environment

Since the Education of All Handicapped Children Act of 1975, P.L. 94-142, federal legislation has required that students with disabilities be educated with their nondisabled peers to the maximum appropriate extent. Removal from the regular education setting should only occur when a student with a disability cannot be successful in the regular education classroom, even with supplementary aids and services. In order to implement the least restrictive environment (LRE) mandate, a continuum of alternative placement options for students with disabilities has emerged. This continuum ranges from full time placement in a general education classroom (least restrictive educational environment) to instruction provided in a homebound or hospital instructional program (most restrictive educational environment). A student's "least restrictive environment" is individually determined by the IEP or placement committee.

Inclusion

Many changes are occurring in the field of special education as researchers and educators combine knowledge regarding effective school practices and recent research about educating students with disabilities. The design of special education programs has moved progressively from segregated and separate programs toward a concept of neighborhood schools and unified school and special education curriculum. Inclusion is the manifestation of a belief and value system that embraces the philosophy of "belongingness." In the education environment this means that students with disabilities belong in classrooms with their typically developing peers so that as adults they can belong in society. Because the federal law does not define inclusion, at this time definitions vary widely (National Center on Education Restructuring and Inclusion, 1994; Rogers, 1993). Lipsky and Gartner (1995) referred to inclusion as:

> providing to all students, including those with significant disabilities, equitable opportunities to receive effective educational services, with needed supplementary aids and support services, in age-appropriate classes in their neighborhood schools, in order to prepare student for productive lives as full members of society. (p. 36)

Some inclusion models incorporate a student with disabilities into the general education classroom throughout the day, whereas other models combine this with part-day, self-contained classroom instruction. Advocates for "full inclusion" envision inclusion as all special education students being taught in general education classrooms all of the time, and encourage the dismantling of the dual systems that exist in the structure of the present delivery systems. Although some definitions refer to students being educated in their neighborhood schools, others define inclusion as simply the least restrictive environment. The definition of inclusion used by a state department of education or local education agency (LEA) often will determine how inclusion is implemented. However, a school district may indicate that it provides for inclusive education when the actual practice may be that students with disabilities are physically present in neighborhood schools, but remain in separate classrooms.

The inclusion movement has caused schools to reexamine outcomes for students with disabilities, education program design, and service delivery models. Recent case law decisions have reinforced the principles of LRE and the right of students to an inclusive education, regardless of the severity of their disability (Blackstone, 1995b). The result has been to change some of the traditional forms of special education service delivery. For example, the traditional role of the special education teacher has been to provide specialized instruction to students with disabilities in the context of a special education classroom. This role is changing to one in which the special education teacher provides training in specialized instructional techniques to general education teachers and provides support for students with disabilities in the context of the general education classroom. Also, more special education teachers are team teaching with their general education colleagues.

The impact of inclusion on general education teachers is that classroom teachers are becoming more involved with students with disabilities and becoming more responsible for the education of those students. Placement of students with severe disabilities in general education classrooms is becoming more common. As a result of the inclusion movement, there is increased collaboration among special education and general education personnel. Additionally, there is more sharing of expertise and resources between general and special education.

The inclusion movement also impacts programs for students with AAC needs and their service providers. The implications for these students are that these students are more likely to be included in general education environments; and the speech-language pathologist or augmentative communication specialist will need to provide classroom support for the student, his or her peers, and general education teacher with regard to the student's augmentative communication system.

ORGANIZATIONAL STRUCTURES AND CONSTRAINTS

There is considerable variation in the organizational structures for delivering AAC services. Factors that influence the design of service delivery systems include the philosophy of the state education agency, geographical boundaries, and demographics. This section examines three different public school service delivery models that are representative of the major types of delivery systems, including a regional rural model, a metropolitan model, and a statewide model. The discussion then turns to some of the constraints to AAC delivery that cut across these models.

Service Delivery Models

Regional Rural Model

In 1988, the Texas Education Agency began providing funding to 20 regional education service centers (ESC) in order to assist public schools in providing assistive technology devices and services for students with disabilities. The provision of AAC services in public schools is supported through this program. The ESCs provide (a) technical assistance; (b) training in the assistive technology services components of the Individuals with Disabilities Education Act (IDEA, the amended version of the Education for All Handicapped Children Act of 1975); (c) training for school district personnel, students, and families; (d) access to an equipment loan bank; (e) assistance in the development of networks for interagency coordination; and (f) assistance in program evaluation to school districts located within their geographical boundaries. The AAC service delivery model of one of the rural ESCs is described here. This education service center is located in the west Texas area and provides services to 33 school districts located within a geographical area approximately the size of the state of Indiana. The school districts range in size from an average daily attendance of 28 to 24,000. Some of the school districts are located in remote areas.

Rural school districts often face challenges in providing AAC services due to a lack of related service personnel, a lack of financial resources, and a lack of access to training and evaluation centers. At the regional level, the ESC has attempted to address these challenges by providing training for school district personnel, on-site technical assistance, and an equipment loan library. First, the ESC has been able to provide ongoing AAC training opportunities at the regional level. For school districts in this area, this means that training opportunities are available within a 2 to 3 hour drive as opposed to a 6 to 8 hour drive. Furthermore, the ESC is able to provide on-site consultation with school staff when requested. This assists districts in accessing the needed expertise (AAC, physical therapy, or occupational therapy) when that expertise is not available locally. Finally, schools have access to a short-term equipment loan program. This allows school districts the opportunity to assess or have a trial period with a device without incurring the expense of purchasing or leasing the device. Once a team has completed the assessment process or has recommended a specific device, the school district is responsible for obtaining the device for that student.

In an effort to address the provision of AAC services at the local level, school districts in the rural west Texas area have established local AAC teams. School districts identify a core team which is given the responsibility of becoming knowledgeable regarding the field of AAC. This team usually consists of a special educator, a speech-language pathologist, and an assessment specialist. Typically, the team will not have direct access to the services of an augmentative communication spe-

cialist; thus, it is critical for the local district team to develop expertise in the area of AAC.

Once the team is identified, training becomes an ongoing process. The team participates in a training program that is provided by the ESC and is designed to increase knowledge and competencies related to the field of AAC. The training consists of two levels. Level I consists of a 30 hour (6 day) training program. The outcomes of Level I training are to develop a transdisciplinary team to serve as a resource for the district; to increase knowledge and competencies regarding the law, AAC assessment strategies, AAC systems (low tech and high tech), positioning issues, and intervention strategies; and to develop a team approach for the AAC assessment process. All Level I team members are required to attend all Level I training sessions and to participate in a guided student assessment.

Level II training allows the teams to target individual team or district needs, and to focus on the development of AAC competencies. Each Level II team develops a team action plan which focuses on the implementation of AAC services for its district. This action plan may identify structure needs or skill needs. For example, a team may identify a structure need such as the lack of district policy regarding AAC, and target that need in the action plan. The team may also identify a skill need such as the need to learn AAC assessment strategies for students with severe/profound disabilities. The training design for Level II teams is customized for each district.

Administrative support at the local district level is critical to the success of this service delivery method. An administrator should be responsible for overseeing the AAC team. For small districts, this administrator will usually be the special education director. In order for this service delivery method to be effective, the administrator must support ongoing training opportunities for the team, and provide opportunities for the team to meet and function as a team. The administrator should see that policy and procedures related to the provision of AAC services are established. The administrator should also be willing to reduce responsibilities in other areas so that appropriate time can be devoted to AAC tasks.

One advantage of small, rural districts is that the AAC population will also be small. According to Blackstone (1990c), demographic studies of the school age population indicate that approximately 0.4% of the school age population will be nonspeaking or require AAC services. For some districts, this may mean a total of one to three students. So the "good news" is that the team will be able to concentrate their efforts on those few students. One disadvantage of this service delivery method is that the team will also have other responsibilities in addition to functioning as the AAC resource team. In addition, they will lack the depth and breadth of experience that professionals who encounter a large number of students who are nonspeaking acquire.

Metropolitan Model

In the state of Maryland, there is no centralized system for the delivery of augmentative communication services. Services are determined on a county-by-county basis. Montgomery County Public Schools is located in an affluent urban area within an hour's distance of Washington D. C. and Baltimore, Maryland. This school district has a total student population of approximately 117,000 and a special education population of approximately 14,000. Montgomery County has a team of professionals identified to provide assistive technology and augmentative communication services to students in their county.

Although a separate department of assistive technology or augmentative communication has not been established, the departments of physical therapy, occupational therapy, and speech-language pathology designate staff and monies from their budgets in order to provide this service. The team consists of three full-time speech-language pathologists, a full-time special educator, a part-time occupational therapist, and a part-time administrator. The team has developed a mission statement and has established operational procedures. In addition, the team has developed a "small-but-growing" bank of equipment to use for diagnostic and short-term trial purposes.

The need to provide a high tech communication system is determined on a case-by-case basis. If a recommendation is made for a long-term high tech communication system, the school district provides a low tech system and/or the loan of the best available high tech device until funding can be obtained for the purchase of a personal device. Funding options that are pursued by the team and family include Medicaid, private insurance, and community groups or service organizations.

In order to increase the knowledge base regarding AAC and to increase services for students, the team began to devote much more of its time to the training of staff at a system-wide level. The team implemented a trainer-of-trainers model, so that staff could go back and train other staff members. This model has proved to be a successful way to jump start knowledge of assistive technology and AAC. Initially, 25 staff members were targeted for the training. This group was selected based on their leadership qualities and ability to replicate the training for peers. Training was targeted 3 days prior to the beginning of school and also occurred periodically throughout the year. This approach was replicated the following year with a new group. As a result of 2 years of training, a core group of staff members is more knowledgeable regarding AAC and serves as resources across a large number of schools. In the third year, the team shifted to an open enrollment training model. Workshops open to all are scheduled across the school year. Brochures describing the workshops and registration forms are sent to a growing database of staff who are using assistive technology. Topics for workshops are selected based upon the results of a yearly staff survey. In the public school setting, the reality is that it is often the teacher assistants who are responsible for the day-to-day maintenance of communication systems and implementation of AAC intervention. Therefore, training efforts are also targeted to paraprofessional staff.

Montgomery County Public Schools permits professional leave for the AAC team. Local resources available to help support the Montgomery County team include the Center for Technology in Education and the Maryland Technology Assistance Program. The Center for Technology in Education is a partnership of the Maryland State Department of Education and the Johns Hopkins University. The center is partially funded by federal funds and grant monies. The Center for Technology in Education is located in the Baltimore area and provides professional training opportunities in the areas of assistive technology, augmentative communication, and instructional technology. The Maryland Assistive Technology Partnership is also located in Baltimore and provides information and training in the areas of assistive technology including augmentative communication. Another source of support is through the Maryland Augmentative Communication Association (MACA). This organization sponsors an annual AAC conference and technology fair and provides opportunities to network informally with other AAC professionals in the state.

Statewide Model

The state of Pennsylvania has a well-developed system for the delivery of augmentative communication services to public school students (ages 3 through 21). In 1984, the Pennsylvania Department of Education used federal funds to establish the Pennsylvania Assistive Technology Center (PATC). One of the center's functions was to assist public schools in the delivery of augmentative communication services. Components of this program include an equipment loan program, training for local augmentative specialists, and information dissemination. The PATC is now known as PennTech.

The PennTech equipment loan program provides for short-term equipment loans, long-term equipment loans, and maintenance of an equipment exchange program. The short-term equipment loan program provides device loans for a 4 week period. This equipment is provided for the purpose of student evaluation and trial intervention. The long-term loan component provides equipment that is assigned to a specific student for the duration of the student's educational program. Recently established agreements between the Pennsylvania Department of Education and the Medical Assistance Program in Pennsylvania have enabled PennTech to provide equipment for students who are exiting the educational program. If students are eligible for the Medical Assistance program, this agreement allows PennTech to bill the Medical Assistance program for reimbursement of the device. If approved, the ownership of the device is transferred to the student. The third component of the program is the equipment exchange component. Equipment may be returned to the program if a device is no longer appropriate for a student or the student leaves the educational system. This equipment is then upgraded and redistributed to other students.

PennTech concentrates training efforts on the development of local Assistive Technology Statewide Support Initiative (ATSSI) Specialists. Early on, PennTech realized that the development of local district expertise was a critical component of effective service delivery. The local directors of special education identify staff members who are then trained to serve as the district's ATSSI specialists. Training is provided for the ATSSI specialists in the form of workshops and on-site technical assistance. In addition, PennTech has developed videotaped training materials. Training and services provided by the PennTech program are free of charge to all state residents.

Information dissemination is accomplished through the distribution of Factsheets. Additional support is provided through the maintenance of toll-free hotlines. Services of PennTech have expanded to include the early intervention and transition age population. The PennTech Program is recognized nationally as a model program.

Service Delivery Constraints

Irrespective of the service delivery model, providing AAC services to students in public schools presents common challenges. Many issues exist in the implementation of AAC services in the educational environment, including logistical, financial, attitudinal, and knowledge barriers.

Logistical Barriers

Logistical barriers such as time and staff constraints are realities that must be addressed by the school. The provision of AAC services is a time-consuming process. Time is needed in order to assess the AAC needs of students, to design and create communication systems for students, and to provide AAC training and intervention. Learning to program various communication devices can also be a very time-consum-

ing process. The time-intensive nature of providing AAC services should be taken into consideration when assigning caseloads. For larger school districts, an augmentative communication specialist may be designated and available for help. For small school districts, an augmentative communication specialist may not be available.

Financial Barriers

The cost of providing AAC devices and services is often an issue. High tech communication systems are expensive. As discussed later in this chapter, the recommendation of a communication system cannot be based on cost. Instead, an AAC system recommendation must be based on student need. School districts are not obligated to fund "state of the art" AAC systems if that communication system is not appropriate for the student. School districts are obligated to provide an AAC system that is appropriate for the student. In funding AAC systems, school districts can use special education funds or pursue other funding sources such as Medicaid, private insurance companies, local service clubs, or vocational rehabilitation programs. Readers should refer to Chapter 9 for more information about funding.

Attitudinal Barriers

Attitudes of communication partners and others regarding AAC impact the use of the system by the student. If family members and communication partners are supportive and express positive attitudes, then the likelihood of the student's use of AAC will be increased. However, if their attitudes are negative and AAC is not valued, then the frequency of use will probably decrease (Silverman, 1989).

Knowledge Barriers

Lack of knowledge regarding AAC can create an implementation barrier. To provide

AAC services (e.g., evaluation, training, intervention), professionals need to be knowledgeable of AAC assessment strategies, AAC communication systems, and intervention strategies. In order to support a high tech communication system, the school staff will need to be able to program and troubleshoot the system and train others in its use. Most professionals receive little or no training in AAC as part of their preservice program. In addition, many universities do not offer courses in AAC. Most professionals will need to rely on training opportunities such as conferences or workshops in order to increase their knowledge regarding AAC. Schools located in metropolitan areas will have more access to these types of AAC training opportunities. Additional resources for accessing AAC information include professional materials such as AAC journals, AAC books, and videotapes that have been developed for AAC training purposes. The identification of a statewide or regional network of AAC service providers can also be an invaluable source of information and support to families and professionals. Several states have established chapters of the United States Society for Augmentative and Alternative Communication (USSAAC). The benefits of membership to a chapter of USSAAC usually include a newsletter, training opportunities, and a membership directory.

THE TEAM ASSESSMENT PROCESS

Chapters 5, 6, and 7 provide an extensive discussion of AAC assessment strategies and the assessment process. The following section highlights some of the significant aspects of assessment strategies and processes that are unique to the school environment.

The goal of the AAC team is to conduct an assessment in order to recommend an AAC system that can meet the immediate communication needs of the student and to develop intervention strategies to facilitate the student's progress toward the use of an appropriate AAC system in various school environments. The assessment will be informal as there are no standardized assessments for this purpose. The AAC team will need to have knowledge not only of assessment strategies for communication system recommendations, but also assessment strategies that facilitate the integration of the system into school, home, community, and work environments. The assessment should be conducted at the school so that the student will be in a familiar environment. At minimum, the student's parent, teacher, related service providers, and speech-language pathologist will be expected to participate. The assessment may occur as a single event, or may occur over a period of time depending on the number of team members involved.

The need for school districts to have an identified process for providing AAC services is essential. New regulations regarding assistive technology are addressed in IDEA. Therefore, it is recommended that each school district have an AAC team identified and policy and procedures in place. School administrators should take a proactive role in the development of policy and procedures regarding AAC. Specifically, policy and procedures should address the district's provision of AAC devices and services as defined by IDEA. Policy and procedures provide assurance that services are delivered in an equitable and systematic manner, and that the presumptive denial of services has not occurred.

AAC Teams in School Settings

Many factors influence the provision of AAC services in school settings. In addition to communication needs, students requiring AAC services may also have positioning, mobility, access, and vision or hearing issues. As a result, it is not possible for one person to have all the knowledge and information needed to provide AAC services. School districts are encouraged to identify an AAC resource team and to utilize a team approach in the provision of AAC services to students. The synergy of the team in terms of knowledge and experience will ensure more appropriate recommendations and services for students with AAC needs. In addition to the student and family members, the school AAC team should comprise professionals from a variety of disciplines, including a speech-language pathologist, a special educator, a general educator, an augmentative communication specialist, an assistive technology specialist, a physical therapist, an occupational therapist, an assessment specialist, and a vision specialist, among others.

It is highly recommended that the function of the team be based on the concept of the "fluid team" model. This model advocates that the members of the AAC team are determined by the individual needs of the student. Thus, all team members do not have to be involved in every evaluation or decision but are available if needed. In the educational environment, the primary team members will typically include the teacher, the special educator, the speech-language pathologist, the augmentative communication or assistive technology specialist, and teacher assistants, as well as the student and family members. Depending on the student's needs, the physical and occupational therapists may be included as primary team members or supportive team members. The assessment specialist, vision specialist, and audiologist may function as supportive team members, working with the primary team members for those students requiring their services. Finally, one team member should be designated as the coordinator. This will ensure that procedures are followed and that someone is ultimately responsible for all aspects of AAC service delivery.

Once AAC team members have been identified, training should be provided in all aspects of AAC service delivery. It is also important that the roles of the various team members be defined. Roles have been defined for the speech-language pathologist, physical therapist, and occupational therapist providing AAC services; however, the roles of the other team members, including the role of the teacher, need additional delineation (American Speech-Language-Hearing Association, 1989; Locke & Mirenda, 1992; Reed & Bowser, 1991).

School System Assessment Models

The delivery methods of AAC assessment services may vary among school districts. Service delivery options may include (a) a team specifically dedicated to providing AAC services, (b) professionals identified as having AAC expertise who are contacted when needed, (c) contract services using AAC consultants, or (d) contract services with an evaluation center. Large school districts may have AAC teams dedicated to the provision of AAC assessment services. Small school districts may call upon the services of identified professionals from within the school system or the school itself who have AAC expertise. This team may function only when there is a need to provide an AAC assessment. When assessment services are provided by persons from within the school, there is the advantage that the team will be familiar with the student and will be available to monitor student progress and support the use of the system in the school and home environments. The weakness of this method is balancing AAC assessment responsibilities against other professional responsibilities.

Some districts may not have a team identified. In these instances, the district either needs to contract with consultants to provide this service on-site or to contract with an evaluation center to provide the AAC assessment. The benefits of the on-site consultant model are that the local district staff can be involved in the assessment process. This gives the evaluators the opportunity to assess the student in natural environments and to assess opportunity barriers. The weakness of this method is that, once the assessment is completed, the team is not available to provide ongoing support to the local school district staff.

If a district must contract with an evaluation center to provide AAC assessment, the student may be taken to the evaluation site for this service. The strength of this type of assessment method is that the team is very skilled and the evaluation is very thorough. There are several weaknesses associated with this method. When the evaluation occurs at the evaluation site, the local district staff may not be involved in the assessment process and the evaluation does not occur in the student's customary environment. In addition, opportunity barriers are difficult to assess. Furthermore, the evaluation occurs usually as a one-time event, and the local district staff may lack the ability or commitment to implement the recommendations of the evaluation.

Familiarity with a variety of assessment models will be helpful. The Pennsylvania Assistive Device Center assessment model (Haney & Kangas, 1987), the Developmental Levels Assessment Model (Larson & Woodfin, 1989), the Augmentative Communication Skills Inventory (discussed in Chapter 5), and Every Move Counts (Korsten, Dunn, Foss, & Francke, 1993) are models that the team may find helpful in devising assessment strategies.

Referral

The AAC assessment process typically begins with a referral. The referral process should be clearly explained and disseminated to all school administrators, general and special educators, and parents. Any student with special needs who has an IEP or who has been referred to special education may be referred to the AAC team for an assessment. Also, AAC needs should be considered routinely as part of the process of initial referral to determine eligibility for special education. If any deficits are noted in the area of communication, this may be an indication that AAC assessment may need to be pursued at this point. Or, a referral for an AAC assessment may occur as part of a comprehensive individual assessment or may be recommended by the IEP committee at an annual review of the student's IEP. Figure 15–1 presents a sample referral form.

A referral form should be completed and sent to the identified AAC team coordinator in order to initiate the assessment process. The referral form should assist in focusing the direction of the assessment process by clearly stating the reason for the referral. Also, concerns related to IEP issues need to be addressed in the referral. A brief description of the cognitive, communication, and physical abilities of the student will be helpful in establishing the direction of the assessment process. Vision or hearing deficits as well as behavioral issues should be described. This information will assist the AAC coordinator in determining which team members will need to participate in the assessment, appropriate assessment strategies, and what equipment will be needed to conduct the assessment.

After the AAC coordinator has received the referral, the AAC coordinator will be responsible for organizing the details of the actual assessment. The coordinator will ensure that the necessary school permission forms are obtained and that notifications of assessment have been sent. The coordinator will compile background information, the current IEP, related service reports, vision and hearing reports, and speech-language reports. The coordinator then disseminates this information to appropriate team members.

REFERRAL FOR AUGMENTATIVE COMMUNICATION CONSULTATION

Student Name:	Date of Birth: ID#
School/Program: Grade:	Parents' Names:
School Phone: Best Times to Call:	Address:
Teacher:	
Speech Language Pathologist:	Home Phone: Best Times to Call:
OT: PT:	Parents' Work Phone:
Person completing form:	Date:

GENERAL INFORMATION:

Reason for referral:

Primary language spoken in home:

Significant medical information and diagnoses:

Status of hearing and vision:

EDUCATIONAL INFORMATION:

Learning situations and techniques that motivate the student:

Student's learning style:

Behaviors which interfere with learning:

Recent psychological information:

Figure 15–1. AAC referral form (Montgomery County Public Schools, Rockville, MD 20850).

MOTOR SKILLS:

Does the student walk independently?

Does the student have good seating/wheelchair positioning? Describe:

Describe gross and fine motor strengths and limitations:

Head control: Arm and hand control:

Can the student point? No ____ Yes ____ Accuracy maintained on what size symbols? _____

Can this student discriminate : Objects? _____   Photographs? _____
                                Black/white drawings? _____   Letters/numbers? _____

COMMUNICATION SKILLS:

Describe current means of communication and give examples:

At school

At home

If verbal, what is the student's percentage of intelligibility

To familiar listeners?

To unfamiliar listeners?

What augmentative methods have been attempted and with what results?

Can the student read? No _____   Yes _____   Grade Level _____

Can the student independently spell?   No ____   Yes ____

                                Words ____   Phrases/Sentences ____

SOCIAL/BEHAVIORAL INFORMATION:

Describe peer interaction:

Describe interaction with adults:

Figure 15-1. *(continued)*

Prior to actual assessment, the school team may meet to determine the disciplines that need to take part in the assessment, and to plan the assessment strategies. Assessment strategies may include a review of the student's records, school staff interview, parent interview, observation of the student in natural environments, and individual assessment. Positioning issues may need to be addressed first in order to ensure appropriate assessment in other areas, and to determine the most appropriate access method for a student. For instance, proper positioning may increase range of motion in upper extremities or improve head control for an individual. Again, these issues, as well as other aspects of the assessment process, are discussed in detail in earlier chapters.

IMPLEMENTATION AND INTEGRATION

AAC in the IEP

Once the initial assessment has been completed, and the team has identified the AAC needs of the student, agreement on skills to target in the IEP must be reached. The team should meet prior to the actual IEP meeting in order to negotiate priority areas. It is important that team members reach consensus on which AAC skills will be targeted for instruction in the IEP. The AAC goals developed by the team must be submitted to and approved by the IEP committee prior to implementation. AAC devices and services must be addressed in the student's IEP as special education, supplementary aids and services, or as a related service. An example of an AAC goal addressed in an IEP is as follows: "During the classroom circle time activity, Susan will use her AAC system to make choices, greet classmates, and respond to questions in 7 of 10 trials."

AAC Action Plans

Once the team has determined which AAC skills will be targeted in the IEP, an action plan for implementing the recommendations should be completed. According to Blackstone (1995a), action plans are consensus-building tools and provide a measure of accountability. This plan should include suggestions for integrating AAC into functional and instructional activities. A sample action plan is presented in Figure 15–2. The AAC team will assist in acquiring the recommended communication system and in providing the necessary training to the classroom staff in order to implement the action plan.

AAC Curriculum Integration Plans

After the AAC skills are targeted, a curriculum integration plan should be developed. This plan reflects the synthesis of each discipline's goal into the context of meaningful activities. Blackstone (1995a) referred to this participation plan as the team's map of daily activities. The team should strive to develop plans that facilitate the development of functional communication skills, not just address the operational use of the device. The team should target the communication opportunities that occur in the student's natural environment for AAC instruction. In this way, the student will learn not only how to use the device but also how to communicate. For example, the team may target the appropriate initiation of and response to greetings as opportunities for device instruction. The result would be that opportunities to practice this goal would be integrated into the student's morning routines. If a goal is to increase the student's ability to ask questions using his or her device, then this skill could be targeted during a science activity or during a discussion about a new book.

AAC ACTION PLAN

STUDENT: Jane Smith

SCHOOL: LBJ Elementary

DATE: 3/3/96

AGE: 5

AAC TEAM MEMBERS: Sherry Smith, Augmentative Communication Specialist; Shelley Brown, Speech/Language Pathologist; Jane Nelson, Special Education; Sally Black, Kindergarten Teacher; and Cynthia Branham, Teacher Assistant.

PURPOSE: Jane will be transitioning into a regular kindergarten classroom in the fall. This Action Plan is designed to facilitate her transition into the regular kindergarten environment.

RECOMMENDATIONS:	PERSON(S) RESPONSIBLE:	BEGINNING DATE
1. Training will be provided to the kindergarten teacher in the use and maintenance of Jane's AAC device.	Sherry Smith, AAC Specialist	August, 1996
2. Vocabulary needs for the kindergarten environment will be identified.	Shelley Brown, SLP Sally Black, Kindergarten Teacher	May, 1996
3. Overlays will be developed for the kindergarten classroom.	Shelley Brown, SLP Cynthia Branham, Teacher Asst	August, 1996
4. Three classroom activities will be "engineered" for Jane.	Shelley Brown, SLP Jane Nelson, Special Education Sally Black, Kindergarten Teacher Cynthia Branham, Teacher Asst	August, 1996
5. The kindergarten staff will be trained in Aided Language Stimulation techniques. These techniques will be applied across the three engineered classroom activities.	Shelley Brown, SLP Jane Nelson, Special Education Sally Black, Kindergarten Teacher Cynthia Branham, Teacher Asst	August, 1996

Figure 15–2. A sample AAC action plan addressing the transition of a student from a preschool program to a kindergarten classroom.

Figure 15–3 provides a format for outlining the integration of AAC into the student's educational day. It links classroom activities with AAC objectives, delineates high tech as well as low tech AAC systems, and specifies the degree of support that is needed to assist the student with the task. It also identifies staff responsible for supervising, as well as implementing the AAC objectives within the curriculum. Although teaching assistants skillfully carry out educational activities and AAC strategies with students, it is ultimately professional staff who must assume responsibility for the AAC objectives and make sure that these objectives are being appropriately addressed. All too often, instructional assistants shoulder too much of this. The format of the curriculum integration plan provides a mechanism for ensuring ample communication opportunities tied to specific AAC goals.

AAC as Supplementary Aids and Services

A supplementary aid or service refers to instances when equipment, such as an AAC device or service, such as an AAC consultation, facilitates placement of a student in a general education setting, whereas the removal of that AAC device or service would result in the student being served in a more restrictive setting. For example, if a student can participate in group discussions and answer teacher questions with a voice output communication system, but without the system the student has no means of expression and cannot participate in the classroom discussions, then AAC can be addressed as supplementary aids or services.

AAC and Related Services

Federal legislation defines related services as those that may be required to assist a child with a disability to benefit from special education. Thirteen services are identified as related services in IDEA; however, the law states that this list is not exhaustive. These services are audiology, occupational therapy, physical therapy, psychological services, medical services for diagnostic or evaluation purposes only, school health services, transportation services, counseling services, speech-language pathology, social work services, parent counseling and training, recreation therapy, and early identification and assessment of disabilities in children. In order for a student to use an AAC system efficiently, training will be needed. This training may be addressed as a related service. Related services must specify the annual goal, amount of time, and the service provider.

Related services traditionally have been provided as "pull-out" services; however, this service delivery model is changing to one in which related services are being provided in the classroom. The related service providers identify the classroom activities in which the related service goal can be integrated. The related service goal is then targeted in the context of that activity. For example, an AAC goal such as increasing the speed and accuracy of row column scanning could be addressed in an art activity. The student would participate in an art activity with peers by using an AAC system to provide directions to a partner and to make choices (color, shape, texture) in order to complete an art activity. A speech-language pathologist or an occupational therapist might be identified as the service provider and target this time for providing AAC intervention as a related service.

To the maximum extent possible, AAC goals and objectives should be integrated into the student's daily routine and general education classroom. When AAC intervention is provided using an integrated service delivery model, the results are that students are more likely to use their AAC systems in an interactive manner and across communication environments.

AAC Curriculum Integration Plan

Student: _____ School: _____ Date: _____

Date: _____

Activity or Class	AAC Objective	Student's Task	Low Tech Strategies	High Tech Strategies	Level of Support I/IS/V/P	Supervising Staff	Implementing Staff

I = Independent; IS = Independent with set up assistance; V = Verbal prompts; P = Physical assistance

Figure 15-3. AAC curriculum integration plan.

Follow-up Services

The recommendation of a communication system and the acceptance of an action plan and curriculum integration plan do not mean the end of AAC assessment or intervention. Instead, it signals the beginning of the follow-up component of AAC services. AAC team members should provide follow-up support to the classroom staff through routine visits to the classroom. Ongoing assessment that results in modifications to a student's action plan when needed is critical to the student's successful use and integration of a communication system in all environments.

Observation of the student's use of the communication system in the natural environment (classroom, home, community, or work) and with natural communication partners will provide the team with information to determine when modifications in the system or the action plan are needed, and when to integrate the communication system into new activities and environments. Issues that usually need to be addressed in this phase of service delivery include: solving technical problems with the communication system; updating vocabulary to meet the needs of new communication environments; training new communication partners; monitoring changes in student abilities that would necessitate a change in the communication system; and evaluating the effect of the communication system on the communicative competence of the student.

IMPLEMENTATION STRATEGIES

Best Practices

AAC services in public schools should be designed and delivered in a manner consistent with identified best practices for educational programs and AAC service delivery. A summary of these best practices appears in Table 15–1. This section will discuss the application of these best practices in the context of providing AAC instruction in the public school setting.

Emphasis on Functional Outcomes

There is strong support for the implementation of a functional curriculum model in educational programs for secondary students with severe disabilities (Brown et al., 1979; Falvey, 1989). A functional curriculum model emphasizes the acquisition of skills that will increase a student's independence in a variety of environments such as home, school, community, and work. Ecological inventory strategies and discrepancy analysis procedures are utilized as tools to determine the content of the instructional program. The ecological inventory strategy is used to identify environments and activities in which the student is expected to participate. The discrepancy analysis procedure is used to identify where discrepancies in student performance occur in relation to the activity. The use of these tools helps target instructional goals that are of value now and in the future, that are age-appropriate, and that increase social interaction opportunities.

Students with severe disabilities often require AAC devices and services in order to attain communicative competence. Because the use of a functional curriculum model is recognized as a best practice in educational program design for students with severe disabilities, the use of this model should be applied in the design of AAC instruction for this population of students. The use of this model can help ensure that functional communication goals are emphasized in AAC instruction. Blackstone (1990b) identified the teaching of functional communication goals as a characteristic associated with exemplary preschool programs. In addition, the teaching

Table 15-1. Best practice indicators for AAC instruction.

Indicator	Reference
1. Emphasis on functional outcomes	Blackstone, 1990a; 1990b Calculator & Jorgensen, 1991
2. Emphasis on chronological age appropriateness	Blackstone, 1990b
3. Emphasis on instruction in natural settings	Blackstone, 1990a, 1990b, 1990c Calculator & Jorgensen, 1991
4. Emphasis on teaching communication as an embedded skill	Blackstone, 1990b Calculator & Jorgensen, 1991
5. Emphasis on training communication partners	Blackstone, 1990b Calculator & Jorgensen, 1991
6. Emphasis on a collaborative approach to service delivery	Blackstone, 1990c Calculator & Jorgensen, 1991
7. Emphasis on integrated programming	Blackstone, 1990a Calculator & Jorgensen, 1991
8. Emphasis on student evaluation	Calculator & Jorgensen, 1991

Source: Compiled from Blackstone (1990a, 1990b, 1990c) and Calculator and Jorgensen (1991).

of functional skills was recognized as a best practice for AAC intervention with adults who have severe developmental disabilities (Blackstone, 1990a).

According to Blackstone (1990a), demographic studies indicate that 75% of the school age population who could benefit from AAC will have mental retardation. The functional communication outcomes for AAC intervention in public schools should be to improve the student's ability to meet everyday communication needs and to increase communication independence in a variety of natural settings. The importance of addressing functional communication skills for students with severe disabilities cannot be overemphasized. The acquisition of functional communication skills facilitates access to a wider variety of environments. The lack of functional communication skills contributes to placement in more restrictive environments. Calculator and Jorgensen (1991) stressed that AAC services that target functional,

educationally relevant outcomes are a necessary component for enhancing the ability to include students with AAC needs in general education classrooms.

Emphasis on Chronological Age Appropriateness

The importance of using chronologically age appropriate activities and materials has been established as a best practice in the educational program design for students with severe disabilities (Brown et al., 1979; Falvey, 1989). It is important that AAC plans utilize activities and materials that are chronologically age appropriate as well (Blackstone, 1990a). The risks of utilizing materials and activities that are not chronologically age appropriate will be discussed next.

One risk of using activities and materials that are not chronologically age appropriate in AAC instruction is that the student may not be motivated to participate in the activity. A second risk is that inappropriate materials and activities may not provide opportunities for social interaction with age appropriate peers in an inclusive environment. AAC instruction should center around activities in which same age, typically developing peers participate. A third risk is that the use of inappropriate materials and activities can negatively impact the perceptions and expectations of the typically developing peers. The use of age appropriate materials and activities may help avoid further stigmatization and may improve perceptions regarding the student's competency.

Emphasis on Instruction in Natural Settings

The location of where instruction occurs is a critical component in the educational program design for students with severe disabilities (Brown et al., 1979; Falvey, 1989). One of the learning characteristics of students with severe disabilities is the lack of or difficulty in generalizing learned skills. Therefore, the use of isolated AAC therapy models in which students are "pulled out" of natural settings is not recommended. Blackstone (1990c) identified "pull out" therapy as a practice that was "not working" relative to AAC intervention. Students may acquire communication skills in a one-to-one, isolated intervention model; however, these skills may not generalize to other communication partners or to other environments. Therefore, it is recommended that communication skills be taught in the context of natural routines, in natural environments, with natural stimuli (Calculator & Jorgensen, 1991).

For example, a student in a preschool program can receive AAC instruction during circle time, snack time, independent play time, and during self-care routines. Another student in a general education elementary classroom might receive AAC instruction during language arts. This student can learn to use her AAC system to retell a story. Responsibilities for AAC instruction in these situations would be shared among the teacher, instructional assistant, and speech-language pathologist. A third student, who is receiving community-based instruction, receives AAC instruction at his work site. In this setting, the job coach and the speech-language pathologist would share the responsibility for his AAC instruction.

Emphasis on Teaching Communication as an Embedded Skill

In the past, instructional programs were often designed to teach isolated skills at discrete times (e.g., 9:00–9:30 Motor Skills; 9:30–10:00 Communication Skills). For students with severe disabilities, this type of program design did not result in the desired outcomes. Often, the students could master the acquisition of the skill but could not demonstrate functional use of the skill in the context of naturally occurring activities.

For students with severe disabilities to demonstrate communication skills that are functional, AAC instruction should occur throughout the day in naturally occurring activities as opposed to being relegated to specific times. According to Van Dijk (1967), language is embedded in all activities and communication skills should not be taught in isolation of other developmental areas. Teaching AAC goals that are embedded in the student's daily activities and routines with natural communication partners is recognized as a best practice for AAC intervention (Blackstone, 1990a; Calculator & Jorgensen, 1991).

For example, if the AAC goal is for the student to indicate a preference when presented a two-item choice, then this skill would be targeted for instruction throughout the day. The student's daily activities would be analyzed to identify the natural opportunities where choice-making could occur. The school staff would share the responsibility for AAC instruction. Choice-making opportunities might be provided by the music teacher during music, the speech-language pathologist during snack time, the classroom teacher during circle time, the teacher assistant during lunch, and classroom peers during cooperative learning activities. In this way, the student will have opportunities to practice this skill throughout the day and with different communication partners.

Emphasis on Training Communication Partners

AAC instruction should not be considered the responsibility of only one person. Any communication partner should be considered an instructor (Calculator & Jorgensen, 1991). This will enable the student to have more communication opportunities and to increase the likelihood of skill generalization. In the school setting, possible communication partners include the classroom teacher, the special education teacher, the classmates, the teacher assistant, the bus driver, the speech-language pathologist, and any other school staff member the student might encounter on a routine basis.

Blackstone (1990a) identified the involvement and training of natural communication partners as a best practice in AAC intervention. All communication partners should be trained to provide communication opportunities for a student, to recognize a student's communication signals, and to implement AAC instruction. Training for these communication partners might occur informally by modeling appropriate interactions with the student. More formal training may be required in order to address the operational maintenance of the AAC system. This training could occur as an inservice to school staff prior to the beginning of school. Training may also be provided in the form of classroom consultation visits. In addition, training will need to be provided for the communication partners in other environments (e.g., home, community, and work).

Emphasis on a Collaborative Approach to Service Delivery

Educational goals, including AAC goals, should be determined by a team that is composed of professional staff, parents, and the student. Blackstone (1990c) identified the use of a team approach in AAC intervention as a practice which "works" and the lack of a team approach as a practice which is "not working." Instructional priorities should be determined by team consensus and not by each discipline in isolation. Calculator and Jorgensen (1991) recognized the use of a collaborative model to establish educational goals as a best practice for integrating AAC instruction into the general education classroom.

Classroom staff are often the team members who can identify the communication needs of the student in regard to classroom participation. The parents are the team members who can identify the communication needs of the student in the home and community environments. The student will also have preferences that will need to be considered. Team meetings should be scheduled at a time that permits teacher participation. Parents may also be able to participate in team meetings if their schedule permits. If not, parental input can be obtained through phone interviews, home visits, or meetings at a mutually determined location (restaurant or library).

Parents have definite opinions regarding communication goals for their children. For example, during a team meeting a parent identified a communication need for her child in the home and community environments. In the home environment, the parent expressed a desire for the child to be able to express discomfort and to indicate the source of discomfort (feeding tube, leg braces, or asthma). In the community environment, the parent wanted the student to be able to use her AAC system to interact with members of her church. This information was incorporated into the decision-making process and AAC goals were developed to address the areas that were important to the parent.

Emphasis on Integrated Programming

Collaborative decision making should result in an integrated instructional program. In designing an integrated program, the first step is to identify the activities that are being targeted for instruction. Next, the activities are analyzed to identify the most appropriate opportunities to integrate the AAC goals. The result is a program in which AAC goals are targeted for instruction within the context of naturally occurring activities and not taught as isolated skills. Blackstone (1990b) recognized the integration of AAC goals into existing activities as a characteristic associated with exemplary preschool programs. Calculator and Jorgensen (1991) identified the use of an integrated therapy model as a means to promote AAC instruction in a general education environment.

Emphasis on Student Evaluation

In order to determine the success of AAC instruction, routine student evaluations are necessary. Students in public schools who are eligible for special education and use AAC have an IEP in which AAC goals are addressed. This IEP is reviewed at least once annually. During this annual IEP review, the student's progress on the IEP goals is reviewed and new goals are established. Every 3 years the student must receive a comprehensive assessment in order to reestablish eligibility for special education services. Although the annual and triennial evaluations are required by law, AAC evaluations should be ongoing. It is only by monitoring student performance that the effectiveness of AAC instruction can be monitored. If a student is not making progress in achieving AAC goals, then AAC instruction will need to be changed.

If the goal of AAC instruction is to promote communication success in the home, school, community, and work environments, then the evaluation of the results of AAC instruction should be based on the student's communication performance in those natural settings. Evaluation of AAC goals should be based on how well a student uses an AAC system to interact with and influence the behavior of communication partners in different settings. The evaluation should not be based on how well a student can use an AAC system to interact with a therapist in a therapy room. Evaluation strategies should include observation of the student using the AAC system in natural settings and interviews with classroom staff and parents. Calculator and Jorgensen (1991) considered the use of this method of evaluating the effectiveness of AAC intervention to be a best practice for integrating AAC into the general education classroom.   .

INTERVENTION STRATEGIES FOR DIFFERENT AGE LEVELS

Infants and Toddlers

The process of developing communicative competence begins at birth. As a result, the need for early AAC intervention is critical. AAC intervention programs for infants and toddlers should focus on strategies that (a) support the development of natural speech, (b) promote active participation in the communication process, (c) increase communication opportunities, (d) provide receptive language training, (e) provide expressive language training, and (f) support the development of emergent literacy skills.

Strategies to Support the Development of Natural Speech

One of the challenges of implementing AAC is the concern that the use of AAC will impede the development of speech or that the child will simply choose to use AAC instead of speech. There is anecdotal evidence to support the fact that the implementation of AAC strategies can facilitate the development of natural speech (Burkhart, 1987; Silverman, 1989). According to Silverman, the use of augmentative communication does not appear to reduce motivation for speech communication and in some children seems to facilitate speech. At this early age, it is advised not to make exclusionary decisions regarding the acquisition of speech. Intervention strategies that focus on the use of AAC and the development of natural speech are recommended (Blackstone, 1990b).

Strategies to Promote Active Participation in the Communication Process

As part of the developmental process, infants cry in response to a physiological need such as to be fed or to be changed. The parent interprets the cry as communicative and attempts to meet the need of the infant by feeding or changing the infant. As a result of having the need met, the infant ceases crying, which is reinforcing to the parent. Eventually, the infant begins to smile, establishes eye contact, and vocalizes in response to interactions with the parent. Again, this reinforces the parent, who continues to engage in communication interactions with the infant.

Through this interactional process, the infant becomes aware that he or she can control the environment and others by crying, smiling, or vocalizing. This awareness is referred to as contingency awareness. Schweigert (1989) stated that the awareness of nonsocial contingencies (objects) and social contingencies (people) is necessary for future learning. The awareness of social contingencies is particularly critical for the development of communication skills.

Infants with disabilities may have delays in or absence of typical infant behaviors such as crying, smiling, eye gaze, or vocalizations. For the parent, this results in the lack of readability and predictability of the infant's behavior. *Readability* refers to the parent's ability to interpret the communicative intent of the infant's behavior. *Predictability* refers to the infant's response to the parent's reinforcement of the communication attempt. This creates a disturbance in the typical parent-infant interaction pattern which may cause the parent to have fewer interactions with the infant. This results in decreased opportunities to establish contingency patterns in parent-child interactions. The consequence of this for the infant with a disability may be that contingency awareness is not established. When contingency awareness is not established, the infant does not learn that he or she can control the environment or the behavior of others. The infant may become passive and be at risk for developing learned helplessness. Learned helplessness was described by Seligman (1975) as a condition in which a child lacks motivation to attempt to effect environmental change which leads to feelings of helplessness. Eventually, the infant will no longer attempt to control the environment and may ultimately become depressed. The concomitant effects of learned helplessness can be as serious as the disability.

It is critical to facilitate the development of contingency awareness for infants with disabilities. Interventions should be designed to improve the readability of the infant's behavior, and to teach parents how to read the infant's behaviors and respond in a consistent, contingent fashion.

Strategies to Increase Communication Opportunities.

In order for infants and toddlers to communicate, they need opportunities to communicate. For infants and toddlers, these opportunities typically occur in the context of play, routine care activities, and games such as pat-a-cake. The importance of play in the development of children is well documented. Play provides natural opportunities for the development of communication skills. Infants and toddlers with disabilities may have limited opportunities to engage in play activities and with play materials.

Toys and other play materials may need to be adapted so that they are accessible for the infant or toddler with a disability. Adapting toys for access provides infants and toddlers with disabilities opportunities to play independently, provides topics for communication, and creates a reason to communicate. Burkhart (1980, 1982), Goossens and Crain (1986a, 1986b), and Musselwhite (1986) provided detailed descriptions for adapting toys and other play materials as well as intervention strategies to facilitate the development of communication skills. Professionals working with the infant and toddler population will find these resources invaluable.

Routine care activities such as eating, bathing, dressing, and toileting occupy a large portion of the day. These activities can also be structured so that they provide many communication opportunities for the infant or toddler. These routines should be made as predictable as possible. This will allow the infant or toddler to become familiar with the activities and begin to anticipate what occurs next. Fingerplays, songs, nursery rhymes, and games such as pat-a-cake or peek-a-boo also provide communication opportunities for the infant and toddler.

Strategies to Provide Receptive Language Training

Major emphasis should be placed on receptive language intervention for the infant and toddler population as this is the natural time for learning language. The training should be provided in the context of routine care activities and play activities. Activities that occur frequently or are highly motivating to the child should be targeted for communication intervention. After the activity is targeted, vocabulary associated with the activity is identified, and a script is developed that describes the activity incorporating the target vocabulary (Goossens, Crain, & Elder, 1992). Receptive language training can be provided through techniques such as aided language stimulation or the total communication approach. In aided language stimulation, the facilitator "talks" through the activity while pointing to appropriate picture symbols on the communication display as the child is engaged in the activity. In a total communication approach, the major concept words are simultaneously spoken and signed. The benefits of these strategies are that they provide a language-rich experience for the child, opportunities to see AAC systems modeled in the context of an activity, and a predictable routine for language learning. Parents can easily be trained to use these approaches. Figure 15–4 shows a communication display that was developed for providing aided language stimulation during bath time—a routine care activity. A sample script for providing aided language stimulation during bath time is provided in Table 15–2.

Strategies to Provide Expressive Language Training

Early expressive language skills training should focus on ensuring that the infant or toddler has a means of gaining attention, expressing acceptance, and expressing re-

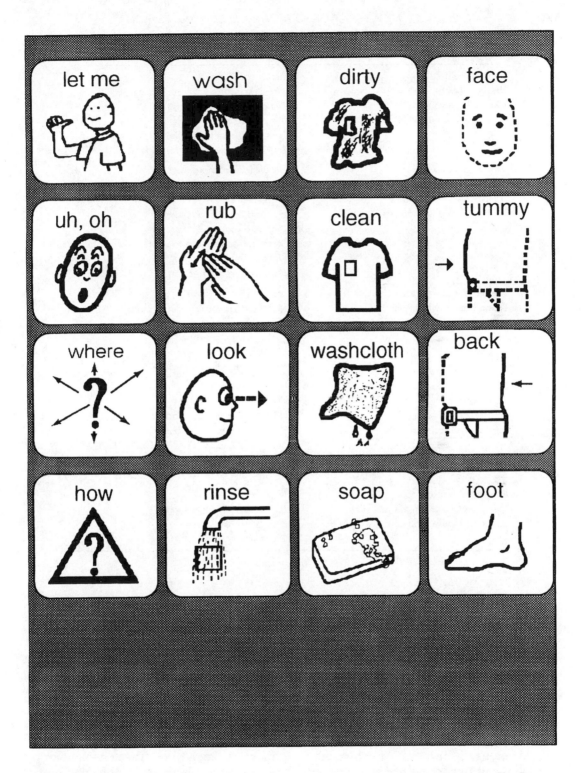

Figure 15–4. A topic miniboard for providing aided language stimulation during bath time. The Picture Communication Symbols © 1981, 1985, 1990 are used with permission of the Mayer-Johnson Company.

Table 15–2. A sample script for providing aided language stimulation during bath time.

Look at you!	(script continues)
Your're all *dirty*.	Now, I'm gonna wash your *face*.
Gotta clean you up.	No more *dirty face*.
How did you get so *dirty*?	We *rubbed* all the *dirt* off!
	Let's *rinse*, *rinse* that *soap* off.
	Look! You have a *clean face*!
We need *soap*.	Uh, oh! Look at those *feet*!.
Gotta have soap to get you *clean*.	Gotta *wash* those *feet*!
Uh, Oh! Where's the *soap*?	Those *feet* are *dirty*!
Where could that *soap* be?	How did they get so *dirty*?
Oh, here it is.	We need *soap*.
	Let me *rub* some more soap on this *washcloth*.
	Dirt's all gone!
	Now those *feet* are clean.
We need a *washcloth*.	Look at your *tummy*!
Gotta have a *washcloth*.	HOW did your *tummy* get so *dirty*?
Where's our *washcloth*?	Let me *wash* that *tummy*.
Look, here it is!	Gotta have more *soap*.
	Gotta *rub* that *dirt* off.
	We want that *tummy clean*!
Look at your *face*!	Let me see your *back*.
Your *face* is *dirty*!	Uh, oh! Your *back* is *dirty*!
How did your *face* get so *dirty*?	How did you get your *back* so *dirty*?
Let me *wash* your *dirty face*.	We have to *wash* your *back*.
	We need more *soap* on this *washcloth*.
	Now, let me *rub* your *back*.
	Gotta make it *clean*.
Uh, oh! We need *soap*.	Now, *let me* see.
Need some *soap* on this *washcloth*.	Let me *rinse* off all this *soap*.
Let me *rub* some soap on this *washcloth*.	Look, all the *dirt's* gone!
	You're all *clean*!

jection. Infants and toddlers with disabilities may function at a nonsymbolic level. Nonsymbolic communication includes the use of gestures, vocal sounds, eye contact, body movement, and facial expressions to convey a message. Siegel-Causey and Downing (1987) defined communication at a nonsymbolic level as the transmission of a message without the use of symbols (words, signs, graphics). Any behavior that the infant or toddler has may be used as a method of communication. Crying is a behavior that is used to gain attention or to express rejection. Smiling or a relaxed muscle tone are behaviors that can be used to express acceptance.

It is important that parents and other communication partners are taught to interpret these behaviors as communicative and to respond to them accordingly. As these behaviors are reinforced as communicative by the parent, the infant or toddler can begin to use these behaviors in a more discriminating fashion. The parent or communication partner can then respond more selectively to the behaviors and begin to shape them into more acceptable forms or more refined signals.

All communication partners need to be made aware of how the infant or toddler communicates. A communication diary may be one way to inform communication partners of the child's communication repertoire. This diary might describe the behavior that the child uses and the message that is being communicated. For example, the diary might indicate that when the child rubs his or her eyes this means that the child is tired and wants to be put in bed.

Some children may never be able to transition to a symbolic system; therefore, it is imperative to consider nonsymbolic communication as a viable AAC strategy (Siegel-Causey & Downing, 1987). Communicators who function at the nonsymbolic level need to be able to express needs, communicate likes and dislikes, make choices, and indicate protests. In nonsymbolic communication more of the burden is placed on the communication partner to acknowledge and interpret the message than in communication exchanges with symbolic users. For these children, efforts should be made to refine and expand their nonsymbolic system and to train potential communication partners. Once the infant or toddler has acquired a system of nonsymbolic communication, strategies to facilitate transition to a symbolic system should be considered.

Strategies to Support the Development of Emergent Literacy Skills

It is important for infants and toddlers with disabilities to participate in home literacy experiences and environments which can provide the foundation for literacy learning. Light and Kelford Smith (1993) identified discrepancies that may exist in home literacy experiences of children with disabilities. These discrepancies can be addressed by increasing parental awareness of the importance of literacy experiences for infants and toddlers with disabilities. Print-related materials such as alphabet blocks, pictures of nursery rhyme characters, and books can be made available and accessible in the infant and toddler environment. Parents may need to incorporate positioning techniques into bookreading experiences so that the infant or toddler can see the text of the book as it is being read. Also, parents need to understand the importance of repeated readings of the same book to the infant or toddler. Finally, because parental expectations of literacy seem to be a powerful predictor of literacy acquisition, parents need to be made aware of the importance of providing literacy experiences for young children with disabilities. No child should be considered too disabled to benefit from literacy experiences (Koppenhaver & Pierce, 1992).

Preschool Programs

AAC needs that were identified for the early intervention population (infants and toddlers) remain appropriate for the preschool population. In addition, the following AAC strategies should be considered: strategies to support ongoing AAC training, strategies to facilitate preschool literacy experiences, and strategies to facilitate transition to general education programs.

Strategies to Support AAC Training

Receptive and expressive language training can be provided in the preschool classroom during naturally occurring routines. A systematic means of providing this training is to engineer the classroom for communication (Goossens, Crain, & Elder, 1992). Engineering the classroom for communication is a process that ultimately allows the child to be immersed in communication training opportunities throughout the entire school day—not just at specific, isolated times targeted for communication.

Engineering the classroom for communication is an approach that requires that the classroom staff and the speech-language pathologist work collaboratively to design a classroom environment that supports the use of AAC systems. Goossens et al. (1992) described a six phase process for engineering a classroom to promote AAC and to identify strategies for receptive and expressive language training with AAC systems. The six phases for engineering a classroom are listed in Table 15–3. These phases address the physical preparation for engineering the classroom environment.

Identifying Classroom Routines and Activities. In the first phase of the engineering process, classroom routines and activities are identified. These routines and activities are then prioritized based on frequency of occurrence and motivational value. For example, in order to begin the process of engineering her preschool classroom for communication, Mrs. Brown created a list of all the activities and routines that occurred in her classroom on a daily or weekly basis. This resulted in a list of 15 activities. In order to determine which activities she would engineer first, she rated the activities in regard to how often the activities occurred and on motivational appeal to the students. From the master list of 15 activities, she identified three activities to begin the engineering process. She selected circle time because it was an activity that occurred on a daily basis and held high appeal to the students. For the second activity, she chose washing hands because this activity occurred multiple times throughout the day. Finally, she selected music time because even though this activity occurred only three times a week, it was an extremely motivating activity for the students.

Identifying Core Vocabulary and Message Sets. In the second phase, core vocabulary and message sets associated with the routine or activity are identified. Next, based on importance to the activity, the vocabulary list is rank ordered. In the example of Mrs. Brown, classroom staff brainstormed possible vocabulary and messages that would be needed during circle time, washing hands, and music activities. It was determined that for the circle time activity the student names, a greeting, days of the week, and vocabulary associated with the daily schedule would be needed. For the washing hands activity, the staff developed a list of 36 words or messages that could be used during this

Table 15–3. Steps in engineering the classroom for communication.

1. Identify and prioritize classroom activities.
2. Generate message or vocabulary sets associated with the activities.
3. Identify AAC selection techniques and symbol display formats.
4. Create the communication displays.
5. Incorporate supplemental AAC symbols.
6. Make the displays and supplemental systems accessible for the student.

Source: From Engineering the Preschool Environment for Interactive Symbolic Communication: 18 Months to 5 Years Developmentally (p. 17), by C. Goossens, S. Crain, & P. Elder, 1992, Birmingham, AL: Southeast Augmentative Communication Conference Publication Clinician Series. Copyright 1992 by Southeast Augmentative Communication Conference. Adapted with permission.

activity. The staff then rank ordered the list based on vocabulary critical to the activity and the frequency of use. In the same manner, a generic vocabulary list for the music activity was generated. Specific vocabulary for songs was predetermined by the lyrics.

Determining Methods of Access to AAC Systems. In phase three, the physical abilities of the students are considered in order to determine how the child will access the communication display. In a classroom setting, the challenge is to provide access to communication displays for students with a wide range of physical abilities. There are four factors that should be considered during this phase of the engineering process. One factor to be considered is the student's physical abilities. Some students will be able to access a 16- or 32-location communication display using their hands. Students who are more severely physically impaired may need to have access to eye gaze communication displays. The reader is referred to Chapters 5 and 7 for more information on this topic. A second factor to be considered is that students may use different types of access methods depending on the activity. For example, a student may be able to use a 16-location display when being held in the teacher assistant's lap on the floor during circle time; whereas, a rotary scan display might be needed for the times the student is positioned in a sidelyer. A third factor to be considered is the need to ensure that the student's view of the activity is not obstructed by the display. The fourth factor is whether or not the display permits access to the manipulatives or materials being used in the activity. The display should not only provide the student access to the communication display but also promote participation opportunities with peers or materials.

Creating Communication Displays. In phase four, the communication displays are made based on individual student need.

Making the communication displays can be a very time- consuming task. After the core vocabulary has been identified, the symbols must be selected to represent the vocabulary. The symbols must then be arranged and affixed to the display. Depending on the needs of the class, the teacher may want multiple displays of a single activity and multiple formats of a single activity.

Three methods for making the displays are discussed here. The first is to use commercially available books of picture symbols. This is a multistep process that involves copying, coloring, cutting, and attaching the symbols to the display. This is a very labor intensive method. The second method is to use a computer program such as the Boardmaker or Boardbuilder program (Mayer-Johnson Company) to create the display. The use of these programs can eliminate several steps in the process as well as the paper waste associated with the first method. The third method is to use the communication display books that have been developed by Goossens, Crain, and Elder (1994a, 1994b). Parents or other volunteers may be willing to make communication displays for the classroom. The school staff should identify and use all available resources to assist in this task.

Adding Supplementary Vocabulary. Phase five involves the addition of supplemental vocabulary to the core vocabulary of the communication display. The addition of supplemental vocabulary may be needed to expand the vocabulary available for an activity, or to customize generic overlays. For example, Mrs. Brown decided to use a generic communication display for her cooking activities. In order to customize the overlay to the activity of making a peanut butter and jelly sandwich, she chose to add supplemental vocabulary to the generic display. The supplemental vocabulary was added to the generic display via a Velcro strip which was attached to the side of the display. If the class was making pudding, she would add the supplemental vocabulary for that activity. By doing this, she eliminated the need to create a specific communication display for every food option.

Storage and Placement of AAC Displays in the Classroom. In phase six, storage options for the communication displays and symbols are determined. The basic rule is that the AAC display must be readily accessible to the staff and students when it is time for the routine or activity. Thus, communication displays addressing play and toy activities would need to be stored near the play center, communication displays addressing music activities would need to be stored near the music center, and toileting displays would need to be stored in the bathroom or toileting area.

Once the physical preparation of the environment is in place, the intervention strategies must be addressed. Goossens et al. (1992) emphasized the importance of implementing intervention strategies that are interactive in nature. Aided language stimulation is the strategy utilized to address receptive language training. In order to provide effective aided language stimulation, facilitators may find it helpful to have a script or dialogue to follow. These scripts provide structure and consistency in routine for both the staff and the student. The education staff can develop their own scripts, or take advantage of the predeveloped displays and play scripts that have been developed by Goossens et al. (1994a, 1994b).

Engineering a Classroom for Communication: A Practical Example

During the 1994–95 school year, Barbara Anderson, a special educator, began the process of engineering her special education classroom for aided augmentative communication training. Mrs. Anderson teaches in a small school district which is located in a rural area. The instructional arrangement of Ms. Anderson's classroom is primarily self-contained; however, the students do have opportunities to be included with other students. The students in this classroom have cognitive, physical, and communication disabilities. The six students in this classroom range in age from 3 to 13 years old. All of the students are nonverbal and require AAC. Support staff for this classroom included two teacher assistants and a speech-language pathologist.

Prior to the implementation of this approach in her classroom, Barbara and the speech-language pathologist attended a 2-day training workshop on "Engineering the Pre-school Environment for Communication" presented by Sharon Crain, one of the developers of this approach. This training provided information regarding the theoretical principles and rationale for engineering a classroom for communication. It also provided information regarding the six-phase process for developing the needed communication displays and materials; practice in developing an activity script and in aided language stimulation techniques; and an opportunity to "make and take" classroom communication displays. At the end of the second day of training, Barbara left with materials and techniques ready for classroom implementation. Later in the year, Barbara and the speech-language pathologist were given release time in order to visit another school district which had been implementing this approach for 2 years.

After attending the workshop, Barbara, with the help of the teacher assistants, began making communication displays based on various student access methods (one student used eye gaze, the others were able to use direct selection) and various classroom activities. By the end of the 1994–95 school year, the staff had created displays for approximately 75% of the classroom activities. Assistance in obtaining materials in order to develop the communication displays (lexan, tempo loop fabric, contact paper) were provided by the regional Educational Service Center.

Initially, Barbara targeted three classroom activities in which she began to incorporate the aided language stimulation techniques. She selected her circle time routine, lunch, and cooking activities. All three activities were selected because of their motivational value for the students and their frequency of occurrence. One of the communication displays used during her circle time activity is shown in Figure 15–5. The communication display that was developed for use during lunch time is shown in Figure 15–6. The communication display that was designed for a specific recipe the class enjoyed is shown in Figure 15–7. By the end of the year, most of their classroom activities (e.g., bathroom, brushing teeth, play) were also being targeted for AAC intervention. In addition to using the nonelectronic communication displays in AAC intervention, Barbara also had access to a Dial Scan (Don Johnston Developmental Equipment), a Wolf (Adamlab), and an adapted tape recorder with loop tapes. She also used strategies and materials from *Storytime* (King-DeBaun, 1989) to combine emergent literacy and AAC instruction.

Barbara shared information regarding this intervention approach with the students' parents during parent conferences and classroom visits. She explained the reasons the approach was being implemented in the classroom, demonstrated aided language stimulation techniques, and encouraged the parents to use the techniques at home. Barbara also provided the parents with a set of communication displays for use at home. She sent notes home with the students which told the parents what activities occurred during the day at school. She encouraged the parents to use the communication displays to talk to the students about the activities that occurred each day at school.

As a result of engineering her classroom, Barbara stated that she learned that AAC intervention is much more effective when motivating activities such as cooking and music activities were targeted for instruction instead of basic needs (eat, drink, bathroom) which have traditionally been a major focus of early communication training. Additionally, she stated that the use of this approach facilitated a more child-directed approach. She indicated that once she and other classroom staff had become proficient in aided language stimulation techniques and had communication displays available in the classroom, the AAC intervention was simply a matter of overlaying the intervention on the naturally occurring activity. This allowed the staff to be able to follow the child's lead rather than having the child participate in a teacher-directed intervention.

For some students, the use of aided language stimulation techniques may be all that is needed to facilitate the expressive use of the communication displays. For other students, specific expressive language training strategies will be required. A variety of strategies, discussed next, are employed to address expressive language training, including the use of templates, nonverbal juncture cues, light cues, and sabotage.

Training Strategies for Aided Language Stimulation

Templates. During expressive language training, a facilitator may chose to limit vocabulary items available to a student. Templates may be used to cover symbols on a communication display until the facilitator decides to incorporate the vocabulary into expressive training. If more than one student is using the same AAC display, templates customized for the unique needs of each child can be created. A paper or card stock template can be placed on top of the communication display. As vocabulary

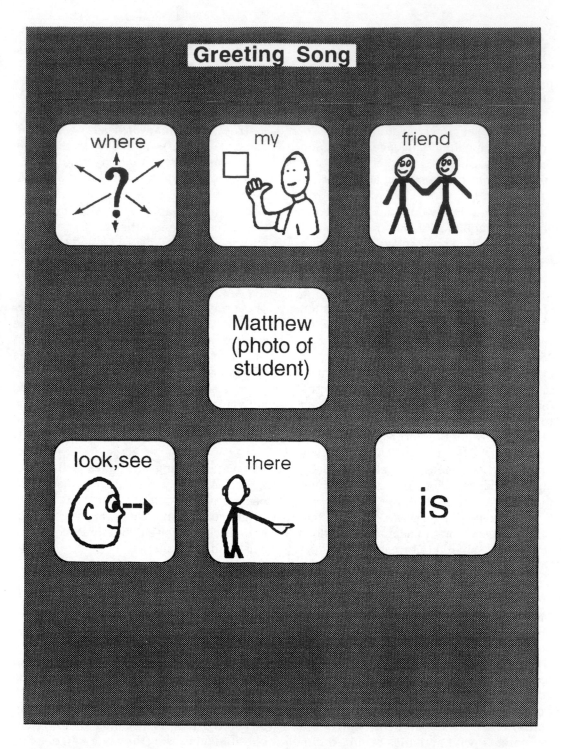

Figure 15–5. A communication display developed to accompany the *Greeting Song*, which was a part of Mrs. Anderson's circle time routine. The Picture Communication Symbols © 1981, 1985, 1990 are used with permission of the Mayer-Johnson Company.

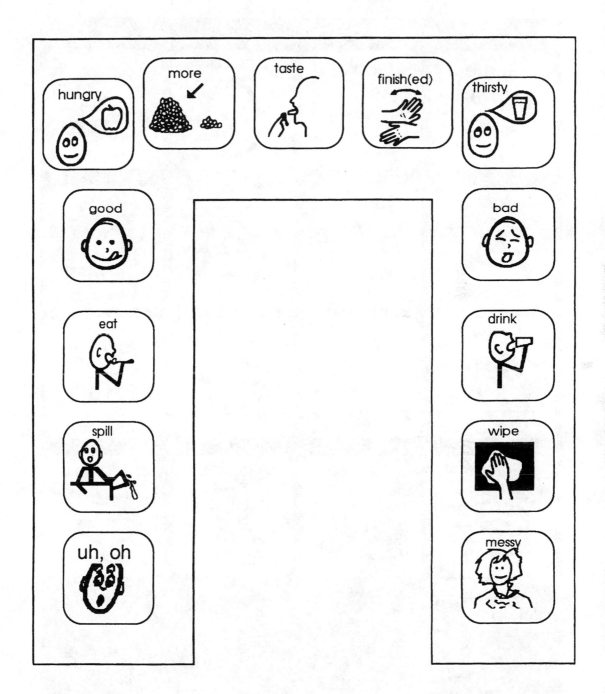

Figure 15–6. A communication display designed for a student who used eye gaze. Mrs. Anderson or the teacher assistants provided aided language stimulation while assisting the student during lunch. The Picture Communication Symbols © 1981, 1985, 1990 are used with permission of the Mayer-Johnson Company.

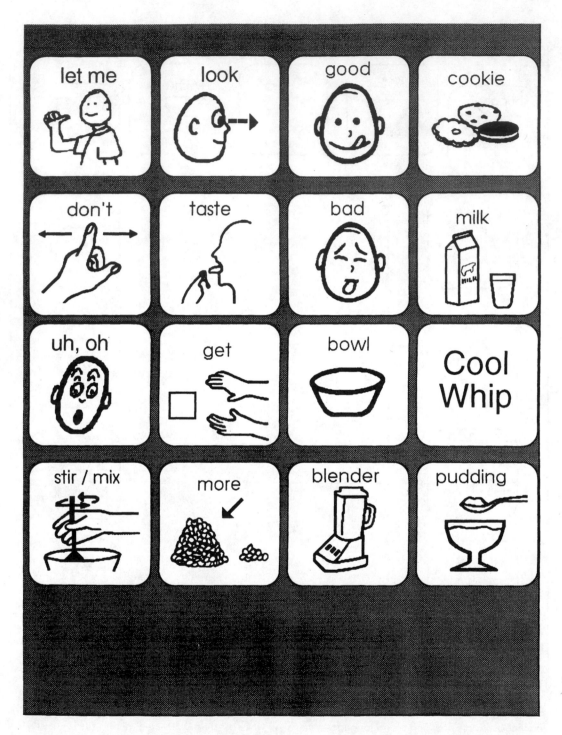

Figure 15–7. A communication display designed for a specific recipe, Dirt Pudding, made during the weekly cooking activity. The Picture Communication Symbols © 1981, 1985, 1990 are used with permission of the Mayer-Johnson Company.

is presented to the child, locations are cut out of the template to expose the picture symbols of that vocabulary. Duct tape or adhesive notes can also be used for quick coverage of symbols.

When using templates with voice output communication systems, a thicker material such as cardboard may need to be added to the paper template in order to prevent the access of the nonexposed location. If the voice output system is being used by only one child, then the facilitator can program the device for only the vocabulary items that are being exposed to the child. Several new AAC devices have "hide" functions that allow a teacher to temporarily disable keys.

Nonverbal Juncture Cues. Goossens et al. (1992) defined a nonverbal juncture cue as a nonverbal signal (achieved via facial expression, gesture, body posture) performed by the facilitator that precedes the highlighting of a symbol on the communication display. Through the use of this technique, the facilitator is "setting the stage" for a communication opportunity. . As the student becomes familiar with a routine, the student begins to anticipate the communication opportunity associated with the activity. During the course of established routines, the facilitator may pause and provide a nonverbal juncture cue such as a gesture or a facial expression. This provides the student an opportunity to initiate the "anticipated" communication prior to the facilitator highlighting the symbol.

Light Cues. An effective training strategy for cognitively older students is the use of light cues to prompt a communication response (Goossens et al., 1992). In this technique, the facilitator uses a small, hand-held penlight or squeeze flashlight. When a communication opportunity occurs, the facilitator cues the student by shining the light on the appropriate symbol on the communication display. This technique permits the student to partici-

pate in a communication exchange without direct verbal cues from the facilitator. The light cues can be systematically faded as the student begins to initiate spontaneous expressive use of the communication system.

A hierarchy of light cues has been delineated by Goossens et al. (1992). A constant light cue provides the highest level of prompt for a student. At this level, the light cue is provided until the student selects the target symbol. The next level of prompt is the momentary light cue. At this level, the targeted symbol is highlighted for only 2 seconds. The search light cue is the least level of prompt provided when using the light cue technique. When providing the search light cue, the facilitator briefly scans the light across all or a portion of the communication display. For some students, the use of light cues alone may facilitate spontaneous expressive use of a communication display or device. For other students, this strategy must be combined with other prompts.

Sabotage Routines. Sabotage routines are used to "set the stage" for communication opportunities. After the students are familiar with the routines associated with the activities, sabotage strategies are inserted into the routines. Sabotage strategies are similar to changing the ending to a familiar story, in that they tend to encourage a reaction or response to the break of the routine. Goossens et al. (1992) identified five types of sabotage strategies, including incorrect item, omitted step, incomplete action, incorrect action, and mischievous action.

For example, during a tooth brushing activity the facilitator might pick up the hairbrush (incorrect item) instead of the toothbrush in order to elicit the response of "No, toothbrush." An example of a sabotage routine integrated into a bubble blowing activity might have the facilitator bring the bubble wand to her lips but not blow (omitted step) to encourage the targeted message of "blow" from the student. A sabotage routine during a dressing activity might have the facilitator putting on only one sleeve of a shirt (incomplete action) in order to cue a response of "No, you forgot to finish." An example of a sabotage routine during a cooking activity might have the facilitator put the carton of milk in the oven (incorrect action) instead of the refrigerator in order to encourage a response of "no, don't," "uh, oh," or "in the refrigerator." A sabotage routine combined with a helping doll could have the helping doll "eating" someone else's snack during snack time (mischievous action) in order to encourage a response of "stop" or "no, don't."

Training Staff and Parents. Engineering the classroom for communication requires a commitment of staff, time, and budget. It is recommended that, once the decision is made to engineer a preschool classroom for communication, the educational staff receive intensive training in this process. The educational staff will need to acquire skills in aided language stimulation techniques as well as in the expressive strategies (nonverbal juncture cues, light cues, and sabotage). It is important that the school staff participate in this training as a team. This will help the team understand the outcomes and benefits of implementing this approach in a preschool classroom.

Members of the educational team should also include family members. Parents should be provided information regarding the process of engineering a classroom, and the expected outcomes to be gained from this type of environment. Information can be provided to parents in a variety of formats, including distribution of a parent newsletter, professional articles, videotape of classroom activities, or by encouraging classroom visits. Parent training opportunities should be provided in which the parents can acquire skills in the training strategies being used in the classroom so that these strategies can be extended to the home environment. Schools may encourage parent involvement in the engineering process by having parent meetings in which the parents can "make and take" communication displays for the home environment, or "make and leave" communication displays for the classroom environment. Parent training and involvement as team members are critical components in the success of an AAC intervention (Musselwhite & St. Louis, 1988).

Engineering Neighborhood Preschool Settings for AAC

Although some young children receive services in self-contained, special education preschool classrooms, there is concern that this does not always constitute the least restrictive environment. As a result, there is more of a movement toward providing services in neighborhood preschool programs. Recent research on preschoolers with disabilities in inclusive settings indicates improvement in play behaviors and more time spent interacting and verbalizing with peers (Guralnick, 1981; Nisbet, 1994).

Engineering the general education preschool setting for AAC is the same in principle as that of the self-contained special education setting, though realistically the extent of AAC immersion may differ as only one child rather than all children are being targeted for AAC use. When developing communication systems designed to provide communication opportunities for a child who relies on AAC, the steps remain the same as previously discussed. First the classroom routines and activities will need to be identified and prioritized. Then the core vocabulary, message sets, and supplemental vocabulary to support these activities must be delineated. The methods by which the child will communicate and the types of communication displays are differentiated based on the abilities of the individual child. The storage and placement of the communication displays in and around the classroom are determined by the nature of the classroom activities.

A critical difference in the neighborhood preschool setting as opposed to the special education setting is the degree to which human resources are available. In special education settings, teachers and therapists may meet regularly or informally to keep pace with AAC plans. In the neighborhood preschool, the bulk of the daily responsibility will rest with the teacher and a teaching assistant. Related services and AAC specialists are often consultative and ongoing classroom support through team involvement is usually limited. It is important to be sensitive to this. Creating overlays that address routine daily classroom activities should be a first priority. Low tech or simple digitized voice output devices that are quick and easy for staff to program should be made available. Although high tech voice output devices should not be excluded from these settings, training and on-site support to keep pace with programming needs should be carefully planned.

When training new staff in a local preschool, principles of AAC should be outlined. Aided language stimulation techniques should be modeled to new staff, who will need training in how to use communication boards to facilitate receptive as well as expressive language. One of the greatest benefits of inclusion for children who use AAC is the added advantage of typical peer interactions. Typical peers should be encouraged to use the same strategies for communication as teaching staff. It is a wonderful sight to see a preschooler hold up two crayons and naturally incorporate AAC strategies by saying to his or her classmate who is physically disabled and nonspeaking, "Look at the color you want me to use."

Strategies to Facilitate Preschool Literacy Experiences

Preschool programs for children with disabilities should provide opportunities for participation in emergent literacy activities. Emphasis should be on creating literacy experiences that are positive in nature, developmentally appropriate, and designed so that the child with a disability can be an active participant. It is important that preschool children with disabilities participate in both reading and writing experiences.

For preschool children with AAC needs, it is important to provide emergent reading activities that include participating in shared bookreading experiences and integrating the child's AAC system into the bookreading experience. During shared bookreading experiences, it is important that the child with a disability be positioned so that the child can see the text as it is being read, hear repeated readings of stories, and have opportunities to choose which story he or she would like to hear. Books may need to be adapted so that children with motor impairments can more easily manipulate the book, turn the pages, or independently access a book.

A child's AAC system can be easily integrated into bookreading experiences. A generic "story" communication display (see Figure 15–8) can be used to provide aided language stimulation during bookreading experiences or a custom overlay (see Figure 15–9) may be created based on the story. The text of the story can be coded by placing picture symbols on the pages of the story. The repetitive or predictable lines of a story or even pages of the story can be programmed into a voice output communication device. The child can then read lines or pages by matching the symbols coded on the page to the symbols on the device. This not only provides the child with a method of reading a story, but also provides the educational staff an

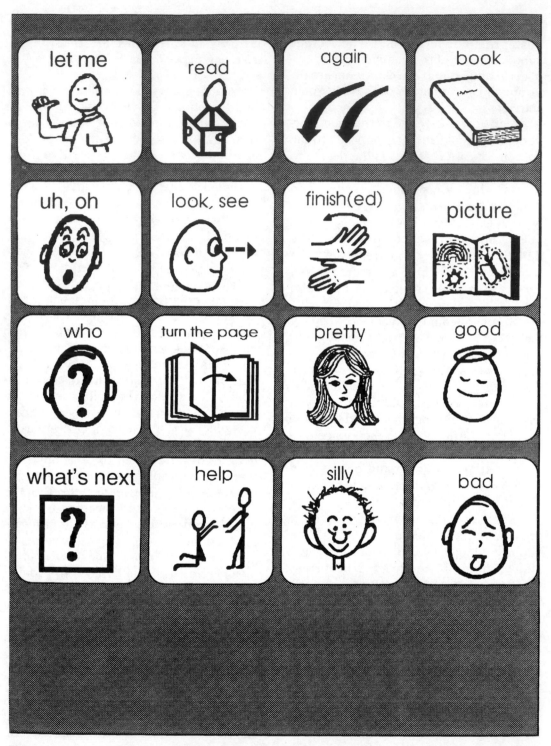

Figure 15–8. A topic miniboard (generic) providing aided language stimulation during a bookreading activity. The Picture Communication Symbols ⁻ 1981, 1985, 1990 are used with permission of the Mayer-Johnson Company.

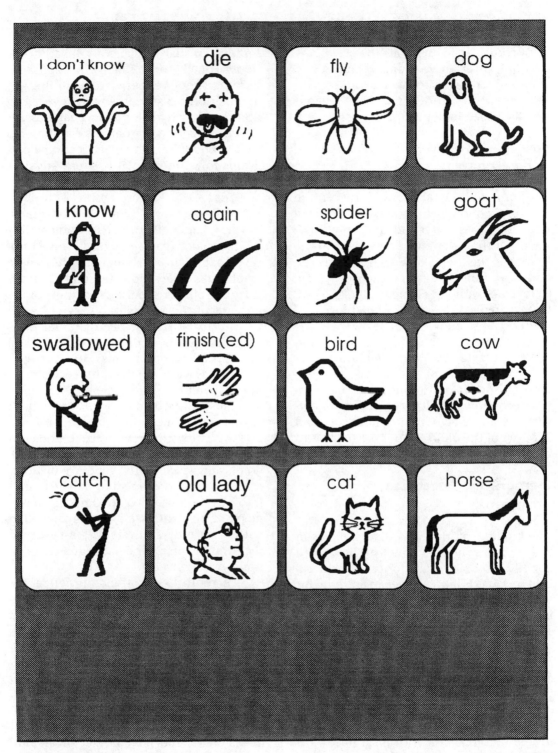

Figure 15–9. A communication display developed specifically for the story *I Know an Old Lady Who Swallowed a Fly*. The Picture Communication Symbols ° 1981, 1985, 1990 are used with permission of the Mayer-Johnson Company.

opportunity to incorporate the use of AAC in a fun, interactive manner. Literacy issues and strategies to facilitate literacy development for students with AAC needs are discussed in detail in Chapter 8.

Strategies to Facilitate the Transition to Kindergarten

The immediate goal of AAC intervention for a preschooler who is nonspeaking is to provide an AAC system that meets the needs of that student. This means a system that has been designed so that the child can quickly begin using the system to interact with peers and family. The AAC team also needs to look toward future AAC needs. The team needs to be aware of the classroom and curriculum requirements of kindergarten, so that the child's communication system will be adequate to meet the needs of the kindergarten educational environment. It is critical that kindergarten staff receive training in the use and support of the child's AAC system prior to receiving the child in class.

Elementary Education Programs

The implementation of AAC techniques in the public schools cannot be limited to specific disability categories. Consideration of AAC should be given to any student who is nonspeaking or has limited speech intelligibility. AAC gives students with disabilities in public school settings access to the general education classroom and curriculum, and it facilitates the development of literacy skills.

Recent studies have questioned educational practices for students with disabilities. Segregated versus inclusive classrooms for students with disabilities are being critically examined. Early research on segregated as compared to inclusive classrooms is demonstrating improved academic, behavioral, and social outcomes

for both special and general education students (Blackstone, 1995b). Research regarding school experiences and literacy acquisition for students with severe disabilities has revealed discrepancies between educational programs for students who are nondisabled and educational programs for students with severe physical disabilities who are nonspeaking (Berninger & Gans, 1986; Kelford-Smith, Thurston, Light, Parnes, & O'Keefe, 1989; Koppenhaver & Yoder, 1990). These studies highlighted major discrepancies in the educational experiences of students with severe disabilities. They indicated that students with disabilities spent a disproportionate amount of time in related services such as physical therapy, occupational therapy, and speech therapy rather than in instructional programs; students with disabilities were less likely to receive reading instruction from a certified reading specialist who would be familiar with both regular and remedial reading techniques; and students with severe disabilities did not receive the benefit of systematic programs and access to the general education curriculum. Studies such as these call into question whether the underachievement of students who are nonspeaking with severe disabilities was a result of the disability itself or of inadequate educational experiences.

Currently, educational practice for students with disabilities at the elementary level is undergoing scrutiny. It is a time of change and unease as educators and families attempt to create new methods of educational programming. AAC specialists need to be prepared to deliver services in a variety of settings, from general education to self-contained classrooms. Though the settings will vary, the AAC needs of students are analyzed on an individualized basis. The process of determining a student's unique AAC needs remains the same regardless of settings. The greater challenge to AAC teams is delineating cre-

As part of the process of AAC implementation, it is important to examine the student's school environment. The AAC team can determine how AAC will facilitate classroom participation by analyzing what is required of all students, identifying communication discrepancies that occur for the child with a disability, and targeting how AAC can assist in the elimination of the discrepancies. A model for this pro-cess was developed by Beukelman and Mirenda (1992). They advocated the use of the Participation Model to facilitate the inclusion of students with AAC needs into the general education classroom and the regular curriculum.

The Participation Model is a planning tool that the AAC team uses to provide a more systematic approach to the inclusion of a student with AAC needs into the general education classroom. The Participation Model is a process in which a team analyzes the four components of classroom participation (integration, social participation, independence, and academic participation). The team also analyzes opportunity and access barriers in the educational program. The Participation Model is discussed in more detail in Chapter 5.

General Education Classroom Settings

When students who use AAC systems are included in general education classrooms, it is important to continue to provide AAC instruction that is activity-based and integrated into classroom routines. A teacher's decisions regarding curriculum adaptations for students in an inclusive setting follow a logical decision-making process that takes into consideration the student's IEP goals and general education units of study (Villa & Thousand, 1995). Table 15–4 provides major steps in the integration of AAC into the general education classroom. AAC objectives must be clearly defined, along with expectations for the student's participation. Each period in the student's day should be examined relative to AAC goals and strategies for enhancing participation. Within each unit of study, the general education curriculum should be analyzed to identify critical learning objectives and to delineate compatible AAC strategies. Low tech as well as high tech strategies should be selected based on issues of practicality, yet should strike a balance with the long-term AAC development needs of the individual student. For example, although a low tech digitized device may be easiest to program for a morning unit on the birthday of Dr. Martin Luther King, the student's high tech communication device should also be incorporated into the school day, as use of this AAC device is in the long-term interest of the student. Material and equipment adaptations

Table 15–4. Steps in engineering the classroom for communication.

1. Identify and prioritize classroom activities.
2. Generate message or vocabulary sets associated with the activities.
3. Identify AAC selection techniques and symbol display formats.
4. Create the communication displays.
5. Incorporate supplemental AAC symbols.
6. Make the displays and supplemental systems accessible for the student.

Source: From Engineering the Preschool Environment for Interactive Symbolic Communication: 18 Months to 5 Years Developmentally *(p. 17), by C. Goossens, S. Crain, & P. Elder, 1992, Birmingham, AL: Southeast Augmentative Communication Conference Publication Clinician Series. Copyright 1992 by Southeast Augmentative Communication Conference. Adapted with permission.*

should be selected based on student need and not on the preferences of staff. The results of lessons carried out with a student should be evaluated daily, over time, and across multiple measures. Determining what the student learned, what the student retained, and skills that are being generalized are issues that should be addressed as part of outcome evaluations.

The engineering concepts that were implemented in the preschool classroom can also be applied to the general education elementary classroom. Classroom events will need to be identified and prioritized; core vocabulary and message sets will need to be delineated; communication displays will need to be designed; and ready access to communication systems will need to be ensured.

The AAC team should make sure that the student has access to communication displays that allow for socialization as well as participation in content area instruction. The student will need numerous communication boards to meet the demands of the curriculum. Communication displays should be organized in ways that help the student keep pace with classroom events and academic subjects. Specific pages for math or social studies will be needed, but displays will also be needed that allow for ordering lunch or for socialization (e.g., to talk about the weekend or a sports event.) A communication page that allows the student to ask for specific types of help may also be useful (e.g., "I need spelling help," "I don't understand," "Repeat the directions," "What do I have for homework?").

The classroom staff should be trained in how to set up the AAC system for the student and should expect the student to use the AAC system throughout the day. It is not enough for the student to have access to the device only during class time. Recess and lunch room opportunities are equally important communication opportunities. Natural peer supports should also be considered. Typical peers are a terrific source of support to students who use AAC systems, helping to set up their communication overlays and using AAC strategies to communicate on social and academic topics.

Keeping pace with vocabulary for AAC overlays is a constant race against time. In some instances, the classroom staff may take the responsibility for adding new vocabulary to the AAC system. At the elementary level, there is usually someone (a special educator or speech-language pathologist) who acts as case manager and helps monitor the communication needs of the student and the AAC system. However, no one person can manage all the responsibilities associated with a student's AAC system. To make AAC an integral part of the educational day, the teacher, the teaching assistant, and related service staff will need to share the workload. Communication among school staff and advance planning are keys. Staff should anticipate upcoming curriculum units in order to plan and design new overlays and program vocabulary into communication devices.

School principal support is also an important variable. Principals need to be aware of the time required to keep pace with a student's communication needs. Team planning time, time to adapt materials, time to create overlays, as well as time to program devices must be factored into the school week.

Self-Contained Special Education Classrooms

Not all students with AAC needs are mainstreamed today into general education classrooms, although the trend is toward more and not less inclusion (Blackstone, 1995b). This may be due to a lack of school initiative or the preference of the family. Some families of children with disabilities still prefer the more protective setting of a special school or a self-contained special education classroom. Although it has opened many doors for students with disabilities, the philosophy of inclusion remains controversial, and its implementation is often problematic due to lack of resources. In the meantime, parents need to be informed of the classroom options for their child and take into consideration LRE issues.

The success of any classroom depends on the people involved. Self-contained special education classrooms in elementary schools have a responsibility and an opportunity to provide AAC immersion. The techniques for this are the same as those described in the section on preschool settings. Although classroom activities will differ, the steps remain the same. The local school team in collaboration with AAC specialists must first identify and prioritize classroom routines and activities and then begin to select vocabulary in order to design AAC overlays.

Another element that should remain the same is the use of curricular themes. Irrespective of whether the student is in a self-contained special education or general education classroom, the team can use the general education curriculum as a guide in the development of lessons that integrate AAC goals and strategies. For example, a science unit on plant growth may have simplified vocabulary as well as activity variations. Rather than a focus on photosynthesis, the focus can be on labeling parts of a plant and learning that plants need air and water to grow. All students, even those with moderate to severe disabilities, need breadth of information. Relating IEP AAC goals to modified curriculum goals ensures the integration of AAC across the school day and provides variation in topics for communication. It also wards against the likelihood that the student's day will be driven by the clock and focus only on isolated skill development (e.g., fine motor time, communication time).

Once classroom routines, activities, and curriculum are identified and prioritized, core vocabulary and message sets will need to be delineated. AAC selection techniques for different activities throughout the day will need to be identified. For example, a rotary dial scan may be used during math activities, whereas the student's AAC device will be needed during science and social studies. Low tech communication boards may be used during recess, whereas digitized voice output devices which are quick and easy to program may be used during morning opening activities. The AAC Action Plan and the curriculum integration formats discussed earlier in this chapter (Figures 15–2 and 15–3) can assist in the planning process.

The design and creation of communication displays is generally a shared responsibility among local school staff. One advantage of special schools is that in-house teams are often accustomed to working together and daily communication is possible. The best way to keep pace with a student's need for updated communication displays is to share the workload. For example, the classroom teacher may take responsibility for organizing vocabulary in keeping with upcoming curriculum themes. The speech-language pathologist may help refine the message sets and define the layout of symbols, and the teaching assistant may assist with device programming or the construction of new communication boards. It is advisable to try to begin this process 2 to 3 weeks prior to the start of a new curriculum unit. It is always helpful to introduce new communication overlays and to provide in advance some direct training to the student using the new overlays.

Facilitating the Acquisition of Literacy and Math Skills Using AAC Systems

Acquisition of literacy skills is crucial for any student's academic and vocational success. For a student who will rely on an AAC system in order to communicate, the acquisition of literacy skills provides the means to communicate original ideas, thoughts, and feelings instead of what has been programmed into the device by someone else. In order for students with AAC needs to become literate, they need access to literacy materials, access to literacy instruction, and integration of AAC into literacy instruction. Chapter 8 provides a detailed discussion of literacy issues and AAC intervention strategies.

Augmentative communication systems are potent tools for students with AAC needs in the literacy acquisition process. The use of augmentative communication systems provides a means for students to participate actively in the reading process and to connect oral language to print. The augmentative communication system should be integrated into the informal and formal reading experiences of the student. Through the use of communication systems, students who use AAC devices have a means of actively participating during reading experiences, and also have writing opportunities (Koppenhaver, Evans, & Yoder, 1991).

Many of the symbol systems that are utilized in AAC feature both the printed word and a graphic symbol. The graphic component may serve as a means to help the student connect the spoken word to the printed word. Over time the graphic component can be faded so that the symbol will eventually be replaced by only the printed word. This may be helpful in the development of a sight word vocabulary.

In order to participate in and meet the demands of the general education curriculum, it is important to be able to write. Some students may require access to a means to facilitate written expression. Some students may need access to a computer with appropriate writing programs in order to facilitate written expression. Other students may be able to interface the AAC system with a computer or printer in order to have written output. Some students may have an AAC system that has a built-in printer.

The use of the AAC system should be integrated into all subject areas, including math. The first step in using the AAC system to facilitate participation in math is to provide appropriate content and concept-

related vocabulary. The student can use a number display to participate in counting activities, to identify numbers, to sequence numbers, and to match objects to numbers. Students can also use math displays to indicate which operation ($+$, $-$, $\times$, $/$) would be performed in a math problem. Another way in which students can use the number display is to indicate the solution sentence for a math problem.

Secondary Education Programs

The transition from elementary to secondary education and the transition from school to work represent times of great foreboding for students with AAC systems. During the elementary years, AAC systems may be going well and gaining momentum; however, this can sometimes be totally lost when the student transitions to a middle school or high school program. In many cases, the student's service providers change during this transition. The student has all new teachers and new related service professionals. Without careful transition planning between the elementary and secondary staff, the AAC system will go unused or communication strategies will be introduced that are unfamiliar to the student and momentum will be lost. The student may be put in the position of having no one who can support the AAC system, or having to change methods of communication.

Logistical Constraints at the Secondary Level

Another challenge at the secondary level is that of managing all the classroom transitions that occur throughout the day in a secondary program. Students usually change classrooms for each subject period. This presents the logistical challenge of having the student and the AAC system move from room to room. If the student cannot manage the AAC system without assistance, then the AAC team will need to delineate who is responsible for setting up the AAC system throughout the day.

The transition to middle or high school is a time when students are expected to function more independently. For the student who relies on AAC, this should not translate into watered-down, simplistic AAC set-ups in the name of independence or time management. For example, eye gaze or 20 questions strategies should not be substituted for the use of the student's voice output device simply because it is easier for staff to set up. This constitutes an opportunity barrier.

It is critical for secondary staff to understand the long-term implications of AAC use. It can take many years for a student to become proficient with an AAC device. Voice output devices provide the individual who is nonspeaking with a means to control communication, whereas communication strategies such as 20 questions or asking yes/no questions rely on the skill and interest of a communication partner. As the student transitions from school to work, he or she cannot rely on the availability of trained communication partners. Independence through voice output adds to the student's communicative competence. But this will not happen if the goals of AAC are considered secondary to needs of the middle school or high school environment.

Transition Planning and Training

In order to ensure a smooth transition from elementary to secondary programs, the AAC team should carefully plan the transition. A member of the AAC team or the student's case manager should visit the secondary campus and talk with the teachers and speech-language pathologist who will be receiving the student. This visit will help the receiving team identify potential barriers and provide information that will help both teams prepare for the transition. If possible, the visit should occur in the spring, prior to the fall transition.

Another strategy that facilitates a smooth transition is for the elementary and secondary teams to get together prior to the student's transition. This provides an opportunity for the elementary staff to share what has been developed for the student and to answer the questions raised by secondary staff. If a joint meeting is not possible, the elementary staff can develop a transition video of the student that explains the AAC system and shows samples of the student using the AAC system in various classroom activities.

The AAC team will need to assess the secondary environment in order to develop new communication displays and program new vocabulary into the communication device for these new environments. Training will need to be provided for the secondary staff prior to the beginning of the school year. The secondary staff will need to learn low and/or high tech communication strategies, how to program new vocabulary, and how to maintain the AAC system. Someone at the secondary level will need to assume the responsibility for being the AAC system manager. This is especially critical in the secondary environment. When no one takes responsibility for a student's AAC system, then the system is underutilized, or there is no consistency in how the AAC systems are used. The role of the AAC case manager is to ensure appropriate use of the AAC system in different classes, and that current use of the AAC system is consonant with stated IEP goals. Secondary team meetings will need to be scheduled on a regular basis in order to plan new vocabulary and assignment modifications.

Self-Contained Secondary Settings

Some secondary students with severe developmental disabilities who use AAC systems may continue to need a structured, supportive environment in which AAC instruction is provided. These students may be included in general education classes for part of the day or they may receive most of their education in a self-contained classroom setting. The engineering approach can be continued at the secondary level in school and work environments. Elder and Goossens (1994) discussed the process for engineering work and living environments to support AAC systems for adolescents and adults who have severe developmental disabilities.

The process for engineering a living or work environment for interactive symbolic communication is similar to the process described earlier for preschool and elementary environments. First, the daily routine is analyzed in order to identify opportunities for communication interaction, and message sets are developed. Next, communication displays are made and stored in readily accessible locations. Finally, interactive training strategies are provided in the context of natural environments and activities. For students with severe developmental disabilities, training often occurs outside of the classroom in home, work, or community settings. The focus of the curriculum is usually on the acquisition of functional life skills.

Functional Curriculum Models and AAC

The content of educational and communication programs for older students with severe developmental disabilities is often based on a functional curriculum model. The activities that are targeted for instruction are based on four domains: the domestic domain, the recreation and leisure domain, the vocational domain, and the community domain (Brown et al., 1979).

The domestic domain consists of activities that relate to functioning in the home or living environment. Examples of activities in this domain include meal preparation, doing laundry, and self-care activities. The recreation and leisure domain is a very critical programming area for adults and adolescent students with severe disabilities. Typically, these individuals have large amounts of spare or "down" time. Examples of activities that could be targeted for instruction in this domain include learning how to play games, or participating in community activities such as bowling or going to the library.

The vocational domain emphasizes learning work skills or work-related skills. Instruction might focus on janitorial skills, skills for working in a fast food restaurant, or working in a motel. Instruction for the vocational domain will often be provided at the actual work site in the community. The community domain focuses on skills that are needed in order to access services in the community. Examples of activities that could be targeted for instruction include going shopping, ordering a meal in a restaurant, or learning how to access local transportation. This instruction usually is provided in the community as well.

Again, the first step in the design of the student's AAC system is to identify and prioritize activities. According to Elder and Goossens (1994), functional curriculum activities for AAC should be prioritized based on their frequency, motivational value, and whether or not the activity is part of the student's educational or rehabilitation plan. Activity-based communication boards are preferred to generic communication boards, which are too general to foster meaningful communication exchange. It is very important to select activities that are interactive in nature. Putting on makeup or washing clothes may be more solitary activities and not require communication boards, whereas discussing with peers what video to rent, going to the doctor, or discussing the weather are more interactive. Message sets are then developed for the targeted activities.

Message sets for older students who use AAC systems are primarily phrase based. The type of symbols, size of symbols and their arrangement on the overlay will depend on the motor and visual skills of the individual student. Generally, it is helpful to arrange the layout of vocabulary in keeping with the natural order of the activity.

Aided language stimulation techniques using a scripted-dialogue approach are used to facilitate communication interaction. Strategies such as the shadow light cues, expansion/exclusion templates, and sabotage techniques are used in conjunction with the scripted-dialogue approach (Elder & Goossens, 1994).

Portability is an important issue for students with disabilities in a functional curriculum. Domestic, recreation-leisure, vocational, and community goals are best exercised in the community setting. For these students, classroom engineering is less applicable. Making communication displays readily accessible in work or home environments is a more age-appropriate focus. Smaller, more lightweight voice output devices such as the WalkerTalker, the MessageMate, or the Pocket Talker are easy to carry in community settings and are easy to program. Carrying straps and mounting systems for wheelchairs, walkers, or motorized scooters should be designed as needed.

Transition Services

The ultimate goal of the educational system is to prepare all students to be independent, productive members of society. This is a challenging goal for students without disabilities; however, for students with disabilities this presents an even greater challenge to the educational system. One of the expected outcomes is that students will leave the educational system with skills to enter the work force. This outcome should also hold true for students with disabilities.

Work is considered an important and valued component of our society. The ability to work and be employed provides not only monetary rewards but also personal rewards such as an improved quality of life and self-esteem. Public school service providers need to be knowledgeable about legislation that affects transition, as well as vocational opportunities for students

with disabilities. Laws that are directly related to the provision of services for assisting individuals with disabilities in becoming employable are The Individuals with Disabilities Education Act (IDEA), The Rehabilitation Act, The American with Disabilities Act, and The Medicaid Act. The reader is referred to Chapter 9 for more information on these federal statutes.

IDEA Mandated Transition Services

IDEA specifically addresses the provision of transition services for students with disabilities. Transition services are described as activities that promote movement from school to postschool activities. Postschool activities may include postsecondary education, vocational training, integrated employment, supported employment, continuing and adult education, adult services, independent living, or community participation. Transition services must be addressed in the IEP for students in special education at age 16, or can be identified earlier if decided by the IEP committee. Transition services are determined on an individual basis and may include instruction, community experiences, the development of daily living skills, the development of employment or related objectives, or a functional vocational evaluation. Agencies that provide adult services are expected to be involved in the transition process before the student leaves the educational system. The intent is to eliminate service gaps which have historically occurred for students with disabilities.

School to Work AAC Transition Issues

For students transitioning to work, AAC systems and services need to be addressed early as part of the transition process. Issues to be addressed include (a) the acquisition of a dedicated AAC system, (b) communication proficiency with the AAC system, (c) integration of the communication system into community experiences, (d) provision of employer awareness training, and (e) the identification of a back-up AAC system.

In the final 2 or 3 years of public school, the goal of the AAC team is be sure that students will matriculate owning and operating their AAC systems to the best of their abilities. Funding AAC devices and services becomes a major obstacle once students leave the educational system. Blackstone (1990c) warned that after age 21 it becomes very difficult to find AAC service providers.

The key to a successful transition of services to the adult world is to start early. If the communication device was on loan from the school system, then securing another device is critical. If the team is recommending a change in device, then the device should be obtained with sufficient time prior to graduation to create the necessary overlays and train the user. If a device is obtained too late, then the individual may leave the school system without becoming proficient in its use. Because there is often significant fragmentation and delays in the provision of adult services, there may be insufficient resources available to help with AAC training once the student leaves school.

It is critical to establish service connections to adult agencies for students with AAC needs prior to when they exit the school system. It is very difficult to establish these services once students are in the community. Finding and funding service providers for adults who require AAC support in the community is often very challenging.

AAC Training in Real Life Settings

As the individual who relies on AAC prepares for the transition to work, the AAC team should collaborate with the family, job coach, and vocational counselor to create overlays that will assist the individual in the school-to-work transition. Work-related, community-related, home-related, and recreation-related overlays should be updated to meet upcoming communication needs. Opportunities to practice the use of these overlays in their real life settings is an important step. Whenever possible, it is highly beneficial for school staff to acquaint the employer or supervisor, as well as fellow workers, with how best to interact with an individual using various AAC systems. AAC systems should include low tech communication systems that will serve as a back-up when high tech devices are not operational. Although the transition to work marks the end of the school years, it is the start of a new AAC chapter in the life of a nonspeaking individual. Chapter 17 provides more information regarding implementing AAC in adult program settings.

CONCLUSION

There are many students in the public schools who could benefit from AAC. Unfortunately, not all students who need AAC receive these services. Although there has been an increase in information regarding the field of AAC and legislation to support the provision of AAC in public schools, there are still many barriers to overcome. School districts need to strive to make the provision of AAC services a routine part of the child-centered educational process (i.e., referral-evaluation-IEP development-implementation-review) for any student who has unmet verbal or written expression needs.

Providing AAC services in the educational environment presents unique challenges. In order to meet the needs of students who require AAC and to fulfill the assistive technology requirements of IDEA, public schools need to have access to professionals who are knowledgeable about AAC. Courses in AAC should be required in preservice programs for special educators, speech-language pathologists, physical therapists, and occupational therapists.

AAC service delivery models will vary among school districts, depending on size and geographical location. Essential components of the service delivery models should include a team approach, family involvement, intervention in natural environments, and intervention integrated in natural contexts. Public schools should try to eliminate "pull-out" programs as a service delivery method for students receiving AAC services. Traditional service delivery methods are often ineffective for AAC intervention (Blackstone, 1990c).

In order for students with severe communication disabilities to receive a "free, appropriate, public education" and be meaningfully included in the least restrictive environment, access to AAC devices and services must be provided. AAC devices and services need to be provided early in preschool programs, so that young students with AAC needs can experience the power of communication in controlling their environment. In addition, they will need an AAC system in place so that they can enter the regular school program with their peers.

Students with AAC needs will require ongoing support and intervention throughout their elementary and secondary years. As students prepare to transition from school to postschool activities, the school and adult service agencies need to be sure that AAC devices and services will be provided once the student exits the school system.

AAC offers much promise and hope for students with severe communication disabilities, and their parents. The acquisition of an AAC device is not sufficient to fulfill the promise. It is the administrators and service providers who will determine if the promise of AAC will become a reality.

REFERENCES

American Speech-Language-Hearing Association. (1989). Competencies for speech-language-pathologists providing services in augmentative communication. *ASHA, 31*, 107–110.

Berninger, V., & Gans, B. (1986). Assessing word processing capability of the nonvocal, nonwriting. *Augmentative and Alternative Communication, 2*, 56–63.

Beukelman, D., & Mirenda, P. (1992). *Augmentative and alternative communication: Management of severe communication disorders in children and adults.* Baltimore, MD: Paul H. Brookes Publishing Co.

Blackstone, S. (1990a). In pursuit of opportunities and interdependence. *Augmentative Communication News, 3*(3), 1–4.

Blackstone, S. (1990b). Early prevention of severe communication disorders. *Augmentative Communication News, 3*(1), 1–5.

Blackstone, S. (1990c). Populations and practices in AAC. *Augmentative Communication News, 3*(4), 2–4.

Blackstone, S. (1995a). AAC teams. *Augmentative Communication News, 8*(4), 1–3.

Blackstone, S. (1995b). What's the verdict? *Augmentative Communication News, 8*(5), 1–4.

Brown, L., Branston, M., Hamre-Nietupski, S., Pumpian, I., Certo, N., & Gruenwald, L. (1979). A strategy for developing chronologically age-appropriate and functional curricular content for severely handicapped adolescents and young adults. *Journal of Special Education, 13*, 81–90.

Burkhart, L. (1980). *Homemade battery powered toys and educational devices for severely handicapped children.* (Available from author, 6201 Candle Court, Eldersburg, MD 21784.)

Burkhart, L. (1982). *More homemade battery devices for severely handicapped children with suggested activities.* (Available from author, 6201 Candle Court, Eldersburg, MD 21784.)

Burkhart, L. (1987). *Using computers and speech synthesis to facilitate communicative interaction with young and/or severely handicapped children.* Wauconda, IL: Don Johnston Developmental Equipment, Inc.

Calculator, S. N., & Jorgensen, C. M. (1991). Integrating AAC instruction into regular education settings: Expounding on best practices. *Augmentative and Alternative Communication, 7*, 204–214.

Elder, P., & Goossens, C. (1994). *Engineering daily living and vocational training environments for interactive symbolic communication: Adolescents and adults who are moderately/severely developmentally delayed.* Birmingham, AL: Southeast Augmentative Communication Conference Publication Clinician Series.

Falvey, M. (1989). *Community-based curriculum: Instructional strategies for students with se-*

vere handicaps. Baltimore, MD: Paul H. Brookes.

Gartner, A., & Lipsky, D. K. (1987). Beyond special education: Toward a quality system for all students. *Harvard Educational Review, 57,* 367–395.

Goossens, C., & Crain, S. (1986a). *Augmentative communication assessment resource.* Wauconda, IL: Don Johnston Developmental Equipment, Inc.

Goossens, C., & Crain, S. (1986b). *Augmentative communication intervention resource.* Wauconda, IL: Don Johnston Developmental Equipment, Inc.

Goossens, C., Crain, S., & Elder, P. (1992). *Engineering the preschool environment for interactive symbolic communication: 18 months to 5 years developmentally.* Birmingham, AL: Southeast Augmentative Communication Conference Publication Clinician Series.

Goossens, C., Crain, S., & Elder, P. (1994a). *Communication displays for engineered preschool environments: Book 1.* Solana Beach, CA: Mayer-Johnson Company.

Goossens, C., Crain, S., & Elder, P. (1994b). *Communication displays for engineered preschool environments: Book II.* Solana Beach, CA: Mayer-Johnson Company.

Guralnick, M. (1981). The social behavior of preschool childen at different developmental levels: Effects of group composition. *Journal of Experimental Child Psychology, 31*(1), 115–130.

Haney, C., & Kangas, K. (1987). The assessment and evaluation of clients for augmentative communication systems: The Pennsylvania model. *Planning, implementation and assessment of students in a statewide assistive device center.* Harrisburg, PA: Pennsylvania Department of Education.

Kelford Smith, A., Thurston, S., Light, J., Parnes, P., & O'Keefe, B. (1989). The form and use of written communication produced by physically disabled individuals using microcomputers. *Augmentative and Alternative Communication, 5,* 115–124.

King-DeBaun, P. (1989). *Storytime: Stories, symbols and emergent literacy activities for young, special needs children.* Acworth, GA: Creative Communicating.

Koppenhaver, D., Evans, D., & Yoder, D. (1991). Childhood reading and writing experiences of literate adults with severe speech and motor impairments. *Augmentative and Alternative Communication, 7,* 20–33.

Koppenhaver, D., & Pierce, P. (1992). Literacy and AAC: Communicating every which way we can. *Proceedings of the 13th Annual Southeast Augmentative Communication Conference,* pp. 71–93. Birmingham, AL: Southeast Unlimited Communications.

Koppenhaver, D. A., & Yoder, D. E. (1990). *Classroom interaction, literacy acquisition, and nonspeaking children with physical impairments.* Paper presented at the biennial meeting of the International Society for Augmentative and Alternative Communication, Stockholm, Sweden.

Korsten, J. E., Dunn, D. K., Foss, T. V., & Francke, M. K. (1993). *Every move counts: Sensory-based communication techniques.* Tucson, AZ: Therapy Skill Builders.

Larson, J., & Woodfin, S. (1989). *Augmentative communication: A developmental levels framework for assessment and intervention.* Austin, TX: The Live Oak Center for Communication Disorders.

Light, J., & Kelford Smith, A. (1993). Home literacy experiences of preschoolers who use AAC systems and of their nondisabled peers. *Augmentative and Alternative Communication, 9,* 10–25.

Lipsky, D., & Gartner, A. (1995). Common questions about inclusion: What does the research say? *Exceptional Parent, 25*(8), 36–39.

Locke, P., & Mirenda, P. (1992). Roles and responsibilities of special education teachers serving on teams delivering AAC service. *Augmentative and Alternative Communication, 8,* 200–214.

McLaughlin, M. J., & Warren, S. (1992). *Issues and options in restructuring schools and special education programs.* College Park, MA: University of Maryland at College Park & Westat, Inc.

Musselwhite, C. (1986). *Adaptive play for special needs children: Strategies to enhance communication and learning.* San Diego, CA: College-Hill Press.

Musselwhite, C., & St. Louis, K. (1988). *Communication programming for persons with severe handicaps.* (2nd ed.). Boston: College-Hill Press.

National Center on Education Restructuring and Inclusion. (1994). *National Survey on In-*

clusive Education (Summary). New York: The Graduate School and University Center, The City University of New York.

Nisbet, J. (1994). Education reform: Summary and recommendations. *The national reform agenda and people with mental retardation: Putting people first* (pp. 151–165). Washington, DC: U.S. Department of Health and Human Services.

Reed, P., & Bowser, G. (1991). The role of the occupational and physical therapist in assistive technology. *Tech Use Guide Using Computer Technology*. Reston, VA: The Center for Special Education Technology.

Rogers, J. (1993). The inclusion revolution. *Research Bulletin*. Bloomington, IN: Phi Delta Kappa.

Schweigert, P. (1989). Use of microswitch technology to facilitate social contingency awareness as a basis for early communication skills. *Augmentative and Alternative Communication, 5*, 192–198.

Seligman, M. (1975). *Helplessness: On depression, development, and death*. San Francisco: W. H. Freeman.

Siegel-Causey, E., & Downing, J. (1987). Nonsymbolic communication development: Theoretical concepts and educational strategies. In L. Goetz, D. Guess, & K. Stremmel-Campbell (Eds.), *Innovative program design for individuals with dual sensory impairments* (pp. 15–48). Baltimore: Paul H. Brookes Publishing Co.

Silverman, F. (1989). *Communication for the speechless* (2nd ed.). Englewood Cliffs, NJ: Prentice-Hall.

Van Dijk, J. (1967). The non-verbal deaf-blind child and his world: His outgrowth toward the world of symbols. *Proceedings of the Jaarverslag Instituut voor Doven,* 1964–1967 (pp. 73–110). Sint-Michielsgestel, Netherlands.

Villa, R. A., & Thousand, J. S. (Eds.) (1995). *Creating an inclusive school*. Alexandria, VA: Association for Supervision and Curriculum Development.

Wang, M. C., Reynolds, M. C., & Walberg, H. J. (1994). Serving students at the margins. *Educational Leadership, 52*, 12–17.

Life Stories

Bill's AAC Story: Team Collaboration

Nancy Underhill and Nancy Horne with Denise DeCoste

Bill's AAC story began when he was a 4-year-old student in a public preschool setting. His major deficit at the time was expressive language. He had little understandable speech. Even in context, much of what he had to say was unintelligible and impossible to comprehend. However, Bill was an active communicator; he had a highly developed gestural system, could mimic actions, and used facial expressions as a means of communication. In the classroom, Bill was beginning to show signs of frustration and "acting out" behaviors when he was unable to communicate. Clearly, Bill needed additional means to express his thoughts, needs, and feelings. Though his teachers perceived that Bill was cognitively normal, there were no test data available to confirm their feelings.

INTERVENTION STRATEGIES: TRADITIONAL SPEECH AND LANGUAGE THERAPY

Bill had been enrolled in a half-day early intervention program at his neighborhood elementary school since he was 3 years old. He had been receiving speech and language services 2 hours each week, concentrating on improving his verbal skills. Even with a year and a half of intervention, he could only produce five consonants: /b/, /d/, /p/, /n/, and /w/. Bill used vowels with these consonants in his attempts to communicate, but his productions consisted mainly of strings of unintelligible syllables. No diagnosis was attributed to Bill's lack of intelligible speech. He had also been taught a limited number of signs. By age 4, when Bill was making little to no progress in the acquisition of new speech sounds and his frustration with his inability to communicate was clearly growing, an assessment for augmentative communication was requested by the school team.

AAC ASSESSMENT: A SEQUENTIAL PROCESS

AAC assessment began in the natural context of Bill's preschool environment with the classroom teacher and the assistive technology specialist. It began by observing Bill communicating within individual and group activities. Although Bill was highly interactive in various classroom activities, his ability to make himself understood was clearly limited.

598

Classroom staff were consulted on communication play topics and vocabulary scripts that would be communicatively powerful and of high interest to Bill. Using selected topics, Bill was assessed for his ability to identify symbols, to understand symbol categories, for his ability to sequence symbols in a meaningful manner, for his ability to follow a series of directions, and for interest in voice output AAC devices. Bill quickly demonstrated his understanding of abstract symbols and was able to sequence three to four symbols to generate a sentence. Bill was also tested for knowledge of letters and sight words. He was able to recognize a few letters and sight words.

Additional data regarding Bill's response to various AAC systems was obtained during routine classroom activities over the next few weeks. AAC strategies were introduced to Bill on a trial basis in naturally occurring situations and data were collected on his performance. For example, picture communication symbols paired with written classmates' names were put on Language Master cards. Using the voice output of the Language Master, Bill was able to correctly call out the names of his peers during group activities. Small picture communication boards were developed for art, snack time, favorite play toys, feelings, weather, and animals. Initial picture communication boards included a limited set of symbols. For example, the snack board included four food choices, three drink choices, "more," "finished," and "thank you." Bill quickly mastered these boards, so more symbols were added. However, Bill found these to be limiting. He would frequently point to the communication board and then shrug his shoulders and shake his head "no," as if to say "what I want to tell you isn't here."

Next, Bill was introduced to an electronic voice output device called the DigiVox, which had been programmed with words and phrases for 36 picture symbols. Bill was highly motivated by the addition of speech. He was able to quickly visually scan the 36 symbols and correctly select his target symbol. However, it soon became clear that Bill needed a communication device with enough memory to allow for more vocabulary expansion. A DynaVox was secured on loan for a period of several weeks for assessment and evaluation purposes. Bill quickly learned how to locate his favorite symbol page: the "tool page." There was an activity station in the classroom supplied with plastic tools, and Bill used the DynaVox to interactively play there with his classmates. After only 2 weeks of classroom practice with the DynaVox, Bill took it to a classroom of fourth and fifth graders, showed them how it worked, answered questions using the device, and told them the "Humpty Dumpty" nursery rhyme using magnetic board pieces for visual effects, and the device for voice output.

FINAL RECOMMENDATIONS

Bill's AAC assessment data were reviewed by the school team and the assistive technology specialist. The results were shared with his family. Over time, as Bill demonstrated increased success with AAC, his family's interest in AAC was heightened. The DynaVox was the recommendation of choice and methods to obtain a DynaVox for Bill were discussed with the family. The school system was able to purchase a DynaVox for Bill to use as part of a long-term loan. The team also felt that Bill should continue to use his gestural language, sign language, and low tech communication boards for special situations, such as muddy playgrounds.

TRAINING AND IMPLEMENTATION STRATEGIES

Beginning use of the DynaVox occurred in the classroom with familiar topics and academic themes. Vocabulary planning for the device was a collaborative effort among school staff working with Bill. Training sessions were scheduled before or after school. Initially, short, frequent sessions were best. Ongoing programming for the DynaVox was a joint effort with the teacher, teaching assistant, and speech-language pathologist. All had important roles in fostering Bill's initiation of communicative interactions. In this case, Bill primarily used the DynaVox at school; his family chose not to use the DynaVox at home, preferring to use low tech communication routines that worked for them in their home environment.

Bill learned quickly and efficiently how to use the communication techniques that were presented to him. This was by design, carefully planned and monitored. Communication techniques were modeled to staff during planning sessions, and modeled with Bill during classroom activities. For example, using a "stacking the deck" technique, Bill's device was programmed with information on a topic no one else had in the classroom. Bill's peers were then encouraged to ask him questions on this topic. In this way, Bill's use of the AAC system and interactive communication with his peers was developed simultaneously. This technique went a long way toward building respect for Bill's abilities on the part of his classmates. There was a concerted effort on the part of the team to avoid situations where Bill would use his AAC device with only his teaching assistant and other adults.

THE UPS AND DOWNS OF AAC

Because Bill had no physical disabilities resulting in motor access problems and because he was cognitively normal, his AAC story may seem less complicated than others. However, two recurring problems demonstrate that even in relatively straightforward AAC situations, the nature of AAC consultation is anything but linear. One rec-curring problem arose when school staff had difficulty keeping pace with Bill's voracious need for new vocabulary. Lack of planning and programming time often interfered so that there were times when Bill did not have access to the language he needed to participate fully on different academic topics. Students using picture symbol devices are constrained by the vocabulary adults provide them. With bright students, it is very hard to keep pace with their vocabulary needs. Eventually, Bill would need to be taught how to access all the Dynavox vocabulary stored within the device, in an effort to provide him with more control to express novel thoughts. Special topic pages would continue to be organized based on Bill's interests and on educational curriculum content.

A second and related problem occurred whenever there was staff turnover. Each year Bill had a new teacher, at times, a new teaching assistant, and occasionally, new therapists. Sometimes long-term substitutes entered the picture due to illness or maternity leave. Each time this occurred, staff training was critical to Bill's ongoing communication success. When staff were not adequately trained, Bill's communication effectiveness declined. New vocabulary was not programmed into his device, his device was often not charged, and in general, the need for device repairs increased.

The need for ready access to input from the assistive technology specialist and the need for team collaboration was critical during these transition periods. Occasionally, staff changes resulted in team members who did not work as well together. When this occurred, there was less continuity in Bill's use of AAC because vocabulary design and device programming did not keep pace with the classroom curriculum. It was important to work out these difficulties in order to foster a team approach to AAC and to stress that AAC responsibilities do not rest with the speech-language pathologist alone. When this occurred, administrative support was crucial. Principals who communicate a child-centered philosophy where the needs of the student must be shared by all staff have a powerful influence on the integration of AAC in the school environment.

However, success breeds success. Little by little, staff learned to value Bill's need for AAC. Often, Bill was his own best advocate, as staff learned to appreciate the power of voice output. Bill's success with AAC required a team process with cooperation, planning, and shared workloads as the crucial ingredients. Regularly scheduled meetings were held with staff to discuss progress and to plan for the next steps in Bill's AAC development. Persistence to meet ever-changing circumstances on the part of Bill and the entire school team was a key factor throughout the AAC assessment and intervention process.

KEY POINTS TO REMEMBER

- When traditional speech and language treatment fails to meet communication needs, then AAC strategies must be considered.
- AAC assessment uses informal strategies to evaluate abilities in natural settings, such as the classroom, or as needed in one-on-one interactive settings.

- To involve the student initially, the vocabulary must be powerful. Find the student's interest, and use this information to build communication overlays.
- AAC assessment is a sequential process. Trial periods using selected AAC devices are needed to determine best systems and strategies.
- Trial periods with careful documentation will avoid costly mistakes. Loan, borrow, or rent communication devices before making final recommendations.
- Multiple AAC strategies, both low tech and high tech, are needed to meet communication needs across a wide variety of situations.
- Training and implementation plans are an integral part of the AAC intervention process. Ongoing consultation and technical support is critical.
- No one person can do it all; responsibilities must be shared. The school team needs to establish a clear delineation of responsibilities with regard to the student and the device: who will charge it, who will program it, how will vocabulary be selected, how will it be transported from class to class, and so forth.
- Success with student use of an AAC device can only occur as part of a team effort, which requires team cooperation, collaboration, and planning. Administrative support is crucial.

Chapter 16

AAC IN THE HOSPITAL SETTING

Sharon L. Glennen

ospitals are intimidating places for most people. Medical staff tend to "do to" patients rather than "work with" patients (Beukelman & Mirenda, 1992). The very word *patient* implies a passive, nondominant relationship with medical staff. Patients frequently enter hospitals with medical conditions or treatments that result in the inability to communicate to medical staff or family. Whether the nonspeaking condition is temporary or permanent, patients often feel frightened, angry, and powerless in the medical setting, feelings that can impede the recovery process. Providing augmentative and alternative communication (AAC) systems for persons who are unable to communicate is an important aspect of patient care in the hospital setting.

There are several different types of hospital settings that require AAC services. The first is the acute care hospital. Individuals are admitted for acute medical needs and are discharged as soon as they are medically stable. Inpatient stays can range from a single day to several months, depending on the individual's medical condi-

tion. The acute nature of various medical conditions often makes it difficult to provide AAC services in this setting. The second setting is the rehabilitation hospital. Patients in rehabilitation hospitals are medically stable, yet in need of therapy services in order to return home or to other facilities. Individuals are typically admitted for longer periods of time (1 week to several months) and are alert and able to participate in ongoing training programs. Finally, patients who cannot return home are admitted to chronic care hospital settings such as nursing homes or specialized chronic care hospital units. Some chronic care facilities specialize in certain medical conditions such as ventilator-dependent patients. Individuals are admitted for lengthy stays and vary in their ability to participate in ongoing therapy programs.

This chapter will focus on providing AAC services in the acute care medical setting. The chaotic nature of large acute care hospitals, the difficulty of working with persons who are not medically stable, and the brief amount of time that individuals are admitted to the hospital makes the provision of AAC services difficult for professionals in this setting. Although the focus is on acute care, many aspects of service delivery in this setting also apply to rehabilitation and chronic care hospital settings. For more information on working with adults in need of AAC rehabilitation services, please refer to Chapter 13.

THE ACUTE CARE SETTING

Acute care hospitals are systematically run in a chaotic manner. Individuals are often unavailable for services because of medical testing or family visits. Sometimes they are too fatigued to participate in service delivery. An acutely ill person can have 40 or more professionals involved in his or her care. Because care occurs 24 hours a day across three staff shifts, staff training is often difficult, if not impossible. Professionals who provide AAC services in this setting will need to be flexible yet aggressive throughout the service delivery process.

Hospitals are organized into units. Each unit specializes in the care of a certain type of patient. In a large teaching hospital, there can be over 20 different hospital units. Each unit has its own nursing staff, attending physicians, resident physicians, and support personnel. Some smaller units may share staff. Hospital specialists such as speech-language pathologists, occupational therapists, respiratory therapists, or neurologists may be assigned to a particular unit or may float across multiple units. Patients are assigned a charge nurse for each shift who is responsible for most care. Patients with intensive care needs may have multiple nurses assigned for care; those with lesser needs may share a charge nurse across several patients. It is not unusual in large hospitals for different units to have different management, teaming, charting, and patient care approaches.

DESCRIPTION OF THE POPULATION

Individuals admitted to an acute care hospital often have fluctuating medical, cognitive, and motor conditions. Those who are admitted with cerebral vascular accidents, spinal cord injury, degenerative diseases, closed head injury, open head injury, or cancer are often unable to communicate verbally during all or part of their hospital stay. For most individuals, the inability to speak is only a temporary byproduct of their medical condition. AAC may only be necessary for 1 or 2 days until their medical condition improves.

Due to the fluctuating nature of various medical conditions, providing AAC services to individuals with acute illness is often difficult. Medical concerns always have to be the primary focus of the hospital stay. Patients who are nonspeaking often cannot be seen for services until they are medically stable. During the early stages of hospitalization, they often cannot tolerate lengthy evalution or intervention sessions. Sessions may only last 10 or 15 minutes because of fatigue, pain, or confusion.

HOSPITAL STAFF

Many hospital professionals are not communication oriented when interacting with patients. Ashworth (1978) observed interactions between nurses and patients who were unable to speak due to medical conditions. She noted that most of the interactions were short-term instructions, commands, or physical care yes/no questions. Only 7% of the observed communications were longer and informative. Because hospital personnel are not focused on communication, many staff fail to refer nonspeaking individuals who are in need of AAC intervention. In a large teaching hospital, 75% of the referrals to the speech and language department were initially for swallowing evaluations, not communication. However, upon completing the swallowing evaluation, many individuals were also found to be nonspeaking (Mitsuda, Baarslag-Benson, Hazel, & Therriault, 1992).

Many hospital professionals are unaware of AAC intervention techniques. Within the author's hospital, patient referrals tend to cluster from specific units that have used our services in the past and realize the importance of AAC for persons who are nonspeaking. Other units rarely refer patients. Sometimes a unit that has been referring steadily will suddenly stop referring patients due to a personnel change. The physician or nurse who knew about our services left the unit and new staff were not trained to refer. AAC professionals will need to inform hospital staff repeatedly about the communication needs of patients and referral procedures for AAC services.

Because of the number of hospital professionals involved in patient care, the potential number of team members who need to be part of the AAC communication process is large. A brief review of potential team players in the hospital setting is listed here.

Physician

The physician often makes the initial written referral for AAC services. Physicians also make medical decisions that can change an individual's communication status. For example, the physician may decide to perform a tracheostomy, or may decide to provide ventilation. When AAC professionals want to use interventions that have medical implications, the physician will need to approve the decision. For example, the speech-language pathologist may want to deflate a cuffed trach tube during therapy sessions to provide the patient with an opportunity to speak. This intervention would need to be approved by the physician. Finally, physicians can provide guidance on specific medical information that is crucial for the patient to communicate to others. This information is then used in the development of the AAC system so the person can better communicate medical needs.

In a large teaching hospital, many physicians can be involved in a single person's care. The attending physician is board certified and in charge of supervising all medical practice on the hospital unit. Resident physicians often serve as the patient's primary doctor under the supervision of the attending physician. Finally, interns often accompany residents or other doctors, but do not provide medical care without direct supervision. In a teaching hospital, residents and interns often rotate between assignments. The resident may be working on a particular unit for the first time, or may be getting ready to leave the unit for another assignment. Specialists such as cardiologists, neurologists, pulmonary physicians, physiatrists, orthopedists, or otolaryngologists see patients when requested. They typically see patients for brief visits to complete medical evaluations or interventions. Specialists may make a single consultative visit or make frequent bedside visits to monitor an individual's medical status. Because of this constant rotation of physicians, AAC professionals need to make sure that medical staff are continually trained in communication interventions for a particular individual.

Nurse

Although the physician makes the initial referral for AAC services, it is often the nurse who asks the physician to make the referral. In some hospitals, nurse practitioners can make the written referral directly. Nurses are the staff members directly involved with ongoing care. Patients are assigned a primary nurse, who is responsible for overseeing all daily care. Depending on medical need, nurses can be assigned to a single person or have several assignments. Primary nurses are typically registered nurses who have completed bachelor or associate degree programs. There is a different primary nurse for each shift. Because nurses cannot work 7 days a week, the primary nurse can change from day to day. Most hospitals try to keep some continuity in primary nurse assignments in order to improve patient care. In addition to the primary nurse, there may be nursing aides who provide patient care under the direction of the primary nurse.

Because the nurse is the professional who spends the most time with the patient, it is important that the nursing staff be trained in AAC interventions. The nurse is usually present during visits from other medical professionals or family members. Therefore, the nursing staff often has the responsibility for training other professionals, family members, or visitors in how to implement AAC strategies. Nurses are also invaluable resources for planning vocabulary on AAC systems. They can assist in exchanging information between the AAC team and the physician or family. In the author's experience, the success or failure of AAC strategies in the hospital is almost always dependent on successful training and participation of the primary nurse.

Respiratory Therapist

Respiratory therapists are graduates of specialized training programs that teach the provision of respiratory care to patients in the medical setting. Individuals who are intubated, ventilated, or on oxygen are seen by the respiratory therapist. Most respiratory therapists are trained to consider medical health when making decisions about respiration. They are rarely trained to consider communication as a factor in the decision-making process (Mitsuda et al., 1992). The AAC specialist will need to consult with respiratory therapists to request changes in medical care that will improve communication. This can involve changes in ventilator settings, or in the type of trach tube being used. The respira-

tory therapist or physician should be present any time changes are made to a patient's ventilator or trach for communication purposes. For example, if an individual is changing to a one way trach speaking valve, the respiratory therapist should be present during the initial session. The physician will need to approve all decisions made by the respiratory therapist and the AAC specialist before implementation.

Occupational Therapist and Physical Therapist

These two professionals work with individuals as soon as they are medically stable. The physical therapist and the occupational therapist both monitor skin integrity and provide active range of motion along with passive range of motion exercises to bed-bound patients. The occupational therapist uses splints to prevent joint contractures, and teaches activities of daily living (ADLs) such as dressing, shaving, or eating. The physical therapist trains individuals to make position transfers, and to ambulate. Both specialists are important team members in the AAC process and provide the AAC professional with information regarding optimum patient positioning for AAC. In addition, the occupational therapist is often involved in assessing fine motor abilities for accessing AAC strategies. Both the occupational and the physical therapist should be consulted when planning vocabulary for AAC systems.

Recreation Therapist/ Child Life Specialist

In most large hospitals, as soon as a patient is medically stable, recreational therapists, or child life specialists, will begin to see the patient for bedside visits. When the person is able to leave the bed for short periods, the recreational therapist may see him in a larger recreational area. Recreational therapists are frequently the first link in providing individuals with a sense of normalcy during the hospital stay. At bedside, recreational therapists may play videos or music, may help write letters, or play games. The recreational therapist often provides individuals with an opportunity to communicate about nonmedical needs and issues. These specialists need to be taught how to communicate using a patient's AAC system, and should be consulted to develop appropriate vocabulary for recreational activities.

Social Worker

The social worker can provide the AAC specialist with information about the individual's background and family. Because it is sometimes difficult to make direct contact with family members in a large hospital setting, the social worker's information may be used as a substitute to develop vocabulary for an initial AAC system. The social worker can also provide information about the individual's adjustment to the hospital and medical condition. Finally, the social worker is often involved in determining discharge plans. The AAC professional can work with the social worker to plan for communication needs following discharge from the hospital.

Family

The family is often a forgotten component of AAC service delivery in the hospital. The social worker can provide the AAC specialist with information about family dynamics and the family's ability to cope with the patient's medical condition. Whenever possible, the family should be consulted in the vocabulary planning process. In addition, family members need to be trained to communicate using the AAC system.

Speech-Language Pathologist

In most hospital settings, the speech-language pathologist is the primary provider of AAC services. The speech-language pathologist evaluates, plans AAC interventions, consults with medical staff about plans for AAC, trains medical staff and family how to use the AAC system, and monitors use of AAC strategies during the hospital stay. Speech-language pathologists who work in acute care settings need to be knowledgeable about traditional forms of AAC such as direct selection and scanning communication systems. They also need to be knowledgeable about communication options for patients with ventilators and tracheostomies. Specific information about AAC evaluation and intervention procedures in the hospital setting will be described in the next sections of this chapter.

REFERRAL AND INITIAL AAC SCREENING

Referral Procedures

Individuals are referred for AAC services by the physician or sometimes by the nurse practitioner. Nursing staff are often the primary professionals who initially identify persons in need of referral. As stated previously, many nurses are not focused on communication issues in acute care medical settings. They may require training to make them aware of an individual's potential communication needs. Nurses need to be provided with simple criteria for referral that can be applied easily across patients and medical conditions.

Mitsuda et al. (1992) developed simple AAC referral criteria for nursing staff in their acute care hospital facility. Nursing staff and other medical personnel were then trained to follow the referral guidelines. The referral process involved the following sequence of questions and decision responses:

- Is the individual alert for short periods of time?
- Can the individual follow a simple one-

step command (i.e., blink eyes, squeeze a hand, move a foot on verbal command)?

Those persons who were alert and able to follow a one-step command were candidates for referral. Patients who were not alert or were unable to follow a simple command were monitored by the nursing staff until their conditions changed. For those who could follow a simple command, nursing staff were trained to refer the following categories of patients for AAC services:

• Persons who were intubated, ventilated, or trached.
• Persons who did not have respiratory interventions, yet were unable to communicate intelligibly using speech.

AAC Screening Procedures

Once the referral for AAC services is made, the speech-language pathologist initially completes a quick bedside screening. The screening serves several purposes: it reviews the success of existing communication strategies, determines if the individual is mentally and medically able to benefit from further AAC intervention, and identifies those persons who are in need of further evaluation. For many acute care patients, the initial AAC screening may be the only time they are seen by the speech-language pathologist. The person may be discharged, or may have a sudden change in communication status before a more formal evaluation can be completed. Decision-making procedures for an initial AAC screening based on the work of Mitsuda et al. (1992) are presented in detail below.

Patient Alertness

If the individual is asleep, fatigued, or appears disoriented, the screening is deferred until a later time. If family members are present, or the nurse is available, they can be interviewed to determine when the person is typically alert, and to obtain further information about current communication abilities.

Production of Yes/No Responses

Those who are alert and oriented can be seen by the AAC professional to find a motor response that is reliable for yes/no responding. Many times individuals will develop their own method for yes/no responding prior to being seen for AAC services. Nursing staff can often provide this information. Whenever possible, nonverbal movements that are used naturally for yes/no responses such as head nods should be used. These naturally occurring responses are readily understood by others without extensive training. Thumbs up/thumbs down and smile/frown are also easily understood by others if head nods are not reliable. If these naturally occurring gestures are not feasible, other methods of responding should be considered. Eye blinks (e.g., yes = one blink; no = two blinks), eye gaze (e.g., yes = eyes up; no = eyes down), raising fingers, or squeezing a hand are other possible methods of yes/no communication. Some patients may be unable to make consistent motor responses. These patients should be seen at a later time in consultation with the occupational therapist or physical therapist.

Listnener Comprehension of Communication Methods

Once a yes/no method of communication is developed, it should be practiced several times during the screening to make sure that the patient is aware of how to produce the yes/no response. Nursing staff and family members should be shown the system and asked to interact with the person for a brief period of time to make sure that they can clearly understand yes/no responses. Finally, the yes/no system should be recorded on a communication protocol which is posted prominently in the individual's room. Communication protocols are instructions for other medical staff regarding the AAC system. Information regarding the yes/no system or any other communication interventions are written onto the protocol. A copy of the communication protocol should also be placed in the front of the patient's medical chart and written into chart notes. It is helpful to write the protocols on brightly colored paper with large print so they are noticed by others. The protocol should be written in easy to understand language with step-by-step instructions. If needed, photographs or drawings of how to use the AAC system are attached. Figure 16–1 shows an example of a communication protocol.

COMMUNICATION PROTOCOL FOR

JANE DOE

1) JANE USES <u>EYEGAZE</u> TO ANSWER <u>YES/NO QUESTIONS</u>.

    Yes = Jane Will Look Up
    No = Jane Will Look Down

2) <u>SPELLING</u>: JANE USES A <u>COMMUNICATION BOARD</u>.

You will need to ask a series of yes/no questions using an alphabet board to help Jane choose letters for spelling messages.

Jane will use a "yes" eye gaze to choose letters when spelling her messages.

Specific instructions for using the communication board with Jane are written on the back of the board.

The communication board can be found hanging at the foot of her bed. Be sure to put it back in the same location when you are finished.

      If you have questions call: Sue Smith
                           Speech Language Pathology
                           KKI Building
                           Beeper #06743

Figure 16–1. Sample communication protocol.

Cognitive Status for Further Intervention

Persons who have just been admitted to an acute care hospital are not candidates for lengthy evaluations. During the initial visit, a brief screening of cognitive abilities is used to determine quickly if the individual has the potential to communicate complex information. Dowden, Honsinger, and Beukelman (1986) developed a simple cognitive status screening tool to use with intensive care patients who are nonspeaking. Most of the questions are designed to be answered with yes/no responses. The last two items of the screening require responding to motor commands. The commands that are listed can be varied, depending on the individual's physical abilities. Table 16–1 outlines the screening questions.

Children who are nonspeaking can also be screened using similar methods. Yes/no orientation questions will need to be adapted to match the child's developmental age. *The Children's Orientation and Amnesia Test* (COAT) (Ewings-Cobbs et al., 1984) is a cognitive screening measure that can easily be adapted for yes/no questions with children. Yes/no questions derived from the General Orientation section of the COAT can be substituted for those listed in Table 16–1. Questions might include: Is your name _____? Are you _____ years old? Are you in the _____ grade? and Do you have a brother/sister?

Dowden et al. (1986) collected data on the success or failure of AAC interventions based on a individual's cognitive status as determined by a screening tool. Persons who did not score well on the screening frequently were unable to use any AAC strategies successfully. It is suggested that individuals who are unable to respond correctly to at least two yes/no screening items are not candidates for further AAC intervention. Those patients should be monitored over time by the nursing staff for improvements in cognitive status. Those who are

Table 16–1. Cognitive screening tool for acute care patients.

Attending Behavior:
- Responds to Spoken Name.
- Responds to "look at me."

Orientation Questions:
- Is your name _____?
- Is the current year _____?
- Is _____ your home town?
- Are you married?

Single Step Commands:
- Close your eyes.
- Open your mouth.

Source: "Serving Nonspeaking Patients in Acute Care Settings: An Intervention Approach" by P. Dowden, M. Honsinger, and D. R. Beukelman, 1986, *Augmentative and Alternative Communication*, 2, p. 26. Copyright 1986 by Williams and Wilkins. Reprinted with permission.

unable to respond correctly should also be screened by an audiologist to rule out the possibility of hearing loss.

Beyond Yes/No Communication

Individuals who are cognitively alert are often ready for a more sophisticated system of communication which will allow them to communicate more than yes/no responses. Nursing staff and family members are interviewed to determine the communication needs of the person. If possible, the individual is also interviewed using the established yes/no system. This portion of the screening is similar to the needs assessment process presented at length in Chapter 5. In the hospital setting the needs assessment process should review the individual's physical environment (e.g., bedside, wheelchair, ambulatory), medical interventions (e.g., oxygen masks, nasogastric tubes), potential communication partners, and possible messages that will need to be communicated to others (Dowden et al., 1986).

Another factor to be considered is the temporary nature of most nonspeaking medical conditions in the hospital. For example, a person may not be able to speak due to an endotracheal tube. Yet the tube is expected to be removed within 24 hours. The speech-language pathologist may elect to delay implementation of a more complex system until after the tube has been removed. At that time, the person can be re-screened to confirm that verbal communication has returned and is intelligible to others. All of these factors should be considered when deciding to move beyond a simple yes/no communication system in the acute care hospital setting.

AAC INTERVENTION APPROACHES IN THE HOSPITAL SETTING

Individuals who are candidates for further AAC intervention will need to be evaluated. The goal of the evaluation process is to develop a method of communication that is easy to use, independent from listener assistance, and close to natural communication. The key to successful AAC outcomes in the hospital setting is simplicity. Any technique that requires extensive learning on the part of the communicator or listener is not practical within the acute care hospital setting and will be frustrating for both communication partners.

Fried-Oken, Howard, and Stewart (1991) collected retrospective information from five adults who were temporarily unable to speak during their hospital intensive care admissions. Across all five adults there was a preference for simple communication systems that could be used independently. Electronic communication systems were frequently mentioned as being difficult to learn and were judged unsatisfactory by most participants. Communication methods that involved a listener positioning equipment or required the listener to par-

ticipate in message formulation were also judged as unsatisfactory.

AAC interventions in the hospital setting can be divided into three categories based on the individual's motor capabilities (Dowden, Honsinger, & Beukelman, 1986). The initial screening usually provides information regarding which category is appropriate. Further evaluation is needed to develop a specific intervention approach within the chosen category. The AAC intervention categories are:

- Oral and Modified Speech Approaches: used with individuals who have good oral motor skills.
- Direct Selection Approaches: used with individuals who have poor oral motor skills, but good fine motor abilities.
- Scanning/Switch Access Approaches: used with individuals who have poor oral motor and poor fine motor abilities.

The next section of this chapter will review communication options within each of the three AAC intervention categories.

ORAL AND MODIFIED SPEECH APPROACHES

Individuals who have good oral motor abilities are candidates for oral and modified speech interventions. This type of intervention is preferred because it most closely resembles natural speech. Persons who are intubated with nasal endotracheal tubes or have tracheostomies are candidates for these approaches. These approaches are used frequently within acute care settings. Dowden, Beukelman, and Lossing (1986) collected retrospective data on 50 nonspeaking persons admitted to acute care settings in the University of Washington Hospital. Of the patients reviewed, 49% were found to benefit from oral and modified speech intervention approaches.

Endotracheal Tubes

Many critically ill patients are intubated with endotracheal tubes in the emergency room. These tubes are inserted whenever a patient will need ventilator assistance for respiration. Endotracheal tubes may remain in place for only a few hours or for several days. Because of the risk of laryngeal stenosis, a tracheostomy is performed if respiratory difficulties will continue past 7 to 10 days. Tracheostomy is also performed to reduce the costs of medical care. Individuals who are intubated need to be cared for in intensive care and critical care units of the hospital. Patients with tracheostomies can be moved to other hospital units or discharged from the hospital (Kirchner & Astrachan, 1988).

Endotracheal tubes can be inserted either orally or nasally. Oral endotracheal tubes can be inserted and removed quickly. They are typically used during the emergency stage of patient care. Because the tube is inserted into the patient's mouth, the patient will be unable to mouth words or speak to others. Persons with oral endotrach tubes will need a direct selection or switch/scanning method of AAC.

Nasal endotracheal tubes are used when the individual is past the emergency stage. The tube passes through the nasal opening into the pharyngeal area, and beyond the vocal folds into the trachea. Patients with nasal endotracheal tubes have the potential to mouth words, but are unable to phonate because the vocal folds are blocked by the tube. Buccal speech (e.g., using air from the cheeks as a sound source) or an electrolarynx are appropriate interventions for these patients. More information about electrolarynges is presented later in this chapter.

Tracheostomy

Tracheostomy is a surgical procedure that creates an opening in the trachea between the second and third tracheal ring. The opening created during surgery is called a stoma. Tracheostomy tubes, commonly referred to as trach tubes, are placed into the stoma to keep the airway open, and to facilitate the delivery of oxygen or moisturized air through the trach tube to the lungs. It is estimated that over 48,000 temporary tracheostomy procedures and 6,000 permanent tracheostomies are performed annually (Pokras, 1987, in Tippett & Siebens, 1995).

Some patients who are incapable of independent respiration require ventilators to provide oxygen in addition to the tracheostomy. Individuals who are medically stable can often be weaned off the ventilator until they are breathing room air through the tracheostomy. However, the process of weaning a patient from the ventilator can take days or weeks. Other patients remain on ventilation for lengthy periods of time, or can remain on ventilation for the rest of their lives. In 1990, it was estimated that there were over 11,419 patients who were chronically dependent on ventilators in the United States (American Association for Respiratory Care, 1991).

There are many communication options for individuals with tracheostomies. The options vary according to the type of trach tube being used and the presence of ventilation. The physician and respiratory therapist will make medical decisions regarding trach tubes and ventilation. However, they may not consider the person's communication status as part of the decision-making process (Mitsuda et al., 1992; Tippet & Siebens, 1995). The speech-language pathologist should also be a part of the decision-making team.

Trach Tube Components

The trach tube consists of several parts (see Figure 16–2). The outer cannula is the outside tube that keeps the stoma open. An inner cannula rests inside the outer cannula and delivers air through the tube into the

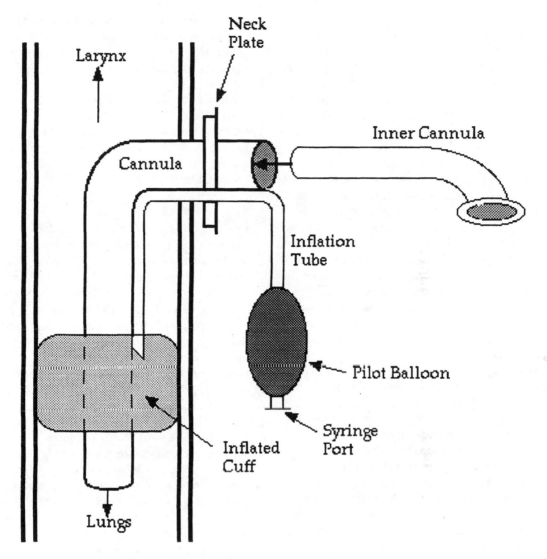

Figure 16–2. Cuffed tracheostomy tube components.

trachea. Trach tubes are classified as cuffed or cuffless trachs. A cuff is a small inflatable soft plastic ring attached to the cannula. Inflation of the cuff blocks the trachea completely to prevent aspiration and to prevent air escaping from the airway. Cuffed trachs have an inflation tube exiting the trach at the neck opening. The cuff is inflated and deflated using the inflation tube. A syringe is typically used to inject air to inflate the cuff. Maintaining the cuff at the appropriate level of inflation is important. Excessive pressure causes tracheal wall difficulties, insufficient pressure increases the chances of aspiration.

Cuffless trachs do not have the cuffed ring, and therefore do not block the potential flow of air through the upper airway. Typically, persons who are not ventilator dependent and are not at risk for aspiration are candidates for noncuffed trachs. More recently, Tippet and Siebens (1995) advocated using noncuffed trachs or temporarily deflating the cuff on cuffed trachs with ventilator-dependent patients. Although the primary purpose of the cuffed trach is to protect the lungs from aspiration, most cuffed trachs create an imperfect seal that can leak secretions. The continued pressure on the trachea from the cuff contributes to desensitization of the trachea and laryngeal musculature. This decreases the individual's protective cough mechanism when aspirations do occur. Secretions that pool on top of the cuff have also been noted to cause inflammation of the tracheal wall (Siebens, Tippett, Kirby, & French, 1993). Continued inflation of the cuff interferes with blood flow to the musculature. Over time, necrosis, tracheomalacia (softening), scarring, or granulation can occur to the tracheal and laryngeal area (Tippett & Siebens, 1995). Based upon these negative impacts, cuffless trach tubes or deflation of the cuff for extended periods are advocated for the majority of patients with tracheostomies (Tippett & Siebens, 1995).

Patients who are medically stable can move from using a trach tube to using a tracheo-stoma button. Trach buttons are short outer cannulas that are simply used to keep the stoma open. There is no other attached tubing or cuff. Trach buttons are used with patients who are not ventilator dependent, and may only need the trach for certain conditions such as frequent suctioning. Patients who are being weaned toward closure of the tracheal opening also use trach buttons. The trach button can be occluded with a closure plug for increasing periods each day until the person is able to tolerate breathing normally.

Communication Options for Persons with Tracheostomies

There are many modified speech communication options for individuals with tracheostomies. The options vary according to the type of trach used, and the presence of ventilation. As stated previously, decisions regarding the trach tube, ventilation, and communication options are made by the speech-language pathologist in conjunction with the physician, nurse and respiratory therapist.

Options for Cuffless Trachs

Cuffless trachs do not block the flow of air from the lungs past the vocal folds. Because the trach is positioned below the vocal folds, there is nothing to block phonation from occurring. During respiration, the majority of air will flow out of the stoma opening which impedes the ability to phonate. However, if the stoma is blocked in some manner, airflow is directed upward past the vocal folds. Phonation and speech then occur in a natural manner. The stoma opening can be occluded in several ways. Simply placing a finger over the outer cannula during exhalation will block the stoma opening and force the air upward. If a patient cannot do this independently, nurses and family members can be trained to occlude the opening. Because of hygiene issues, sterile gloves should be worn when occluding the stoma with a finger.

One way speaking valves can also be used to occlude the stoma opening. These valves are placed over the outer cannula. Their design allows for the inhalation of air through the trach tube, but blocks the exhalation of air through the tube. Use of a one way speaking valve bypasses the need to occlude the stoma manually. These valves are frequently used by persons who have the ability to manually occlude the trach because it frees up their hands to do other tasks.

There are several different types of one way speaking valves available (see Figure 16–3). Most use either a moving ball that blows back and forth to open and close the valve opening or a circular membrane that is pushed back and forth during respiration. The Passy Muir valve consists of a circular flap that rests in a closed position and is blown open to allow for airflow during in-

One Way Speaking Valves

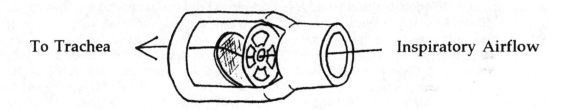

To Trachea ← Inspiratory Airflow

Circular Membrane Valve

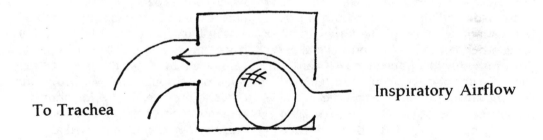

To Trachea — Inspiratory Airflow

Hopkins Ball Valve

Figure 16-3. One way speaking valves.

spiration (Passy, 1986). The Hopkins one way speaking valve consists of a ball mechanism that is sucked toward the cannula during inspiration, allowing for airflow. During exhalation the ball is pushed forward to close off airflow out of the cannula (French, Siebens, Kummell, Kirby, & Eisele, 1984).

Before recommending use of a one way speaking valve, individuals should be evaluated by the team to determine their candidacy. Respiratory and laryngeal status should be evaluated by occluding the cannula manually during expiration. The resulting attempts to phonate should be evaluated to determine if the individual will be able to phonate without shortness of breath, inspiratory stridor, significant effort, or altered voice quality. If good phonation is achieved, then use of a one way speaking valve is indicated (Tippett & Siebens, 1995).

Options for Cuffed Trachs

When a cuffed trach is inflated, the cuff completely fills the tracheal area, blocking the flow of air from moving upward past the vocal folds. Individuals can mouth words but cannot achieve phonation without using other methods. There are several options for achieving phonation that can be tried. These options can only be attempted with the authorization of the physician and respiratory therapist. One method is to partially or totally deflate the trach tube cuff. Because of the risk of aspiration, cuff deflation should only be done by medical staff who are trained in the procedure. Deflation is done in conjunction with suctioning to remove any secretions that may have pooled in the trachea above the cuff. Once the cuff has been deflated, using the occlusion methods mentioned previously (e.g., manual blocking, or a one way speaking valve) pushes the airflow upward past the vocal folds, resulting in natural phonation. Some patients will only be able to have their cuffs deflated for a brief time; others may be medically ready to have the cuff de-

flated for longer periods. As stated previously, the cuffed trach should be deflated whenever possible because of negative medical impacts.

A fenestrated trach can also be used. Fenestrated trachs have small openings in the upper posterior area of the outer cannula (see Figure 16–4). This opening is above the level of the cuff. When the inner cannula is in place, air does not reach the outer cannula, or the fenestration opening, which blocks air from moving upward past the vocal folds. When the inner cannula is removed and the trach tube is occluded, air can flow through the fenestration opening and phonation can occur. To achieve maximum phonation, the cuff can also be partially or totally deflated. Fenestrated trachs can have numerous problems (Tippett & Siebens, 1995). The small opening is often blocked by secretions, and it is difficult to place the cannula so that the opening allows for unobstructed airflow.

Talking trachs are specially designed cuffed trachs that have an extra air tube which courses over the upper portion of the outer cannula. Air can be directed through a fenestration opening for phonation. Talking trachs have fully inflated cuffs and inner cannulas that direct the patient's exhalations out through the trach opening. In order to provide airflow for phonation, a separate external air catheter line sends an outside source of compressed air through the fenestration opening. The external air line is manually regulated by occluding an opening on the side of the catheter. Because the airflow source is external, phonation can occur during both inspiration and exhalation. Talking trachs are used for individuals who cannot tolerate cuff deflation, or who are at great risk for aspiration. Patients who cannot occlude the catheter independently will need to rely on nursing staff or family to perform the occlusion process manually. The same weaknesses noted for fenestrated trachs are duplicated when attempting to use talking trachs. In

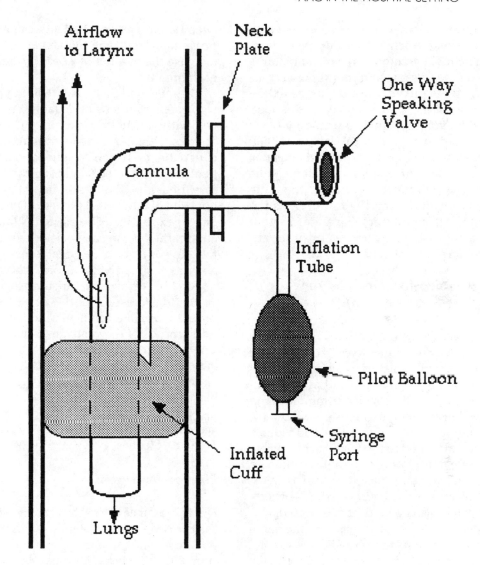

Figure 16–4. Fenestrated tracheostomy tube components.

addition, the compressed air source alters voice quality, and may audibly leak around the stoma opening. Tippett and Siebens (1995) noted that they had only limited success with talking trachs in their rehabilitation setting.

Ventilators

Ventilators are primarily used for patients with spinal cord injuries that result in respi-

ratory inefficiency or failure. Spinal cord injuries at a C3 level or above will result in complete ventilator dependence for respiration (Mitsuda et al., 1992). Ventilators are also used when patients have lower cervical and high thoracic spinal cord injuries which result in respiratory difficulties due to weaknesses of the intercostal and abdominal muscles. Patients with muscle weakness due to neuromuscular disease often require ventilators toward the end stages of their disease. Patients are attached to ventilators by endotracheal tubes, or trach tubes.

The most common type of ventilator is the Volume Cycle ventilator (Mitsuda et al., 1992). Air is pushed into the lungs until a predetermined tidal volume level is met. The tidal volume equals the amount of air exchanged in each breath. Using tidal volume as a maximum cutoff prevents pushing excessive air into the lungs, which can be damaging over time. For an adult, the ventilator is set to deliver 10 to 14 breaths per minute. All ventilators have alarms that ring when pressure changes or other airway obstructions occur.

Communication Options for Ventilator Dependent Patients

Speech-language pathologists will need to work closely with the physician, nurse, and respiratory therapist to maximize the communication potential of ventilator dependent patients. The specific communication method prescribed depends on the type of tube being used to deliver air. Individuals who are attached to the ventilator by an endotracheal tube will not be able to phonate as the tube extends past the vocal folds. Direct selection or scanning methods of communication will need to be considered.

Persons who are attached to the ventilator by a trach tube are candidates for oral or modified speech approaches. Trach tube procedures that were outlined previously in this chapter also apply to ventilator dependent patients. Talking trachs, deflation of cuffed trachs, and one way speaking valves are all options that will provide ventilator dependent patients with laryngeal phonation. When using cuffed trachs, patients will need to learn to time voicing for speech with the exhalation cycles of the ventilator. Manipulations to ventilator settings can increase the time available for speaking on each cycle. These manipulations include decreasing air flow rates during exhalation and reducing pause time between breath cycles. Patients can also improve speaking time by talking quickly to increase the number of words produced on each breath.

Tippett and Siebens (1995) advocated using cuffless trachs or deflating cuffed trachs with downsized cannulas (Shiley or Jackson Number 6) for ventilator dependent patients. To achieve phonation, the patient is taught to speak during the inspiratory phase of the ventilator. This is the opposite of the normal process of phonating during expiration. The patient is taught to control the opening and closing of the vocal folds to vary glottal resistance. Instructions such as "tighten your throat," "hold your breath," or "push down" are used to achieve adduction (closure) of the vocal folds. In order to facilitate communication, the inspiratory phase of the ventilator is lengthened. The tidal volume level of the ventilator is also increased to compensate for cuff deflation air leakage from the glottis. This procedure has been used successfully to restore communication in ventilator dependent patients across multiple studies (Bach & Alba, 1990; Tippett & Siebens, 1995).

Electrolarynges

Electrolarynges are external sound sources that provide voicing for individuals who are unable to phonate but have good articulation abilities. Electrolarynges can be used with persons with nasoendotracheal tubes or cuffed trach tubes that cannot be deflated. They can also be used with those who have sustained vocal fold damage and are unable to phonate. There are two types of electrolarynges: neck placement and oral.

Neck-type electrolarynges have a flat surface that is placed on the neck in a position that provides good sound resonation (see Figure 16–5). A button on the electrolarynx is pushed to generate vibrations for phonation. When the button is pushed, the patient mouths words to talk. There are many models of neck-type electrolarynges

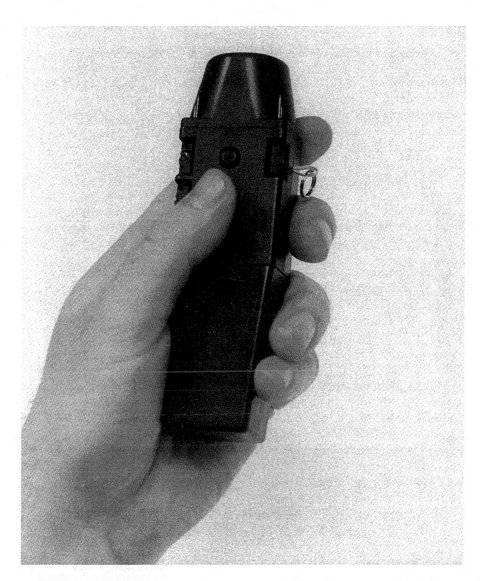

Figure 16–5. Denrick 2 neck placement artifical larynx. Photo courtesy of Luminaud Inc.

available. Using a neck-type electrolarynx requires good upper extremity strength. The individual needs to hold the electrolarynx in place against the neck and push the on/off button. Sometimes a communication partner can be trained to hold the device and push it on and off. Using a communication partner to operate the electrolarynx is difficult and usually does not result in a good outcome.

Oral electrolarynges consist of a plastic tube that is attached to the vibration source and inserted into the mouth (see Figure 16–6). The exact positioning of the tube varies with each individual. The user pushes a button on the electrolarynx to generate the vibration tone. Oral electrolarynges are useful for those who cannot use neck-type devices due to neck injuries or braces. Luminaud has developed a remote-

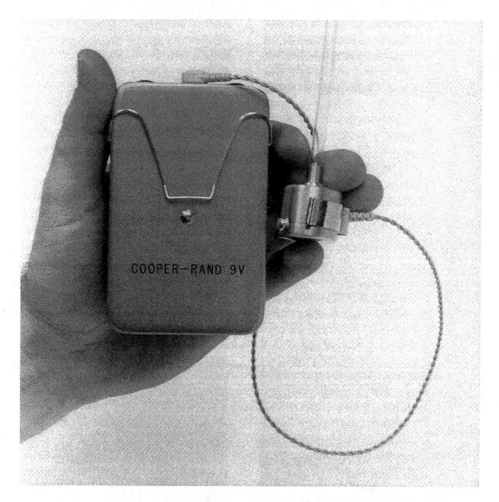

Figure 16-6. Cooper Rand intra-oral artifical larynx. Photo courtesy of Luminaud Inc.

switch version of the oral electrolarynx for individuals who do not have the upper extremity strength to hold the device in place and push the tone button. An adaptive switch (see Chapter 3) is attached to the electrolarynx to control the tone button. The plastic tube can be attached to a headband or eyeglasses to keep it within reach of the user's mouth. Luminaud also manufactures a pneumatic switch version of the oral electrolarynx. By sipping and puffing into the plastic tube, the tone source is turned on and off. This eliminates the need for a separate switch for tone activation.

DIRECT SELECTION COMMUNICATION APPROACHES

When individuals do not have adequate oral motor control to consider use of oral and modified speech approaches for intervention, consideration should be given to developing a direct selection AAC system. Within the acute care setting, it is important that any AAC intervention be simple, independent, fast, and require minimal learning on the part of the communicator or listener (Fried-Oken et al., 1991). Direct selection communication methods are used almost as frequently as oral and modified speech approaches in the acute care hospital setting. Dowden, Beukelman, and Lossing (1986) found that 46% of their acute care patients required direct selection communication methods.

Handwriting

Handwriting is often used as a direct selection communication method because no learning is needed for the patient or listeners. During the AAC evaluation the team will need to determine if the individual's handwriting is legible throughout all positioning situations. In addition, fatigue from handwriting needs to be reviewed. Writing with pen and pencil on paper will work for individuals who can apply sufficient pressure to the writing instrument, and can write in an upright position. If an upright position is not possible, pens are available in office supply stores with pressurized ink that will write in any position. Writing aids such as a Magic Slate, which does not require pressure and can also be used when upside down or supine are also options (Mitsuda et al., 1992).

Direct Selection Communication Boards

Individuals who cannot write legibly may benefit from simple low technology communication boards. Direct selection methods of accessing the boards can include finger pointing, pointing with an adapted pointer, or eye gaze, among others. Persons with good literacy abilities are candidates for alphabet spelling boards. The alphabet boards can be arranged in an ABC order, or a QWERTY (computer keyboard) order. The user should be interviewed to ask which ordering is preferred. In addition to letters, the board should also have available spelling assistance messages such as

"end of word," "end of sentence," "start over," "backspace," and "mistake." Spelling messages on a low tech communication board can be a cognitively intense process for the communicator and listener who must remember what was previously spelled to construct messages mentally. Teaching the listener to use a Magic Slate board or paper to write down letters and messages as they are being spelled can improve communication and reduce the number of message breakdowns.

Eye gaze boards should be considered for patients who cannot directly select using other methods. One method of easily using direct selection to communicate with eye gaze boards is to use a moving eye gaze board technique (see Figure 16–7). Letters of the alphabet or other symbols are arranged on a clear piece of plexiglass with each symbol approximately 1½ to 2 inches apart. The communicator fixes his or her eye gaze on the selected symbol and visually tracks the item as the listener moves the board. The listener moves the board until the communicator's and listener's eye gaze lock together through the board. The symbol that they are both looking at is the selected item. This technique is fast, efficient, and not fatiguing for the communicator. During the evaluation, the team will need to determine if the patient has the visual tracking skills necessary to successfully use the technique.

Phrase or sentence message boards, or picture symbol boards, can be used when alphabet spelling is not feasible. Phrase boards should not be used when patients are capable of spelling, as they are often perceived by patients as being too limiting (Fried-Oken et al., 1991). Phrase boards should be considered when individuals do not have sufficient motor skills to access a board with the complete alphabet, or cannot spell to communicate. When developing phrase or picture communication boards, medical staff, family, and the patient should be interviewed to develop a

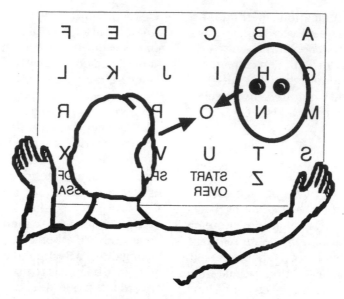

Figure 16–7. Moving eye gaze board. The communicator fixates eye gaze on the desired symbol and maintains eye gaze on the symbol as the board is moving. The listener moves the board until both individual's eyes lock through the board on the same symbol.

list of necessary phrases. If needed, separate boards can be made for specific situations. For example, one board might be used by the nursing staff to attend to medical needs, and a separate board is used by the family to talk about friends, home, and other issues.

Encoding communication systems require the individual to learn a coding system to communicate messages to others. Chapters 3 and 4 in this text discuss various encoding methods at length. Encoding methods require both the communicator and listener to learn the coding system. Because this method requires learning on the part of both parties, it is often a last resort to be used when alphabet spelling is unfeasible, and the individual wants to communicate more messages than a simple phrase board will allow. Eye gaze, eye blinks, or finger wiggles, among others, can be used to indicate the codes. Table 16–2 lists an encoding system for using eyeblinks to communicate. If an encoding system is used, the code should be posted prominently

Table 16–2. Eye blink encoding system.

Number of Eyeblinks	Message
1–1	I'm in pain.
1–2	My head.
1–3	My back.
1–4	My neck.
2–1	My stomach.
2–2	My legs.
2–3	I'm tired.
2–4	Please turn me.
3–1	I'm nauseous.
3–2	I'm hot.
3–3	I'm cold.
3–4	Tell me what is happening.
4–1	Talk to me.
4–2	I need suctioning.
4–3	Leave me alone.
4–4	When is my family coming?

where all parties (including the patient) can easily refer to it.

SCANNING COMMUNICATION OPTIONS

AAC scanning methods should only be considered for acute care patients when other approaches are not feasible. Most individuals can be provided with a direct selection AAC system, or can benefit from oral and modified speech interventions. Only 5% of acute care hospital patients will require AAC scanning methods for communication (Dowden, Beukelman, & Lossing, 1986). As stated previously, most individuals who are critically ill do not want to use complex communication systems that require extensive learning (Fried-Oken et al., 1991). This rules out the use of switch-activated electronic AAC systems for most individuals in acute care settings. Instead, low technology scanning communication approaches that can be implemented easily should be considered.

Low technology AAC scanning approaches require maximum listener participation in the communication process. Fried-Oken and her colleagues (1991) found that patients did not like communication methods that required listener assistance because the listeners were often not trained in the communication procedures. To ensure success with a low technology scanning

AAC system, the AAC specialist will need to provide extensive training for listeners to make sure that the system is used properly. Scanning communication methods require frequent monitoring by the AAC specialist to make sure that all parties continue to communicate with a mininum of message breakdowns or frustration.

Twenty Questions

A crude form of scanning communication is to simply ask the patient multiple yes/no questions until the necessary information is communicated. This method requires limited learning on the patient's part. However, the individual is dependent on the listener to ask the right questions. For example, the person may want to discuss a particular family member. If the nurse fails to ask the right questions to narrow down the topic to that family member, a communication breakdown occurs. In order to improve the 20 questions approach, communication partners should be given guidance for developing the questions. Partners should be trained to start with broad topics and work down to narrow topics. Table 16–3 provides an example.

Low Tech Scanning AAC Approaches

In order to provide the individual with more control over communication topics,

Table 16–3. A guided approach to 20 questions in the medical setting.

Do you want to discuss your . . .				
Level 1:	condition	family	leisure activities	
What LEISURE activity do you want?				
Level 2:	radio	write letter	television	game	other
What do you want to watch on TELEVISION?				
Level 3:	Cartoon	Video	Soap Opera	News	Comedy
What NEWS show do you want to see?				
Level 4:	ABC	CBS	NBC	CNN	

other methods of scanning should be considered. A low technology method of scanning communication is to train the listener to verbally scan choices on a communication board. This can be done using an alphabet board, phrase board, or picture board. The patient responds with yes/no responses to indicate choices during the scanning process. For example, the listener would point to pictures on a communication board and verbally ask "Do you want to watch television, listen to the radio, write a letter, read a story?" and continue until the user makes a choice.

Trade-offs between making a low tech scanning system easy to use, versus fast and efficient, will need to be made. A linear method of scanning, in which every item on the communication board is reviewed in an established order, is cognitively the easiest method of scanning through choices. However, this method does not work well for more than a few choices. Individuals who will be scanning through the entire alphabet or through more than 20 symbol choices will need to use row column methods of scanning to speed up communication. For row column scanning, the listener will need to be trained to verbally indicate each row, then to verbally scan through items in the selected row. For example, the listener would ask "Is the letter in the first row? the second row? the third row? the fourth row?" Once the row is selected, the listener would ask "A? B? C?" until the desired letter is selected.

Vocabulary and symbols for a low tech scanning boards are developed similarly to the direct selection approaches already described in this chapter. Because scanning is a slow method of communication, messages that will be communicated frequently should be arranged so that the listener scans them first. Phrase or picture boards should have urgent messages such as "something hurts," or "I need the bedpan" placed in the upper left corner. Because scanning methods of communication are slow, individuals who are capable of using

an alphabet board may also want to have phrase symbols for frequently communicated or emergency messages. The communication board can be arranged with emergency phrases on one side and an alphabet display on the other. The listener needs to be trained to first ask "Do you want to spell a message, or do you want one of your phrases?" The alphabet should be arranged with vowels and frequently used consonants toward the upper left corner of the scanning display.

IMPLEMENTATION OF AAC IN THE ACUTE CARE HOSPITAL SETTING

The final aspect of service delivery in the hospital setting is actual implementation of the recommended AAC system. The AAC specialist can develop an exceptional AAC communication system, yet see the system fail if it is not implemented properly. Poor implementation leads to a lack of communication opportunities and frequent communication breakdowns which can be extremely frustrating for acutely ill patients. Fried-Oken et al. (1991) provided the following quote from one of their AAC patients who was temporarily nonspeaking in the intensive care hospital setting:

They'd get frustrated. My mom would try to figure out what I was saying and she'd get sorta nervous. That would pretty much be the end of our attempt because I'd realize she wasn't picking up on my message so I'd stop. Normally that was the end of our visit. She'd get so frustrated she'd say "well I guess maybe I should go." Then she'd leave and never know that all I was telling her was thank you for coming. (p. 49)

Staff and Family Training

Staff and family training is an essential component of implementing any AAC system in the hospital setting. Prior to training listeners, the AAC specialist should make sure that the patient understands and can successfully use the recommended method of communication. If the person's ability to use the AAC system is inconsistent, other communication methods should be considered. Once a consistent method of communication is found, all staff and family members need to be trained to implement the AAC system.

In a large acute care hospital, it is impossible for the AAC specialist to individually train every medical staff person, family member, or visitor who will come into contact with the patient. This inability to train all listeners in the individual's environment makes it essential that any recommended AAC communication system be intuitively simple and easy to use. However, no matter how simple the communication method appears to be, the following staff and family training steps should be completed.

Train Key Personnel and Family Members

It is important that key medical staff and family members be trained to implement the communication system. The primary nurse and the nursing assistant responsible for the patient's care need to be directly trained. Because of shift changes, medical staff from each shift will need to be shown how to use the AAC system. Trying to conduct training during shift changes is often difficult. Nurses have paperwork and other essential tasks to complete as they begin and end each shift. AAC professionals should try to arrange time to train staff separately on the two day shifts (e.g., 7:00 to 3:00, and 3:00 to 11:00). Because most AAC professionals will not be available during the 11:00 to 7:00 night shift, they will need to rely on nursing staff from earlier shifts to train the night shift. In a large hospital, a logsheet that indicates which medical staff have been trained to use the AAC system is helpful. The logsheet can list the name of

the person trained, the date training occurred, the person's role (e.g., nursing assistant, social worker), and the name of the person who provided training. If possible, the logsheet should be posted by the AAC communication protocol.

Key family members also need direct training. If family members have not been available during evaluation visits, the social worker or primary nurse can provide information on who visits frequently and who needs to be trained. If needed, appointments can be made to meet family members at specific times to provide direct training. Family members can also be asked to sign the logsheet if they are trained by other staff.

AAC Communication Protocols

Figure 16–1 in this chapter presented an example of a communication protocol. As stated previously, protocols are posted at the patient's bedside and in the medical chart. Protocols should be visually vibrant to attract the attention of medical staff and visitors. Protocols can be printed on brightly colored paper, using large print, cartoons, drawings, or photographs to illustrate communication methods. Instructions should be clear yet brief. Information regarding whom to contact for more information about using the AAC communication system should be written on the protocol. More detailed information about the communication protocol can be written into the medical chart.

Label AAC Communication Equipment

All AAC communication equipment needs to be labeled with the patient's name, room number, and information regarding how to use the equipment. Large pieces of equipment such as communication boards can have the AAC communication protocol attached directly to the back of the device. Smaller pieces of equipment can have simple labels attached which refer the listener to the communication protocol. The equipment should also clearly state where to return the device upon discharge from the hospital, or if the equipment is the property of the patient.

Make Back-Up Copies of Everything

During a lengthy hospital stay, patients are often transferred from one unit to another and between rooms within hospital units. Every time a new room assignment occurs, the potential to lose communication equipment occurs. In addition, individuals who are not bedbound have the potential to misplace AAC equipment as they are taken to different hospital departments or recreational areas. AAC professionals in acute care hospital settings should always make back-up copies of AAC communication protocols, and direct selection or scanning communication boards.

Continued Implementation

Individuals in acute care hospital settings are in a state of medical transition. This means that their communication abilities often change during the course of their hospital stay. The speech-language pathologist will need to be in daily contact with nonspeaking patients during the hospital stay. Daily contact is needed to monitor implementation of the existing AAC communication system, and to determine when the system needs to change. Every time a change in communication status occurs, the speech-language pathologist will need to repeat staff and family training steps that were reviewed previously in this chapter.

Although some individuals will regain verbal speech during the inpatient stay, others will be medically ready for discharge while remaining nonspeaking. The speech-language pathologist will need to determine an appropriate discharge plan. Individuals who are moving into other less acute hospi-

tal settings can be followed by speech-language pathologists in that setting. Prior to or at the time of discharge, the hospital AAC specialist should make attempts personally to contact professionals at the new facility to make sure that they receive information regarding the patient's communication needs and abilities. If staff at the new facility are unfamiliar with AAC techniques, they can be referred to other resources for consultative assistance as needed. Nonspeaking persons who are discharged to other hospital facilities have the opportunity to have their communication skills monitored over time. Some of these individuals will gradually gain verbal speech over a lengthy rehabilitation process and will not require AAC on a long-term basis.

Individuals who are directly discharged home also have the potential to gain verbal speech over time. They will need to be referred to a facility that can provide them with ongoing speech therapy services following discharge. Children are usually referred to their school system. Adults will need to be referred to outpatient speech therapy programs. These persons should also be simultaneously referred to an outpatient program or educational team that specializes in AAC. The AAC specialists can monitor the individual's improvements in verbal speech over time, and can make recommendations for implementing an AAC system for long-term use if needed.

At the author's hospital, we provide AAC services on both an inpatient and outpatient basis. When nonspeaking inpatients are discharged from the hospital, we contact speech-language pathologists in the community who will be providing direct services to discuss the AAC system, and to discuss the individual's potential to improve spoken communication. If needed, we arrange to go to the speech-language pathologist's facility to provide more extensive training.

The nonspeaking person is then followed through our outpatient clinic. If we expect speech abilities to improve, we contact the outside speech-language pathologist or family members by phone at certain time intervals to follow progress. Individuals who have not made adequate progress over time are brought back to the outpatient clinic, or referred to other facilities for evaluation of long-term AAC needs. If we do not expect speech abilities to improve, we set up outpatient follow-up appointments at our facility at the time of discharge, or refer the individual to other AAC programs that can evaluate and recommend AAC systems for use on a long-term basis.

SUMMARY

Providing AAC services in an acute care hospital setting requires a different professional approach than other AAC settings. The patient's constantly changing medical condition, the chaotic nature of acute care hospitals, and the large number of medical staff interacting with the individual make service delivery challenging. AAC specialists need to be flexible, aggressive, and creative to implement appropriate AAC strategies within this setting. A guiding philosophy of AAC practice in the medical setting is to "keep it simple." AAC approaches need to be as close to natural speech as possible, easy to use for both the communicator and listener, and require minimum listener participation. This chapter reviewed modified speech, and low technology AAC approaches that are appropriate for communication in the acute care medical setting. Use of high technology AAC approaches is not recommended and results in frequent frustration for both the communicator and listener (Fried-Oken et al., 1991). At times, medical staff, patients, and families will specifically request glitzy high tech AAC systems. AAC professionals will need to counsel that "less is more" for communication within acute care medical settings.

REFERENCES

American Association for Respiratory Care. (1991). *A study of chronic ventilator patients in the hospital.* Dallas: AARC.

Ashworth, P. (1978, February). Communication in the intensive care ward. *Nursing Mirror,* 34–36.

Bach, J. R., & Alba, A. S. (1990). Tracheostomy ventilation: A study of efficacy with deflated cuffs and cuffless trachs. *Chest, 97,* 679–683.

Beukelman, D. R., & Mirenda, P. (1992). *Augmentative and alternative communication: Management of severe communication disorders in children and adults.* Baltimore, MD: Paul H. Brookes.

Dowden, P., Beukelman, D. R., & Lossing, C. (1986). Serving nonspeaking patients in acute care settings: Acute care outcomes. *Augmentative and Alternative Communication, 2,* 38–44.

Dowden, P., Honsinger, M., & Beukelman, D. R. (1986). Serving nonspeaking patients in acute care settings: An intervention approach. *Augmentative and Alternative Communication, 2,* 25–32.

Ewing-Cobbs, L., Levin, H. S., Fletcher, J. M., McLaughlin, E. J., McNeely, D. G., Ewert, J., & Francis, D. (1984). *Assessment of posttraumatic amnesia in head injured children.* Paper presented to the International Neuropsychological Society.

French, J., Siebens, A., Kummell, J., Kirby, N., & Eisele, J. (1984). Preserving communication and airway clearance in tracheostomized children and adults. *Archives of Physical Medicine and Rehabilitation, 65,* 651.

Fried-Oken, M., Howard, J., & Stewart, S. R. (1991). Feedback on AAC intervention from adults who are temporarily unable to speak. *Augmentative and Alternative Communication, 7,* 43–50.

Kirchner, J. A., & Astrachan, D. I. (1988). Tracheostomy as an alternative to prolonged intubation. In M. J. Bishop (Ed.), *Problems in anesthesia.* Philadelphia: J. B. Lippincott.

Passy, V. (1986). Passy-Muir speaking valve. *Otolaryngology—Head and Neck Surgery, 95,* 247–248.

Mitsuda, P., Baarslag-Benson, R., Hazel, K., & Therriault, T. (1992). Augmentative communication in intensive and acute care unit settings.

In K. M. Yorkston (Ed.), *Augmentative communication in the medical setting.* (pp. 5–57). Tuscon AZ: Communication Skill Builders.

Siebens, A. A., Tippett, D. C., Kirby, N., & French, J. (1993). Dysphagia and expiratory air flow. *Dysphagia, 8,* 266–269.

Tippett, D., & Siebens, A. A. (1995). Preserving oral communication in individuals with tracheostomy and ventilator dependency. *American Journal of Speech Language Pathology, 4,* 55–61.

Life Stories

Danielle's AAC Story: A Rehabilitation Journey

Beth Reckord with Sharon L. Glennen

Danielle's AAC story began years before she lost the ability to speak. An inner city teenager, she faced many urban challenges including poverty, lack of education, and lack of family structure. Like her mother, Danielle became pregnant and gave birth to a daughter at the age of 15. Shortly after the birth of her child, she had a cerebral vascular accident, or stroke, which completely changed her life. In one afternoon, she lost the ability to walk, talk, and take care of herself or her young child.

AAC IN THE INTENSIVE CARE UNIT: BASIC COMMUNICATION NEEDS

Danielle first came to our attention when she was in the intensive care unit of the hospital. She had extreme weakness in all extremities with limited movements of her legs and arms. She had a tracheostomy with a cuffed trach tube and was using a ventilator which left her unable to vocalize. Severe oral muscular weakness made it difficult for her to move her tongue or lips for feeding or communication. A nasogastric tube was inserted for feeding because of the danger of choking and aspiration. Despite these setbacks, Danielle immediately smiled when we joked with her about the TV show she was watching.

During the initial assessment in the intensive care unit, the goal was to develop a simple method of communication that Danielle could use to communicate basic needs to others. Physically, her only movements were eye gaze, eye blinks, and smiling. She was quickly taught to smile and frown to answer yes/no questions. Eye gaze was used to evaluate her ability to use symbols for communication. A quick screening found that she had good reading abilities and was able to spell common single words. Danielle was given an eye gaze communication board which required the listener to follow her gaze to spell messages. Danielle immediately used the eye gaze system to spell words to her mother. Through use of the eye gaze system, she was able to ask her mother questions about her family and her daughter's care.

AAC IN THE REHABILITATION HOSPITAL: CHANGING STRATEGIES OVER TIME

Two weeks later, Danielle was transferred into the rehabilitation hospital. Although she was no longer dependent on the ventilator, she had a cuffed trach and severe oral motor weakness which prevented her from communicating. She still was unable to move her arms or legs. The immediate goal was to get her up and out of bed on a regular basis, and to establish a routine of active rehabilitation and education. For the first few days, staff at the hospital were trained to use the eye gaze board with Danielle, and were shown her yes/no system of communication. These communication methods were posted for staff and visitors on a brightly colored note over her bed. A copy of the note was also placed in the front of her medical chart to constantly remind hospital staff about her communication methods. As Danielle grew stronger and was able to remain in a wheelchair for extended periods of time, we began exploring other methods of communication.

During the first 2 weeks of rehabilitation, Danielle's ability to move her head improved. It was noted that she had no difficulty turning her head to watch others, and could use head nods to answer yes/no questions. The Assistive Technology Team worked with Danielle's regular rehabilitation therapists to assess her ability to use either a head stick or light pointer for communication. Danielle did well with both devices, but preferred the light pointer since it looked more normal. She was given a laser light pointer to use. We were able to attach the light pointer to a custom head band that held it in place at midline on top of her head.

It was still unclear if Danielle's speech would return. It was also unclear whether she would regain any functional use of her arms or legs. The team decided to use the light pointer as an interim communication tool, and to hold off on developing any final recommendations. An alphabet communication board was made and placed on an upright easel on Danielle's wheelchair tray. In addition to the alphabet, the board also had functional phrases and sentences that could be communicated with a single selection of the light. Danielle was able to use the light pointer to communicate with others, to point to people and objects in the hospi-

tal, and to participate in school lessons provided by the hospital's teacher. Using the light pointer and the communication board, she began meeting daily for counseling sessions with the social worker. Danielle was able to use her communication system to discuss the impact of her disability and to begin the emotional journey that is a necessary part of the overall rehabilitation process.

Four weeks into her hospital stay, it was clear that Danielle's rehabilitation progress would be slow. It was decided to loan her a Light Talker augmentative communication system to provide her with voice output. The Light Talker can be set up to use an optical light pointer to select symbols. Because Danielle was able to spell, the system was set up with an alphabet display and a few single key messages for important information that needed to be communicated quickly. Danielle enjoyed having the ability to speak through the electronic communication system even though she did not like the synthesizer's voice quality. Using the Light Talker, Danielle was able to begin communicating with family members over the phone on a regular basis.

Although Danielle adjusted quickly to the new device, the process of upgrading from a low tech to high tech approach was difficult for hospital staff. When Danielle used the low tech laser light pointer, staff usually remembered to put it on. They sometimes forgot to get the alphabet board to use with it, but Danielle could use the bright red light beam of the pointer to show them the board across the room. The Light Talker added a new level of complexity for hospital staff that made implementation difficult. The device had to be charged nightly. There were many mornings when Danielle would arrive for therapies with the Light Talker only to discover that the system hadn't been charged. The optical pointer of the Light Talker doesn't actually shine a beam of light, which added a significant drawback. It couldn't be used to point to anything except the Light Talker itself. Danielle lost the ability to easily point to objects and persons in her room. The optical pointer also had to be plugged into the Light Talker device in order to work. There were several times when Danielle was wearing the optical light pointer, and had the Light Talker mounted on her wheelchair yet was unable to communicate because a nurse or therapist forgot to plug in the light pointer!

These difficulties were overcome in several different ways. After repeated episodes of not charging the Light Talker, Danielle's speech-language pathologist took over responsibility for charging the system overnight. This meant that Danielle lost access to the device each evening at 5:00, and couldn't use it again until the next morning. Her previous low tech system with the laser light pointer was used for communication during the evenings. The problem of providing Danielle with access to the laser light pointer when using the Light Talker was solved by creating a special mounting headband that held both pointing devices at midline. Danielle could point to objects in the room using the laser light pointer and still access the Light Talker using the optical light pointer. It took some getting used to, especially when she would see two lights shining in parallel on the Light Talker display.

The problems of plugging in the optical light pointer and correctly placing her equipment on the wheelchair were addressed in a series of staff trainings. Every nursing shift and each team therapist was shown how to set up the Light Talker system. Finally, Danielle's family was also trained so they could make sure the system was in place. Step-by-step instructions for setting up the system were posted over her bed on neon pink paper, on the back of the LightTalker device, and in the medical chart. Despite intensive staff and family training, there were still many times when components of her system were not set up correctly, and Danielle was unable to communicate using the Light Talker.

After 10 weeks in the rehabilitation hospital, Danielle began to develop movement in the fingers of her left hand and forearm. Working with her occupational and physical therapists, we were able to use a mobile arm support, or sling, to position her left forearm. With the sling's support, she was able to move her hand across the surface of a Touch Talker and computer keyboard to type messages. She initially had some difficulty producing enough pressure to make key selections. A splint was made by her occupational therapist to provide her with additional index finger and thumb stability. The computer and Touch Talker were loaned to Danielle and used regularly in occupational therapy as a motivating method of increasing her arm and hand function. The transition from the Light Talker to the Touch Talker took several weeks. As she gained strength in her arms, she was eventually able to use the Touch Talker without the mobile arm support.

At the end of 16 weeks of hospitalization, Danielle was using the Touch Talker for all communication activities. She could also point to objects in her environment using her left hand. This increase in physical ability made it possible for Danielle to take responsibility for her communication equipment. At night, she could point to a list of instructions above her bed to remind the nurses to charge the device. In the morning, she could point to the device to request placing it on her wheelchair tray. Staff noticed that she was communicating more frequently and using longer messages. She also began using unaided gestures to wave hello, signal "okay" and respond with a thumbs up/thumbs down response to others. As her success at communication increased, her overall affect improved. She began actively participating in her rehabilitation and made significant progress each day.

During this time, Danielle's tracheostomy was plugged for gradually increasing amounts of time. She began attempting to vocalize words to communicate. Because of severe oral and respiratory weakness, her initial attempts were only weak nasal vowels. Other than intonation, it was impossible to determine what she was attempting to say. Her speech-language pathologist began working to improve her articulation abilities. After several more weeks, Danielle's trach tube was removed and the tracheostomy was allowed to close. Over time, she acquired the ability to produce the sounds "l" and "n" and the occasionally intelligible phrase "I don't know." It was still unclear if she would ever communicate using speech as her primary mode of communication.

Prior to her stroke, Danielle had dropped out of school after the ninth grade. During her hospital stay, she did well in her educational classes and decided that after leaving the hospital she would return to school. The assistive technology team began to evaluate Danielle's long-term communication and educational technology needs. Danielle was introduced to an IBM compatible laptop computer adapted with a MultiVoice speech synthesizer, EZ Keys (a word prediction software program with AAC communication features), and Word Perfect (word processing software). By this time, she had no difficulty using her left index finger to type letters on the keyboard. Because her typing speed was slow, use of the word prediction features of EZ Keys was assessed. Danielle had the opportunity to use this system on loan for 3 weeks during her hospital stay. Over time, it was discovered that word prediction actually slowed Danielle's typing speed down. The length of time it took her to visually scan the word prediction lists was slower than the length of time it took her to simply spell the words. In addition, although she could access the entire keyboard, her access time was slowest for the numbers row, which is used frequently with word prediction. Danielle continued to use EZ Keys because it had AAC features that made it easy to switch from

word processing to communication activities. However, the word prediction features of the program were turned off.

Five months after Danielle was first admitted to the rehabilitation hospital, it was time to begin preparing for her discharge. It was determined that she would need an AAC system for communication, an adapted computer for completing written assignments at school, and a power wheelchair for mobility. Prior to this point in the rehabilitation process, Danielle's AAC devices, computer equipment, and wheelchairs were provided to her on loan from the hospital's Assistive Technology Department. Thus, it was possible to give her multiple pieces of equipment designed to meet different technology needs. Now that she was being discharged, the reality of funding equipment needed to be considered in making final recommendations. Because of funding constraints, it was decided that a laptop computer would be adapted to meet both communication and educational needs.

An Invacare Action Arrow power wheelchair controlled with a left side joystick was also recommended. The laptop computer and power wheelchair then needed to be integrated. After considering several options, Danielle decided that she wanted her laptop computer attached to the power chair using a fold-down wheelchair mounting system. She wanted the option of using her computer without needing a tray placed on the wheelchair. The fold-down features of the mount also made it easy to transfer her in and out of the chair. The process of funding all of this equipment through Danielle's health insurance was initiated.

AAC IN THE COMMUNITY: TRANSITION STRATEGIES

Six months after her stroke, the process of transitioning Danielle back into high school was initiated. Meetings were held with the special education team at her neighborhood high school to begin the school transition. Because Danielle came from a poor neighborhood, the high school had relatively few resources to adapt the curriculum. A majority of her teachers had never used a computer and felt uneasy integrating a computer into their courses. There were concerns about Danielle's laptop computer being taken by other students. A one-to-one aide was needed to go with Danielle from class to class and to monitor her technology equipment. Finally, the high school building was old and could not easily be adapted to make all classes accessible. Class locations were moved so that Danielle could independently move from class to class.

Although funding for Danielle's equipment was initiated, it would be several months before funding was authorized and equipment could be ordered. Danielle's team had to develop an interim plan for the 2 to 3 months that she would be without her equipment. Working with the schools, a laptop computer was obtained for her use at the high school. It did not have a speech synthesizer or software for communication. This allowed her to meet her educational needs but was not ideal for communication. A simple communication board consisting of the alphabet and 100 commonly used words was developed as an interim communication tool. Multiple copies of the board were made and laminated for her use.

Danielle's transition into her home also required the efforts of her rehabilitation team. Danielle lived in a row house that was not wheelchair accessible. Long before her discharge from the hospital, the social worker worked with Danielle's family to find accessible housing. Unfortunately, the waiting lists were lengthy. Plans were made to adapt her existing house as an interim measure. Row homes were built years before anyone considered the need for accessibility. Narrow hallways, small openings between rooms, and steep staircases are typical in many of these inner-city homes. There was no way that a power wheelchair could be used. It was decided that the power chair would need to stay at school, and a manual wheelchair would be found for her use at home. Unfortunately, Danielle's health insurance would only pay for one wheelchair. We adapted a used manual wheelchair that had been donated to the hospital for her use at home. Finally, Danielle's row home was built years before current electrical codes were in existence. There were no grounded three pronged outlets available for plugging in a laptop computer, and the family frequently blew fuses when trying to use multiple appliances in the home. The landlord was contacted and special wiring was installed in one room so that Danielle's computer could be recharged. Multiple batteries for the computer were ordered so that she could use the computer while the other batteries were charging.

It would be nice to say that once Danielle was discharged and received her own AAC equipment and power chair, she rode off into the sunset and did not need the assistance of the hospital's assistive technology team. The reality was that her assistive technology complications were only beginning. Two months after discharge, Danielle received her power wheelchair and AAC laptop computer. She received the power chair first. Her one-to-one aide at school came to the hospital to learn how to set up and charge the chair. Two weeks later, the aide was transferred and Danielle was left with constantly changing substitute aides for 1 month. During this period, the power chair wasn't used. Fortunately, Danielle was continuing to come to the hospital for outpatient therapies after school. As soon as we were alerted to the situation, a special meeting was called at her school to resolve the problem. A new permanent aide was appointed within 1 week, and training took place at school to teach the aide and Danielle how to set up and charge the chair. Over the next year, Danielle went through four different aides and the training process was repeated several times. Danielle eventually became comfortable enough with her wheelchair system that she was able to show her aides and teachers how to charge and set it up.

Danielle's IBM compatible laptop computer was implemented 1 month after she received the power chair. The laptop system consisted of the computer, an external MultiVoice speech synthesizer, EZ Keys software, a Diconix portable printer, and Daessy fold-down wheelchair mount. The initial implementation took place in two stages. Because the equipment needed to be mounted to her power wheelchair, Danielle was seen at the hospital so that the adaptive equipment specialist could assist with mounting the system. The mounting system for the computer was attached to the right side of her wheelchair so that it wouldn't interfere with her joystick controls on the left side. One difficulty was determining where to position the attached speech synthesizer. After exploring several options, it was attached behind her wheelchair seat. Danielle and her mother were taught how to charge all of the components, how to connect the components, and how to use the software installed in the system. Because Danielle was still returning regularly to the hospital for therapies, her speech-language pathologist planned to use the system in therapy and train more advanced features of the software over time.

A separate initial training session was arranged for Danielle's school. The assistive technology specialist met with Danielle's one-to-one aide, several of her teachers, and the school system's AAC team to train them how to implement the laptop computer. This was the beginning of several sessions spent at Danielle's school to resolve issues surrounding use of the AAC system. These sessions were collaborative efforts between Danielle, the hospital's assistive technology team, and the school

system's AAC team. The hospital team knew Danielle's family and were able to mediate any issues that required family involvement. The school team knew the teachers and therapists at the school. They were able to steer Danielle into classes with teachers who would be open to implementing the AAC system, and also provided additional staff training for the teachers.

Despite all of this hand-holding and training, problems with the AAC system occurred. Danielle's family did not always take responsibility for charging the system overnight. She often came to school with a dead computer which needed recharging before it could be used. This was resolved by purchasing a separate charger and extra battery for the school to use. Danielle often came to school with components missing from her AAC system. For example, the computer might arrive, but the speech synthesizer would be left behind. Danielle was given a checklist of components to make sure that everything was packed into the carrying case each morning. Although this did not entirely resolve the problem, it placed the responsibility with Danielle, not others. Finally, the problem of staff changes, especially her one-to-one aide, and changing classes across semesters required frequent retrainings. Over time, Danielle became familiar with her equipment so that she could show others how to charge and connect the components.

At home, Danielle did not have access to her power chair. She spent most of her time in the manual chair, or seated on a couch. Because there was no AAC wheelchair mount for the manual chair (her insurance would not fund two mounts), Danielle had to use the laptop system at the kitchen table or hold it in her lap. Because of these difficulties, Danielle used the system to complete her homework and play games, but did not rely on it for communication. Extra low tech communication boards were made for her use at home.

AAC IN TRANSITION

During the next year, Danielle was seen every 2 months at her school by the assistive technology team so that we could troubleshoot any difficulties with her AAC system. She also continued to be seen weekly for speech, physical, and occupational therapy at the hospital. During this time she continued to make gains in upper extremity function. By the end of her first year, Danielle had regained functional use of her right hand and was able to access the laptop computer using both hands. This significantly increased her keyboarding speed. She also regained enough use of her left hand to begin writing with paper and pencil. Over time, her handwriting became more legible, though it was still slow and laborious.

Danielle's speech also changed. She was able to make additional consonant sounds, her speech was louder, and her vowel approximations were good. Her speech was still hypernasal, and her hypotonic oral motor tone reduced articulation intelligibility, but in limited contexts she could be understood. As her family grew accustomed to her speech, she began using that modality of communication at home most of the time. The low technology alphabet-word communication board was used to clarify messages when needed. Because Danielle's family was still having difficulty coordinating her laptop computer between home and school, the decision was made to keep the computer at school full-time during the week, and to only send it home on weekends or long holidays.

During the second year after her stroke Danielle continued to improve physically. As her physical skills and endurance increased, her desire to use the laptop computer for educational or communication needs decreased. She began to insist to her teachers and aides at school that she did not want it mounted on her wheelchair. She wanted to sit at a desk and write using paper and pencil like other students in her class. For a while she used the laptop computer placed on a desk or table surface, but eventually decided not to use it regularly. Her writing speed had improved and she was easily able to write short answers and sentences to complete class assignments. When lengthier assignments were given, she continued to use the laptop to write.

As Danielle's speech improved, her aides were able to understand her most of the time. Although many of her teachers and fellow students were still unable to understand her, the aides began "translating" Danielle's messages, which decreased her motivation to continue with the laptop computer AAC system. As Danielle's second year in school progressed, she gradually phased out using the laptop computer for communication purposes. The alphabet-word board was used to clarify messages with her aides, and to communicate with those who did not understand her speech.

LIFE AFTER AAC

It is now 3 years since Danielle's life-changing stroke occurred. Although her speech is still hypernasal and often unintelligible, Danielle now considers speech to be her primary method of communication. The communication board is rarely used, but is needed when she speaks to strangers or to others who do not know her well. She continues to come for speech therapy services at the hospital in hopes that her speech will improve even more. Physical improvements have also occurred in other areas. She is now able to walk for short distances using a cane for support, and can complete most activities of daily living independently. The power chair is still used for community outings and at school to get from class to class. Danielle's writing abilities have also improved. She is able to write easily using her left hand, and only uses the laptop computer to type major papers. The EZ Keys software program and MultiVoice synthesizer were removed from her computer, and she now uses it simply as a word processing device.

Danielle is now a senior in high school and will graduate this spring, the first member of her immediate family to ever achieve this goal. She is unclear about her plans after graduation. Although jobs and educational opportunities through the vocational rehabilitation system have been discussed, she is undecided about her future. If she forgoes job training and chooses to remain at home, she will probably not require further AAC services. However, if she does decide to enter a job training or educational program, her AAC needs will need to be evaluated for those environments. Although she no longer requires AAC in her current situation, Danielle's AAC story is one that will continue to evolve.

KEY POINTS TO REMEMBER

- Implementing AAC strategies in a hospital setting is difficult because of constant changes in staff. Simple strategies that require a minimum of equipment or knowledge work best.
- Individuals with acquired disabilities require frequent changes in AAC strategies until their conditions stabilize. Low tech AAC strategies, equipment loans, or rental equipment should be used initially to prevent unnecessary purchases of equipment.
- AAC clients are clients for life. As individuals transition from one setting to another, intensive services are usually needed to ensure successful AAC outcomes. Even then, success does not come easily.
- When individuals need more than one type of assistive technology, AAC needs have to be integrated with other technology needs. Because of funding limitations, a single system may need to perform multiple functions.
- The patient's home and community environments need to be thoroughly evaluated before making AAC recommendations. A high level of detailed information is necessary to prevent failed outcomes. For example, Danielle's AAC system would have failed from the start (or been short circuited!) if the electrical wiring in her home had not been changed. Without a home visit and a checklist designed to double-check electrical circuits, we would have missed this crucial piece of information.
- Whenever possible, empower the AAC consumer with responsibilities for taking care of equipment. The consumer is more motivated than others to make sure the equipment is charged and used properly.
- Across all areas of assistive technology, individuals decrease their reliance on technology as their ability to function independently increases. When applied to communication, individuals will use whatever speech abilities they have to communicate and prefer using speech rather than their AAC systems.
- When an individual is recovering from an acquired disability, it is difficult to strike a balance between immediate needs and long-term recovery projections. Although Danielle eventually learned to speak and did not need an AAC system, AAC was a crucial component of her recovery process for the first 2 years after her stroke. Although Danielle's AAC system was eventually retired, it was a necessary and appropriate device to meet her communication needs during her first 2 years out of the hospital. Professionals need to be aware that technology may eventually be set aside as the individual recovers.

Chapter 17

AAC FOR ADULTS WITH DEVELOPMENTAL DISABILITIES

Elizabeth M. Delsandro

The world of adults with developmental disabilities has been changing for many years. Prior to World War II, institutions were widely accepted lifelong residences for individuals with mental retardation (Stroud & Sutton, 1988). The deinstitutionalization movement transitioned many long-term residents from institutions to less restrictive community environments as part of the movement toward normalization (Stroud & Sutton, 1988). The principles of normalization are defined as a normal rhythm of the day, a normal rhythm of the week, a normal developmental life cycle, a range of choices, living in the world of two sexes, and the right to economic standards (Bernstein, Ziarnik, Rudrud, & Czajkowski, 1981).

With the trend toward normalization, the total environment of adults with developmental disabilities has changed. Integration within the community has expanded opportunities for adults with developmental disabilities and in turn has created additional needs. Specifically, the communication needs of adults with developmental disabilities have changed with the introduction of new programs, new living arrangements, and new communication partners in the community. Despite the trend toward normalized community placements, professional staff in these new environments have difficulty facilitating communicative interactions with adults with developmental disabilities who have the ability to speak. Adults with developmental disabilities who use augmentative and alternative methods of communication (AAC) are even less likely to participate in appropriate communicative exchanges. This chapter outlines the environment of adults with developmental disabilities who use AAC, reviews their communication needs within existing program environments, and proposes changes to improve those environments for communication.

THE EXISTING ENVIRONMENT

Although residential and vocational placements for adults with developmental disabilities have become more normalized over the years, individuals continue to reside and work in settings that are a step or two removed from complete independence. This lack of independence makes most AAC consumers reliant on others to facilitate communicative interactions between peers, professional staff, and the community. In order to make appropriate and functional AAC recommendations, it is important to understand the typical residential and work environments.

Residential Environments for Adults with Disabilities

Residential settings for consumers have changed in response to deinstitutionalization and the movement toward a least restrictive environment. Researchers have studied the process of movement within institutional residential settings (Altman & Cunningham, 1993) and movement from residential facilities to community settings (Lakin, Krantz, Bruininks, Clumpner, & Hill 1982). Between 1977 and 1987 the number of residents with mental retardation in facilities with more than 300 residents was reduced by 52 percent, from 143,000 to 69,000 (Lakin, Bruininks, Chen, Hill, & Anderson 1993). This trend is continuing as evidenced by the steady closure of many state institutions for the disabled.

Residences are classified into categories of institutional facilities and community facilities. State institutions, hospitals, correctional or training facilities, and nursing homes are examples of institutional facilities. Group homes, foster homes, and semi-independent living are classified as community facilities. Living arrangements outside of the traditional options for residence include houses, apartments, retirement homes, and boarding or rooming homes (Altman & Cunningham, 1993).

Small group homes and foster homes have been identified as the two fastest growing models of residential living arrangements for adults with disabilities (Chen, Bruininks, Lakin, & Hayden, 1993). A group home is defined as a residence with staff providing care, supervision, and training for one or more persons with disabilities (Chen et al., 1993). Group homes provide training in daily living skills, recreational opportunities, and a supportive environment for increased independence (Seltzer & Krauss, 1987). A foster home is typically a licensed residence in which individuals are accepted into a pre-existing household (Seltzer & Krauss, 1987). The level of specialized training for care providers and the level of habilitation services available for residents vary in foster and group homes.

Day Programs for Adults with Developmental Disabilities

Hill, Lakin, and Bruininks (1984) described four types of day placements for individuals with mental retardation. For younger individuals, these include public and private schools. For adults, vocational-work-training programs, day activity centers, and home-based training are available. Vocational-work-training programs provide vocational activities within a full-time supervised program. Vocational activities are often confined to jobs that require repetitive sorting, packaging, or cleaning such as collating forms, packing cassette tapes into plastic cases, or cleaning windows. Clients are paid for their work at these facilities. Day activity centers offer a full-time program without vocational services. Clients may participate in leisure activities, make crafts, or watch television. Many adult centers offer both vocational and day programs with clients assigned to different programs depending on skills.

Individuals who function in the profound range of mental retardation and also have motor, sensory, or behavior impairments have not traditionally participated in community-based vocational tasks (Rusch, Hughes, Johnson & Minch, 1991). Rather, individuals with severe disabilities have traditionally been placed in day activity centers and sheltered vocational workshops. The Vocational Rehabilitation Act Amendments of 1986, Public Law 99-506, authorized demonstration programs to extend supported community employment to individuals with severe disabilities (Black & Meyer, 1992).

In a supported employment setting, an individual receives support to be employed in the community from an employment training specialist or job coach. Individuals usually secure supported employment jobs in food service, light industry, or other service occupations. Positions in food service might consist of dishwashers, bus persons, and general kitchen laborers. Positions in light industry include assemblers, janitors, groundskeepers, and warehouse workers. Jobs in laundry, health care, clerical, or retail settings are classified as service occupations (Rusch, Wilson, Hughes, & Heal, 1994). Supported employment has several levels of supervised training. Some individuals initially receive intensive training on the job with gradual fading as work skills improve. When possible, the job coach or training specialist turn day-to-day supervision over to the employer. The job coach might check in on a weekly or monthly basis to make sure that employment is proceeding smoothly and to troubleshoot any difficulties. In contrast, many individuals with disabilities require ongoing daily supervision in the work setting. A cleaning crew in a hotel might be staffed by several adults with disabilities who are supervised by a supported employment job coach.

The move toward normalization has theoretically improved opportunities for interactive communication by placing AAC users into community-based settings. In reality, facilitating communication in these settings requires intensive planning, staff training, and structured implementation. The next section will review the AAC team and methods of designating team responsibilities.

AAC TEAM MEMBERS

Consumers

The consumer is an adult with a developmental disability. Consumers usually reside in an institutional or community facility and participate in day programs such as vocational-work-training programs, day activity centers, or home-based training. In both the residential and day programs, direct care providers give some level of supervision.

Direct Care Providers

Direct care providers directly supervise the consumer in a designated program. Direct care providers can have different titles in different settings. For example, a residential counselor is the direct care provider in residential programs. The job coach is considered the direct care provider in supported employment programs.

AAC Support Service Providers

Primary AAC support service providers are speech-language pathologists, augmentative communication specialists, or other professionals who provide consultative services related to implementation of AAC systems across a consumer's environments.

The Community

Members of the community play an important role in the successful implementation of a consumer's AAC system. A cashier at the local grocery store, an employee at the fast food restaurant, and a woman at the senior center are all potential communication partners for an adult consumer using AAC.

Establishing Primary Team Contacts

The AAC specialist needs to be familiar with the consumer's total environment prior to implementation of an augmentative communication system. The total environment typically consists of a place of residence; a day, vocational, or supported employment program; community activities; and leisure activities. Knowledge of the total environment assists the AAC specialist in determining the communicative needs of both the consumer and listeners in the the consumer's programs. Often two separate agencies operate the consumer's residential and day programs, which makes collaboration and continuity for implementing an AAC system challenging.

Identifying a primary AAC contact person for each program is crucial. Due to high staff turnover in programs for adults with developmental disabilities, an individual at the supervisory level rather than the staff level serves as a practical primary contact person. The primary contact person should have both direct daily interaction with the consumer and supervisory responsibilities over direct care providers within a designated program. For example, a residential supervisor and a day program director are suitable contact persons for the home and vocational programs. Figure 17–1 presents a form that is designed to identify the consumer's programs and primary AAC contact persons for each program. A copy should be given to each primary contact person to encourage collaboration between the consumer's programs, with updates to the form reviewed annually.

IDENTIFYING AAC NEEDS

Once an AAC system is implemented, the primary contact person for each program will have responsibility for organizing ongoing vocabulary planning, encouraging implementation of the AAC system, and recognizing the training needs of both the consumer and direct care providers. The needs of both the consumer and the consumer's programs can initially be identified

through interviews with primary contact persons and observations of the consumer within program environments.

Interviewing Primary Contact Persons and Direct Care Providers

Interviews with primary contact persons, conducted by an AAC specialist, provide information about the consumer's current communication skills, the success of the consumer's current communication system, communication demands placed on the consumer, and potential communication partners across environments. In addition, the interview should address the typical daily routine of the consumer. When possible, primary contact persons from each environment should be interviewed. The primary contact's perceptions of the consumer's communication skills, and potential opportunities for communication may differ across environments. Perceptions and knowledge of AAC systems will affect the overall success of a consumer's communication system. A sample interview form is available in Figure 17–2. The first section of the form identifies existing methods of communication and their effectiveness. The second section attempts to determine routine activities that may require use of AAC to facilitate communication.

Consumer Routines

Knowledge of consumer routines assists in determining what type of communication system is suitable within the environment. It also helps to identify potential communication partners and gives a structure for generating and organizing AAC vocabulary.

For example, Chris, an adult with moderate mental retardation and mild cerebral palsy, lived in a group home with two peers and attended a vocational program. The initial augmentative communication assessment revealed that Chris would probably

AAC NEEDS ASSESSMENT
PRIMARY CONTACT PERSON FORM

Focus: This form is designed to identify the components of a consumer's AAC environment and primary contact persons in each environment. This form should be updated annually.

Name of Consumer: _____ Date: _____

AAC Specialist: _____ Phone: _____

Program Name	Address	Telephone Number	Primary Contact Person
Residential Setting:			
Day Program Setting:			
Other:			

Figure 17-1. Augmentative and alternative communication (AAC) needs assessment primary contact person form.

<table>
<tr><td colspan="2" align="center">**Augmentative and Alternative Communication Needs**
KENNEDY KRIEGER INSTITUTE</td></tr>
<tr><td>Consumer:_____</td><td>Date:_____</td></tr>
<tr><td colspan="2">Informant:_____</td></tr>
<tr><td colspan="2">Relationship to consumer:_____</td></tr>
<tr><td colspan="2">Agency/Program:_____Telephone:_____</td></tr>
</table>

Focus: This form is designed to obtain information about the consumer's augmentative communication needs.

1. Current methods of communication:

Method of Communication	Description	Vocabulary Size	Level of Effectiveness
speech			
vocalizations			
sign language			
gestures or pointing			
head nods			
eye gaze			
facial expression			
augmentative communication system			
other:			

Figure 17-2. Augmentative and alternative communication needs interview form.

Augmentative and Alternative Communication Needs

Consumer:_____   Date:_____

2. The Consumer's Daily Routine: List the consumer's routine activities in the order they occur during a typical day. Briefly describe the activity and the people that communicate with the consumer during the activity.

Activity	Description	Communication Partners

benefit from use of a picture symbol AAC system to clarify his verbal messages to direct care providers in his group home. After interviewing his primary contact person, it was determined that Chris's morning routine consisted of showering, brushing his teeth, shaving, blow drying his hair, getting dressed, eating breakfast, and making his lunch. Chris was able to complete all of these morning activities with minimal assistance from direct care providers. The primary contact person indicated that he rarely interacted with direct care providers or peers during morning grooming activi-

ties. Breakfast and lunch preparation included interactions between Chris, his peers, and his direct care providers. Staff typically initiated conversations with Chris about the breakfast menu, choices for lunch, and the weather. From the interview, it was determined that Chris needed messages in his picture communication system related to breakfast, making lunches, and conversing about the weather or other current events. Messages for grooming activities were not needed due to Chris's level of independence and the limited interactive qualities of these activities. Because the number of symbols needed for the morning routine was small, it was decided to place the pictures into a small wallet-sized AAC communication system.

Observation of the Consumer

Observations of the consumer within the natural environment provides the AAC specialist with vital information about the interactive nature of the program environments. Moreover, observations reveal the communication needs of the consumer within the routine environment. An AAC specialist needs to evaluate the overall appropriateness of consumer activities and communication demands within designated activities. The consumer's ability to meet communication demands within designated activities should also be addressed. In addition, the level of support provided by staff to facilitate interactions within routine activities should be identified. Ideally, the consumer should be observed interacting across several routine daily activities.

Interviews with primary contact persons and observations of the consumer help to identify both the communication needs of the consumer and the need for change within the consumer's programs. Environmental issues that negatively impact implementation of AAC systems in programs for adults with developmental disabilities are common. For example, adult consumers in day vocational programs often work in large noisy warehouse rooms which make communicative interactions difficult, if not impossible. Neglect in making communication changes for both the consumer and the consumer's program will likely lead to failed outcomes when AAC systems are implemented. The next identifies common issues related to implementation of AAC in adult program settings and proposes methods for resolving them.

COMMON COMMUNICATION ISSUES

Opportunities for Choice Making

The opportunity to make choices or indicate preferences adds significantly to one's quality of life. A typical adult without disabilities makes many choices throughout a routine day. The complexity of choice-making depends on factors such as the individual's skill level, interests, and lifestyle. The freedom to make basic, everyday choices is taken for granted by adults without disabilities. In programs for adults with developmental disabilities, direct care providers often assume the role of choice-maker for the consumer. Notably, opportunities for choice-making by AAC consumers are frequently limited by demanding time contraints placed on direct care providers and the lack of an effective means of communication for the consumer.

When creating choice-making opportunities, direct care providers need to be familiar with the consumer's verbal and nonverbal means of effectively indicating a choice. Reaching toward or touching a preferred object is an example of nonverbal choice-making. For a consumer who does not discriminate between pictures but can recognize objects, a direct care provider can simply hold up two to three objects and ask the consumer which is preferred. Introducing picture symbols increases the array of choices available to a consumer at any given time. Picture symbols can be arranged into category-based displays or activity-based displays. Category-based communication systems are primarily designed for simple choice-making. For example, an array of food picture symbols can be organized on a page for the consumer to select items from a menu. Although category-based displays are useful in the choice-making process, after the menu is selected the consumer has nothing else to say. In contrast, activity-based communication boards are designed to facilitate multiple types of messages specific to a designated activity (Elder & Goossens, 1994). For example, picture symbols of actions, descriptions, foods, utensils, and feelings specific to the activity of food preparation can be organized onto a single page to promote a wide variety of communication messages. Adults who are capable of using a large number of AAC picture symbols usually require communication systems that combine category- and activity-based vocabulary. Examples of category-based and activity-based communication boards for doing the laundry are shown in Figure 17–3 (a & b).

Josh was an adult with autism, moderate mental retardation, and a severe behavior disorder characterized by brief episodes of aggressive and destructive behavior. He resided in a group home with two other individuals and a team of direct care providers. His communication consisted of a limited number of signs, approximations of some single words, and gestures. Josh's opportunities for choice-making in this environment were severely limited. Every month, residents of the group home were

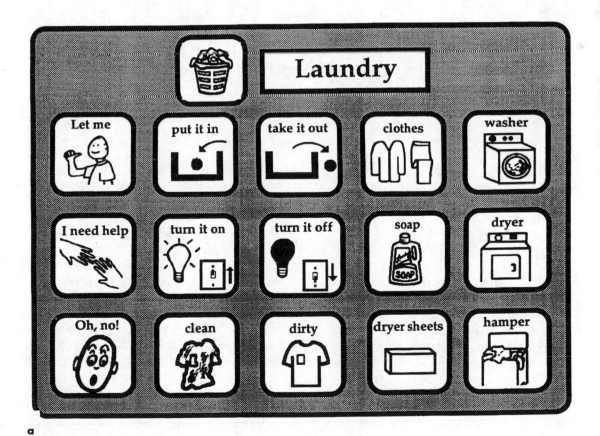

Figure 17–3. Communication boards for laundry activities, **(a)** is activity-based,

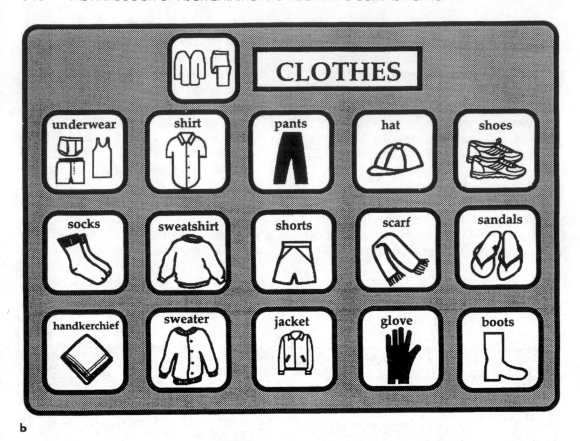

b

Figure 17-3. *(continued)* **(b)** is category based. Symbols courtesy of Boardmaker (Mayer-Johnson,

accompanied to a movie selected by the direct care provider. On one occasion at the local movie theater, when the direct care provider handed Josh a soda, he pushed the soda out of her hands. After this episode, Josh's leisure activities were modified. To avoid conflicts, Josh was not taken to the movie theater, but encouraged to participate in solitary activities such as walking in the park.

A wallet AAC system composed of multiple category-based or choice-making boards was created for Josh by his speech-language pathologist. The wallet contained a limited number of picture symbols depicting Josh's interests and daily needs. In the beginning, he required constant visual models to point to picture symbols for choice-

making. Although Josh did not initiate choice-making with the picture symbols, his imitation of models provided by direct care providers was a positive prognostic indicator. Josh's house counselors were encouraged to add picture symbols to Josh's wallet as his interests and needs changed. Staff continued to model use of the AAC wallet within the routine context of Josh's daily schedule. Ongoing participation of the house counselors in the AAC planning and implementation process helped them to take over "ownership" of the AAC system from the speech-language pathologist. Ownership by the staff strengthened the investment of direct care pro-viders in the success of the AAC system. Six months later, Josh also began taking ownership responsibilities for his AAC wallet. He refused to leave the house without the wallet and occasionally would initiate requests using the picture symbols. He gradually established an effective means of communicating simple requests to his direct care providers. Over a relatively short period of time, Josh replaced some of his maladaptive behaviors with more socially acceptable means of communication through picture symbols. As Josh progressed, he was eventually able to add socially based leisure choices to his AAC system, such as choosing to attend the movies, or selecting his snacks at the movies. Plans were made to add activity-based communication pages to his AAC system to develop higher level communication skills within preferred activities.

A choice-making system composed of photographs, line drawings, or picture symbols can promote improved opportunities for consumers to indicate their wants and needs in a socially acceptable manner. The availability of category-based or activity-based communication boards often serves as a visual reminder for direct care providers to present choice-making and other communication opportunities.

Establishing a Routine

Most adults are guided by some type of routine in their lives. Routines can be large-scale, such as leaving home, going to work, and coming home. They can be detailed, such as taking a work break, getting change for the soda machine, buying a soda, drinking the soda, throwing the can away, and returning to work. A lack of routine is an inconsistent or erratic sequence of activities across a day. Unscheduled events frequently inhibit a consumer's transition from one activity to another. Some consumers become frustrated or anxious when unable to predict upcoming events. Knowledge of daily routines provides consumers with additional structure to facilitate communication. A consumer who

knows that break time follows a period of working can use that knowledge to ask a superviser when the next break will occur.

A schedule of routine events across the day needs to be available to both consumers and direct care providers. A schedule of events can be reviewed with the consumer at designated times during the day. For example, each morning the direct care provider can announce the daily schedule of activities during breakfast. Upon completion of each activity, direct care providers can announce the next activity. For example, after breakfast, a direct care provider announces "We are finished with breakfast, it's time to clean up." Use of a picture schedule can strengthen the individual's recall of daily or weekly events and provide necessary structure for consumers as well as direct care providers. Picture schedules are particularly helpful for new staff members. Picture schedules can be created with different levels of detail and designed for individual or group use. Sample picture schedules are shown in Figure 17–4. A mini-picture schedule can easily be contained in a small wallet communication book. Picture schedules can also be enlarged and located on the wall or table surface in highly visible areas in a residential or vocational setting. Large schedules can be used by multiple consumers and can also provide visual cues to direct care providers to assist them in scheduling the consumer's routines.

Availability of Appropriate Activities

Observations of adults using AAC engaging in routine activities provides information about the level of appropriateness and the interactive nature of each activity. A common issue in programs for adults with developmental disabilities is a lack of age-appropriate activities in leisure, daily living, and vocational areas. Schleien, Olson, Rogers, and McLafferty (1985) identified

DAILY PICTURE COMMUNICATION SCHEDULES

Daily Home Schedule: Leisure Options

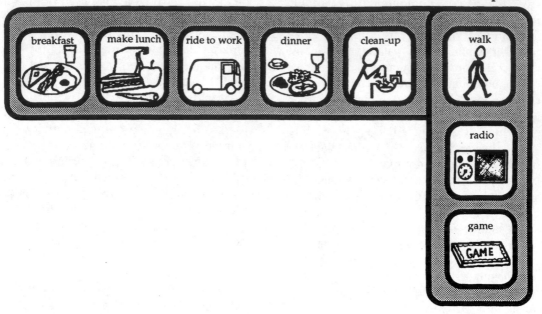

Daily Work Schedule:

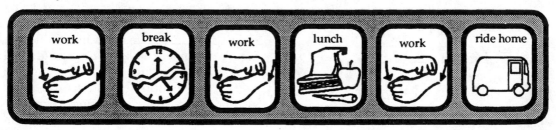

Figure 17–4. AAC picture communication schedules. Symbols courtesy of Boardmaker (Mayer-Johnson, 1994).

the need to develop leisure skills that are age-appropriate, community-based, and facilitate community integration. These criteria are listed with other characteristics of appropriate activities in a checklist format in Table 17–1. Additional features of preferred activities include interactions between more than one individual, including peers without disabilities, a clear goal for the activity with outlined step-by-step procedures, an end product when the activity is completed, and adaptations of the activity for sensory, motor, or cognitive disabilities. Inappropriate selection of activities can lead to both consumer and staff boredom. Of course, many activities that are suitable for a given individual do not possess all of these preferred characteristics. Examples of appropriate activities for adults with developmental disabilities are listed in Table 17–2. These include leisure activities, daily living activities, and vocational activities.

Table 17–1. Checklist of preferred characteristics of activities for adults with developmental disabilities.

1. Is the activity age appropriate?
2. Is the activity functional?
3. Was consideration given to the individual's interests and abilities?
4. Was the activity easily adaptable for cognitive, sensory, and motor disabilities?
5. Did the activity involve two or more individuals?
6. Were peers without disabilities integrated into the activity?
7. Did the activity encourage collaborative group efforts?
8. Were there clear objectives for the activity?
9. Were there sequenced concise steps to complete the activity?
10. Did the activity result in a concrete end product?

Table 17-2. Activities in adult program settings.

LEISURE ACTIVITIES	DAILY LIVING ACTIVITIES	VOCATIONAL ACTIVITIES
amusement park	shopping for household items	packing boxes
bowling	shopping for groceries	preparing and mailing
church	shopping for clothes	sorting books
fair	shopping for household items	busing tables
library	riding the bus	washing dishes
hobby groups	riding the metro	wiping tables
parties	cleaning the house	greeting customers
sporting events	dressing	greeting co-workers
vacation	laundry	collecting trash
picnics	grooming	cleaning offices
restaurants	packing lunches	collating

Choice-making by the consumer is a critical communication component when selecting appropriate activities. Realistically, a consumer's schedule of daily activities consists of nonpreferred neutral activities that must be completed and preferred activities that may or may not be required. For most adults, daily chores such as cleaning the dishes are not preferred activities. To increase motivation and communication opportunities, the consumer can be given a choice between two or three jobs. Although the activities themselves are still unmotivating, the consumer is given some empowerment through making a choice. A consumer can be involved in selecting some, but not all, of the daily activities. For example, cleaning the dishes is often a required chore that is completed after every meal without exception. However the individual can still be given the option to clear the table, wash dishes, load the dishwasher, dry dishes, or put dishes away. A simple AAC system such as a choice board can be established that allows consumers to select activities when appropriate. If a group of individuals is involved, they can alternate selecting activities. For example, John selects group bowling on Saturday, and Dave selects a group walk in the park on Sunday.

Active participation of direct care providers in planning activities also helps to promote ownership and staff investment in the activities. This staff ownership helps secure a direct care provider's concern for the success of an activity. Multiple factors must be considered when selecting activities including the age of the individuals, disabilities, and skills (see Table 17–1). Selection of preferred activities that involve interactions with others is important for implementation of AAC systems. Direct care providers often require assistance in determining whether appropriate and frequent communication opportunities are being offered within an activity. One method of increasing staff awareness regarding appropriate activities is to have direct care providers evaluate existing activities using the preferred features checklist presented in Table 17–1. If needed, videotapes of existing activities can be made and evaluated by a team of direct care providers. Staff completion of the interactional activity checklist will increase awareness of the need to select activities that facilitate interactive communication opportunities.

Structure in a Given Activity

Predictibility and structure are required components of activities that facilitate communication. An unstructured activity is one that lacks basic components such as concise sequenced steps and an end product. Without consistency and structure, the predictability of a task is shattered. To compensate for a lack of structure, direct care providers often dominate the interaction and may actually complete tasks for consumers. When direct care providers fail to provide assistance during unstructured tasks, consumers often become passive or frustrated. In worst case scenarios, consumer boredom and frustration leads to maladaptive behaviors such as disruption, aggression, or self-injury.

Performing a basic task analysis is one method of assisting direct care providers in recognizing the clear components of an activity; the steps within the activity that consumers can independently achieve; and the steps in the activity that may require assistance. A task analysis is the process of sequencing an activity into its component steps. First, the objective or goal for the activity needs to be established. The goal should reflect the consumer's interests, chronological age, and program routine. The goal is recognized as what the consumer is striving to achieve within the activity. The steps toward completion of the activity then need to be defined. To assist in determining the steps for achieving a goal, peers without disabilities should be observed performing similar tasks. The activities can later be adapted for the capabilities of the consumer. Once the goal and steps have been defined, a written protocol for the activity can be created by a program supervisor. A written protocol is designed to clearly outline the consumer's objective or goal and the means or steps to achieve the targeted goal. Figure 17–5 is an example of a written activity protocol. Because of high staff turnover in programs for adults with developmental disabilities, written protocols help guide new direct care providers in consistently structuring consumer activities to enhance the use of AAC.

The use of written protocols helps to provide consumers with consistent structure in communication activities. For consumers who need to use AAC, written protocols specifying actual use of the system should be written into the Individual Habilitation Plan (IHP). An IHP is a formal

CONSUMER ACTIVITY PROTOCOL

ACTIVITY:	Greeting customers at work
CONSUMER:	Sam Johnson
CONTACT PERSON(S):	Pat Jones (Job Counselor) (410) 872-9872
GOAL:	Sam will greet customers using a variety of message choices available on his Voice Pal.
MATERIALS:	Voice Pal augmentative communication device programmed with four greeting messages.

STEPS:

1) Before going to the front of the store, Sam's aide should prepare him to greet customers as they enter. Sam will have four social messages available to him on the Voice Pal. The aide should model how to interact with customers by pointing to a message on Sam's Voice Pal. The aide and Sam should practice by role playing greeting customers for ten minutes.

2) After practicing, Sam and the aide should move to the work area at the front of the store. Sam will be provided with a table and chair. The Voice Pal should be placed on the table in front of Sam. The aide should initiate greetings by using the Voice Pal to greet customers. After three to four models, the aide should encourage Sam to push message keys on the Voice Pal to greet customers.

3) Initially, Sam's aide will show him what button to push. Sam should be prompted to use a variety of messages to greet customers. Sam should also be instructed to look at the customer and smile after pushing a message on the Voice Pal. Hopefully, Sam will be reinforced by customers who respond to his greetings. Sam's aide should intermittently provide Sam with verbal reinforcement throughout the shift (i.e., "Nice job, Sam!" or "Way to go, Sam!").

4) As Sam begins to push buttons more frequently, the aide should let him initiate greetings independently. If he is able to initiate 8 out of 10 greetings successfully without cueing, the aide should step back from the table and simply observe from a few feet away.

Figure 17–5. Augmentative and alternative communication consumer activity protocol.

written plan of habilitation similar to the Individualized Education Plan (IEP) written for students in school. Written protocols provide structure for direct care providers to implement AAC systems within functional activities. Unfortunately, some direct care providers and program supervisors perceive and treat use of AAC devices as part of speech therapy. The AAC systems are used during designated weekly speech times and placed aside on a shelf during naturally occurring activities. Even with the support of written protocols, direct care providers may still need hands-on demonstrations to learn to model use of an AAC system for a consumer.

Assistance Available to a Consumer during an Activity

The level and quality of consumer supervision available from direct care providers vary widely across adult programs. The frequency, type, and quality of communication prompts that can be provided by direct care workers need to be considered. This information is helpful for predicting the level of support a consumer would receive when an AAC system is introduced.

For example, Rachel was an adult with moderate mental retardation, minor neuromotor dysfunction, visual impairments, and a severe dysarthria of speech resulting in an expressive communication disorder. She independently walked without assistance but was not always steady on her feet. She was able to complete many functional living skills independently. During the initial AAC evaluation, Rachel's direct care providers were interviewed regarding the level of support that they could provide. Rachel resided in an apartment with three peers and one residential direct care provider. This direct care provider spent much of her time assisting another resident who had more severe physical disabilities. She indicated that she would be able to prompt Rachel to use an AAC sys-

tem, but would not be able to spend extensive time assisting her with the device. During the day, Rachel worked for a company that maintained indoor plants for large businesses as part of a supported employment program. She was part of a group of six employees supervised by a single direct care provider. AAC system portability and ease of use were primary requirements mentioned by Rachel's supported employment coach.

An AAC evaluation revealed that Rachel could successfully use a large vocabulary of picture symbols to interact with others. She was able to combine two to three picture symbols in a concrete manner to relay messages when given a verbal prompt. Due to minor neuromotor dysfunction, Rachel was unable to isolate her fingers to access picture symbols smaller than 1 inch in size. In addition, her visual impairment impeded her ability to visually scan and locate small picture symbols. It was determined that Rachel needed an AAC system that would provide her with a limited number of large-sized symbols on a single picture display yet would support her need for a large vocabulary. High tech static display AAC devices such as the AlphaTalker, or Macaw were ruled out because Rachel would not be able to change the device pages independently, and could not rely on direct care providers to consistently change the pages for her. High tech AAC systems with more vocabulary on a single static display used small symbols that could not be visually or physically accessed by Rachel. When consideration was given to Rachel's active work responsibilities, high tech dynamic display AAC devices such as the Dynavox were also ruled out due to portability issues.

Through further investigation, it was determined that Rachel would benefit from use of a small picture communication notebook. Activity-based picture symbol pages were mounted on cardboard with page dividers to make them easier to turn. A carrying strap was attached so that Rachel could wear it over her shoulder like a purse. The AAC notebook provided her with independence to select communication topic pages and was lightweight for easy portability.

The AAC evaluation process needs to consider the consumer's communication needs and potential, and the level of support available from direct care providers. Although Rachel was certainly capable of using more sophisticated AAC devices, the lack of support from her direct care providers was a primary factor in determining the type of AAC system that would work best in her existing environments. Ultimately, the goal is to provide the adult consumer with the least restrictive communication environment or necessary amount of support. In other words, the goal is to develop an AAC system that can immediately be used independently by the consumer. This does not mean that the existing level of support provided in Rachel's environment was appropriate. However, changing the amount of support provided by direct care providers is a major systems change process that could take months or years in the adult program environment. Rachel needed an AAC system that would be successful for her immediately.

AAC systems can be planned with built-in features that assist adult consumers to use their communication aids independently. Table 17–3 provides a list of features to consider when developing picture communication systems. Features include using picture symbols that are instantly recognized by the consumer; making the symbols large enough to be easily accessed or seen; reducing the number of symbols on a single page to decrease assistance needed to find a particular symbol; placing frequently used symbols in consistent locations across AAC display pages; and color coding symbols to assist in visual discrimination. These AAC features apply when implementing both high tech and low tech strategies. Selection and design of specific AAC features is always based on the consumer's skills, communication needs, and the ability of the consumer's environment to implement the system.

Interactions Between Consumers and Peers

Interactions between adults with developmental disabilities and age-related peers who are nondisabled are frequently limited. Interactions are often restricted by the

Table 17–3. AAC system features designed to increase communication independence.

- Use symbols that are immediately recognized.
- Picture symbols are sized and arranged for independent access.
- Fewer picture symbols are shown on a single communication page.
- Consistent locations are used for frequently occurring symbols..
- Color coding is used to assist with visually scanning multiple symbols.
- Sharp figure-ground color contrasts are used to assist with visual scanning of symbols.
- If multiple pages of picture symbols are required, they are arranged so the individual can independently select and change pages.
- Systematic organization of multiple picture pages is used to assist with locating symbols.
- Picture symbol cues are provided as a guide to search through multiple pages of symbols.
- Portability features are added such as a carrying strap, key ring, or carrying case.

limited availability of integrated programs for adults with developmental disabilities. Adults with developmental disabilities typically reside with other adults with similiar skill levels. They also participate in day or vocational programs specifically geared toward adults with intellectual and physical limitations. Frequently, direct care providers in a group home or a day program are an adult consumer's closest nondisabled communication partners. Direct care providers often act as bridges or buffers between adult consumers and age-related peers in the community. This intervention can sometimes enhance interactions, but typically tends to limit direct interactions with community peers. Less visibility and interaction within the community restricts opportunities to increase general public awareness and acceptance of individuals with developmental disabilities, obstructs the development of meaningful relationships, and impedes the chance for future participation in community activities.

The case of Jim illustrates the need to increase direct interactions with peers in the community. Jim was an adult with mental retardation. He could not speak and engaged in mild self-injurious behaviors. Jim interacted primarily through facial expressions, gestures, and basic picture communication. He resided in a group home with three other adult males and a rotating staff of two residential counselors. On weekends, the group frequently traveled to a nearby restaurant for dinner. Because one of the residential counselors was highly familiar with all of the adults, she typically encouraged the group to find a booth and sit down. Then she proceeded to order everyone's meals at the counter. Although the residential counselor was helpful in ordering the adults' meals, Jim was not provided with an opportunity to make a menu choice through pointing or interacting with employees at the restaurant. Additionally, restaurant employees were denied direct interaction with Jim.

This scenario did not support public awareness and acceptance of Jim or his disability.

An initial step toward integrating adults with developmental disabilities and AAC systems into the community is to increase visibility within typical social activities. This provides members of the community with direct experiences interacting through alternative means of communication. Direct care and support service providers need to identify a consumer's communication abilities and to develop opportunities and means for the consumer to successfully interact during community activities.

Jim's residential counselor unintentionally made the mistake of making choices for Jim and limiting his interactions with community peers. Jim was not given the opportunity to make a meal selection or to interact with the cashier at the restaurant. Both Jim and the cashier may have mutually benefited from this interaction. Providing Jim with this community experience would not have required much planning. A simple menu containing photographs of food and drink selections at the restaurant could have been shown to Jim. While at the counter, his counselor could have asked "Jim, would you like a hamburger or a cheeseburger?" while simultaneously pointing to the photographs. If a picture menu was not available, the counselor could request the restaurant cashier to show Jim the actual foods for him to select through a hand reach. Through basic adaptations in the environment, Jim would be able to meaningfully interact with other adults in the community. In addition, the restaurant cashier would have become familiar with AAC and might learn to recognize that adults with special needs can actively and successfully participate in everyday community activities.

This type of community activity can be adapted for differing levels of communication skills. For example, a consumer who is unable to discriminate between a choice of more than one object or picture can be taught to hand a premade menu card or request strip to a store clerk. A direct care provider who was highly familiar with the consumer's likes and dislikes could prepare a request card or menu card prior to the visit to the store. A sample request card for the drug store is shown in Figure 17–6. This type of system should be avoided if the consumer is capable of actively making choices. A generic "request card" can be used for multiple community activities. The request card can be constructed with laminated cardboard, a strip of velcro, and a set of picture symbols or written words that are velcroed to the card. During bowling, a consumer could hand a request card to the cashier which states "I would like size 8½ shoes, please." Consumer requests can also be pre-recorded onto portable, single message AAC devices such as the Attainment Two Talker, Enabling Device's Talking Switch Plates, or Ablenet's Big Mack. Developing basic AAC options can provide many opportunities for consumers with significant intellectual impairments to actively participate in community activities.

Community Awareness

Although integration of children and adults with developmental disabilities is becoming more frequent, not all individuals in the community feel prepared to interact with a consumer using AAC. Integration of consumers within everyday community activities such as shopping increases the visibil-

REQUEST CARDS

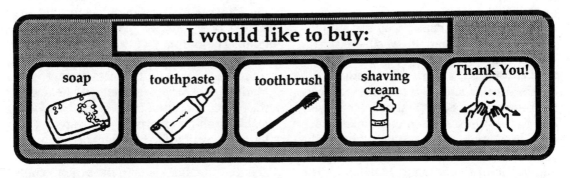

Figure 17–6. Request card used to ask for items in a drug store. Symbols courtesy of Boardmaker (Mayer-Johnson, 1994).

ity of individuals with developmental disabilities. However, the community may need additional assistance to interact with adults who use AAC. A short-term strategy for facilitating interactions between employees of an establishment and AAC consumers is to prepare the employees immediately prior to the interaction. For example, direct care providers for Jim, the consumer profiled in the previous section, might have briefly described his menu request system to the cashier before sending him up to the restaurant counter. A long-term strategy to enhance community interactions is to consult with the management of a frequented establishment such as a local restaurant or grocery store. This meeting should focus on forming relationships with the establishment and increasing employee awareness of AAC.

Local programs and organizations can be contacted and asked if they are interested in integrating adults with special needs. Consumers can participate in community activities on a weekly or bimonthly basis. Consumers can be paired with individuals in the community who have similar interests through a buddy system. For example, Mildred was an older woman with cerebral palsy and mild to moderate mental retardation. She communicated using one to two word spoken utterances which were intelligible with careful listening. She supplemented her speech with gestures, and a picture communication book. The AAC system was typically used to establish a topic of communication. After the topic was established, Mildred relied on her speech. Mildred attended a day program which focused on increasing independence in daily living and leisure activities. Mildred was independent in all activities of daily living such as toileting, eating, and communicating basic needs to others. Mildred especially enjoyed participating in arts and crafts activities in her day program. Observation of Mildred revealed that she readily initiated interactions with staff members

during these activities. Unfortunately, staff members were often busy assisting other clients who were more physically or intellectually challenged than Mildred. Mildred enjoyed the leisure activities provided by her day program, but was hindered by limited opportunities to socialize with adults who demonstrated similar or higher skill levels.

Mildred was placed in a day program that` did not meet her social needs. Just as professionals have learned that children benefit from the least restrictive environment, Mildred also needed an environment that would provide her with appropriate opportunities for communication and socialization. Mildred's day program supervisor decided that she was a candidate for participating in arts and crafts activities at a local senior center. Initially, Mildred visited and toured the center. She appeared interested and one visit per week was organized for the following month. Mildred was paired with a nondisabled peer who was related in age and interests. Prior to sending Mildred to the senior center, her assigned peer was invited to the day program. The purpose of this meeting was to introduce Mildred to her new friend, and to train the peer how to best interact with Mildred. A separate meeting was held with the director of the senior center who was also told about Mildred's AAC system. This initial consultation between peers in the community and Mildred's day program ensured that her visits to the senior center were a success.

A variety of factors should be considered before introducing consumers into least restrictive environments. In review, consumers should show an interest in community programs, and more importantly, community programs need to be interested in meeting consumer needs. The program should be aware of the individual's level of independence, communication abilities, and general interests. This is to ensure that the program is equipped with adequate staff and can make adaptations as needed. To aid in the transition from a highly supported program to a least restricted program, the consumer can be placed with a companion or partner with similar interests. In addition to the peer companion, other community participants also need to be educated about adults with developmental disabilities. The education process can range from formal training to gradual learning through natural interactions. Choosing the appropriate educational training process is usually dependent on the number of adults with developmental disabilities who will be introduced into the community activity. A single consumer can often be introduced into a community program gradually, with minimal peer training. If groups of consumers participate in community programs without support from direct care providers, then formal peer training is necessary.

Overall, programs for adults with developmental disabilities need to provide daily activities and leisure opportunities involving interactions between consumers and their nondisabled peers. Schleien and Mustonen (1988) suggested that progress toward the development of a meaningful and satisfying lifestyle for individuals with developmental disabilities is burdened by programs that offer segregated and diversional recreation opportunities. AAC specialists and direct care providers need to serve as advocates for providing least restrictive communicative environments for adults with developmental disabilities.

Uneven Interactions Between Consumers and Peers

Uneven interactions between adult consumers and direct care providers result in a lack of communicative initiations from consumers, limited social conversations from direct care providers, and frequent use of verbal commands by direct care providers. Direct care providers often assume the role of commanding or directing

tasks rather than facilitating interactions. Verbal interactions between direct care providers and adults with developmental disabilities frequently consist of commands or directions such as "Come here," "Pick it up," or "Put it over there." In turn, the adult consumer often adopts a passive role in communication.

Regardless of the individual's level of understanding, it is important to treat the consumer as an adult. Staff should try to avoid discussing sensitive issues in front of the consumer. Direct care providers should use conversational starters or language that encourages the consumer to reciprocate or engage in the interaction. For example, every adult prefers to participate in conversations that revolve around interests, past memories, or daily activities. In order to facilitate interactions, the direct care provider's familiarity with the consumer's language comprehension and expressive means of communication is critical. For example, a consumer may have an adapted sign for "more, please." The communication attempt may be ignored or misinterpreted by direct care providers who are unfamiliar with the consumer. New staff need to receive training regarding a consumer's AAC skills.

Uneven interactions between consumers who use AAC and direct care providers also occur in the work environment. As consumers make the transition into supported work settings in the community, employee supervisors and peers become important partners in the interaction process. Adult AAC users often lack the social-communication skills to ensure positive adjustment to the work environment. Ferguson, McDonnell, and Drew (1993) found that co-workers without mental retardation initiate interactions or conversations significantly more often than employees with mental retardation. This lack of social interaction with co-workers can result in the failure to develop meaningful relationships in the workplace. Lignugaris-Kraft, Salzberg,

Rule, and Stowichek (1988) found that employees value the following social-vocational skills in other employees: following directions, obtaining information prior to performing a task, providing job-related information to others, and offering assistance to co-workers. In some cases, the consumer may not have the means to meet the social-vocational demands of a job due to an ineffective or absent AAC system. It is important that consumers using AAC receive intensive intervention when entering employment settings. A major portion of this intervention needs to focus on training employee supervisors and peers how to facilitate appropriate interactions in the work setting.

PLANNING AND IMPLEMENTING AAC SYSTEMS

Consideration of the Daily Routine

The consumer's interests and daily routines are essential in determining the content and organization of an AAC system. Most adults with developmental disabilities lead highly structured lives with minimal variation in activities from day to day. It is important that the vocabulary developed for an AAC system provide the individual with the support necessary to interact within this daily structure. However, the process of learning to use this vocabulary functionally is difficult for adults who have never been able to clearly communicate their needs to others. As an example, consider Megan, an adult diagnosed with autism and moderate mental retardation. Megan resided in a group home with two other adults. Her two peers communicated through spoken language. Megan communicated through a combination of idiosyn-

cratic gestures and sign language. Interviews with staff who knew her well found that she had approximately 10 sign gestures that were used consistently. On occasion, Megan engaged in self-injurious or destructive behavior when her gestured messages were misinterpreted or unclear to her peers and direct care providers. In addition, Megan's peers and direct care providers were not always familiar with her sign language.

Megan was referred to an AAC specialist who determined that Megan had the skills to functionally use a simple picture-based communication system. Initially, Megan's direct care providers wanted an AAC system with functional messages such as "eat," "drink," and "bathroom." Because the concept of using pictures for communication would be new for Megan, staff were counseled to initially develop a simple AAC system that would be highly motivating for her to use. For a trial period, a picture communication wallet containing five pages of picture symbols was provided for Megan to use. Each page contained three symbols related to a highly motivating topic or activity. In developing Megan's picture-based AAC system, direct care providers in the group home were interviewed about her daily routine and special interests. Observations of Megan's peers during communicative exchanges were also instrumental in planning appropriate messages for Megan's communication system. Over a 1-month trial period, direct care providers modeled use of the picture communication wallet with Megan.

As Megan and her direct care providers grew accustomed to communicating through picture symbols, pages related to Megan's daily routine were implemented. The activity-based pages of the wallet were organized in their naturally occurring sequence across a routine day. The organization of the AAC wallet assisted both Megan and her direct care providers in rapidly locating a page for a designated activity. The organization of the wallet also aided Megan in transitioning from one activity to another. Introduction of an AAC system played a role in reducing the frequency of Megan's maladaptive behaviors. An increase in Megan's positive adaptive behaviors, including communication skills, resulted in improved relations with peers in her group home.

Generating Vocabulary for a Communication System

Vocabulary is one factor that can affect the consumer's and the direct care provider's motivation to use an AAC system. AAC vocabulary should reflect the individual's interests, needs, and routines. As indicated previously in Megan's case, direct care providers often have difficulty making the distinction between choosing vocabulary to meet their own needs versus vocabulary the consumer is motivated to communicate. Direct care providers need to be reminded that the AAC system is a means for the consumer to interact with others and not a tool for direct care providers to instruct the consumer.

With appropriate daily routine activities established, the communication demands of each activity need to be identified. This process assists the AAC specialist in planning the vocabulary and guiding the organization of an AAC system. The AAC specialist determines what communicative intents are required to interact during a designated activity. A worksheet for identifying communication requirements within a single activity is available in Figure 17–7. The worksheet lists categories of communication requirements with an area for describing the situation that occurs when the communication attempt is needed. When making vocabulary decisions, the AAC specialist needs to consider the communication demands or opportunities available within each activity, the con-

sumer's skills, and the level of support that can be provided by direct care providers.

From a basic interview, category-based communication symbol pages can be developed. A snack page containing items such as cookies, cupcakes, potato chips, popcorn, and soda is an example of a category-based communication page. Category-based communication pages are typically limited to choice-making. As previously mentioned in this chapter, choice-making is only one component of communication. AAC systems developed primarily with category-based pages are useful for some adult consumers who need a method of clarifying communication topics. Consumers who communicate primarily through spoken language and have some unintelligible speech can use category-based communication pages to clarify spoken words. Consumers who demonstrate difficulty recalling words may also use category-based communication pages as a self-prompting system for generating spoken language.

An activity-based AAC symbol page contains multiple messages related to a designated activity or topic. In addition to choice-making, consumers can socially interact, direct the actions of others, and ask questions through use of an activity-based communication board. Activity-based communication boards provide the user with most of the necessary vocabulary for a given activity in a single location. This organization serves to speed up the communication process within an activity by eliminating the process of hunting for symbols across multiple communication pages. In order to provide adult consumers with rapid interactive communication while maintaining vocabulary depth, most AAC systems need a combination of category- and activity-based communication pages.

Messages for designated activities can be generated through scripting. The focus of scripting is to capture messages that are typically produced during a designated

COMMUNICATION REQUIREMENTS	
Focus: To identify the consumer's required communication needs along with examples of how the consumer is currently meeting communication requirements within an activity.	

Consumer: _____   Date: _____

Activity: _____

COMMUNICATION REQUIREMENTS	EXAMPLES
1. To socially interact.	
2. To engage in turn-taking.	
3. To gain the attention of others.	
4. To request assistance.	
5. To request objects.	
6. To request actions.	
7. To direct others' actions.	
8. To ask questions.	
9. To respond to questions.	

Figure 17–7. Activity communication requirements form.

activity (Elder & Goossens, 1994). Scripting an activity leads to the development of activity-based communication pages. Scripting involves documenting the sequence of events and transcribing the interactions of individuals engaged in a designated activity. To facilitate natural interactive situations, direct care providers can develop scripts by observing and documenting messages of adults without special needs engaged in leisure activities. For example, a group of staff might go to the bowling alley and record the events that occurred and typical messages that were communicated to develop a bowling script for group home residents. Figure 17–8 presents a form designed to facilitate the scripting process. Scripting provides direct care providers with experience in recognizing the pronouns, social messages, verbs, descriptor words, prepositions, and nouns necessary for an individual or group of individuals to interact during a targeted activity.

Systematic Organization of Vocabulary

An AAC system should be flexible enough to adjust to the user's changing interests and needs. The physical setup of vocabulary in an AAC system needs to be systematically organized to possess the qualities of reduplication and flexibility. Systematic organization of a communication system allows for the addition of new vocabulary with the least amount of disruption to the existing setup. For example, many adult consumers learn to identify symbols on their communication boards according to the placement of the pictures. Through frequent use of their communication systems, they learn that the symbol located in the lower corner gets them one object, and the symbol in the upper corner gets them another object. When changes are made to the AAC system, it is important that these location and placement cues are maintained from one system to another. If learned picture symbols are moved or changed, the consumer may require additional training and prompts to relearn independent use of the AAC system. Systematic organization of vocabulary or messages applies when developing a simple communication board and when developing complex multilevel AAC systems.

Systematic organization of an AAC system positively affects a direct care provider's ability to facilitate use of the system. For example, Vicki's direct care providers were involved in the development of a communication wallet with 25 pages of messages. Each page was related to a single activity. Pages were organized into sections such as activities of daily living, vocational tasks, and leisure. Because Vicki was not familiar with the vocabulary in her newly acquired communication system, the topic for each page was written near the edge so that her direct care providers could quickly flip through to find appropriate pages. The following weekend, Vicki, her one-to-one aide, and two peers from the group home traveled to the movie theater and stood in line to order a snack. Vicki unsuccessfully pointed toward an item in the glass display case. The movie clerk was unable to interpret Vicki's request. As a team member in planning the AAC system, Vicki's one-to-one aide opened the wallet to the leisure section and found the page related to the movies. Vicki's aide then pointed to two pictures of snacks and asked her what she wanted. Because of the systematic organization of the communication wallet and the direct care provider's involvement in planning the AAC system, an interactive opportunity was provided for Vicki.

Category-Based Communication Boards

A category-based communication system is primarily designed to promote choice-making opportunities for a consumer. Choice-making is only one facet of commu-

The Kennedy Krieger Institute
Department of Assistive Technology

ACTIVITY SCRIPTING

Consumer: _____ Activity: _____

Focus: This worksheet is designed to assist in planning activity-based communication overlays. While observing peer interactions, record the sequence of events in order and the vocabulary that was used during the activity. Vocabulary concepts are organized as they typically appear on a communication overlay.

Script Events in Sequence	People Pronouns	Social	Actions	Descriptors Prepositions	Objects
1)					
2)					
3)					
4)					
5)					
6)					

Figure 17-8. Activity scripting form. *Note:* From *Assistive Technology: The Predictive Assessment Process*, by S. Glennen, E. Delsandro, U. Radell, and S. Schiaffino, 1995, paper presented at the Closing the Gap Conference, Minneapolis, MN. Reprinted with permission.

nication. The physical organization of a single category-based page depends on the consumer's needs and skill level. Within a category-based page, vocabulary may be organized by columns, rows, or groups. A consistent setup of vocabulary is beneficial for both the consumer and direct care staff, specifically for quickly accessing messages during communicative exchanges. Even when individuals are not familiar with the location of a targeted message, direct care staff can have increased success in locating messages if the vocabulary setup is consistent across pages. A category-based communication page can be organized in alphabetical order or in sub-category groups. Examples of both methods of organization are shown in Figures 17–9 and 17–10.

If the category-based pages are part of a larger AAC communication book or wallet, the entire array of pages needs to be

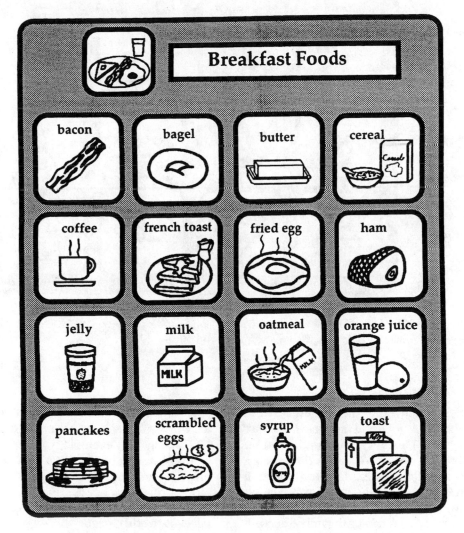

Figure 17–9. Category-based AAC communication board arranged alphabetically. Symbols courtesy of Boardmaker (Mayer-Johnson, 1994).

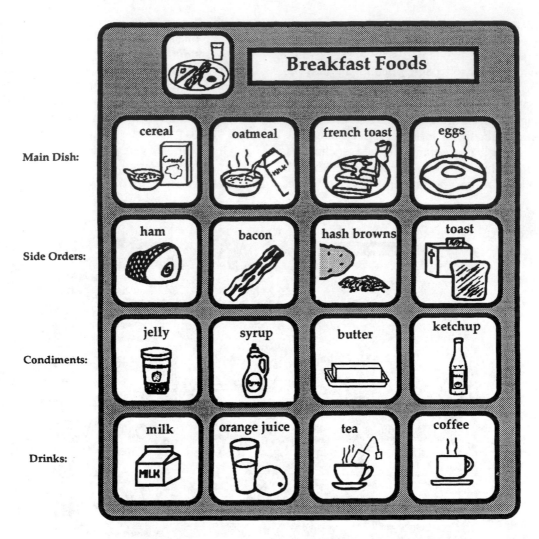

Figure 17-10. Category-based AAC communication board arranged into breakfast food subcategories. Symbols courtesy of Boardmaker (Mayer-Johnson, 1994).

logically sequenced. If the consumer is not independent in locating messages, the category-based pages can be organized in alphabetical order to assist direct care staff in rapidly locating targeted pages. If the user is able to independently search through the pages to locate messages, category-based pages can be organized according to the individual's cognitive schema for remembering page ordering. Many con-

sumers do well when their AAC system pages are sequenced as they are needed during a typical day. For example, the first page is clothing and grooming items related to getting dressed, the second page is breakfast foods, the third page is items to pack into lunches. An additional method of locating pages is to add category-based picture symbol cues on the edges of each page, and to color-code the pages. For example, foods can be printed on green paper, clothes on yellow paper, and people on white paper.

Activity-based Communication Boards

An activity-based communication page contains multiple messages related to a designated topic or activity. As previously mentioned, an activity-based communication page allows a person to socially interact, direct the actions of others, comment, ask questions, and make choices. Once vocabulary or messages for an activity have been generated through scripting, strong consideration to the physical organization of a single activity-based page needs to be made. The physical organization refers to how concepts or messages are arranged on a page. The physical organization of symbols should remain constant across all pages whenever possible.

An activity-based communication board can be logically organized with columns for pronouns and people, verbs or actions, descriptor words such as adjectives and adverbs, directional words or prepositions, and objects. Elder and Goossens (1994) have published several books which consist of premade, activity-based communication boards for adult consumers with coordinating scripts for implementation. Activities include cleaning, grooming, work, and community leisure. The boards come in different formats which vary by the number and size of symbols available.

Activity-based scripting, described previously and outlined in Figure 17–8 is used to develop the vocabulary that is needed for each communication board. Once an initial vocabulary list is developed through direct observation of the activity, direct care staff can review the list to add any missing vocabulary or concepts. In addition, an AAC professional should review the list to determine if additional interactional vocabulary such as social greetings, action words, or descriptive terms need to be added.

Once the listing of vocabulary has been developed, the messages need to be organized. Visual representation of vocabulary is important for multiple direct care providers. A handout designed to show others how to organize picture communication symbols into activity-based formats can be helpful and can be placed in the consumer's permanent file for future reference. Figure 17–11 is an example of an activity-based communication board arrangement based on a modified Fitzgerald Key format suggested by Elder and Goossens (1994). This handout gives direct care providers a systematic map to follow when developing new communication pages for an individual's AAC system.

Modeling AAC Within the Natural Context

Once an organized AAC system is developed, the next step is implementation of the communication program. Both the consumer and direct care staff may not recognize the power of an AAC system and may not know how to implement the system within daily routines. Most direct care providers have little training, if any, in how to facilitate language in natural contexts. Because of limited skills in this area, supervisors often develop highly contrived AAC training programs. AAC professionals will need to demonstrate how to use an AAC system through natural language modeling in the consumer's environment. Teaching natural language modeling is beneficial to both the AAC user and direct care staff.

Modeling use of the communication system should always be conducted within the natural routine environment. Promoting AAC use in the natural environment promotes the consumer's generalization of communication skills. For example, modeling AAC use in the grocery store demonstrates to the individual that a picture communication wallet can be used to direct peers to retrieve shopping list items, make choices about snack foods, and to interact with the cashier.

Activity-Based Communication Board Design

Consumer: _____   Date: _____

Activity: _____

The layout shown below should be used when new communication boards are created for this consumer. Organize picture symbols into each vocabulary category.

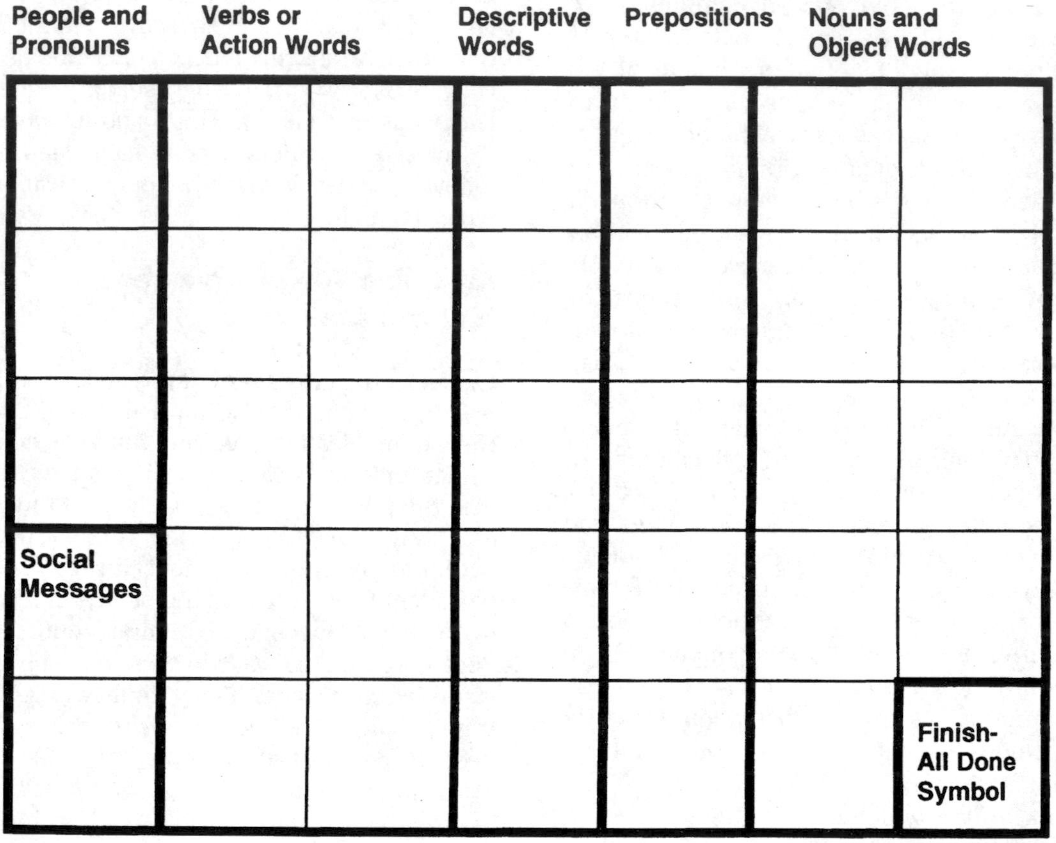

People and Pronouns	Verbs or Action Words	Descriptive Words	Prepositions	Nouns and Object Words	
Social Messages					
					Finish- All Done Symbol

Figure 17–11. Activity-based communication board design based on the Fitzgerald Key format.

The process of teaching direct care providers to use natural language modeling techniques usually requires direct intervention from AAC specialists. For example, every evening after dinner while his peers were watching a popular game show, Dan and his residential counselor Jenna would sit at the kitchen table for 20 minutes of "speech time." Jenna would ask Dan to point to named pictures in his pic- ture communication wallet. This task con- centrated on identification of picture sym- bols but failed to focus on functional use of the symbols. "Speech time" served as an added chore in both Dan's and Jenna's busy schedules. Jenna failed to see the value of "speech time" as Dan never used his AAC wallet except for these training periods. Dan enjoyed interacting with Jenna during "speech time" but would frequently get up and walk over to his peers to see what was on television.

Dan's speech-language pathologist suggested creating a symbol page specifically for the televised game show. The page contained social messages, actions, and comments that would allow Dan to spend time with his peers and interact through use of his AAC system. The speech-language pathologist came to Dan's home on a weekly basis over a 6-week period to meet with Dan and Jenna. During these sessions, videotapes of the game show were played on television. Jenna was shown how to model use of the communication symbols for Dan. They began to spend their evening "speech time" sessions watching the game show with the other residents. After Jenna mastered modeling language during the game show, new AAC activity boards were developed for Dan. Each time a new activity was added, Jenna and Dan received direct training from the speech-language pathologist, who would show Jenna how to model use of the AAC system in each situation. Jenna found that using a naturalistic approach to communication did not disrupt the general routine of the day. In addition, both Jenna and Dan were motivated to use the AAC system in interactive situations rather than in noncommunicative, nonfunctional, repetitive tasks.

When consumers are not independently using AAC systems, modeling is crucial to the success of the system. Individuals who are learning how to interact through pictures will require direct modeling. Modeling assists the individual in learning the location of vocabulary on picture communication displays, teaches the meaning of vocabulary through natural situations, and teaches the user when to interact with specific symbols. Traditionally, AAC modeling has been provided by facilitators who directly point to pictures using their fingers. Elder and Goossens (1994) proposed using light cues to assist consumers in pointing to targeted picture symbols. Light

cues can be provided by flashing a small penlight or flashlight onto the targeted symbol. Light cues call attention to a specific symbol without obstructing it. Light cues are also a less direct method of cueing that visually separates the cue from the person providing the model.

Through use of light cues or direct pointing models direct care providers can interactively highlight picture communication symbols within the context of an activity. Communication board models are given when the direct care provider is discussing the activity (i.e., the direct care provider states "I'm going to *Pour* [light cue] the *Milk* [light cue] into the *Bowl* [light cue]). Models are also used to help the individual select communication symbols during an activity (i.e., the direct care provider asks "Do you want to *Pour* [light cue] or *Stir* ? [light cue]). Use of light cues or other models should be gradually faded as the individual becomes more independent interacting through pictures.

Direct intervention from an AAC specialist can be used to train direct care providers how to model communication within natural contexts. However, the AAC user comes into contact with many different direct care providers. In addition, frequent staff turnover in adult program agencies makes it difficult to maintain appropriate natural AAC training programs. A videotape that demonstrates the consumer participating in natural activities while direct care providers model use of the AAC system can serve as a powerful staff training tool. The videotape should demonstrate how the individual uses the AAC system and how direct care providers can provide modeled prompts.

USE OF HIGH TECH AAC SYSTEMS

Up to this point, this chapter has focused on the use of simple AAC systems. The examples that were reviewed discussed the use of simple picture communication boards, communication books, communication wallets, and use of single symbols taped to specific locations in the natural environment. Although the emphasis of the chapter is on simple AAC systems, some adults with developmental disabilities use high tech AAC devices with voice output. Because of funding limitations, the use of high tech devices is less prevalent among developmentally disabled adults when compared to children. However, as more school-aged children with experience using high tech devices reach the age of 21 and enter adult programs, the use of AAC systems with voice output will hopefully become more common.

Due to the nature of programs for adults with developmental disabilities, implementation of high technology AAC devices is challenging. High rates of staff turnover, poorly trained staff, and a lack of collabo-

ration between residential and day programs make it difficult if not impossible to ensure quality AAC outcomes when high tech devices are used. This section will address specific issues related to the implementation of high technology AAC devices in adult program settings.

Training Direct Care Providers

Similar to the implementation of simple AAC communication boards and books, when high tech AAC systems are introduced representatives from both residential programs and day programs need to be trained. Training should involve individuals from direct care and supervisory levels to limit the impact of future staff turnover. Because high tech AAC devices are complex, training needs to be conducted over several sessions. Training can be divided into the sections presented in Table 17–4.

Table 17-4. Basic training areas for implementing high tech AAC systems.

SKILL AREA	EXAMPLES
General Maintenance	• charging the AAC system • cleaning the display or device • transporting the device
General Operation	• adjusting the volume • adjusting the viewing angle • connecting device components
General Programming	• storing messages • erasing messages • changing levels or pages
Vocabulary Generation	• consideration of the consumer's interests • consideration of the consumer's routines • activity scripting
Vocabulary Organization or Set-up	• category-based communication overlays or pages • activity-based communication overlays or pages
Modeling Use of the Device	• implementing the device in naturalistic settings • use of light cues or other models
Designating Responsibilities	• Responsibility Checklist

These include reviewing general maintenance and operation of the device, how to program messsages into the system, developing vocabulary, deciding how to organize the vocabulary, modeling use of the AAC system, and designating responsibilities for care and maintenance of the device. The process of developing vocabulary and modeling use of the AAC system is similar for both simple AAC communication boards and high tech AAC systems. Vocabulary organization varies, depending on the features of the high tech AAC device being used. What is unique to high tech AAC systems is the process of maintaining, operating, and programming the device.

Maintenance of an AAC device is critical to the overall functioning of the system. If not charged or charged improperly, the device will not be available for use. If a consumer is not capable of independently charging his or her own equipment, designated direct care providers need to be responsible for this duty. To assist direct care providers in this process, a charging schedule should be developed. Use of a charging schedule is especially helpful when many different direct care providers are involved with the consumer. To implement a charging schedule, an area in the residential or day program should be designated as the charging area. A charging schedule is then posted in the area. Direct care providers initial and date the schedule each time they plug the AAC device in for charging or unplug the device following charging.

One difficulty encountered when so many different direct care providers are involved is designating who will program and oversee basic operation of the AAC system. If too many staff members attempt to program the system, the potential for disorganized vocabulary increases. Although more than one staff member can be trained to program an AAC device, it is recommended that a single direct care provider take responsibility for ongoing device programming. Similarly, a single direct care

provider should be responsible for troubleshooting difficulties with the AAC system. Typically, one person is trained to complete both tasks. Due to daily demands and time constraints in the consumer's environment, direct care providers do not have time to consult AAC device manuals for operation and programming instructions. In addition, some manuals are complex and difficult to interpret. The AAC specialist needs to provide the designated direct care provider with written minitraining instructions for operating and programming the AAC device. In addition, simple programming instructions can be placed directly on the device for easy access by the designated direct care provider. Minitraining instructions can include directions for programming messages, erasing messages, changing pages or levels, attaching switches, and troubleshooting when the system does not work properly.

Implementation of a high tech voice output AAC device is a complex process in most environments. Many responsibilities have to be met to maintain the system. Responsibilities need to be coordinated across environments and with designated individuals from the consumer's programs. Common AAC system responsibilities include the following:

- Charging the equipment.
- Contacting the manufacturer about equipment concerns.
- Planning vocabulary.
- Developing picture displays for the device.
- Daily setup of the equipment.
- Ongoing staff training.
- Transportation of the equipment.
- Developing a low technology backup AAC system.

It is helpful to designate specific team members who will be responsible for each of the areas listed. Figure 17–12 is an AAC

```
┌─────────────────────────────────────────────────────────┐
│        Augmentative and Alternative Communication         │
│                 Responsibility Checklist                  │
│                                                           │
│                 Kennedy Krieger Institute                 │
└─────────────────────────────────────────────────────────┘
```

Consumer: _____ Date: _____

List all AAC team members.

Name   **Relationship**   **Phone Number**

_____

_____

_____

_____

_____

List all AAC equipment and identifying information.

Equipment Description   **Serial Number**   **Company Phone No.**

_____

_____

_____

_____

Figure 17–12. AAC responsibility checklist form. *Note:* From *Assistive Technology: the Predictive Assessment Process,* by S. Glennen, E. Delsandro, U. Radell, and S. Schiaffino, 1995, paper presented at the Closing the Gap Conference, Minneapolis, MN. Reprinted with permission.

These AAC responsibilities will be covered by the following persons:

Responsibility   Person Responsible

1) Charging the system.   _____

2) Contacting the company/vendor
   to address equipment concerns.
   (See page 1 for company contacts).   _____

3) Planning AAC system vocabulary

   a. For the home   _____

   b. For the school/day program   _____

   c. For the community   _____

   d. Other: _____   _____

4) Developing picture displays.   _____

5) Programming the AAC system.   _____

6) Daily set-up of equipment components.
   (e.g., head stick, switch, splints, mount)   _____

7) Ongoing staff training.   _____

8) Safe storage of equipment
   when not in use.   _____

9) Transportation of the AAC system.   _____

10) Providing back-up equipment when
    the primary system is not functioning.
    (e.g., a picture communication board)   _____

Responsibility Checklist that can be used to designate these team responsibilities (Glennen, Delsandro, Radell, & Schiaffino, 1995). The first page lists names and phone numbers for all team members. The AAC equipment is listed along with serial or identification numbers, and phone numbers of the manufacturer. The second page lists each responsibility area and identifies who is responsible for each item. Each team member should receive a copy of a responsibility checklist. This checklist should be placed in the consumer's permanent file, and stored in the AAC device carrying case or instruction manual. Because of frequent staff turnover, the checklist needs to be updated every 6 to 9 months.

CONCLUSION

Providing AAC services for adults with developmental disabilities is challenging. Developing an AAC system in adult program environments requires evaluating the communication needs and potential of nonspeaking individuals, and evaluating the ability of the program to implement an AAC system. In most cases, strong preparation of staff in the environment will lay the groundwork for implementation of augmentative communication systems. In order to ensure a successful outcome, relationships need to be established between the AAC professional and adult program agencies at administrative, supervisory, and direct care provider levels. Through systematic training within the consumers' environment, AAC systems can be incorporated into the daily lives of adults with developmental disabilities. In summary, AAC specialists need to view the individual consumer and the AAC system within the context of the whole environment.

Many nonspeaking adults in programs for developmentally disabled individuals were previously placed in institutional settings. They have entered community-based environments with little experience engaging in successful interactions. Because underlying pragmatic communication skills are missing, and direct care staff support for communication is limited, it is often difficult to achieve positive AAC outcomes. In the next decade, with advancements in knowledge and availability of AAC technology, a generation of children who successfully communicate using AAC will grow into adults with developmental disabilities. As they gradually assimilate into adult programs, the use of AAC systems in these environments will increase. There will be an obligation from AAC professionals and adult program administrators to ensure that the communication gains made in childhood transfer into successful integration of AAC into the adult community.

REFERENCES

Altman, B. M., & Cunningham, P. J. (1993). Dynamic process of movement in residential settings. *American Journal on Mental Retardation, 98*, 304–316.

Bernstein, G. S., Ziarnik, J. P., Rudrud, E. H., & Czajkowski, L. A. (1981). *Behavioral habilitation through proactive programming.* Baltimore: Paul H. Brookes.

Black, J. W., & Meyer, L. H. (1992). But does it really work? Social validity of employment training for persons with very severe disabilities. *American Journal on Mental Retardation, 96*, 463–474.

Chen, T. H., Bruininks, R. H., Lakin, C. K., & Hayden, M. (1993). Personal competencies and community participation in small community residential programs: A multiple discriminant analysis. *American Journal on Mental Retardation, 98*, 390–399.

Ferguson, B., McDonnell, J., & Drew, C. (1993). Type and frequency of social interaction among workers with and without mental retardation. *American Journal on Mental Retardation, 97*, 530–540.

Elder, P. S., & Goossens, C. (1994). *Engineering training environments for interactive augmen-*

tative communication. Birmingham: Southeast Augmentative Communication Conference Publications Clinician Series.

Glennen, S., Delsandro, E., Radell, U., & Schiaffino, S. (1995). Assistive technology: The predictive assessment process. Paper presented at the Closing the Gap Conference, Minneapolis, MN.

Hill, B. K., Lakin, C. K., & Bruininks, R. (1984). Trends in residential services for people with mental retardation. *Journal of the Association for Persons with Severe Handicaps, 9,* 243–250.

Lakin, C. K., Bruininks, R. H., Chen, T. H., Hill, B. K., & Anderson, D. (1993). Personal characteristics and competence of people with mental retardation living in foster homes and small group homes. *American Journal on Mental Retardation, 97,* 616–627.

Lakin, C. K., Krantz, G. C., Bruininks, R. H., Clumpner, J. L., & Hill, B. K. (1982). One hundred years of data on populations of public residential facilities for mentally retarded people. *American Journal of Mental Deficiency, 87,* 1–8.

Lignugaris-Kraft, B., Salzberg, C. L., Rule, S., & Stowitchek, J. (1988). Social-vocational skills of workers with and without mental retardation in two community employment sites. *Mental Retardation, 26,* 297–305.

Mayer, T. & Johnson, R. (1994). *Boardmaker.* Solana, CA: Mayer-Johnson.

Rusch, F. R., Wilson, P. G., Hughes, C., Heal, L. (1994). Matched-pairs analysis of co-worker interactions in relation to opportunity, type of job, and placement approach. *Mental Retardation, 32,* 113–122.

Rusch, F. R., Hughes, C., Johnson, J. R., & Minch, K.E. (1991). Descriptive analysis of interactions between co-workers and supported employees. *Mental Retardation, 29,* 207–212.

Seltzer, M. M., & Krauss, M. W. (1987). *Aging and mental retardation: Extending the continuum.* Washington, DC: American Association on Mental Retardation.

Schleien, S., & Mustonen, T. (1988). Community recreation and persons with disabilities. In S. Schleien & M. T. Ray (Eds.), *Community recreation and persons with disabilities: Strategies for integration* (pp. 67–82). Baltimore: Paul H. Brookes.

Schleien, S., Olson, K., Rogers, N., & McLafferty, M. (1985). Integrating children with severe handicaps into recreation and physical education programs. *Journal of Parks and Recreation Administration, 3,* 74–78.

Stroud, M., & Sutton, E. (1988). *Expanding options for older adults with developmental disabilities.* Baltimore: Paul H. Brookes.

Life Stories

Wayne's AAC Story:
Pictures at an Exhibition

Sharon L. Glennen

Many adults with severe communication impairments are able to communicate adequately within the context of their structured group home and day programs. With few opportunities for choice-making or for participating in spontaneous unstructured events, the need for AAC may not be immediately apparent to program staff. Wayne's AAC story illustrates the potential for adults with developmental disabilities to improve their communication when AAC strategies are applied in adult program settings.

Wayne was a 26-year-old adult when he was referred to our outpatient hospital program for augmentative and alternative communication (AAC) services. Initial background information indicated that he had mild cerebral palsy, severe mental retardation, characteristics of pervasive developmental disorder (PDD), maladaptive behaviors, and a severe expressive communication impairment. He attended public schools up until the age of 21, always in self-contained classrooms for individuals with severe retardation. Following his graduation from school, Wayne stayed home for 3 years because waiting lists to enroll in area programs for adults were lengthy. At the age of 24, he finally obtained a coveted placement in a group home and adult day program. Initially staff focused on providing Wayne with a routine daily structure, in-creasing his independence within that daily structure, decreasing his anxiety about new situations, and improving his behavior.

The initial referral for AAC services was made 2 years after Wayne had enrolled in the adult program. Wayne's adult day program coordinator, Susan, felt that he had the potential to improve his communication skills and possibly transition into a community job through a supported employment program. Wayne's group home, which was operated by a different agency, initially did not know that he had been referred for AAC services. The first assessment goal was to make sure that both agencies were involved in the AAC evaluation process. Wayne's residential manager, Cindy, was invited to the initial session, which was held at the day program. Wayne lived in a rural community located over 2 hours away from the hospital AAC program. Prior to scheduling Wayne's evaluation, Susan and Cindy were made aware that the speech-language pathologist could evaluate and provide AAC guidance, but the adult program staff would need to carry out any AAC recommendations.

THE INITIAL AAC EVALUATION

Wayne's AAC evaluation was held at the day program. Representatives from his day program and residential program were present. The initial staff interview focused on the effectiveness of Wayne's current methods of communication. Staff indicated that he had learned to use sign language, and could sequence together simple phrases in sign such as *I + go + bus*. He was also frequently using speech to communicate. His IHP (Individualized Habilitation Plan) goals were focused on teaching him to simultaneously sign and speak at the same time. His speech was extremely dysarthric, but staff indicated that they were usually able to understand him. Wayne also had savant-like artistic skills. He had the ability to crudely draw objects and rooms (never people or animals). When not understood, Wayne would sometimes draw a picture of what he was attempting to communicate. Cindy, his residential manager, then surprised everyone by pulling an Intro Talker voice output AAC device out of a bag. She stated that it had been purchased for Wayne during his last year of school. She was not sure who recommended the device nor that Wayne had ever used it. She reported that Wayne never used the device at the group home.

In discussing Wayne's existing communication abilities, it became clear that everyone who knew him felt they were able to understand him. Staff repeatedly stated "I understand him most of the time, and if I don't, he will work to make himself understood." Staff frequently stated that "other people" had difficulty understanding Wayne. More specifically, they were concerned that strangers and community peers would not understand his speech or signs. In summary, staff who knew him felt that his communication skills were functional within a structured, self-contained adult program. However, he needed to improve his communication abilities to move independently into community settings.

Wayne was then evaluated. His receptive language abilities scattered from a 4 to 6 year age level. Expressively, he was able to use speech and sign gestures to communicate. However, the quality of each modality was not always effective. Because of his physical disability, his signs were often poorly formed approximations. His speech was extremely dysarthric and difficult to understand out of context. In order to demonstrate his unintelligibility to program staff, Susan was asked to participate with Wayne in intelligibility testing. He was asked to name pictures from the *Expressive One Word Picture Vocabulary Test* using speech and sign gestures. Susan was instructed to repeat back what Wayne had named. In this single word context, Wayne was less than 44% intelligible. Staff who observed this intelligibility testing repeatedly stated that they realized for the first time just how unintelligible his speech and signs were when contextual cues were removed.

Wayne's drawing abilities were remarkable. During a conversation about a van breakdown that had occurred the previous day, he was able to draw pictures of the van, a tire, a telephone, and a wrench to supplement his speech and signs. Finally, Wayne's use of the Intro Talker was reviewed. Miraculously, the device was still working. It had been programmed long ago with one display of 32 messages. Wayne was easily able to use the device to communicate functional messages. However, considering that his receptive language abilities were at a 4 to 6 year age level, the 32 messages on the Intro Talker were limiting.

By the end of the evaluation it was clear that Wayne's ability to communicate effectively could be improved. What remained to be answered was how, with whom, and in what settings. The first decision was to continue with use of sign language, speech, and drawing as Wayne's primary communication methods in the group home and adult day program settings. The second decision made by the evaluation team was that Wayne would need to learn to use a picture-based AAC system to achieve independent communication in the community. However, in order to learn community-based communication skills, the picture-based AAC system would initially need to be trained in his existing structured environments. Staff were instructed to "sabotage" Wayne's communication in the home and adult day program by periodically pretending that they did not understand his messages. During those instances, Wayne would be prompted to use his picture-based communication system.

The next questions concerned the type of picture-based AAC system to recommend. Voice output devices such as the Liberator, and Dynavox were considered, but because the systems were large and heavy the team felt they were impractical for Wayne to carry in community settings. Other small voice output systems that weighed less were limited in the number of available messages. The Intro Talker that Wayne already owned could easily be set up to match these capabilities.

It was decided to approach the problem with different solutions for different situations. First, the Intro Talker would be set up to meet Wayne's communication needs during weekly group outings to a fast food restaurant. Vocabulary for the fast food setting was developed during the initial evaluation session. Staff were then shown how to program the device with new vocabulary. IHP goals were developed to train Wayne to use the device in the fast food setting. Second, a small picture communication notebook was recommended. The notebook would have small ½ inch pictures arranged on category-based and activity-based pages. Wayne would use the picture communication book in his group home setting, the adult day program, and during other community outings. Additional IHP goals were written to implement the picture communication notebook. Cindy stated that she had access to Mayer-Johnson's *Picture Communication Symbol* books (see Appendix A). She would work with her staff and Susan's staff to develop most of the symbol pages

for the communication book. Cindy also volunteered to make the picture display for the Intro Talker.

THREE MONTHS: THE FIRST FOLLOW-UP SESSION

Three months after the initial evaluation, Wayne's AAC team gathered at the group home to evaluate his progress. Cindy had made the fast food picture display for the Intro Talker. Wayne was now using the device on a weekly basis to order food. Cindy indicated that he didn't seem to be particularly excited or motivated to use the system. He would use it when prompted by staff, but otherwise tended to revert back to sign language and speech. In looking through data sheets, it was determined that he had only taken the device to a fast food restaurant six times. The team decided to continue with Wayne's IHP goals for the Intro Talker, and to add daily role play practice sessions. Wayne's abilities with the device would be reevaluated in 3 more months.

Cindy had started to develop custom-made communication displays for Wayne's picture symbol notebook. Cindy and Wayne initially worked together to review through symbol choices in the Mayer-Johnson *Picture Communication Symbols* books. However, Wayne would repeatedly select every symbol on the page. When told that he didn't need some of the symbols, Wayne would protest and insist that he wanted all of them. Cindy decided that if Wayne wanted all of the symbols she would simply make him a photocopy of every page in the book. These photocopied pages were arranged in a notebook but staff had not yet begun to implement the system.

Wayne's AAC team decided that the picture notebook was overly large, inefficient, and needed to be thinned down. Staff reviewed the symbol pages and decided which categories could be eliminated and which categories could be decreased in size, and ultimately succeeded in reducing the notebook's pictures by half. During the meeting, staff also brainstormed vocabulary for activity-based pages. By the end of the session, vocabulary displays for four separate activities had been planned. Susan offered to make the activity-based displays for Wayne's notebook. It was decided to implement the book immediately using the existing pictures. New vocabulary displays would be added to the book as they were finished.

SIX MONTHS: THE SECOND FOLLOW-UP SESSION

The second follow-up session took place at the adult day program. Wayne's AAC team gathered together again to reevaluate his progress and to make recommendations for changes to his program. In contrast to the previous session, Wayne had begun to make good progress. His use of the picture communication notebook was reviewed first. Staff stated that after the book had been thinned down, Wayne insisted that the deleted symbols be replaced. The notebook was now in a whopping 3-inch binder with hundreds of photocopied symbols. Despite its overwhelming size, Wayne had grown attached to the notebook and insisted on carrying it everywhere. He was reportedly initiating conversations by sitting down with staff and peers to look through symbol pages in the book.

Wayne had also begun to draw his own symbols in the book. For example, on the vehicles page he drew pictures of the van used by the adult day program, the truck of his favorite residential counselor, and his sister's car. These additional pictures were labeled by staff so other listeners could understand their meaning. Finally, Wayne was beginning to add his art work to the book. He had an obsession for drawing the bathroom of every place he visited. Any time he visited a new location, he would return home and immediately sit down with paper and pencil to draw the bathroom. With prompting, he would also draw additional objects, signs, or other inanimate objects that were observed. His bathroom "gallery" was added to the back of the notebook. Wayne enjoyed looking through these pictures and would point excitedly to a drawing, then supplement by pointing back to picture symbols to discuss the events that occurred or the people who were with him when he was at each location. Staff added extra blank pages to the back of the notebook so Wayne could draw additional symbols or pictures as needed.

Wayne was observed interacting with staff at the adult day program. The picture communication notebook combined with signs and speech made Wayne an extremely effective communicator. He often initiated topics using the picture notebook. Once a topic was initiated, he typically reverted back to speech and signs, but would supplement these modalities with pictures when needed. When asked questions, Wayne would initially respond using speech combined with sign. However, if staff indicated that they did not understand him, he would begin turning through the pages of the book to respond. Wayne was also observed using the book with another peer in his program. The peer, who was verbal, sat with Wayne as they looked through the book's pictures together. Typical of many adults with developmental disabilities, they interacted together expressively with minimal listening to each other. However, staff indicated that prior to using the picture communication book, Wayne tended to ignore his peers and would walk away when they came up to him to interact. The picture communication book provided him with a way to initiate and respond to peer interactions without staff mediation.

The only drawback to Wayne's picture notebook was its large size. Although Wayne was always able to find a symbol to express himself, it often took him a minute or more to look through the book to find the symbol he wanted. However, staff were reluctant to tamper with success. Rather than reducing the number of symbols, it was decided to provide Wayne with a better method of searching through the pages. Pages were organized in sections with notebook dividers. Category-based picture symbols were added to the dividers to help Wayne determine which symbols were found in each section. A topic symbol was added to the outside edge of each page to help him find the page he was searching for within a section. Additional visual cues were added using a highlighter marker to create a border around the edge of each page. Various highlighter colors were linked to different categories or concepts.

Another recommendation was to turn Wayne's "bathroom gallery" into a "memory book" that could be used to initiate conversations more effectively. Wayne's bathroom pictures were slipped into clear notebook page covers. Staff added photographs, ticket stubs, and other memorabilia to each page. In addition, a short description of the event was written by staff and added to each bathroom page. These additional items gave Wayne's listeners cues to discuss past events, and reduced Wayne's need to search through picture symbol pages to comment about an event.

Wayne's use of the Intro Talker was then discussed. Staff had continued with the Intro Talker during role play sessions at the group home, and weekly outings to fast food restaurants. Wayne was now beginning to initiate using the Intro Talker without staff intervention. However, they stated that the device was still limiting. Wayne would rotely order his three food choices, then say Thank you at the end of his order. Staff did not feel that the Intro Talker gave him the ability to truly express himself during community interactions. In addition, staff were having difficulty remembering to charge the Intro Talker so that it was ready to take to the restaurant. There were several times that

the device was brought to the restaurant, only to discover that it needed a charge.

At this point, there were two equally valid directions that could be taken. Some team members wanted to completely abandon the Intro Talker. They wanted Wayne to solely use the picture communication notebook across all community outings. Other team members felt that if the Intro Talker was expanded with additional activity-based community pages, Wayne would begin to see the value of using a voice output AAC system. If the device was used more frequently, then staff would be sure to charge the system on a regular basis. Wayne was asked to make the decision. He was asked if he wanted to continue bringing the Intro Talker to the restaurant, or if he wanted to bring his picture notebook instead. Wayne confused the issue even more by indicating that he wanted both!

A compromise between the two viewpoints was reached. It was decided to try expanding use of the Intro Talker to two additional community settings on a trial basis. Wayne would be given the option to use the Intro Talker or use his picture communication book in each setting. At the end of the next 3 month period, his progress would be reevaluated. The additional settings were selected and vocabulary was planned for the device. Staff were taught how to change pages within the Intro Talker system. Step-by-step instructions were then taped onto the back of the device.

NINE MONTHS: THE THIRD FOLLOW-UP SESSION

Wayne's third follow-up session was held 3 months later. As before, his AAC team gathered to discuss his progress and determine future AAC goals. The changes recommended for his picture notebook system had been implemented with good success. Staff reported that Wayne was able to quickly find appropriate pictures to communicate with others. Wayne had also continued to add to his "bathroom gallery." The addition of pictures and other mementos to the bathroom drawings made it easier for listeners to communicate with him about past events. In fact, Wayne was so enthusiastic about this new section of his communication book that he had dramatically expanded the number of drawings included in its pages. His AAC pictures had to be subdivided into two smaller 2-inch notebooks. The picture symbols were in one book, Wayne's drawings and mementos were in another. This division slightly improved the portability of the AAC system. Staff at the group home were able to convince Wayne to leave the memory AAC book behind on community outings. However, Wayne insisted on bringing both books to the adult day program.

Wayne's use of the Intro Talker was similar to what was seen during the previous follow-up sessions. For the two additional community settings, he had learned to use the device in a rote-sequenced manner to make basic requests. Otherwise, he reverted back to signs, speech, and his picture notebooks. After much discussion, it was decided to temporarily discontinue using the Intro Talker. Wayne would use the other three methods of communication in community settings and in his group home and adult day program. In the future, if Wayne entered a supported employment program, the need to use a voice output AAC system would be reevaluated. It was decided that he would not be seen for another follow-up session until his next IHP meeting 9 months later. Staff from the group home and adult day program would continue to carry out his AAC program until then. For Wayne, a well organized low tech picture communication system proved to be the most effective AAC option at this stage in his life.

KEY POINTS TO REMEMBER

- Many adults live in group homes and attend work programs that are managed by separate agencies. Communication between the two agencies is often poor. When AAC strategies are implemented it is important that representatives from both agencies are involved from the beginning to develop a viable AAC system.

- Speech and language services are usually not available on a regular basis for adults with developmental disabilities. Staff from group homes and adult day programs are often limited in their knowledge of communication, much less their ability to plan and implement AAC programs. Because of funding constraints, a consultative model is recommended. A professional with AAC experience can work with program staff to evaluate clients and develop AAC goals. Program staff are then responsible for carrying out the AAC plan under the guidance of the consultant.

- An AAC consultative model for adult clients with developmental disabilities needs to include frequent follow-up visits during the first few months of program implementation. The final success of Wayne's AAC program was dependent on periodic reassessment of his progress. During each follow-up session, adjustments to his AAC program were made based upon his performance.

- Many adults with developmental disabilities who are nonspeaking are taught sign language during their school years. Once they age out of school they are frequently placed into settings where staff or community peers do not know sign. This is especially true for adults who are placed into community-based job settings. It is important to consider all potential communication modalities at an early age and to train these modalities during the school years when intensive services are available.

- Adults with developmental disabilities are often placed in highly structured settings with limited opportunities for communication. In order to effect AAC changes, program staff need to be made aware of the need for improved communication. Without this awareness, the best designed AAC program will fail.

- The process of developing custom-made picture communication displays is extremely time consuming. Staff who have never gone through the process may not initially realize how much time will be involved in developing the system. A way to divide the work among multiple staff should be devised so that no single person is stuck with all of the copying, cutting, and pasting. Even when computer programs such as Boardmaker (see Appendix A) are used to develop picture displays, the time involved is still extensive.

- Adult consumers need to be involved in making AAC decisions. Wayne's AAC success was in part due to his involvement in the symbol selection process. When decisions were made without his input, he immediately insisted on reverting the AAC system back to his preferences.

- The AAC system should reflect the personality of the user. Wayne's memory album was unusual, yet it was targeted toward his interests and activities. He was enthusiastic about using the memory album to communicate with staff and peers because it contained information about a topic that he enjoyed discussing.

- Wayne fell into the category of individuals who are difficult to match to voice output AAC devices. He was able to walk, and required a lightweight, small portable system. Yet he had extensive vocabulary needs. AAC devices that are small have limited vocabulary capabilities. AAC devices that have more messages and vocabulary are larger in size and weight. Manufacturers have recently become aware of this dilemma and have developed several new picture-based AAC systems that are smaller in size yet have the same capabilities of older larger models (see Appendix A).

- Low tech picture communication systems can often be as effective, if not more effective, than high tech voice output AAC devices. Because of funding constraints, adults with developmental disabilities who have never used picture-based methods of communication can initially be introduced to the modality through low tech approaches. Success with a low tech approach then provides additional justification for the need to evaluate and pursue funding for high tech voice output AAC systems.

Appendix A

AAC PRODUCT DIRECTORY

Sharon L. Glennen

Augmentative and alternative communication (AAC) products have proliferated during the past decade. New products appear rapidly on the market as old products are retired. This means that any publication that attempts to list all possible pieces of AAC hardware and software is at risk of quickly becoming outdated. This appendix lists AAC hardware and software products that were available at the time the book was written. Readers are urged to use this listing as an introduction to the wide variety of commercially available products. Additional information can be obtained directly from vendors (see Appendix B), through comprehensive assistive technology database resources such as Hyper-ABLEDATA on the Internet (see Appendix D), or through the *Closing the Gap* annual product directory (see Appendix D). In addition, the Rehabilitation Engineering Research Center on AAC at the University of Delaware publishes the *Guide to Augmentative and Alternative Communication Devices* (1996) which contains detailed descriptions of AAC devices along with photographs, prices, warranties, and available accessories.

The AAC products listed in this directory are organized into several categories.

These include the following:

- Dedicated AAC devices: hardware specifically manufactured for AAC purposes.
- AAC computer access hardware: hardware used to provide alternative methods of using computers.
- AAC computer software: software products that have AAC capabilities.
- Switches: switches and other simple input devices used to operate dedicated AAC devices and computers.
- Mounting and positioning equipment: hardware used to position AAC devices and switches.
- Symbols and AAC languages: commercially available AAC symbols and language systems.
- Low technology aids: commercially available communication books, boards, and materials for making AAC systems.

The process of determining an appropriate category for AAC products in this appendix was often difficult. For example, there are several software programs that are AAC symbol languages designed for specific dedicated communication systems. These language programs could be categorized as either software, symbol sets, or part of a dedicated AAC communication system. In reality, these products serve all three functions yet the process of cross-referencing products across categories would be overwhelming. The solution was to select the primary function served by these products (in this case, a symbol language) and to list them once under that category.

DEDICATED AAC DEVICES

The AAC devices listed in this category are electronic hardware systems specifically designed for communication. These devices range from simple clock communicators, to single message switches, to complex systems with a myriad of access and language features.

Device/Vendor	Description
4 Compartment Switch with Speech Toys for Special Children/ Enabling Devices	This device has four arm slots that can operate up to four different switch toys. Digitized voice messages accompany switch activation.
Abovo Abovo	This is a small AAC system with an alphabet keyboard display. It has an LCD print display, and can be purchased with a remote LCD display. This device does not have voice output.
ACS ScanPAC with RealVoice ACS Technologies	This system uses abbreviation expansion codes to prestore messages. An Epson portable computer is the heart of the system. It can be accessed using switches, Morse code, joystick, and a light pointer. Voice output is provided through the RealVoice synthesizer which is available in male and female versions.
Action Voice Ability Research	This device is a small hand-held AAC system with 10 message areas. Digitized speech messages can be accessed using direct selection and single or dual switch scanning. Auditory scan prompts can be added to each message area.
Alpha Talker Prentke Romich Company	This dedicated AAC system comes in 32, 8, or 4 location keyboard formats. It can be accessed through direct selection, scanning, or an optical light pointer. The AlphaTalker has up to 25 minutes of digitized speech recording. Picture symbols can be sequenced to increase message choices.
Attainment Talkers Attainment Company	This family of AAC devices consists of direct selection systems with digitized speech. The 15-message version comes with 2 minutes of recording time. Five message systems have either 32 seconds or 2 minutes of recording. The 2-message version has 16 seconds available for recording.
Big Blue Macaw Zygo	The Big Blue version of the Macaw is designed for multiple users. It can be programmed with 33 "per-

sonalities" with up to 32 levels of pages within each personality. Each level has up to 32 keys. Picture symbols can be sequenced to increase message choices on a given level. Direct selection, scanning, and Morse code access are available. Up to 19 minutes of digitized speech can be recorded into each personality with up to 13 hours of saved messages in internal memory.

BigMack
Ablenet

This is a large switch that can be programmed with a single 20 second digitized speech message. It can also control an attached single switch toy. It is available in 5 different colors.

Black Hawk
Adamlab

The Black Hawk consists of 16 keys that are 1-inch square. Up to four different levels can be accessed through direct selection. It comes with 4 minutes of digitized speech recording.

Canon Communicator CC-7P
ACCI, Imaginart

The Canon has been available since 1977. It features a small alphabetical letter display. Messages are printed onto a strip printer. A limited number of messages can be prestored. There is no voice output.

Canon Communicator CC-7S
ACCI, Imaginart

This version of the Canon is identical to the CC-7P model, but adds digitized voice recording for up to 26 messages. A total of 240 seconds of recording time is available.

Cheap Talk 4
Toys for Special Children/
Enabling Devices

This low-cost four-message device comes with 20 seconds of digitized recording time. It is available in direct selection, scanning, and direct switch access models.

Cheap Talk 8
Toys for Special Children/
Enabling Devices

The Cheap Talk 8 has eight message areas with 40 seconds of available digitized speech recording. It is a low cost device that is available in direct selection, scanning, and direct switch access modes.

Clock Communicator
Toys for Special Children/
Enabling Devices

This traditional switch activated clock communicator uses a turning clock hand to point to picture symbols.

Communiclock
Crestwood Company

This is a simple clock dial scanning system that is operated using a single switch.

Companion 401
Luminaud

This small hand-held device has four message keys for digitized recorded speech. It is accessed through direct selection.

Crespeaker
Crestwood Company

This is a small text-to-speech AAC device that can speak up to 100 characters for each message. It was originally designed as an English to Spanish translation system and can be used for that purpose.

Crestalk
Crestwood Company

This small AAC device has an alphabet keyboard. Typed messages appear on a small LCD display. There is no voice output.

Delta Talker
Prentke Romich Company

This new AAC device replaced the Light and Touch Talkers. It can be accessed through touch, scanning, or light pointers. It has both digitized and text-to-speech DecTalk voice capabilities. The keyboard can be configured for 128, 32, 8, and 4 symbols. Symbols can be sequenced to increase message choices. Minspeak AAC language programs can be loaded into the Delta Talker.

Dial Scan
Don Johnston, Inc

Dial Scan is a clock communicator that can be operated using a single switch. The speed and direction of scanning can be adjusted.

Digivox
Sentient Systems Technology

The Digivox has a 48 message display that can be programmed across 8 different levels using digitized speech. Keys can be combined together to create larger keys with fewer messages on each level. Keys can be sequenced together to provide more message choices within a single level. Up to 26 minutes of recording time is available. The Digivox can be accessed through direct selection and scanning options.

Dual Clock Communicator
Toys for Special Children/
Enabling Devices

This low cost clock communicator has seven compartments which can be used with small objects or pictures. A circular cut-out plate scanner or clock hand scanner comes with the system. Switches are used to control the scanning process.

Dynavox 2
Sentient Systems Technology

Dynavox 2 combines a touch screen into a stand-alone AAC system. This version of the device has a monochrome monitor. Over 2,600 DynaSym symbols are available for organization into dynamic display pages. The Dynavox 2 has printed output at the top of the touch screen, and text-to-speech DecTalk voice synthesis. It can be accessed through direct selection on the touch screen or scanning. A unique feature of this device is infrared environmental control capabilities.

Dynavox 2C
Sentient Systems Technology

The 2C model of the Dynavox adds a color display to the basic Dynavox 2 system. Both Dynavox 2 devices have word prediction capabilities through the DynaWrite software program. Digitized recordings can also be used for some messages.

EasyTalk
The Great Talking Box Company

This small AAC device can be accessed using direct selection or scanning. Four levels of 40 messages are available. The keyboard is adjustable into 1, 2,

4, 10, and 20 key layouts. It has 4 or 8 minutes of dig-itized speech depending on the model.

FastTalk
The Possibilities Company

FastTalk consists of words arranged in menus which are accessed using arrow keys on the display of the device. FastTalk can only be accessed using direct selection. The location, size, and arrange-ment of the device's 23 keys cannot be changed.

Finger Foniks
Words+

This unusual hand-held AAC system has phonics sound keys which are sequenced together to create messages. Instead of text-to-speech synthesis, the system offers phoneme-to-speech synthesis. A lim-ited number of messages can also be prestored.

Giant Lightwriter
Toby Churchill, LTD.
Zygo

The Giant Lightwriter has a 22" × 18" alphanumer-ic keyboard. Similar to other voice output versions of the Lightwriter, it has DECtalk speech, a backlit LCD print display, and word prediction and abbre-viation expansion features.

Great Green Macaw
Zygo

The Great Green version of the Macaw is similar to the Green Macaw. It can be configured for up to 40 "personalities" or users with up to 8 levels of pages in each personality. It has an additional 13 hours of internal digitized speech available.

Green Macaw
Zygo

This AAC system has 128 small message areas that can be programmed across eight levels. Keys can be configured into 64, 32, 8, 4, 2, and 1 message areas. Nineteen minutes of digitized recording are available. It can be accessed through direct selec-tion, scanning, and Morse code.

Handy Speech
Consultants for Communication
Technology

This system consists of an IBM-compatible laptop computer, synthesizer, and communication soft-ware. It can be accessed through the keyboard or a single switch.

Hawk
Adamlab

The Hawk is a durable device with nine large direct selection message areas. Digitized speech record-ing is available for a total of 45 seconds of recording time.

Holly.Com
Communication Devices

This device has 8 or 32 message areas that can be accessed using direct selection and linear or row-column scanning. A total of 76 seconds of digitized speech can be programmed onto each overlay. Multiple overlays are stored on computer disks for retrieval.

Language Master 6000-SE
Franklin Electronics

Franklin Electronics manufactures popular hand–held electronic dictionaries. They adapted this ver-sion of the dictionary for use as an AAC system. It provides text-to-speech synthesis of spelled messages and up to 26 prestored phrases and sentences.

Liberator
Prentke Romich Company

The Liberator uses Minspeak AAC language programs. It supports all access methods and has several different key size configurations. The newest version combines Minspeak symbol sequencing with word prediction. The Liberator uses the DECTalk synthesizer for voice output. Printed output is available on a back-lit LCD display and small paper printer.

Light Talker
Prentke Romich Company

The Light Talker is no longer manufactured and has been replaced by the Delta Talker and Liberator. It was accessed through several scanning options or with an optical headpointer.

Lightwriter SL35 & SL5
Toby Churchill, LTD
Zygo

These AAC devices have small alphanumeric keyboards. Both models have backlit LCD print displays. The SL35 model adds text-to-speech voice output through various synthesizers, including DECtalk. The SL35 has word prediction and abbreviation expansion capabilities.

Lightwriter SL4b
Toby Churchill, LTD.
Zygo

The SL4b version of the Lightwriter family of AAC devices has a larger alphanumeric keyboard (13" × 11"). It has voice output, backlit LCD print displays, and abbreviation expansion and word prediction features.

Lynx
Adamlab

This small device has four message keys that can be accessed directly, through multiple switches, or through single switch visual or auditory scanning. Switch-adapted toys or appliances can be connected for additional learning experiences.

Macaw 3
Zygo

The Macaw 3 is similar to the Macaw II. It provides an additional 9 to 19 minutes of digitized recording, Morse code input, and 32 levels of programming.

Macaw II, XL, SC, SC-XL
Zygo

There are nine different versions of the Macaw. These four versions have 32 keys that can be arranged into various configurations. Direct selection and scanning access methods are available in the SC models. The II and XL models support only direct selection access. Up to 8 levels of messages can be programmed and symbols can be sequenced to create additional messages on each level. Digitized recording time ranges from 2 minutes for the II and SC models, to 8 minutes for the XL models.

Message Mate 20
Words+

Message Mate is a small AAC system with twenty ¾ inch message areas. The 20 keys can be combined to make larger key areas with fewer messages. It can be purchased with 20 to 120 seconds of analog recording time. Scanning options are included.

Message Mate 40
Words+

This device is identical to the Message Mate 20 except it has 40 message keys available. Analog voice recording times range from 60 to 240 seconds depending on the model purchased.

MicroVoice
Frame Technologies

The MicroVoice is a small hand-held portable system with 24 message areas. Digitized messages of up to 5 seconds can be recorded into each area.

Nine Compartment Row/ Column Scanner
Toys for Special Children/ Enabling Devices

This simple device has nine compartments that can be used for small objects or picture symbols. A switch is attached to operate row column scanning selections. There is no voice or printed output.

Parrot and Parrot JK
Zygo

The Parrot is a small AAC system with 16 message areas. It can be accessed through direct selection. One minute of digitized recording is available. The JK version of the device can also be accessed using direct switch methods.

Peacemaker and Peacekeyper
Tiger Communication Systems

The Peacemaker, and it's companion Peacekeyper, combine Franklin Electronics' Language Master AAC system with a 66 page picture communication book in a tote binder. The Peacekeyper produces single spoken words, the Peacemaker can speak sentences.

Pegasus Lite
Words+

Pegasus Lite is a dedicated AAC system which uses Words+ Talking Screen software with a dynamic color display touch screen. Text-to-speech synthesized voice and up to 4 hours of digitized speech recording is available. An external CD ROM drive can be attached to run additional programs on the system.

Real Voice
ACS Technologies

The Real Voice is built into an Epson microcomputer system. It has a QWERTY keyboard and built-in synthesizer which comes in male or female versions. Printed output is available on an LCD display and a paper printer. Abbreviation expansion letter codes are used to retrieve lengthier prestored messages.

Round Clock Communicator
Toys for Special Children/ Enabling Devices

These lightweight clock communicators come with a gooseneck mount and universal clamp to attach them to bed railings or wheelchairs. A switch is used to control the scanning process.

Say It All
Innocomp

This system has text-to-speech synthesis through the Clarity synthesizer. Up to 846 different messages can be prestored in the system. Letter or picture symbols can be used on the touch surface but key sizes are limited to ¾ inches. The Say It All can only be accessed using direct selection. Limited infrared environmental controls are available.

Say It All Gold
Innocomp

The Say It All Gold is similar to the original Say It All. The difference is an upgrade to the DECTalk synthesizer with up to nine different voice options.

Say It Simply Plus
Innocomp

Say It Simply Plus has a large 12 × 12 touchpad which can be programmed with up to 762 picture symbol messages. Key sizes range from 1 inch to 12 inches square and are accessed using direct selection. Voice output is provided through the Clarity synthesizer.

Say It Simply Plus Gold
Innocomp

The Gold version of the Say It Simply Plus adds the DECTalk speech synthesizer to the system.

Scan It All
Innocomp

The Scan It All can be operated through single switch scanning or a laser light beam for direct selection. Keyboard configurations can be designed for 2 to 96 symbols. Messages can be prestored using the Clarity text-to-speech synthesizer.

Scan It All Gold
Innocomp

The Scan It All Gold is identical to the Scan It All but adds the higher quality DECTalk speech synthesizer.

ScanLite
ORCCA Technology

ScanLite is a series of simple scanning systems. It comes in different configurations, including a four and six choice linear array, and a flexible array that consists of lights on suction cups that can be attached to variety of objects or pictures.

Scanmate 4
Tash

The Scanmate 4 is similar to the Voicemate 4 from Tash. This version of the device can be accessed using single switch scanning.

Scanmate 8
Tash

Scanmate 8 adds four additional message areas to the Scanmate 4 system. It can be accessed using direct selection and single switch or dual switch scanning options. The eight message areas can each be programmed with 4 seconds of digitized speech.

Sequential Scanner
Toys for Special Children/
Enabling Devices

The Sequential Scanner is a light tech scanning system with two or four object compartments. A switch is attached to control the scanning process.

Shadow Talker
Toys for Special Children/
Enabling Devices

Shadow Talker has four message areas that are activated when a change in light reflection (i.e., a shadow) occurs. Up to 20 seconds of digitized speech recording is available.

SpeakEasy
Ablenet

SpeakEasy is a small AAC system that can be accessed through direct selection or direct switch selection. Twelve message areas can be programmed with up to 4 minutes of digitized speech. The device can be connected to up to two switch toys for simultaneous activation.

Switchmate 4
Tash

This device is a cousin of the Voicemate 4 from Tash. Four messages can be accessed using direct selection, or through four attached switches. Up to 4 seconds of digitized speech can be recorded into each message area.

Synergy PC
Synergy

This dedicated computer system mounts to a power wheelchair. It includes AAC software, environmental controls, and access to IBM-compatible software. Because the device is a custom-made computer, any IBM-compatible AAC software program can be used. Direct selection is available through a touch screen or keyboard, scanning input is also supported. Text-to-speech voice output is available using the DECTalk synthesizer.

Synergy Mac
Synergy

This dedicated computer system is similar to the Synergy PC. It is designed to run Macintosh-compatible software.

Talk Back III, Talk Back VI
Crestwood Company

Talk Back III has three buttons that are pressed to activate digitized speech messages. Up to 20 seconds of recording time is available. Switches can be connected to activate the messages. Talk Back VI has six messages and 60 seconds of recording time.

Talking Switch Plates
Toys for Special Children/
Enabling Devices

These large 5" × 8" plate switches activate messages up to 20 seconds long. They come in a single plate (one message) format, or a rocking plate (two message) format.

Talk Pad
Frame Technologies

This is a low cost system with 4 message areas. The message areas are large colorful buttons built into a plastic case with a large carrying handle. Up to 15 seconds of digitized speech can be recorded into each message area. External switches can be attached for direct switch access.

Touch Talker
Prentke Romich Company

The Touch Talker is no longer manufactured and has been replaced by the Delta Talker and Liberator. For many years it was a popular direct selection system that used Minspeak software applications.

Versascan
Prentke Romich Company

The Versascan is a circular scanning communication system that is accessed with a single switch. Up to 16 symbols can be indicated by scanning lights. There is no output.

Vocal Assistant
Luminaud

This AAC device is a small hand-held system with 16 message areas. Model 1 has 3 seconds of digitized speech available per message. Model II can record up to 6 seconds. Model I is for direct selection, Model II adds single switch scanning.

Voice in a Box
Frame Technologies

This low cost direct selection system comes in 16, 20, and 40 message versions. Each message area has 3.75 seconds of digitized speech recording available. Four external jacks are available to connect switches for direct switch selection.

Voicemate 4
Tash

This small hand-held device has four message areas that can be accessed using direct selection. Up to 4 seconds of digitized speech can be programmed into each area.

VoicePal Plus
AdapTech

VoicePal Plus has 10 message areas that are recorded using digitized speech. Sixty seconds of recording time is available. It can be accessed using direct selection, linear scanning, and multiple switch input.

VOIS 160 with P.A.L.L.S.
Phonic Ear

This device has 128 keys that access preprogrammed single words and phrases and custom vocabulary. Vocabulary is accessed using multiple levels, abbreviation expansion, or picture sequencing. It uses the DECTalk synthesizer.

VOIS 160 with VoisShapes
Phonic Ear

This version of the VOIS 160 organizes vocabulary using American Sign Language features. Sign language components are represented in picture form. Sequencing the components together retrieves the corresponding vocabulary.

Walker Talker
Prentke Romich Company

The Walker Talker was designed for ambulatory consumers and is worn around the waist. It consists of the digitized speech synthesizer, battery pack, and attached 16 symbol keyboard. Picture symbols can be sequenced for multiple messages.

Whisper Wolf
Adamlab

The Whisper Wolf is identical to the Wolf but adds the features of auditory scanning and single switch selection. A private listening earphone can be used by the consumer to listen to auditory choices during the scanning process.

Wolf
Adamlab

The Wolf features text-to-speech synthesis in a 36 key direct selection panel. The panel can be divided into larger key areas if needed. Up to three different user areas can be programmed with over 90 levels of vocabulary. In addition, fixed levels using Wolf CAP predeveloped vocabulary are included.

AAC COMPUTER ACCESS HARDWARE

There are many hardware products that can be used to provide alternative access methods for computers. Computer access is important because many AAC consumers use computers as the operating base for their communication systems. Hardware adaptations are usually necessary to provide a method of motorically accessing the computer. This section of the product directory lists computer access items that have hardware components. There are several products listed here that consist of both hardware and software. However, the software is reliant upon specific hardware to operate properly. Computer access hardware products are designed to operate with different computer operating platforms. Each product is listed for compatibility with Apple IIGS, Macintosh, DOS, and Windows platforms. Like any hardware or software product, the manufacturer or vendor should be contacted for specific information related to system requirements.

Device/Vendor/Platform	Description
Access Now Innocomp DOS, Macintosh, Windows	This expanded alphanumeric keyboard can be accessed using a single switch in scanning modes, or through direct selection with a laser light pointer. Two letter overlays are included.
Adaptive Firmware Card Don Johnston, Inc Apple IIGS	The Adaptive Firmware Card is an access interface for Apple II series computers. Custom setups for switch access, expanded keyboards, Morse code, and direct switch access can be developed for use across most Apple II software programs.
Best Switch Interface Boston Educational Systems and Technology (BEST) DOS	The Best interface provides switch access for users of IBM DOS compatible computers. Up to three switches can be connected. Several software programs written to work with the interface teach cause effect skills and early scanning communication skills.
CommPac Words+ DOS, Windows	CommPac comes in different configurations and can combine a speech synthesizer, touch screen panel, and IBM-compatible Soft Key computer access system into a single unit. It is designed to operate with Words+ software.
Computer Switch Interface Ablenet Apple IIGS	This switch interface installs into the nine pin joystick connector interface on Apple IIGS computers. It can be used with software designed for single switch users.
DADA Entry Tash DOS	This IBM-compatible keyboard emulator provides computer access through a single switch, alternative keyboard, joystick, mouse emulator, or Morse code. Word prediction features and synthesized speech output are available.

DARCI Too
Wes Test Engineering Co.
DOS, Macintosh, Windows

DARCI Too is a keyboard and mouse emulator. It provides computer access through a single switch, Morse code, joystick, and alternative keyboards. It works transparently with all software.

Discover:Board
Don Johnston, Inc
Macintosh, Windows

Discover:Board is a Ke:nx access application for individuals who need an enlarged keyboard. The system comes with a Key Largo keyboard, starter overlays for popular software programs, and the ability to customize overlays for additional applications.

Discover:Switch
Don Johnston, Inc
Macintosh, Windows

This product consists of a Big Red switch that contains the Ke:nx access system software for single switch users. The system has ready-made scanning arrays for commonly used software programs. In addition, custom scanning arrays can be developed. Different switches can be plugged into the unit.

DJ PC Switch Interface
Don Johnston, Inc
DOS, Windows

This switch interface plugs into any unused serial port on an IBM-compatible computer. Four switch jacks are available.

Expert Mouse
Kensington Microware
DOS, Windows

Expert Mouse is a trackball for IBM-compatible computers. It has two buttons that can be adapted for either right or left handed users.

Eyegaze Computer System
LC Technologies/Eyegaze Systems
Windows

This access system uses eye gaze movements to directly select items on a eye gaze keyboard display. Eye movements are "read" by a remote sensor which sends the information to a computer.

EZ Touch
Words+
DOS, Windows

EZ Touch is a touch screen that can be used with most IBM-compatible laptop computers. It connects to the computer through the serial port. The user touches the screen to emulate mouse movements.

Gus! Touch Screen
Gus Communications
Windows

The Gus! Touch Screen is designed for IBM-compatible laptop computers. It is an external touch screen that is placed over the existing laptop monitor and connects through the serial port.

HeadMaster Plus
Prentke Romich
DOS, Macintosh, Windows

This mouse emulation device consists of a headset worn by the user, and a remote control unit placed on a computer monitor. User head movements translate into cursor movements. Attached switches are used to emulate mouse button functions.

HeadMouse
Origin Instruments
Apple IIGS, Macintosh, DOS, Windows

HeadMouse is a pointing system for use with computers. An optical sensor is placed above the computer monitor. Movements of a silver sticker attached to the user are tracked by the sensor to control on-screen mouse movements.

Intellikeys
IntelliTools
Apple IIGS, DOS, Macintosh, Windows

This expanded keyboard attaches to the keyboard port. It works transparently with any software. Six standard keyboard overlays are included. Additional overlay setups can be purchased or custom designed using Overlay Maker software.

Ke:nx
Don Johnston, Inc
Macintosh

Ke:nx is a versatile computer access system that works transparently with all Macintosh software. It supports single switch, on-screen keyboard, alternative keyboard, Morse code, and assisted keyboard access methods. Customized overlays and access configurations can be programmed through the Ke:nx Create portion of the system.

Ke:nx On:Board
Don Johnston, Inc
Macintosh

Ke:nx On:Board combines a Key Largo expanded keyboard with the Ke:nx access system. It is designed for direct selection computer access, especially with Macintosh laptop systems. Custom symbol overlays and computer macros can be created for the keyboard.

Key Largo
Don Johnston, Inc
Apple IIGS, Macintosh

Key Largo is an expanded keyboard. Up to 128 symbol areas can be custom programmed. AAC applications can be created using picture symbol overlays and talking word processing or other software.

LightBoard
Ability Research
Apple IIGS, DOS, Macintosh, Windows

This alternative keyboard is accessed using an optical light pointer. It connects to the computer through an emulation system such as Ke:nx, DARCI Too, DADA Entry, or Words+ EKI.

LipStick
McIntyre Computer Regional Systems Corporation
Macintosh

LipStick is an alternative small joystick that emulates mouse movements. It comes with an on-screen keyboard and word prediction software.

Macintosh Switch Interface
Don Johnston, Inc
Macintosh

This interface connects to Macintosh computers through the ADB connector. Up to five different switches can be attached.

MacMini Keyboard
TASH
Macintosh

The MacMini Keyboard is a small alternative keyboard designed for users with minimal range of motion and good direct selection abilities. It has mouse emulation and keyboard functions.

MiniMorse
Bloorview Children's Hospital
Apple IIGS, DOS, Macintosh

This computer access system uses one to three switches to send Morse code signals. It works transparently with all software.

**Mouse Emulator
and Mouse Mover**
Tash
Apple IIGS, DOS, Macintosh, Windows

This computer interface is designed to emulate mouse movements through attached switches. Up to five switches can be used.

Multiple Switch Box
Don Johnston, Inc
Apple IIGS, Macintosh

This switch box works in conjunction with Ke:nx or the Adaptive Firmware Card. Up to eight switches can be connected to control keyboard actions or mouse movements.

MultiVoice
Mayer-Johnson
Words+
DOS, Macintosh, Windows

MultiVoice is a speech synthesizer which was developed at the Institute of Applied Technology at Boston Children's Hospital. It produces 9 high quality DECTalk voices. MultiVoice is supported by most AAC software programs.

Penny and Giles Joystick
Don Johnston, Inc
Macintosh

This joystick is designed for individuals with physical disabilities and can be used to control mouse functions on Macintosh computers. Separate buttons are widely spaced to control click, double click, and drag operations. A keyguard is available.

Penny and Giles Rollerball
Don Johnston, Inc
Macintosh

The Rollerball is a trackball with features for individuals with physical or learning disabilities. The ball is mounted within a keyguard. The three trackball buttons are widely separated and control click, double click, and drag functions.

Penny and Giles Trackerball
Don Johnston, Inc
Macintosh

The Trackerball is a trackball with adjustable mouse speeds, and mouse movement controls. Separate widely spaced buttons control click, double click, and drag functions. A keyguard is available.

Powerpad
Dunamis
Apple IIGS, DOS, Macintosh

The Powerpad is an alternative expanded key board that can be customized for a variety of picture communication overlays. It has a large 12 × 12 inch surface which can be divided into as few as 1 or as many as 144 programmable areas.

SAM Switch Adapted Mouse
R.J. Cooper
Apple IIGS, DOS, Macintosh

This interface uses a single switch to activate mouse click functions. SAM needs to be combined with Cross Scanner or other software to provide full mouse emulation.

T-Tam
Prentke Romich Company
Apple IIGS, DOS, Macintosh

T-Tam provides a serial connection between the computer and Prentke Romich AAC systems. It provides for text entry and mouse emulation through the AAC device.

Touch in a Box
Carroll Touch
Windows

This computer monitor has a built-in touch screen. Mouse emulation is achieved through touching the monitor.

Touch Screen Mac LT
Synergy
Macintosh

This touch screen can be custom-built into the monitor of a Macintosh Powerbook computer. The user simply touches the monitor to produce mouse emulation movements. A Touch Screen Speak Mac LT version adds an external speaker to the system.

Touch Window
Edmark
Apple IIGS, DOS, Macintosh

The Touch Window mounts on top of existing computer monitors. Monitors with diagonal measurements of 10 to 15 inches can be adapted using this input method. The user touches the computer screen to produce mouse clicks and other mouse functions.

Troll Touch Screens
Troll Technology Corporation
DOS, Macintosh, Windows

Troll Touch Screens are built into existing computer monitors, including laptop systems. The touch screen provides the user with a direct selection method of mouse emulation.

AAC COMPUTER SOFTWARE

With the increased power, speed, and portability of laptop computers, many AAC consumers use computers combined with software and synthesizers for communication. This section of the product directory lists software designed for communication purposes. Some of these programs can be used directly without any other adaptations to the computer. However, the majority of consumers will need to use these software programs in conjunction with computer hardware adaptations. Software programs are written for specific computer platforms. The listings describe whether the program is designed for Apple IIGS, DOS, Macintosh, or Windows operating systems. Many of these programs are designed to operate simultaneously while other programs are also running. For example, a scanning word prediction program is used to simultaneously access a word processing program. Large amounts of random access memory (RAM) are necessary to run more than one program at a time. Manufacturers should be contacted for specific information regarding memory and system specifications.

Device/Vendor/Platform	Description
Adaptive Firmware Card **Custom Scans** Technology for Language and Learning Apple IIGS	These public domain programs contain custom scanning arrays for use with the Adaptive Firmware Card and many popular children's programs on the Apple IIGS platform.
Adult Switch and Touch Window Progressions R. J. Cooper Apple IIGS, Macintosh	These simple programs provide adult-level visuals with simple attention training, cause effect, and one step command skill building progressions. All programs are activated with a single switch.
AFC: Literacy Setups Don Johnston, Inc Apple IIGS	Adaptive Firmware Card setups are available for over 100 programs. Scanning, Touch Window, and expanded keyboard setups are included.
Aladin INCAP Dallas Windows 3.1	This program contains over 1,200 picture symbols that can be arranged into communication board displays for scanning access. Symbol organization is a branching tree structure. Voice output can be added when an external synthesizer card is attached.

AudScan
Words+
DOS

AudScan is a DOS compatible program designed for auditory scanning using single switch input. It has alphabet spelling and abbreviation expansion capabilities. An external speech synthesizer is needed for the computer system.

Aurora 2.0
Aurora Systems, Inc.
Windows

Aurora is a word prediction program that has single key typing features. Abbreviation expansion features are also included. An external speech synthesizer is needed for text-to-speech output.

Biggy
R. J. Cooper
Macintosh

Biggy enlarges the size of the mouse cursor on the computer monitor. It can also alter the color, and replace the mouse arrow with a pointing finger.

Childrens Switch and Touch Window Progressions
R. J. Cooper
Apple IIGS, Macintosh

Attending, cause-effect, and one step commands are trained through simple switch-activated animations.

Clicker Plus
Don Johnston, Inc
Windows

Clicker Plus is a talking on-screen keyboard with text to speech output. Custom dynamic arrays of letters, whole words, or pictures can be developed to access standard software applications.

ClickIt!
Intellitools
Macintosh

This program adapts any software program that requires a mouse click. Hotspots are assigned to the mouse click areas. Scanning arrays for switch users or custom displays for expanded keyboards can be developed to simulate mouse functions.

Co:Writer
Don Johnston Co.
Macintosh, Windows

Co:Writer is a word prediction program designed to reduce keystrokes. It is used in conjunction with word processing programs.

Communication Board Skill Builder
Edmark
Apple IIGS

Edmark's Lesson Maker program was used to create this training program for communication board skills. Children can use a Touch Window or single switch to select pictures.

Communication Series
Dunamis
Apple IIGS

This is a series of separate programs designed to use a PowerPad expanded keyboard with an Apple IIe or IIGS computer. Twelve symbol communication boards can be used on the PowerPad. There are separate programs for feelings, eating, home, and so forth.

Cooperative Electronic Library on Disability
Trace Research and Development Center
DOS, Macintosh, Windows

This CD program contains multiple assistive technology resources including ABLEDATA (a database of products), publication resources, a service delivery directory, and other resources.

Cross Scanner
R. J. Cooper
Macintosh, Windows

Discover:Screen
Don Johnston, Inc
Macintosh

DJ Speech ProPack Modules
Don Johnston, Inc
Macintosh

Doors
Madenta
Macintosh

Dr. Peets Talkwriter
Hartley
Apple IIGS

Dynavox 2
Sentient Systems Technology
Macintosh

Easy Access
Apple Computer Inc.
Apple IIGS, Macintosh

Edmark Lesson Maker
Edmark
Apple IIGS

Expanded Keyboard Emulator
Words+
DOS

Cross Scanner provides single switch access for most software programs. The switch has to be attached through a computer port that provides a mouse click signal.

This program is an on-screen keyboard for Macintosh users. It comes with ready-made keyboard arrays designed for children who need simplified layouts for specific programs. A design program is included to develop custom keyboard layouts.

These text to speech software modules add Macintalk II Pro synthesizer quality to Macintosh computers. The program expands standard Macintosh speech capabilities with additional voices and better pronunciations. Both English and Mexican Spanish versions are available. The modules are designed to work with Don Johnston software.

Doors is an on-screen keyboard program that can be accessed using a single switch, multiple switches, or mouse control device. The software contains word prediction, abbreviation expansion, custom macros, and speech output features.

This program was one of the first talking word processors. Text-to-speech synthesis is provided through an attached Echo II synthesizer unit.

This program uses 2,600 Dynasyms symbols to create a unique system of dynamic picture communication displays. It also contains Dynawrite, a word prediction program with picture symbols. The software is identical to the program that runs in the Dynavox 2 AAC system.

Easy Access is a utility program that is provided free of charge within the system software for later model Apple computers. It has sticky key typing features, auditory beep feedback, key activation delay features, and keyboard controls for the mouse.

Educational lessons can be designed with this software to teach basic picture communication skills. A Touchwindow and Echo synthesizer are needed. Branching, visual prompting, and verbal cues can be added to the lessons.

This software/hardware interface allows for the connection of expanded keyboards to IBM DOS compatible computers. Word prediction, abbreviation expansion, and sticky key typing features are included. An external synthesizer is needed for speech output.

EZ Keys
Words+
DOS, Windows

EZ Keys is AAC software that has word prediction and abbreviation expansion features. The "talk" feature allows the user to chat while continuing to run other applications. Various direct selection and scanning access options are available. An external synthesizer is needed for operation.

EZ Morse
Neil Squire Foundation
DOS

A single or dual switch can be used to encode Morse code signals for keyboard emulation with this program.

EZ Scan
Neil Squire Foundation
DOS

This program uses an on-screen keyboard that is accessed using a single or dual switch for keyboard emulation.

Finish Line for DOS/Windows
Innovative Designs
DOS, Windows

These two separate programs provide word prediction features for most word processing applications.

Five Finger Typist
Mayer-Johnson
Macintosh

This typing tutorial is designed to teach keyboarding skills to individuals who are only able to use one hand. Separate tutorials are available for left or right handed typists. The program is self-paced and progresses through graduated lessons.

Freedom Writer
World Communications
DOS

Freedom Writer is a stand-alone word processing program that can be accessed using several input methods. Whole words are selected from word menus to reduce keystrokes.

GIRO!
Interlexis Technologies
DOS

Giro! is a word processor with word prediction and spell checking features. It is designed to compensate for common spelling errors of individuals with dyslexia.

Gus! Abbreviations for Windows
Gus Communications Inc.
Windows

This program allows the user to create abbreviation expansion macros that can be used across multiple Windows applications.

Gus! Multimedia Speech System
Gus Communications Inc.
Windows

This program creates dynamic display AAC systems on Windows-based computers. A Sound-Blaster Card or GusTalk synthesizer is needed for speech output. It can be accessed through mouse emulators or switch scanning.

Gus! Speak Clipboard for Windows
Gus Communications Inc.
Windows

Speak Clipboard is combined with a Sound Blaster card to provide spoken communication within the Windows computer environment. Users can leave applications to communicate with this program, then return back to their work.

Gus! Talking Keyboard for Windows
Gus Communications Inc.
Windows

Talking Keyboard is an on-screen keyboard that can be accessed using a single or dual switch. It has word prediction and abbreviation expansion features. A speech synthesizer is included in the price.

Half-QWERTY
Matias Corporation
DOS, Macintosh

This utility program is designed for one-handed typists who have already learned keyboard skills.

HandiCHAT
Microsystems Software, Inc.
DOS, Windows

This pop-up utility is combined with a speech synthesizer to provide text-to-speech communication. There is also a screen reader included.

HandiCHATDeluxe
Microsystems Software, Inc.
DOS, Windows

This communication software lets the user store vocabulary into a library of 1,296 items. Abbreviation expansion is used to recall phrases. A synthesizer is needed for spoken output.

HandiCODE
Microsystems Software, Inc.
DOS, Windows

HandiCODE is designed for Morse code access using a single or dual switch. Abbreviation expansion features are included. A separate speech synthesizer is needed for spoken output.

HandiKEY
Microsystems Software, Inc.
DOS, Windows

An on-screen keyboard is accessed using a switch or mouse emulator. Word prediction and abbreviation expansion features are included. It can also be adapted for auditory scanning.

HandiWORD
Microsystems Software, Inc.
DOS, Windows

This program has word prediction and abbreviation expansion features and can be used in conjunction with most popular word processing programs.

HandiWORD Deluxe
Microsystems Software, Inc.
DOS, Windows

This program is similar to HandiWORD. Added features include word prediction with foreign language dictionaries (French, Spanish, German and Italian).

Help U Key
World Communications
DOS

Help U Key adds an on-screen keyboard that can be accessed using a switch or mouse emulation system. It includes abbreviation expansion features.

Help U Keyboard
World Communications
DOS

This on-screen keyboard can be accessed with a mouse emulator or single switch. It has word prediction features.

Help U Type and Speak
World Communications
DOS

Text-to-speech output is provided when a synthesizer is added to the computer. Sticky key typing features provide access for one fingered typists. Word prediction and abbreviation expansion features are included.

Help U Type
World Communications
DOS, Windows

Help U Type is a sticky key typing program for one fingered typists.

Hyper Bliss 3.0
Blissymbolics Communication
International
Macintosh

This scanning communication program uses Bliss symbols. The user selects parts of a symbol which are used to retrieve the entire symbol. Symbols are then combined for communication. Blissymbol prediction features are included.

HyperStudio
Roger Wagner Publishing
Apple IIGS, Macintosh, Windows

This multimedia authoring program is designed for professionals to create branching software lessons. It can be used to design custom communication displays.

I Can Cook Too!
I Can Play Too!
Mayer-Johnson
Macintosh

These two programs consists of dynamic communication boards with vocabulary for common children's games and cooking activities. The digitized voice output is delightful. It can be accessed by a single switch or through mouse emulation.

I-Key
Neil Squire Foundation
DOS

This program has sticky key features for one fingered typists.

IBM Access DOS
IBM Special Needs Systems
DOS

Access DOS provides sticky key features for one fingered typists. It also allows for mouse emulation through a numeric keypad. It is available free of charge.

IntelliKeys Overlay Maker
IntelliTools
Apple IIe, IIGS, Macintosh

Overlay Maker is used to create custom overlays for the Intellikeys expanded keyboard. A picture library of 300 symbols is included.

IntelliPics
Intellitools
Macintosh

Intellipics is an authoring system that can create multimedia educational programs. Communication activities can be created using the system.

IntelliTalk
Intellitools
Apple IIGS, DOS, Macintosh

Intellitalk is a low cost talking word processor. An external synthesizer is needed for DOS or Apple IIe versions.

Key Ability
Meeting the Challenge
DOS

This is a sticky key program for one fingered typists. The user has an option of using a DVORAK left or right handed keyboard layout.

Key Wi
Consultants for Communication
Technology
Windows

This software program incorporates word prediction and abbreviation expansion features. The on-screen keyboard can be accessed with a switch or mouse emulator. A synthesizer is added for speech output.

Key Wiz
Words+
DOS

Key Wiz is identical to the EZ Keys program listed previously, except that voice output features are not an option.

Keycache
OMS Development
DOS, Windows

This word prediction program is used in conjunction with standard word processing programs.

KeyUP
Ability Systems Corporation
DOS

KeyUP has sticky key typing features with one unique option. The software can be configured to only accept keystrokes when the key is released.

Magic Cursor
Madenta
Macintosh

Most mouse emulators require a method of creating a mouse click or pressing the mouse button. Magic Cursor provides an alternative dwell method to produce mouse functions. The user holds the cursor over a particular location for a specified length of time to select the item.

Morse Code WSKE
Words+
DOS

One and two switch Morse code is used to operate this computer access software. Word prediction and abbreviation expansion options are included. For AAC use a separate speech synthesizer is required.

MouseKeys for Windows
World Communications
Windows

This on-screen keyboard uses mouse emulators to select letters and other keystrokes. Word prediction and abbreviation expansion features are included.

Multimedia Access for Students with Disabilities
Emerging Technology Consultants
DOS, Macintosh

This software training program teaches professionals how to adapt computers for individuals with disabilities. Workbooks and other materials are included within the training package.

My-T-Mouse
Future Technologies
Windows

My-T-Mouse is a utility program that works with mouse emulation hardware. An on-screen keyboard with pop-up menus is used to operate the computer. Macros can be created and assigned to keys using the system.

One Access
Consultants for Communication Technology
DOS, Windows

A single switch and on-screen keyboard are used to access word prediction features within this program. The word prediction lists are custom selected for the user.

One Finger
Computers to Help People
DOS

One Finger is a sticky key typing utility for one fingered typists.

PicTalk
UCLA Intervention Program for the Handicapped
Apple IIGS

This preschool picture program is designed to teach AAC skills using a limited set of symbols arranged into branching category displays. A single switch is used to make selections.

Picture Scanner
R. J. Cooper
Apple IIGS, Macintosh, Windows

This scanning program teaches picture matching skills. It includes an authoring component that lets professionals decide which pictures to include and their placement in the scanning array.

Point to Pictures
R. J. Cooper
Apple IIGS, Macintosh, Windows

Point to Pictures begins with cause effect activities and moves into picture matching skills. Professionals can create custom lessons using the picture library. An expanded keyboard or Touch Window is required.

Power Talker
UCLA Intervention Program for
Handicapped Children
Apple IIGS

Power Talker is an authoring system designed to create 16 choice communication boards using a Power Pad expanded keyboard and Echo speech synthesizer.

PowerKey
Dunamis
Apple IIGS, DOS

This program lets users create custom expanded keyboard displays for the Power Pad.

PowerPad Toolkit 4
Dunamis
Apple IIGS

The Power Pad Toolkit 4 is an authoring system for the Power Pad expanded keyboard. It can be used to create talking communication boards when used with an Echo synthesizer.

Predict It
Don Johnston, Inc
Apple IIGS

This word prediction program includes a full featured word processor.

Pro Words Talking Word Processor
Access Unlimited
Apple IIGS

This stand-alone talking word processor requires an Echo synthesizer.

Radar Mouse/Crosshair Mouse
Words+
Windows

This software program uses single switch activation to emulate mouse movements. Radar Mouse uses a radar sweep to select mouse movement locations, Crosshair Mouse uses a row-column scanning sweep across the screen.

Revolving Doors
Madenta
Macintosh

Revolving Doors provides full computer access for single switch users. Word prediction features and customizeable on-screen keyboard layouts are included.

Scanning WSKE
Words+ Inc.
DOS

Scanning WSKE is a switch-operated word prediction program. It can be used to run most DOS programs. An external speech synthesizer provides voice output for communication.

ScreenDoors
Madenta
Macintosh

This on-screen keyboard has word prediction and abbreviation expansion features. There are three different keyboard layouts to choose from. It is accessed using a mouse emulator.

SignWare
SignWare
DOS, Macintosh

This is a tutorial program designed to teach finger spelling and American Sign Language. Other computer-based training programs for foreign sign languages are available.

SofType
Origin Instruments
Windows

SofType is an on-screen keyboard that can be accessed using a mouse emulator.

Speaking Dynamically
Mayer-Johnson
Macintosh

Speaking Dynamically is used to create custom dynamic communication displays for Macintosh users. PCS picture symbols are imported from Mayer-Johnson's Boardmaker program. The symbols can be sized and organized in any manner.

StoryBliss
Blissymbolics Communication
International
Macintosh

StoryBliss is a program that creates custom stories to be read aloud by users of Blissymbols. It was designed to transition Blissymbol users to traditional orthography.

Switch Assessment Program
Assistive Device Center School of
Engineering and Computer Science
Apple IIGS, Macintosh

This program is used to evaluate switch motor access skills. It collects data on switch timing, release, and speed. Joystick or multiple switch arrays can also be evaluated.

Switch Clicker Plus
Don Johnston, Inc
Windows

This Windows program is designed to develop custom scanning arrays for software applications accessed using a single switch. The arrays can consist of letters, whole words, or pictures in a dynamic display.

Talk About
Don Johnston, Inc.
Macintosh

Talk About is a unique AAC application that combines text-to-speech synthesis with prestored text retrieval. Sections of text are organized by interaction categories and user stories.

Talking Junior Writer
Technology for Language and Learning
Apple IIGS

This program is a low cost talking word processor. An Echo synthesizer is required.

Talking Screen
Words+
DOS, Windows

Talking Screen creates dynamic picture communication displays. It can import symbols from a variety of symbol sets, and can use photo and graphic images scanned into the computer. A speech synthesizer is required for voice output.

Talking Text Writer
Scholastic Software
Apple IIGS, DOS

This is a stand-alone talking word processor for children. An external speech synthesizer is required.

Talking Touch Window
Edmark
Apple IIGS

This authoring system uses an Echo synthesizer to create talking picture boards on the computer. A Touch Window is required to access the picture displays.

Telepathic
Madenta
Macintosh

Telepathic is a word prediction program that also provides voice output through the Macintosh Macintalk built-in synthesizer. It can learn foreign words and languages and add them to the word prediction lists.

Turn Talking
R. J. Cooper
Macintosh, Windows

This software program is designed to teach the concept of interactive communication to individuals who are nonspeaking. Up to two users access switches to communicate predeveloped conversations. Pictures can be added to increase comprehension of the conversations.

Wish Writer
Consultants for Communication

Wish Writer is a word prediction program combined with an on-screen keyboard that can be ac-

Technology
DOS, Windows

cessed by single switch users. The program can also be accessed through the keyboard.

Wivik 2.0
Prentke Romich
Windows

Wivik uses an on-screen keyboard that can be accessed using a mouse emulator. Custom or international keyboard configurations can be created.

Wivik WREP
Prentke Romich
Windows

This software is an extension to the Wivik 2.0 program. It adds word prediction and abbreviation expansion features.

Wivik2 with Scanning
Prentke Romich
Windows

This variation of the Wivik programs is designed for single switch access. A separate switch interface box is required.

Word Writer
Prentke Romich Company
Macintosh

This desk accessory program has word prediction features that can be used with any Macintosh application program.

Write Out Loud
Don Johnston, Inc
Macintosh, Windows

Write Out Loud is a talking word processor for the Macintosh. It includes a spell checker, a feature that is missing from many other talking word processors.

SWITCHES AND LIGHT POINTERS

Switches are simple devices that are used to send signals to dedicated AAC systems, switch adapted toys, or computer input systems. The switch plugs into a special access port on the AAC device or toy. Each switch has unique characteristics. The method of activating the switch, the switch size, the amount of force needed to produce an activation, auditory or visual feedback, and other features should be thoroughly reviewed in product catalogs before recommending a particular product. There are several products that adapt the signal sent by the switch. These include timers, which send a switch signal to a device for a specified time period; switch latches, which turn the switch into an on/off signal; and transmitters, which send radio or infrared signals to a receiver when the switch is activated. This section also contains information on light pointers designed to work with simple communication boards or with specific AAC devices.

Device/Vendor

Description

ACS Twinkle Remote Switch
ACS Technologies

The Twinkle switch consists of two small electrodes worn by the user and a remote receiver that interprets signals from the electrodes. Minimal eye movements or lateral head movements generate the switch signals. This switch is designed for individuals with minimal motor movements.

Air Cushion Switch
Prentke Romich Company

The Air Cushion Switch consists of a pneumatic squeeze bladder that activates the switch using puffs of air. It comes in single and dual function versions.

BASS Switch
Don Johnston, Inc

BASS switches are pressure switches with a large (6 × 3 inch) flat surface area. They come in multiple colors. Pictures can easily be attached to the large surface of the switch.

Baton Laser Pointer
Innocomp

This laser light pointer comes with a head gear mounting system. It has a unique sip and puff accessory that turns the light pointer on and off.

Big Red Switch
Ablenet

Big Red has a large 5 inch circular pressure surface. Pressing the surface activates the switch. Auditory feedback is provided. It comes in seven colors.

BlinkSwitch
Innocomp

The BlinkSwitch consists of a sensor attached to eyeglass frames. The sensor monitors changes in light reflection to detect switch activations. As the individual's eye blinks, the skin surface of the eyelid refracts light differently from the eye itself, causing a switch activation.

BS-1 Body Switch
DU-IT Control Systems Group

The BS-1 Body Switch is a push button switch with a 1.5 inch diameter activation surface. It provides an auditory click when pressed.

Buddy Button
Tash

The Buddy Button is a low profile circular switch which is 2½ inches in diameter. The switch provides tactile and auditory feedback when pressed. It comes in seven colors and in unusual designs such as plaid and happy face.

Ellipse
Don Johnston, Inc

The Ellipse series of switches come in different size oval shapes. They have a low profile and auditory click feedback. Different amounts of pressure are needed for the different sizes.

Grip & Puff Switch
Toys for Special Children/
Enabling Devices

Squeezing the grip of this switch will cause air to flow through a pneumatic tube to activate the switch.

Head Switch
Toys for Special Children/
Enabling Devices

The Head Switch has a small surface area with a button cap. Pressing the cap activates the switch.

IST Switch
Words+

This switch can be used in three different modes. The infrared sensor detects changes in reflection, including eyeblinks. The sound sensor detects slight sounds. The touch sensor is activated by slight skin contact.

Jelly Bean Switch
Ablenet

The Jelly Bean has a circular surface that is 2½ inches in diameter. Auditory and tactile feedback is provided when the switch is pressed. It is available in seven different colors.

L.T. Switch
Don Johnston, Inc

This switch is designed for individuals with low tone and limited strength. It only requires ¾ ounces of pressure to activate. An auditory click signals a switch activation to the user.

Latch Box
Creative Switch Industries

Plugging a switch into this latch box changes the switch operation into an on/off activation mode.

Leaf Switch
Toys for Special Children/
Enabling Devices

The leaf switch is a long wire enclosed in a vinyl band. When the leaf switch is moved enough to bend the encased wire, the switch will activate.

Leaf Switch
Zygo

The leaf switch consists of a wire encased in a band of red vinyl. Bending the wire in either direction activates the switch. The Zygo leaf switch comes in short and long lengths.

Lever Switch
Zygo

The lever switch consists of a circular foam pad attached to a long 6 inch lever. Pressing the lever activates the switch.

LightBeam
Ability Research

This light pointer consists of a small red beam light source connected to a battery pack. A single switch can be attached to control turning the light pointer on and off. The beam of light is 2 inches across when shined on items up to 2 feet away.

Lighted Plate Switch
Toys for Special Children/
Enabling Devices

This large surface plate switch has an enclosed light that turns on when the switch is pressed. This visual feedback is helpful for young children learning to activate switches.

LightSwitch
Ability Research

This single switch is activated when a beam of light shines on its sensor. A flashlight, adapted light pointer, or other light source can be used to activate the switch.

LinkSwitch
AdapTech Inc.

LinkSwitch consists of touch sensitive taction pads. The taction pads have adhesive backings which can be attached to objects or placed on top of picture symbols. Touching the pad activates the switch without needing to apply pressure.

Mounting Switch
Don Johnston, Inc

The Mounting Switch is a variation of the lever switch. It consists of a long lever with a circular pad at the end. Pressing the pad activates the switch. It is primarily designed to be activated using head movements. A switch mount is available.

P-Switch
Prentke Romich Company

The P-Switch is designed for individuals with minimal muscular movement. Small sensors are strapped to the body to detect muscle contractions. It can be adjusted for different sensitivities.

Petite Pillow Switch
Toys for Special Children/
Enabling Devices

This soft padded pillow switch is activated by pressure.

Pillow Switch
Tash

The pillow switch has a padded foam surface encased in a soft fabric cover. Pressing the surface activates the switch.

Pinch Switch
Toys for Special Children/
Enabling Devices

The pinch switch is activated with a pincer grasp on either side of the small switch surface.

Plate Switch
Toys for Special Children/
Enabling Devices

Plate Switches come in several different sizes ranging from 3×5 inches up to 8×13 inches. Pressing the plate surface activates the switch. The switches can be purchased with timer, latching, and counter features.

Rocking Lever Switch
Prentke Romich Company
Don Johnston, Inc

This switch consists of a metal plate attached to a switch base. Pressing the plate activates the switch. Some versions are dual switches that use one side to make switch selections and the other side for on/off or other dual switch functions.

Rocking Plate Switch
Toys for Special Children/
Enabling Devices

This large rocking lever switch can activate up to two different toys or devices.

Sensor Switch
Don Johnston, Inc

The sensor switch consists of small sensors that are strapped onto the user. Small muscle movements activate the switch. It is designed for individuals with significant paralysis.

Signal Switch
Toys for Special Children/
Enabling Devices

The Signal pressure switch uses a circular bicycle reflector as the switch surface.

Sip & Puff Switch
Toys for Special Children/
Enabling Devices

This dual switch is activated by sip and puff breathing through a pneumatic tube. A double sip and puff version is available that provides up to four different switch closure possibilities.

Sip and Puff Switch
Prentke Romich Company

Sip and Puff switches are designed for quadriplegics who are able to control respiration functions. The switches have dual capabilities, using the sip and puff to control separate functions.

Snappy Switch
ORCCA Technology

The snappy switch is grasped in the palm. Squeezing the soft foam activates the switch. It provides auditory feedback.

Sound Activated Switch
Invotek

This switch activates when a sound is made. The sound sensitivity and sound duration needed for activation can be adjusted.

Specs Switch
Ablenet

Specs are small 1 inch circular switches that are activated when pressed. They come in seven different colors and provide tactile and auditory feedback.

String Switch
Toys for Special Children/
Enabling Devices

Pulling a string activates this switch.

Switch Latch and Timer
Ablenet
Don Johnston, Inc

This device contains switch latching on/off capabilities and a switch timer.

Taction Pad
AdapTech

Taction pads are adhesive-backed strips of clear material that can be attached to any object or picture. Touching the Taction pad activates the switch. This switch can only be used with AdapTech's AAC and environmental control products.

Talking Laser Beam
Crestwood Company

This red laser beam light pointer comes attached to a child- or adult-sized cap. The name is a misnomer as the beam system itself does not "talk." It can be used with low tech AAC boards. It can also be purchased without the cap.

Twitch Switch
Toys for Special Children/
Enabling Devices

Small muscle movements activate a sensor that is taped to the skin surface. This switch is designed for consumers with paralysis or low tone. It can operate in latched, momentary, or timed modes.

Tilt Switch
Toys for Special Children/
Enabling Devices

This gravity switch is activated when the switch is tilted off-balance.

Tongue Switch
Prentke Romich Company

This dual switch was originally designed for quadriplegics who had enough tongue control to flick the switch up and down. It can also be operated using fingers and requires only light pressure.

Touch Switch
Zygo

The Touch Switch is designed for light pressure. It has a small surface and requires minimal pressure to activate. An adjustment screw can increase or decrease pressure requirements.

Tread Switch
Zygo

Tread Switches are durable metal switches that are pressed down to activate the switch. An audible click feedback is provided.

Ultimate Switch
Toys for Special Children/
Enabling Devices

The Ultimate Switch consists of a spring with an attached ball. Hitting the ball in any direction activates the switch. The switch is entirely coated in a vinyl sheath which increases its durability. It comes with a gooseneck mounting system.

Universal Module
Toys for Special Children/
Enabling Devices

The Universal Module is used with switches. Single and dual switch latching, timers, and counters are features of this switch module.

Vertical Plate Switch
Toys for Special Children/
Enabling Devices

This large switch is mounted at a 45 degree angle in a sturdy base. Pressing the switch causes activation.

Vibrating Plate Switch
Toys for Special Children/
Enabling Devices

The vibrating plate switch has a large 5 × 8 inch surface that vibrates when pressed.

Vibration Switch
AdapTech

This switch senses vibrations to produce a switch activation. The switch can be placed on a table or other surface. Tapping the table activates the switch. Timed or latching features can be adapted for the user.

Viewpoint Optical Indicator
Prentke Romich Company

This optical light pointer generates a small white light beam that is functional up to 3 feet from the light source. It comes with an adjustable headband.

Voice Activated Switch
Toys for Special Children/
Enabling Devices

Sounds can be used to activate this switch. The loudness threshold sensitivity can be adjusted. This switch comes with a timer and can be used in latching modes.

Wireless Switch Link
Bloorview Children's Hospital

This unit consists of a transmitter and receiver. Switches are plugged into the transmitter. Pushing the switch sends a radio signal to the receiver. AAC devices, toys, or other switch activated systems can be controlled through the receiver.

Wobble Switch
Prentke Romich Company

This switch consists of an elongated spring with a small ball attached to the end. Moving the ball in any direction activates the switch.

MOUNTING EQUIPMENT

As part of the AAC evaluation process, professionals determine the best position for AAC devices, computer hardware, or switches. During the assessment, the team usually holds the equipment in place. Once the exact placement is determined, the team then needs to consider how to permanently mount the equipment in the specified position. There are several products on the market that are designed to position AAC devices and switches on wheelchairs or table tops. Some products are made specifically for a particular device, others can be adapted to fit a wide variety of equipment.

Device/Vendor

Description

Communication Station Desk Mount
Sentient Systems Technology

The Desk Mount is designed to position Sentient Systems AAC devices on a desk or table surface. Desk mounts allow the AAC device to be angled and held steady on flat surfaces.

Communication Station Folding Mount
Sentient Systems Technology

This Communication Station Mount attaches Sentient Systems AAC devices to wheelchairs. The fold-down model allows for easy transfers into and out of the chair. The wedge block that attaches directly to the chair is larger than most mounting systems.

Communication Station Rigid Mount
Sentient Systems Technology

This mount is similar to other Communication Station wheelchair mounts. The rigid model swings away from the chair to allow for consumer transfers into and out of the chair.

CPVC Parts Kit
Adamlab

This kit contains CPVC plastic piping, elbow joints, T-joints, and switch plates. The pipes are combined together like Tinker Toys to create eye gaze displays, switch mounts, and mounts for other lightweight systems.

Daessy Desktop Mount
Daedulus Technologies

The Daessy Desktop mount provides a stable base for mounting AAC systems that need to be used at an angle on table or desk surfaces. Mounting plates are available for most commercially available AAC systems.

Daessy Folding Mount
Daedulus Technologies

The Daessy Folding mount can be used with most commercially available AAC systems to attach the device to a wheelchair. The folding design allows for easy transfers into and out of the chair. The mounting base is smaller than most which makes it easier to attach to small wheelchairs.

Daessy MiniMount
Daedalus Technologies

The MiniMount is designed to clamp lightweight AAC devices and switches onto the arm-rest area of a wheelchair.

Dycem Non-Slip Surfaces

Dycem is a nonslip material that can be used on flat surfaces to hold switches or lightweight AAC devices in place. It is available in rolls that can be cut to size, or in precut pads. Dycem is easy to place and can be rolled up and used multiple times. It is available through many ADL, AAC, and occupational therapy catalog sources.

Flexible Mounting Kit
Crestwood Company

This clamp mount consists of a gooseneck arm with a large clip. Lightweight communication boards or plexiglass eye gaze systems can be attached using the clip.

Head Mounting Kit
Don Johnston, Inc

This gooseneck mounting system is designed to attach some Don Johnston switches to wheelchairs. It can be adapted for other switches.

Magic Arm Mounting System
Toys for Special Children/
Enabling Devices

This mounting system is designed to hold switches in place.

Mighty Mount
TASH

This switch mount is designed to attach any switch to a table or wheelchair tray surface.

MS-34 Friction Set
Zygo

This clamping system is designed to position Macaw communication systems. It can be clamped to a wheelchair tray, table surface, or other flat surface.

Quick Release Adapters
Prentke Romich Company

The Quick Release Adaptors are designed for mounting Prentke Romich company equipment to wheelchair mounting systems. They can be used on

Rover Walker
Noble Motion

wheelchair mounts available from PRC, or on mounting systems purchased from other companies.

This lightweight walker has large rubber tires and an attached tray which can be used to hold AAC equipment.

Scoot-A-Bout
CJT Enterprises

This four wheeled small platform is designed for transporting AAC systems that need to be positioned near the floor.

Simplicity
Words+

The Simplicity Mount attaches AAC and computer systems to a wheelchair. The mount has a swing down feature which places it out of the way when the AAC system is not needed, or when the consumer is transferring out of the chair.

Slim Armstrong
Ablenet

Slim Armstrong is a system of parts that can clamp a switch or lightweight device (up to 5 pounds) in position on a wheelchair or table surface.

Switch Mounting Hardware
Toys for Special Children/
Enabling Devices

Enabling Devices has various clamps, switch plates, rods, and tubing available to create custom switch mounts. Components of the mounting system are ordered individually.

UltraStick Adhesive
Ablenet

This reusable sticky adhesive product is useful for positioning switches, communication boards, or other lightweight items on flat or slightly angled surfaces. It holds the items in place without slipping, yet can be easily removed.

Universal Switch Mounting Kit
Don Johnston, Inc

This kit contains rigid, angled, and gooseneck tubing along with several clamps and rods. Consumers use their creativity to make custom mounting systems for switches or other lightweight equipment.

Walk It
for
CJT Enterprises

The Walk It is a two-wheel tripod system designed

children and adults who are able to walk but need assistance carrying their AAC devices. The Walk It can be pulled or pushed to carry an AAC system on an attached tray.

WCMK
Prentke Romich Company

The WCMK was one of the first available wheelchair mounting systems for AAC devices. It is a low cost mounting system that does not have as many points of adjustment or options as later models.

AAC SYMBOL SETS AND LANGUAGES

This category of products is a listing of commercially available AAC picture symbol materials, AAC languages, and products designed to manage vocabulary. The products include a wide range of items including books of symbols that can be photocopied, software clip art programs, sticker sets, premade picture communication boards, and specialized AAC software language programs designed to load into specific AAC devices. Similar to the software listings that preceded this section, software products are listed with the computer operating platform designed to run the program.

Device/Vendor/Platform	Description
AAC Vocabulary Manager Don Johnston, Inc Macintosh	This Hypercard stack assists professionals in managing large vocabularies for AAC users. Frequently used words and category listings are included to assist in developing vocabulary.
Access Bliss Blissymbolics Communication International Macintosh	This program contains all approved Blissymbols in a a system file. Symbols can be retrieved, cut, and pasted into communication boards or other applications.
Blissymbol Component Minspeak Words Strategy Prentke Romich Company	This Minspeak application was written for adult and teen Blissymbol users who are using Prentke Romich AAC systems. Blissymbols and their components are combined into sequences to access 1,000 root words and up to 3,000 messages.
Blissymbols Gallery Don Johnston, Inc Macintosh	This symbol set is used with Ke:nx and Ke:nx On Board to create custom AAC applications. Over 2,500 Blissymbols are available.
Boardmaker (International) Mayer-Johnson Macintosh, Windows	Boardmaker contains the 3,000 symbol PCS library in color or black and white. It is designed to retrieve and size symbols, allowing for cutting and pasting into any drawing application. The software comes with it's own drawing program. Symbol translations are available for 10 languages.
Communic-Ease Prentke Romich Company	Communic-Ease is a Minspeak program that can be used in Prentke Romich AAC systems. Over 500 words and 300 phrases are organized into categorical groupings using multiple meaning picture sequences.
Communication Board Builder Mayer-Johnson Co. Macintosh	A set of 3,000 PCS Symbols are contained in this program designed to create communication boards using Hypercard stacks. The program is easy to use but can only create specific pregridded boards with 1¼ inch symbols.
Communication Displays for Engineered Preschool Environments Don Johnston, Inc Mayer-Johnston Co.	Carol Goossens, Sharon Crain, and Pamela Elder created ready-made PCS communication boards for most preschool topic based activities. Book I has boards which fit 16 symbol and eye gaze systems, Book II has boards for 36 and 32 symbol systems.

Communication Overlays for Engineering Training Environments
Mayer-Johnson Co.

This series of four books by Elder and Goossens is a resource for communication boards designed for adolescents and adults. Over 63 age appropriate activities are represented in the boards. The boards range from 8 symbol overlays in Book I, to 32 and 36 symbol overlays in Books III and IV.

Communication Icon Galleries
Don Johnston, Inc
Macintosh

These symbols can be used within Ke:nx applications to create custom scanning or expanded keyboard communication displays. There are several symbol sets including PCS, Core Picture Vocabulary, Blissymbols Gallery, ComPic, DynaSyms, and Kids in Action.

COMPIC Gallery
Don Johnston, Inc
Macintosh

The COMPIC library of line drawings can be retrieved to create AAC displays using Ke:nx and Ke:nx On:Board.

Core Picture Vocabulary
Don Johnston, Inc

The Core Picture Vocabulary set was designed for young children. The symbols are black and white line drawings that are relatively realistic. The 160 symbols in the set are printed on 2¾ inch cards or are available as stickers.

Core Picture Vocabulary Gallery
Don Johnston, Inc
Macintosh

The 300 Core Picture Vocabulary Symbols are available on CD ROM disk. They can be retrieved for use with Ke:nx and Ke:nx On:Board AAC applications.

Cut & Paste 1000 Dynasyms Book
Poppin and Company

This set of 1,000 black and white Dynasyms symbols comes with three copies of each symbol. The symbols come in three sizes (⅜, ⅞, and 1¼ inches).

Cut & Paste Full Color 1,700 Dynasyms Book
Poppin and Company

This set includes over 1,700 color Dynasyms. Two copies of each symbol are included in the book. Symbols are ⅞ inch in size.

DigiTalk 1
Sentient Systems Technology
Digivox

This program contains premade picture symbol communication displays for preschool children that can be loaded into a Digivox AAC system. The program can be modified after being loaded into the system.

DynaSyms Gallery
Don Johnston, Inc
Macintosh

Over 1,700 symbols from the Dynasyms symbol set are available on this CD Rom disk. The symbols can be accessed for custom applications using Ke:nx and Ke:nx On:Board.

Full Color Self Adhesive Dynasyms Stickers
Poppin and Company

This set of 1,700 color Dynasyms symbols comes in full color stickers. The stickers are ⅞ inch in size.

Gus! Imaginart Symbol Set
Gus Communications Inc.
Windows

This 1,200 symbol library from Imaginart is contained on disk. The symbols can be used within the Gus! Multimedia Speech System to design communication displays for Windows-based computers.

Gus! Mayer-Johnson Symbol Set
Gus Communications, Inc.
Windows

Mayer-Johnson's PCS symbols are contained in this program. The symbols can be used within the Gus! Multimedia Speech System.

Imaginart Gallery
Don Johnston, Inc
Macintosh

Over 1,000 Imaginart Pick 'n Stick symbols are available to create custom AAC applications using Ke:nx and Ke:nx On:Board.

Interaction, Education, & Play+
Prentke Romich Company

IEP+ is written for Prentke Romich AAC devices using Minspeak strategies. It was designed for preschool to early elementary age children and contains over 1,000 words necessary for education, social, and play activities.

Kids in Action Gallery
Don Johnston, Inc
Macintosh

This symbol set includes 400 color pictures of children. The symbols can be used with Ke:nx and Ke:nx On:Board to create custom AAC displays. The realistic pictures show children of different ethnicities.

Language, Learning, & Living
Prentke Romich Company

This Minspeak program is written for teens and adults with learning disabilities using Prentke Romich AAC devices. The program has a large lexicon of prestored words which are accessed using 2 and 3 symbol picture sequences.

Passports to Independence
Crestwood Company

Passports consist of black and white Talking Symbols picture cards arranged into small communication books. Different passport systems are available for specific community needs such as fast food ordering, drug store, or recreation, and so forth.

PCS Gallery
Don Johnston, Inc
Macintosh

The Mayer-Johnson PCS symbol set is available on CD-ROM in this software library. The symbols can be retrieved and used in AAC custom applications with Ke:nx and Ke:nx On:Board.

Pick 'n Stick
Imaginart

Pick 'n Stick symbols are colorful concrete symbols that depict adults and adult activities. The symbols are available in 1½ inch and ¾ inch sizes. There are over 1,000 symbols in the set.

Pick 'n Stick Primary Pack
Imaginart

These 2½ inch concrete color stickers are designed for young children. There are 96 symbols in the set.

Pick 'n Stick on Disk
Imaginart
DOS, Macintosh, Windows

The Imaginart Pick 'n Stick library of over 1,200 symbols is included on these disks. Color and black and white versions of symbols are available. Symbols can be retrieved for copying and pasting into drawing applications to make communication displays.

Picsyms Categorical Dictionary
Poppin and Company

Picsyms are a set of black and white symbols that preceded Dynasyms. The dictionary contains over 800 symbols with rules for creating new symbols for the set.

Picture Communication Symbols
Mayer-Johnson Co.

Picture Communication Symbols is one of the largest picture systems available, with over 3,000 symbols. They are available in notebook form, as stickers, stamps, and clip art software. Both color and black and white versions of the software are available.

Picture Prompt System
Attainment Company

Picture prompts were designed to provide picture cues for adult functional living activities. They consist of colored drawings on laminated cards with matching stickers.

Power in Play
Prentke Romich Company

This Minspeak symbol program is designed for Prentke Romich AAC devices. The program uses eight picture symbols which are combined into multiple meaning sequences to access 400 words, phrases, and songs. It was written for preschool children.

Stories & Strategies for Communication
Prentke Romich Company

Stories & Strategies for Communication was designed for preschool children to participate in early literacy activities. Vocabulary for five different stories and accompanying activities is included. The program is used in Prentke Romich AAC devices.

Super Sticker Set
Attainment Company

This sticker set consists of 576 picture prompt symbols, 588 WordWise symbols, 192 mealtime symbols, and money symbols. Stickers are 1 inch colored drawings. This set was designed for teaching daily living skills.

Symbols
Bill & Richards Software
Macintosh

Symbols requires Hypercard 2.0 to retrieve over 1,000 symbols. Symbols can be cut and pasted into other applications to make communication displays. Morse code, Braille, signs, and other symbols are included.

Talking Pictures
Crestwood Company

Talking Pictures are available in five sets and are oriented to adult communication needs. Symbols are black and white drawings on cards (2½" × 3¼") or smaller (1⅜" × 2") stickers.

Topics to Learn Communication
Prentke Romich Company

TLC is a Minspeak application program for Prentke Romich AAC systems. A 32 symbol overlay is used to access over 500 single words through multiple meaning picture sequences. This program is written for children between the ages of 2 and 10.

Touch 'n Talk Communication Stickers
Imaginart

These 600 black and white symbols are designed for adult hospital communication settings. They come in 1 ½" and 5/8" sizes. They are similar to the color Pick 'n Stick symbol sets.

Unity
Prentke Romich Company

Previous Minspeak application programs had limited carryover from one program to another. Unity is designed to begin with simple, single symbol messages and progress in three stages to multiple meaning sequences. The program is designed to take children from beginning language levels to adult vocabulary. The final level provides access to over 2,100 root words. Unity is written for use in Prentke Romich AAC devices.

Words Strategy
Prentke Romich Company

Words Strategy is a Minspeak application for Prentke Romich AAC systems. It is designed for the teen or adult user who is capable of sequencing words together to construct sentences. Over 2,500 words are organized by picture-grammar label sequences.

WordWise Sticker Set
Attainment Company

WordWise symbols are colored drawings on 1 inch stickers. There are 588 different symbols consisting of nouns, verbs, prepositions, adjectives, and adverbs.

LOW TECHNOLOGY PRODUCTS

Many individuals who need AAC systems benefit from simple nonelectronic communication devices. Families and professionals can make these communication boards, communication books, or picture displays using materials available from office supply, hardware, and art materials stores. However, the process of searching through stores to find the materials, and then assembling the materials, is time consuming. To meet the need for low cost materials to construct AAC systems, several vendors sell products for this purpose.

Device/Vendor	Description
Chain Talk Crestwood Company	Chain Talk is a retractable key chain that can be attached to a belt loop, purse strap, or belt. The key ring comes with vinyl envelopes to insert picture symbols.
Communication Boards Attainment	These plastic communication boards are printed with 20 picture symbols on the front and a QWERTY keyboard on the back. Child and adult versions are available with preselected symbols. A blank board is also available which can be custom designed with symbol stickers.
Communication Books Mayer Johnson	Several different sizes of communication books and wallets are available from Mayer Johnson. The books have clear vinyl pockets for communication displays that are designed to fit page sizes from the Board Maker software program. Key ring attachments are available.
Eye Com Board Imaginart	This clear acrylic communication display can be used to create eye gaze boards.

Eye Gaze Frame
Adamlab

The Eye Gaze Frame is made of CPVC piping. It includes enough Lexan plastic to make three eye gaze symbol displays.

Fold It System
Don Johnston, Inc

The Fold It System communication boards are lightweight denim boards with plastic pockets for picture symbols. Each board has a carrying strap and folds down into a portable size.

Mounting Boards
Crestwood Company

Various sizes of mounting boards for communication displays are available. Boards consist of heavy matboards, vinyl envelope covers, and key rings.

Object Communicator
Crestwood Company

The Object Communicator Plexiglass eye gaze board has shelves that can be used to place up to four different objects. A table stand is available.

Opticommunicator
Crestwood Company

This is a Plexiglass frame for eye gaze communication. A table stand is available to hold it in place.

Pocket Overlays
Imaginart

Pocket Overlays clip to Imaginart's Eye Com Board. It has eight vinyl pockets that can be used to display objects in an eye gaze display.

Pocket Picture Holder
Imaginart

This small communication book fits easily into a pocket or purse. It has 16 picture pockets and is $4\frac{1}{2} \times 3$ inches in size.

Porta Board
Crestwood

Porta Boards come in 2, 4, 6, and 8 sided versions. They are designed to hold Talking Symbols picture cards but can be used with other symbol sets to make AAC communication displays.

Porta Book
Crestwood Company

Porta Books come in several different sizes. They are designed to hold Talking Symbols symbol cards, but can also be used for other symbol systems to make AAC communication books.

Touch 'n Talk Communication Notebook
Imaginart

This notebook comes with dividers for common communication categories. Picture symbols can be arranged into the symbol category sections.

Touch 'n Talk Tote Boards
Imaginart

These lightweight plastic boards have a carrying handle. Picture symbol stickers are placed onto the surface of the board. Two sizes are available.

References

Rehabilitation Engineering Research Center on AAC. (1996). *The guide to augmentative and alternative communication devices*. Wilmington: University of Delaware.

Appendix B

AAC PRODUCT VENDORS AND MANUFACTURERS

Sharon L. Glennen

Appendix A inventoried hundreds of products related to augmentative and alternative communication (AAC). Each product was listed with a description and the name of the vendor or manufacturer. Appendix B is an alphabetical listing of these product vendors. Consumers and professionals are encouraged to contact the vendors to obtain product catalogs along with information regarding new devices. Because many assistive technology companies are small, addresses and phone numbers can change from year to year. Readers are encouraged to review hyper-ABLEDATA or *Closing the Gap* for up-to-date information on vendors (see Appendix D). Several manufacturers have developed World Wide Web sites on the Internet which include information, photographs, and ordering specifics for their products. When available, web addresses are provided for manufacturers.

Ability Research
P.O. Box 1721
Minnetonka, MN 55345
(612) 939-0121
http://www.skypoint.com/~ability

Ability Systems Corporation
1422 Arnold Ave.
Roslyn, PA 19001
(215) 657-4338

Ablenet
1081 10th Avenue, S.E.
Minneapolis, MN 55414
(800) 322-0956
(612) 379-0956

Abovo
96 Rhinebeck Avenue
Springfield, MA 01129
(413) 594-5279

Access Unlimited
3535 Briarpark Drive, Suite 102
Houston, TX 77042-5235
(800) 848-0311
(713) 781-7441

ACCI
280-B Moon Clinton Road
Moon Township, PA 15108
(800) 982-2248

ACS Technologies
1400 Lee Drive Suite 3
Coraopolis, PA 15108
(800) 227-2922
(412) 269-6656

Adamlab
33500 Van Born Road
P.O. Box 807
Wayne, MI 48184
(313) 467-1415

AdapTech
ISU Research Park
2501 N. Loop Drive
Ames, IA 50010
(515) 296-7171

Apple Computer Inc.
1 Infinite Loop
Cupertino, CA 95014-6299
(800) 800-SOS-APPL

Assistive Device Center
School of Engineering and Computer Science
California State University
Sacramento, CA 95819
(916) 278-6679

Attainment Company
P.O. Box 930160
Verona, WI 53593
(800) 327-4269

Aurora Systems Inc.
2647 Kingsway
Vancouver, BC V5R5H4
Canada
(800) 361-8255
http:/ /www.scbc.org/hinet/business/
CoProf/Aurora/aurora.html

Bill & Richards Software
P.O. Box 1075
Litchfield, CT 06759
(203) 567-4307

**Blissymbolics Communication
International**
1630 Lawrence Avenue, W., Suite 104
Toronto, Ontario M6L 1C5
Canada
(416) 242-9114

Bloorview Children's Hospital
Communication and Assistive Technology
25 Buchan Court
Willowdale, Onfario M2J 4S9
Canada
(416) 494-2222

Boston Educational Systems and Technology
63 Forest Street
Chestnut Hill, MA 02167
(617) 277-0179

Carroll Touch
P.O. Box 1309
Round Rock, TX 78680
(800) 386-8241

CJT Enterprises
3625 W. Macarthur Boulevard, Suite 301
Santa Ana, CA 92704
(714) 751-6295

Communication Devices, Inc.
2433 Government Way, Suite A
Coeur d'Alene, ID 83814
(208) 765-1259

Computers to Help People
825 E. Johnson Street
Madison, WI 53703
(608) 257-5917

Consultants for Communication Technology
508 Bellview Terrace
Pittsburgh, PA 15202
(412) 761-6062

Creative Switch Industries
P.O. Box 829
North San Juan, CA 95960
(515) 287-5748

Crestwood Company
6625 N. Sidney Place
Milwaukee, WI 53209
(414) 352-5678

Daedulus Technologies
2491 Vauxhall Place
Richmond, BC V6V 1Z5
Canada
(604) 270-4605

Don Johnston, Inc.
1000 Rand Road, Building 115
P.O. Box 639
Wauconda, IL 60084
(800) 999-4660
(708) 526-2682
http://www.donjohnston.com

DU-IT Control Systems Group
8765 Township Road 513
Shreve, OH 44676
(216) 567-2001

Dunamis
Highway 317
Suwanee, GA 30174
(800) 828-2443
(404) 932-0485

Edmark
P.O. Box 3218
Redmond, WA 98073
(206) 556-8431

Emerging Technology Consultants
5 Bessom Street, Suite 175
P.O. Box 4000
Marblehead, MA 01945
(617) 639-1930

Enabling Devices
385 Warburton Avenue
Hastings on Hudson, NY 10706
(914) 478-0960

Frame Technologies
W681 Pearl St.
Oneida, WI 54155
(414) 869-2979

Franklin Electronics
122 Burrs Road
Mt. Holly, NJ 08060
(800) 525-9673

Future Technologies
1061 E. Flamingo Road, Suite 8
Las Vegas, NV 89119
(800) 551-3926

Gus Communications Inc.
P.O. Box 4362
Blaine, WA 98231
(604) 279-0110
http://www.gusinc.com

Hartley
3451 Dunkle Drive, Suite 200
Lansing, MI 48911
(800) 247-1380

IBM Special Needs Systems
P.O. Box 1328
Internal Zip 5432
Boca Raton, FL 33432
(800) 426-4832

Imaginart
307 Arizona Street
Bisbee, AZ 85603
(800) 828-1376
(602) 432-5741

INCAP Dallas
720 Sparrow Lane
Coppell, TX 75019
(214) 393-1040

Innocomp
26210 Emery Road, Suite 302
Warrensville Heights, OH 44128
(800) 382-8622
(216) 464-3636

Innovative Designs, Inc.
2464 El Camino Real, Suite 245
Santa Clara, CA 95051
(408) 985-9255

Intellitools
55 Leveroni Court, Suite 9
Novato, CA 94949
(800) 899-6687
(415) 382-5959

Interlexis Technologies
1357 MacBeth Street
McLean, VA 22102
(703) 556-0737

Invotek
700 W. 20th Street ENRC
Fayetteville, AR 72701
(800) 576-6661

Kensington Microware
2855 Campus Drive
San Mateo, CA 94403
(800) 535-4242

LC Technologies
9455 Silver King Court
Fairfax, VA 22031
(800) 733-5284
(703) 385-7133
http://lctinc.com

Luminaud
8688 Tyler Road
Mentor, OH 44060
(216) 255-9082

Madenta
9411A-20 Avenue
Edmonton, AB T6N 1E5
Canada
(800) 661-8406
(403) 450-8926

Matias Corporation
178 Thistledown Boulevard
Rexdale, ON M9V lK1
Canada
(416) 749-3124

Mayer-Johnson Co.
P.O. Box 1579
Solana Beach, CA 92705
(619) 550-0084

McIntyre Computer Regional Systems Corporation
22809 Shagbark
Birrmingham, MI 48025
(810) 645-5090

Meeting the Challenge
3630 Sinton Road, Suite 103
Colorado Springs, CO 80907
(719) 444-0252

Microsystems Software Inc.
600 Worcester Road
Framingham, MA 01701
(800) 828-2600
(508) 879-9000
http://www.handiware.com

Neil Squire Foundation
1046 Deep Cove Road
North Vancouver, BC V7G 1S3
Canada
(604) 929-2414

Noble Motion
P.O. Box 5366sm
Pittsburgh, PA 15206
(800) 234-9255

OMS Development
610-B Forest Avenue
Wilmette, IL 60091
(800) 831-0272
(708) 251-5787

ORCCA Technology
218 McDowell Road
Lexington, KY 40502
(606) 268-1635

Origin Instruments
854 Greenview Drive
Grand Prairie, TX 75050
(214) 606-8740

Phonic Ear
3880 Cypress Drive
Petaluma, CA 94954
(800) 227-0735
(707) 769-1110

Poppin and Company
P.O. Box 5439
Arlington, VA 22205
(703) 533-1080

Prentke Romich Company
1022 Heyl Road
Wooster, OH 44691
(800) 262-1984
(216) 262-1984
http://dialup.oar.net/~Pprco/index.html

R. J. Cooper and Associates
24843 Del Prado, Suite 283
Dana Point, CA 92629
(800) RJ-COOPER
(714) 240-1912
http://www.rjcooper.com

Roger Wagner Publishing
1050 Pioneer Way, Suite P
El Cajon, CA 92020
(800) 421-6526

Scholastic Software
730 Broadway, Department JS
New York, NY 10003
(800) 541-5513
(212) 505-6006

Sentient Systems Technology Inc.
2100 Wharton Street, Suite 630
Pittsburgh, PA 15203
(800) 344-1778
(412) 381-4883
http://www.omega.sentient-sys.com

Signware
P.O. Box 521
Cedar Falls, IA 50613
(319) 266-7800

Synergy
68 Hale Road
East Walpole, MA 02032
(508) 668-7424

Tash Inc.
Unit 1, 9l Station Street
Ajax, Ontario L1S3H2
Canada
(800) 686-4129
(905) 686-4129

Technology for Language and Learning
P.O. Box 327
East Rockway, NY 11518
(516) 625-4550

The Great Talking Box Company
2211B Fortune Drive
San Jose, CA 94043
(800) 361-8255
http://www.ourworld.compuserve.com/
homepages/gtb

The Possibilities Company
2103 Burlington Street, Suite 600
Columbia, MI 65202
(800) 566-3333
(314) 474-8066

Tiger Communication Systems
155 E. Broad Street, #325
Rochester, NY 14604
(800) 724-7301
(716) 454-5134

Toby Churchill, LTD.*
102 Christchurch Road
Winchester, Hants S023 9TG
United Kingdom
011-44-962-862340
*U.S. product distributor is Zygo Industries
http://dspace.dial.pipex.com/town/
plaza/rby47/tcl.htm

Toys for Special Children
385 Warburton Avenue
Hastings on Hudson, NY 10706
(914) 478-0960

Trace Research and Development Center
Room S-151 Waisman Center
1500 Highland Avenue
University of Wisconsin
Madison, WI 53705
(608) 262-6966

Troll Technology Corporation
25510 Stanford Avenue
Suite 106
Valencia, CA 91355
(805) 257-1160

**UCLA Intervention Program
for the Handicapped**
1000 Veteran Avenue, Room 23-10
Los Angeles, CA 90024
(310) 825-4821

Wes Test Engineering Co.
1470 N. Main Street
Bountiful, UT 84101
(801) 298-7100

Words+
40015 Sierra Highway, Building B-145
Palmdale, CA 93550
(800) 869-8521
(805) 266-8500

World Communications
245 Tonopah Drive
Fremont, CA 94539
(510) 656-0911

Zygo Industries, Inc.
P.O. Box 1008
Portland, OR 97207
(800) 234-6006
(503) 684-6006

Appendix C

AAC AND ASSISTIVE TECHNOLOGY ORGANIZATIONS

Sharon L. Glennen

There are many organizations that provide services in the field of augmentative and alternative communication (AAC). Some organizations are simply information and referral networks, others provide assessment and treatment services. This appendix lists hundreds of these organizations. The appendix is divided into several sections which are listed here. This resource is by no means all encompassing, nor are the agencies and organizations listed endorsed in any way.

- Section 1: International and National Organizations

- Section 2: State and Regional Organizations
- Section 3: State Technology Related Assistance Programs
- Section 4: State Programs for Infant and Toddlers with Disabilities
- Section 5: State Departments of Special Education
- Section 6: State Medicaid Agencies
- Section 7: State Vocational Rehabilitation Agencies
- Section 8: Social Security Administration (SSA) Regional Offices

Section 1

INTERNATIONAL AND NATIONAL ORGANIZATIONS

Alliance for Technology Access
2173 E. Francisco Boulevard Suite L
San Rafael, CA 94901
(415) 455-4575

This organization is a network of centers across the nation that provide information and training related to assistive technology. Individual centers are listed in Section 2 of this appendix.

American Occupational Therapy Association
P.O. Box 31220
4720 Montgomery Lane
Bethesda, MD 20824
(301) 652-2682

AOTA is the national professional organization for licensed occupational therapists. It has a Technology special interest division.

American Speech-Language-Hearing Association (ASHA)
10801 Rockville Pike
Rockville, MD 20852
(301) 897-5700

ASHA is a professional organization for certified speech-language pathologists and audiologists. It has a special interest division for AAC.

AT&T National Special Needs Center
5 Woodhollow Road Room 1119
Parsippany, NJ 07054
(800) 233-1222

The special needs center assists customers who need to make adaptions to access information resources, including the telephone.

Blissymbolics Communication International
1630 Lawrence Ave. West, Suite 104
Toronto, ON
Canada M2J4S9
(416) 242-2222

This nonprofit organization develops training materials, publications, and customer products for users of Blissymbols.

Council for Exceptional Children
1920 Association Drive
Reston, VA 22091
(703) 620-3660

CEC is an organization for educators with an interest in special education. The Technology and Media (TAM) division sponsors a newsletter and annual conference on the topic of assistive technology.

International Society for Augmentative and Alternative Communication (ISAAC)
P.O. Box 1762 Station R
Toronto, ON
Canada M4G4A3
(905) 737-9308

ISAAC is an international organization for professionals, parents, and consumers interested in AAC. It sponsors a quarterly newsletter and biannual conference. ISAAC members receive discounts on affiliated publications such as the *AAC* journal. Many countries have formed national AAC organizations under ISAAC.

National Association for Hearing and Speech Action
10801 Rockville Pike
Rockville, MD 20852
(800) 638-8255

This is a consumer-oriented organization that works in conjunction with the American Speech-Language-Hearing Association. Information brochures, newsletters, and consumer assistance are provided.

RESNA
1700 N. Moore Street Suite 1540
Arlington, VA 22209
(703) 524-6666

RESNA was originally the Rehabilitation Engineering Society of North America. Over the years, RESNA has broadened its focus and now includes a wide variety of professionals interested in rehabilitation technology. RESNA has an AAC special interest division. RESNA is actively involved in the process of creating a credentialing procedure for assistive technology professionals.

United States Society for Augmentative and Alternative Communication
P.O. Box 5271
Evanston, IL 60204-5271
(708) 869-2122

USAAC is a national branch of ISAAC. USAAC sponsors conferences and a quarterly newsletter. Several states have formed state chapters, including California, Connecticut, Florida, Georgia, Indiana, Maine, Maryland, Minnesota, Missouri, New Hampshire, New Mexico, North Carolina, Ohio, Oklahoma, Pennsylvania, Texas, Utah, Washington, West Virginia, and Wisconsin. Contact USAAC to reach the state groups.

Section 2

STATE AND REGIONAL ORGANIZATIONS

ALABAMA

Augmentative Communication Service
2430 11th Avenue
North Birmingham, AL 35234
(205) 251-0165

ALABAMA

Birmingham Alliance for Technology Access Center
Independent Living Center
3421 5th Avenue South
Birmingham, AL 35222
(205) 251-2223

ALABAMA

Technology Assistance for Special Consumers
915 Monroe Street
P.O. Box 443
Huntsville, Al 35804
(205) 532-5996

ALASKA

Alaska Services for Enabling Technology
P.O. Box 6485
Sitka, AK 99835
(907) 747-3019

ARIZONA

Technology Access Center of Tucson
4710 E 29th Street
P.O. Box 13178
Tucson, AZ 85732
(602)745-5588

ARKANSAS

Technology Resource Center
c/o Arkansas Easter Seal Society
2801 Lee Avenue
Little Rock AR 72205
(501) 663-8331

CALIFORNIA

Assistive Device Center
School of Engineering and Computer Science
Sacramento State University
Sacramento, CA 95819
(916) 278-6601

CALIFORNIA

Augmentative Communication and Technology Services
350 Santa Ana Avenue
San Francisco, CA 94127
(415) 333-7739

CALIFORNIA

Center for Accessible Technology
2547 8th Street 12-A
Berkeley, CA 94710
(510) 841-3224

CALIFORNIA

Computer Access Center
1807 Wilshire Boulevard #202
Santa Monica CA 90403
(310) 829-6395

CALIFORNIA

Rancho Los Amigos Medical Center
Communication Disorders Department
7601 East Imperial Highway 500 HUT
Downey, CA 90242
(310) 940-8116

CALIFORNIA

Special Awareness Computer Center
Rehabilitation Center
2975 North Sycamore Drive
Simi Valley CA 93065
(805) 582-1881

CALIFORNIA

Special Technology Center
590 Castro Street
Mountain View CA 94041
(415) 961-6789

CALIFORNIA

Team of Advocates for Special Kids
100 W. Cerritos
Anaheim CA 92805
(714) 533-TASK

CANADA ALBERTA	Glenrose Rehabilitation Hospital 10230 111 Avenue Edmonton, AB T5G0B7 Canada (403) 471-7971
CANADA BRITISH COLUMBIA	CBI Consultants 2122 Kitchener Street Vancouver, BC V5L2X1 Canada (604) 251-1057
CANADA BRITISH COLUMBIA	Special Education Technology British Columbia Provincial Centre 105-1750 West 75th Avenue Vancouver, BC V6P6G2 Canada (604) 261-9450
CANADA ONTARIO	Blissymbolics Communication International Ontario Federation of Cerebral Palsy 1630 Lawrence Avenue W Toronto, ON M6L1C5 Canada (416) 244-8003
CANADA ONTARIO	Bloorview Children's Hospital Communication and Assistive Technology 25 Buchan Ct. Willowdale, ON M2J4S9 Canada (416) 494-2222
CANADA ONTARIO	Hugh Macmillan Medical Centre Augmentative Communication Service 350 Rumsey Road Toronto, ON M4G1R8 Canada (416) 424-3805
CANADA ONTARIO	Technology Access Clinic Chedoke McMaster Hospital Box 2000 Station A Hamilton, ON L8N3Z5 Canada
COLORADO	Childrens Hospital Assistive Technology Center 1056 E. 19th Avenue #B030 Denver, CO 80218 (303) 837-2559

COLORADO	Colorado Easter Seal Society 5755 W. Alameda Avenue Lakewood, CO 80226 (303) 233-1666
CONNECTICUT	Connsense Special Education Center University of Connecticut 249 Glenbrook Road Box U-64 Storrs, CT 06268 (203) 486-0172
DELAWARE	A.I. duPont Institute Augmentative Communication Program P.O. Box 269 Wilmington, DE 19899 (302) 651-5621
DISTRICT OF COLUMBIA	Rehabilitation Engineering Program National Rehabilitation Hospital 102 Irving Street N.W. Washington, D.C. 20010 (202) 877-1932
FLORIDA	Assistive Technology Educational Network 434 N. Tampa Avenue Orlando, FL 32805 (407) 849-3504
FLORIDA	Computer CITE 215 E. New Hampshire Street Orlando FL 32804 (407) 898-2483
GEORGIA	Georgia Project for Assistive Technology 5277 Ash Street Forest Park, GA 30050 (404) 362-2024
GEORGIA	TechAble 1140 Ellington Drive Conyers, GA 30207 (404) 922-6788
HAWAII	Aloha Special Technology Access Center 1750 Kalakaua Avenue #1008 P.O. Box 27741 Honolulu, HI 96827 (808) 955-4464
ILLINOIS	Northern Illinois Center for Adaptive Technology 3615 Louisiana Road Rockford, IL 61108 (815) 229-2163

ILLINOIS	Technical Aids and Assistance for the Disabled Center 1950 West Roosevelt Chicago, IL 60608 (312) 421-3373
INDIANA	Assistive Technology Training and Information Center 3354 Pine Hill Dr. P.O. Box 2441 Vincennes, IN 47591 (812) 886-0575
INDIANA	Crossroads Rehabilitation Center 4740 Kingsway Drive Indianapolis, IN 46205
INDIANA	Rehabilitation Technology Center 6862 Hillsdale Court Indianapolis, IN 46250 (317) 845-3408
KANSAS	Technology Resources for Special People P.O. Box 1160 Salina, KS 67402 (913) 827-9383
KANSAS	University of Kansas Medical Center Interdisciplinary Technology Center 39th and Rainbow Kansas City KS 66160-7602 (913) 588-7195
KENTUCKY	Blue Grass Technology Center for People with Disabilities 169 N. Limestone Lexington, KY 40507 (606) 255-9951
KENTUCKY	Disabled Citizens Computer Center Louisville Free Public Library 301 York Street Louisville, KY 40203 (502) 574-1637
KENTUCKY	SpeciaLink 36 West 5th Street Covington, KY 41011 (606) 491-2464
LOUISIANA	CATER 731 Park Ave. Mandeville, LA 70448 (504) 626-7088
MARYLAND	Center for Technology in Education Johns Hopkins University School of Continuing Studies 2500 East Northern Parkway

Baltimore, Maryland 21214-1113
(410) 254-8466

MARYLAND   Kennedy Krieger Institute
                    Department of Assistive Technology
                    707 North Broadway
                    Baltimore, MD 21205
                    (410) 550-9519

MARYLAND   Learning Independence through Computers
                    28 E. Ostend Street Suite 140
                    Baltimore, MD 21230
                    (301) 659-5462

MASSACHUSETTS   Children's Hospital
                    Communication Enhancement Center
                    Fegan Plaza 300 Longwood Avenue
                    Boston, MA 02115
                    (617) 735-8392

MASSACHUSETTS   Massachusetts Special Technology Access Center
                    12 Mudge Way
                    Bedford, MA 01730
                    (617) 275-2446

MICHIGAN   Living and Learning Resource Center
                    601 W. Maple Street
                    Lansing, MI 48906
                    (517) 487-0883

MINNESOTA   Courage Center
                    3915 Golden Valley Road
                    Golden Valley, MN 55422
                    (612) 520-0520

MINNESOTA   Gillette Childrens Hospital
                    500 County Road D Suite 12
                    New Brighton, MN 55112
                    (612) 636-9443

MINNESOTA   PACER Center
                    4826 Chicago Avenue South
                    Minneapolis MN 55417
                    (612) 827-2966

MISSOURI   Technology Access Center
                    12110 Clayton Road
                    St. Louis, MO 63131
                    (314) 569-8404

MONTANA   Parents Lets Unite for Kids
                    1500 N. 30th Street
                    Billings, MT 59101
                    (406) 657-2055

NEBRASKA	Barkeley Memorial Center University of Nebraska Lincoln Lincoln, NE 68583 (402) 472-5463
NEBRASKA	Meyer Rehabilitation Institute 600 S. 42nd Street Omaha, NE 68198 (402) 559-5754
NEW JERSEY	Computer Center for People with Disabilities 35 Haddon Avenue Shrewsbury, NJ 07702 (201) 747-5310
NEW JERSEY	The Center for Enabling Technology 622 Route 10 W. Suite 22B Whippany, NJ 07981 (201) 428-1455
NEW YORK	SUNY Buffalo Communication and Assistive Device Lab 120 Park Hall Buffalo, NY 14260 (716) 645-3400
NEW YORK	Techspress Resource Center for Independent Living 409 Columbia Street Utica, NY 13502 (315) 797-4642
NORTH CAROLINA	Carolina Computer Access Center Metro School 700 East Second Street Charlotte, NC 28202 (704) 342-3004
NORTH CAROLINA	Center for Literacy and Disability Studies 730 Airport Road Suite 200 Chapel Hill, NC 27599-8135 (919) 966-7486
NORTH DAKOTA	Pathfinder Training and Information Center ATA Computer Resource Center 1600 2nd Avenue SW Minot, ND 58701 (701) 852-9426
OHIO	Technology Resource Center Inc. 301 Valley Street Dayton, OH 45404 (513) 222-5222

PENNSYLVANIA	PennTech Gateway Corporate Center 6340 Flank Drive Suite 600 Harrisburg, PA 17112 (717) 541-4960
PENNSYLVANIA	The Rehabilitation Institute 6301 Northumberland Pittsburgh, PA 15642 (412) 521-9000
RHODE ISLAND	Tech Access of Rhode Island 300 Richmond Street Providence, RI 02903 (401) 273-1990
TENNESSEE	East Tennessee Special Technology Access Center 3525 Emory Road N.W. Powell, TN 37849 (615) 947-2191
TENNESSEE	Technology Access Center of Middle Tennessee Fountain Square Suite 126 2222 Metro Center Boulevard Nashville, TN 37228 (615) 248-6733
TENNESSEE	West Tennessee Special Technology Resource Center 60 Lynoak Cove P.O. Box 3683 Jackson, TN 38305 (901) 668-3888
TEXAS	Callier Center University of Texas 1966 Inwood Dallas, TX 75235 (214) 905-3137
UTAH	Computer Center for Citizens with Disabilities Utah Center for Assistive Technology 2056 S. 1100 East Salt Lake City, UT 84106 (801) 485-9152
VIRGINIA	Tidewater Center for Technology Access Special Education Annex 3352 Virginia Beach Boulevard Virginia Beach, VA 23452 (804) 431-4095
VIRGINIA	Woodrow Wilson Rehabilitation Center Department of Communication Services Fisherville, VA 22939 (703) 332-7086

WASHINGTON

Children's Hospital and Medical Center
CH &MC, CH-89
4800 Sand Point Way N.E.
Seattle, WA 98105
(206) 526-2104

WEST VIRGINIA

Eastern Panhandle Technology Access Center
P.O. Box 987
Charles Town, WV 25414
(304) 725-6473

WEST VIRGINIA

Project GLUE
Children's Therapy Clinic
2345 Chesterfield Avenue
Charleston, WV 25304
(304) 342-6501

WISCONSIN

Communication Aids and Systems Clinic
S-120 Waisman Center
1500 Highland Avenue
University of Wisconsin Madison
Madison, WI 53705
(608) 263-2522

Section 3

STATE TECHNOLOGY RELATED ASSISTANCE PROGRAMS

State Program	Phone Number
Alabama Statewide Technology Access and Response (STAR) Project	(205) 288-0240 (Voice) (205) 281-2276 (TDD)
Assistive Technologies of Alaska	(800) 770-0138 (Voice/TDD)
American Samoa Assistive Technology Project	(684) 633-1805/2336 (Voice) (684) 233-7874 (TDD)
Arizona Technology Access Program (AZTAP)	(602) 324-3170 (Voice) (602) 324-3177 (TDD)
Arkansas Increasing Capabilities Access Network	(800) 828-2799 (Voice) (501) 666-8868 (Voice/TDD)
California Assistive Technology Initiative	(916) 324-3062 (Voice) (916) 324-7386 (TDD)
Colorado Assistive Technology Project	(303) 420-2942 (Voice/TDD)
Connecticut Assistive Technology Project	(203) 298-2042 (Voice) (203) 298-2018 (TDD)
Delaware Assistive Technology Initiative	(302) 651-6790 (Voice) (302) 651-6794 (TDD)

D.C. Partnership for Assistive Technology	(202) 877-1932 (Voice) (202) 726-3996 (TDD)
Florida Alliance for Assistive Services and Technology	(904) 487-3278 (Voice/TDD)
Georgia Tools for Life	(404) 657-3084 (Voice) (404) 657-3085 (TDD)
Guam System for Assistive Technology	(671) 734-9309
Hawaii Assistive Technology Training and Service Project	(808) 532-7110 (Voice/TDD)
Idaho Assistive Technology Project	(208) 885-3559 (Voice) (800) 432-8324 (TDD)
Illinois Assistive Technology Project	(800) 852-5110 (Voice/TDD In State) (217) 522-7985 (Voice/TDD)
Indiana Accessing Technology Through Awareness in Indiana (ATTAIN) Project	(800) 545-7763 (Voice/TDD)
Iowa Program for Assistive Technology	(800) 348-7193 (Voice/In State) (319) 353-6386 (Voice)
Assistive Technology for Kansans Project	(316) 421-8367 (Voice) (316) 421-0954 (TDD)
Kentucky Assistive Technology Services Network	(502) 573-4665 (Voice/TDD)
Louisiana Assistive Technology Access Network (LATAN)	(504) 342-2471 (Voice/TDD)
Maine Consumer Information and Technology Training Exchange (CITE)	(207) 621-3195 (Voice/TDD)
Maryland Technology Assistance Program	(410) 333-4975 (Voice/TDD)
Massachusetts Assistive Technology Partnership Center	(617) 735-7820 (Voice) (617) 735-7301 (TDD)
Michigan TECH 2000	(517) 373-9233 (Voice) (517) 373-4035 (TDD)
Minnesota STAR Program	(612) 297-1554 (Voice) (612) 296-9962 (TDD)
Mississippi START Project	(601) 987-4872 (Voice/TDD)
Missouri Assistive Technology Project	(816) 373-5193 (Voice) (800) 647-8558 (TDD)
Montana MonTECH	(406) 243-5676 (Voice/TDD)
Nebraska Assistive Technology Project	(402) 471-0734 (Voice/TDD)
Nevada Assistive Technology Collaborative	(702) 687-4452 (Voice) (702) 687-3388 (TDD)
New Hampshire Technology Partnership Project	(603) 224-0630 (Voice/TDD)
New Jersey Technology Assistive Resource Program	(609) 292-7498 (Voice) (800) 382-7765 (TDD)

New Mexico Technology Assistance Program	(505) 827-3532 (Voice/TDD)
New York State TRAID Project	(518) 474-2825 (Voice) (518) 473-4231 (TDD)
North Carolina Assistive Technology Project	(919) 850-2787 (Voice/TDD)
North Dakota Interagency Program for Assistive Technology (IPAT)	(701) 265-4807 (Voice/TDD)
Commonwealth of the Northern Mariana Islands Assistive Technology Project	(670) 322-3014
Ohio TRAIN Project	(614) 292-2426 (Voice/TDD) (800) 784-3425 (Voice/TDD/In State)
Oklahoma ABLE Tech	(800) 316-4119 (Voice) (405) 427-3312 (TDD)
Oregon Technology Access for Life Needs Project (TALN)	(503) 399-4950 (Voice/TDD) (800) 677-7512 (Voice/TDD/In State)
Pennsylvania's Initiative on Assistive Technology (PIAT)	(215) 204-1356 (Voice/TDD)
Puerto Rico Assistive Technology Project	(800) 496-6035 (from U.S. mainland) (800) 981-6033 (Puerto Rico only)
Rhode Island Assistive Technology Access Project	(401) 421-7005 (Voice) (800) 752-8038 ext 2608 (Voice/In State) (401) 421-7016 (TDD)
South Carolina Assistive Technology Program	(803) 822-5404 (Voice/TDD)
South Dakota DakotaLink	(605) 394-1876 (Voice/TDD) (800) 645-0673 (Voice/TDD/In State)
Tennessee Technology Access Project	(615) 532-6530 (Voice) (615) 532-6612 (TDD)
Texas Assistive Technology Partnership	(512) 471-7621 (Voice) (512) 471-1844 (TDD)
Utah Assistive Technology Program	(801) 797-1982
Vermont Assistive Technology Project	(802) 241-2620 (Voice/TDD)
Virginia Assistive Technology System	(804) 662-9990 (Voice/TDD)
Washington Assistive Technology Alliance	(206) 438-8051 (Voice) (206) 438-8644 (TDD)
West Virginia Assistive Technology System	(304) 766-4698 (Voice) (304) 293-4692 (TDD)
Wisconsin WisTech	(608) 267-6720 (Voice) (608) 266-9599 (TDD)
Wyoming's New Options in Technology (WYNOT)	(307) 777-6947 (Voice) (307) 777-7450 (Voice/TDD)

Section 4

STATE PROGRAMS FOR INFANTS AND TODDLERS WITH DISABILITIES

ALABAMA

Early Intervention Program
2129 East South Blvd.
P.O. Box 11586
Montgomery, AL 36111-0586
(205) 281-8780

ALASKA

Early Intervention Services
Department of Health & Human Services
1231 Gambell Street
Anchorage, AK 99501-4627
(907) 277-1651

ARIZONA

ICC for Infants and Toddlers
Department of Economic Security
1717 West Jefferson
Phoenix, AZ 85005
(602) 542-5577

ARKANSAS

Department of Human Services
P.O. Box 1437, Donaghey Plaza
North 5th Floor, Slot 2520
Little Rock, AR 72203-1437
(501) 682-8676

CALIFORNIA

Early Start Program
1600 9th Street, Room 310
Sacramento, CA 95814
(916) 654-2773

COLORADO

Early Childhood Initiatives
201 East Colfax Avenue, Room 301
Denver, CO 80203
(303) 866-6709

CONNECTICUT

Early Childhood Unit
Connecticut Department of Education
25 Industrial Park Road
Middletown, CT 06457-1520
(203) 638-4208

DELAWARE

Management Services Division
Health & Social Services, 2nd Fl., Room 231
1901 North DuPont Highway
New Castle, DE 19720
(302) 577-4647

DISTRICT OF COLUMBIA	Commission on Social Service Department of Human Services 609 H Street, NE, 4th Floor Washington, DC 20002 (202) 727-3755
FLORIDA	Children's Medical Services Department of Health and Rehabilitation Services 1317 Winewood Boulevard, Building B, Room 125 Tallahassee, FL 32399-0700 (904) 488-6005
GEORGIA	Local EI Program Support Division of Public Health 2 Peachtree Street, Room 7-315 Atlanta, GA 30303-3166 (404) 657-2726
HAWAII	Zero-to-3 Hawaii Project Pan Am Building 1600 Kapiolani Boulevard, Suite 1401 Honolulu, HI 96814 (808) 957-0066
IDAHO	Bureau of Developmental Disabilities Department of Health and Welfare 450 West State Street, 7th Floor Boise, ID 83720-0036 (208) 334-5523
ILLINOIS	Early Intervention Program Illinois State Board of Education 100 West Randolph Street, C-14-300 Chicago, IL 60601 (312) 814-5560
INDIANA	Division of Families and Children Bureau of Child Development 402 West Washington Street, Room W-386 Indianapolis, IN 46204 (317) 232-2429
IOWA	Early Intervention Center 133 Education Center University of Northern Iowa Cedar Falls, IA 50614 (319) 273-3299
KANSAS	State Department of Health and Environment 900 S.W. Jackson, 10th Floor Topeka, KS 66612-1290 (913) 296-6135

KENTUCKY

Infant and Toddler Program,
275 East Main Street
Frankfort, KY 40621
(502) 564-7700

LOUISIANA

Office of Special Education Services
Department of Education
P.O. Box 94064
Baton Rouge, LA 70804-9064
(504) 342-1837

MAINE

Child Development Services
State House, Station #146
Augusta, ME 04333
(207) 287-3272

MARYLAND

Maryland Infants and Toddlers Program
One Market Center, Box 15
300 West Lexington Street, Suite 304
Baltimore, MD 21201
(410) 333-8100

MASSACHUSETTS

Early Intervention Services
Department of Public Health
150 Tremont Street, 7th Floor
Boston , MA 02111
(617) 727-5090

MICHIGAN

Comprehensive Program in Health and Early Childhood
Department of Education
P.O. Box 30008
Lansing, MI 48909
(517) 373-2537

MINNESOTA

Interagency Early Intervention Project
Department of Education
Capitol Square Building, Room 927
550 Cedar Street
St. Paul, MN 55101
(612) 296-7032

MISSISSIPPI

Infant and Toddler Program
Mississippi State Department of Health
P.O. Box 1700
2423 North State Street, Room l05A
Jackson, MS 39215-1700
(601) 960-7622
(800) 451-23903

MISSOURI

Section of Early Childhood Special Education
Department of Elementary and Secondary Education
P.O. Box 480
Jefferson City, MO 65102
(314) 751-0185

MONTANA	Developmental Disabilities Division Department of Social and Rehabilitation Services P.O. Box 4210 Helena, MT 59604 (406) 444-2995
NEBRASKA	Special Education Section State Department of Education P.O. Box 94987 Lincoln, NE 68509 (402) 471-2471
NEVADA	Early Childhood Services/DCFS Department of Human Resources 3987 S. McCarren Boulevard Reno, NV 89502 (702) 688-2284
NEW HAMPSHIRE	New Hampshire Infants and Toddlers Program Hospital Administration Building 105 Pleasant Street Concord, NH 03301-3860 (603) 271-5122
NEW JERSEY	Programs for Children with Disabilities 225 West State Street, CN 500 Trenton, NJ 08625 (609) 292-5987
NEW YORK	Early Intervention Program Bureau of Child and Adolescent Health Corning Tower, Room 208 Albany, NY 12237 (518) 473-7016
NORTH CAROLINA	Department of Human Resources 325 North Salisbury Street Raleigh, NC 27603 (919) 733-3654
NORTH DAKOTA	Department of Human Services State Capitol. 600 E. Boulevard Ave. Bismarck, ND 58505-0270 (701) 224-2768
OHIO	Bureau of Early Intervention P.O. Box 118 246 North High Street 4th Floor Columbus, OH 43266-0118 (614) 644-8389
OKLAHOMA	Early Intervention Department of Education 2500 North Lincoln Boulevard, Room 411 Oklahoma City, OK 73105-4599 (405) 521-4880

OREGON	Early Intervention Programs Department of Education 700 Pringle Parkway, S.E. Salem, OR 97301 (503) 378-3598
PENNSYLVANIA	Division of Early Intervention Services Office of Mental Retardation P.O. Box 2675 Harrisburg, PA 17105-2675 (717) 783-4873
RHODE ISLAND	Division of Family Health State Department of Health 3 Capitol Hill, Room 302 Providence, RI 02908-5097 (401) 277-2313 or (401) 277-2312
SOUTH CAROLINA	Division of Rehabilitation Services—Baby Net Robert Mills Complex, Box 101106 Columbia, SC 29201 (803) 737-4046
SOUTH DAKOTA	Office of Special Education 700 Governors Drive Pierre, SD 57501-2291 (605) 773-4478
TENNESSEE	Special Education Programs State Department of Education 132 Cordell Hull Building Nashville, TN 37243-0380 (615) 741-2851
TEXAS	Early Childhood Intervention Program 1100 West 49th Street Austin, TX 78756 (512) 502-4900
UTAH	Children's Special Health Services P.O. Box 142885, BCSHS Salt Lake City, UT 84116-0650 (801)538-6165
VERMONT	Division of Children with Special Needs Department of Health P.O. Box 70 Burlington, VT 05402 (802) 863-7338
VIRGINIA	Infant and Toddler Program Department of Mental Health, P.O. Box 1797 Richmond, VA 23214 (804) 786-3710

WASHINGTON

Birth to Six Planning Project
Department of Social and Health Services
P.O. Box 45201
Olympia, WA 98504-5201
(206) 586-2810

WEST VIRGINIA

Early Intervention Program
Office of Maternal and Child Health
1116 Quarrier Street
Charleston, WV 25301
(304) 558-3071

WISCONSIN

Division of Community Service
Department of Health and Human Services
P.O. Box 7851
Madison, WI 53707
(608) 267-3270

WYOMING

Division of Developmental Disabilities
Herschler Building, 1st Floor West
122 West 25th Street
Cheyenne, WY 82002
(307) 777-6972

Section 5

STATE DEPARTMENTS OF SPECIAL EDUCATION

ALABAMA

Department of Education,
Division of Special Education Services
P.O. Box 302101
Montgomery, AL 36130-2101
(205) 242-8114

ALASKA

Alaska Department of Education,
Division of Special Education
801 West 10th St, Suite 200
Juneau, AK 99801-1894
(907) 465-2971

ARIZONA

Arizona Department of Education,
Special Education Section
1535 West Jefferson
Phoenix, AZ 85007
(602) 542-3084

ARKANSAS

Arkansas Department of Education,
Special Education Section
Education Building, Rm 105-C, #4 Capitol Mall
Little Rock, AR 72201-1071
(501) 682-4221

CALIFORNIA	Special Education California Department of Education 515 L Street, Suite 270 Sacramento, CA 95814 (916) 445-4729
COLORADO	Special Education Services Unit Colorado Department of Education 201 East Colfax Avenue Denver, CO 80203 (303) 866-6695
CONNECTICUT	Bureau of Special Education and Pupil Service Connecticut Department of Education 25 Industrial Park Road Middletown, CT 06457-1520 (203) 638-4265
DELAWARE	Exceptional Children Team Department of Public Instruction P.O. Box 1402 Dover, DE 19903 (302) 739-5471
DISTRICT OF COLUMBIA	State Office of Special Education Browne Administration Unit 26th Street & Benning Rd., NE Washington, DC 20002 (202) 724-4178
FLORIDA	Bureau of Education for Exceptional Students Florida Department of Education 325 West Gaines St., Suite 614 Tallahassee, FL 32399-0400 (904) 488-1570
GEORGIA	Division of Exceptional Students Georgia Department of Education 1952 Twin Tower East Atlanta, GA 30334-5060 (404) 656-3963
HAWAII	Special Education Section Hawaii Department of Education 3430 Leahi Ave. Honolulu, HI 96815 (808) 737-3720
IDAHO	Special Education Section Idaho State Department of Education P.O. Box 83720 Boise, ID 83720-0027 (208) 334-3940

ILLINOIS	Department of Special Education Illinois State Board of Education 100 North First St., E-216 Springfield, IL 62777-0001 (217) 782-6601
INDIANA	Division of Special Education State Department of Education State House, Room 229 Indianapolis, IN 46204 (317) 232-0570
IOWA	Bureau of Special Education Iowa Department of Education Grimes State Office Building Des Moines, IA 50319-0146 (515) 281-3176
KANSAS	Special Education Outcome Kansas State Board of Education 120 East 10th St. Topeka, KS 66612 (913) 296-3869
KENTUCKY	Special Instructional Services Kentucky Department of Education Capitol Plaza Tower, 8th Floor Frankfort, KY 40601 (502) 564-4970
LOUISIANA	Office of Special Educational Services Louisiana State Department of Education P. O. Box 94064 Baton Rouge, LA 70804-9064 (504) 342-3633
MAINE	Division of Special Education Department of Education State House, Station #23 Augusta, ME 04333-0023 (207) 289-5950
MARYLAND	Department of Education Division of Special Education 200 West Baltimore Street Baltimore, MD 21201-2595 (410) 333-2491
MASSACHUSETTS	Program Quality Assurance Department of Education 350 Main Street Malden, MA 02148-5023 (617) 388-3300

MICHIGAN

Office of Special Education
Department of Education
P.O. Box 30008
Lansing, MI 48909-7508
(517) 373-9433

MINNESOTA

Department of Education
811 Capitol Square Building
550 Cedar St.
St. Paul, MN 55101-2233
(612) 296-1793

MISSISSIPPI

Bureau of Special Services
Department of Education
P.O. Box 771
Jackson, MS 39205-0771
(601) 359-3490

MISSOURI

Coordinator of Special Education
Dept. of Elementary and Secondary Education
P.O. Box 480
Jefferson City, MO 65102
(314) 751-4909

MONTANA

Special Education Division
Office of Public Instruction
State Capitol, 1300 11th Avenue
Helena, MT 59620
(406) 444-4429

NEBRASKA

Special Education
Department of Education
P.O. Box 94987
Lincoln, NE 68509-4987
(402) 471-2471

NEVADA

Special Education
Department of Education
400 West King St.
Capitol Complex
Carson City, NV 89710-0004
(702) 687-3140

NEW HAMPSHIRE

Special Education Bureau
Department of Education
101 Pleasant Street
Concord, NH 03301-3860
(603) 271-3741

NEW JERSEY

Office of Special Education Program
Department of Education
225 West State Street, CN 500
Trenton, NJ 08625
(609) 633-6833

NEW YORK	Special Education Services State Education Department 1 Commerce Plaza Education Building, Room 1610 Albany, NY 12234 (518) 474-5548
NORTH CAROLINA	Exceptional Children Support Team Department of Public Instruction 301 N. Wilmington Street Education Building #570 Raleigh, NC 27601-2825 (919) 715-1565
NORTH DAKOTA	Special Education Department of Public Instruction 600 East Boulevard Bismarck, ND 58505-0440 (701) 224-2277
OHIO	Division of Special Education State Department of Education 933 High Street Worthington, OH 43085-4017 (614) 466-2650
OKLAHOMA	Special Education Section Department of Education Oliver Hodge Memorial Building, Room 411 Oklahoma City, OK 73105-4599 (405) 521-3351
OREGON	Office of Special Education Department of Education 700 Pringle Parkway, S.E. Salem, OR 93710-0290 (503) 378-3598
PENNSYLVANIA	Bureau of Special Education Department of Education 333 Market Street Harrisburg, PA 177126-0333 (717) 783-6913
RHODE ISLAND	Special Needs Service Department of Education Roger Williams Building #2209 22 Hayes Street Providence, RI 02908-5025 (401) 277-3505
SOUTH CAROLINA	State Department of Education Office of Programs for Exceptional Children

	1429 Senate Street, Fifth Floor Columbia, SC 29201 (803) 734-8465
SOUTH DAKOTA	Office of Special Education 700 Governors Drive Pierre, SD 57501-2291 (605) 773-3678
TENNESSEE	Special Education Programs Department of Education 132 Cordell Hull Bldg. Nashville, TN 37243-0380 (615) 741-2851
TEXAS	Texas Education Agency William B. Travis Building Room 5-120 1701 North Congress Avenue Austin, TX 78701-2486 (512) 463-9414
UTAH	At Risk and Special Education Services State Office of Education 250 East 500 South Salt Lake City, UT 84111-3204 (801) 538-7706
VERMONT	Family and Education Support Team 120 State Street, State Office Building Montpelier, VT 05620-3403 (802) 828-3141
VIRGINIA	Office of Special Education Services Department of Education P.O. Box 2120 Richmond, VA 23216-2120 (804) 225-2933
WASHINGTON	Special Education Section Superintendent of Public Instruction Old Capitol Building Olympia, WA 98504-0001 (206) 753-6733
WEST VIRGINIA	Office of Special Education Programs Department of Education Building 6, Room B-304 Capitol Complex Charleston, WV 25305 (304) 558-2696

WISCONSIN

Division of Handicapped Children and Public Services
125 South Webster Street
P.O. Box 7841
Madison, WI 53707-7841
(608) 266-1649

WYOMING

Department of Education
Hathaway Building, 2nd Floor
2300 Capitol Avenue
Cheyenne, WY 82002-0050
(307) 777-7414

Section 6

STATE MEDICAID AGENCIES

ALABAMA

Alabama Medicaid Agency
2500 Fairlane Drive
Montgomery, AL 36110
(205) 277-2710

ALASKA

Division of Medical Assistance
P.O. Box H-07
Juneau, AK 99811
(907) 465-3355

ARIZONA

Arizona Health Care Cost Containment
801 East Jefferson
Phoenix, AZ 85034
(602) 234-3655

ARKANSAS

Office of Medical Services
P.O. Box 1437
Little Rock, AR 77203-1437
(501) 682-8292

CALIFORNIA

Department of Health Services
714 P Street, Room 1253
Sacramento, CA 95814
(916) 322-5824

COLORADO

Bureau of Medical Services, DSS
1575 Sherman Street
Denver, CO 80203-1714
(303) 866-5901

CONNECTICUT

Medical Care Administration
110 Bartholomew Avenue
Hartford, CT 16106
(203) 566-2934

DELAWARE

Department of Health and Social Service
Delaware State Hospital
New Castle, DE 19720
(302) 421-4904

DISTRICT OF COLUMBIA

Department of Human Services
1331 H Street, NW, Suite 500
Washington, DC 20005
(202) 727-0725

FLORIDA

Department of Health and Rehab Services
1317 Winewood Boulevard
Tallahassee, FL 32399-0700
(904) 488-9347

GEORGIA

Department of Medical Assistance
2 Martin Luther King Jr. Drive, SE
Atlanta, GA 30334
(404) 656-4479

HAWAII

Department of Human Services
P.O. Box 339
Honolulu, HI
(808) 586-5391

IDAHO

Bureau of Medical Assistance
450 West State Street
Boise, ID 83720
(208) 334-5794

ILLINOIS

Illinois Department of Public Aid
201 South Grand Avenue, East
Springfield, IL 62743-0001
(217) 782-0472

INDIANA

Department of Public Welfare
State Office Building, Room 702
Indianapolis, IN 46204
(317) 232-6865

IOWA

Bureau of Medical Services
Hoover State Office Building
Des Moines, IA 50319
(515) 281-8794

KANSAS

Department of Social & Rehab Services
Docking State Office Building
Topeka, KS 66612
(913) 296-3981

KENTUCKY

Department of Medical Services
275 East Main Street
Frankfort, KY 40621
(502) 564-4321

LOUISIANA	Bureau of Health Services Financing P.O. Box 91030 Baton Rouge, LA 70821-9030 (504) 342-3891
MAINE	Department of Human Services 249 Western Avenue/State House Augusta, ME 04333 (207) 289-2674
MARYLAND	Department of Health and Mental Hygiene 201 West Preston St. Baltimore, MD 21201 (410) 225-6535
MASSACHUSETTS	Department of Public Welfare 180 Tremont Street Boston, MA 02111 (617) 348-5313
MICHIGAN	Department of Social Services P.O. Box 30037 Lansing, MI 48909 (517) 335-5001
MINNESOTA	Department of Human Services 444 Lafayette Road St. Paul, MN 55155-3848 (612) 296-2766
MISSISSIPPI	Division of Medicaid 239 North Lamar Street Jackson, MS 39201-1311 (601) 359-6050
MISSOURI	Department of Social Services P.O. Box 6500 Jefferson City, MO 65102 (314) 751-6529
MONTANA	Department of Social and Rehab Services P.O. Box 4210 Helena, MT 59604 (406) 444-4540
NEBRASKA	Department of Social Services 301 Centennial Mall South, 5th Floor Lincoln, NE 68509 (402) 444-9718
NEVADA	Department of Human Resources 2527 North Carson Street Carson City, NV 89710 (702) 687-4775

NEW HAMPSHIRE

Division of Human Resources
6 Hazen Drive
Concord, NH 03301-6521
(603) 271-4353

NEW JERSEY

Department of Human Services
CN-712, 7 Quakerbridge Plaza
Trenton, NJ 08625
(609) 588-2602

NEW YORK

N.Y. Department of Social Services
40 N. Pearl St.
Albany, NY 12243-0001
(518) 474-9132

NORTH CAROLINA

Division of Medical Assistance
Department of Human Resources
1985 Umstead Drive
Raleigh, NC 27603
(919) 733-2060

NORTH DAKOTA

Medical Operations
Department of Human Resources
State Capitol Building
Bismark, ND 58505-0261
(701) 224-2321

OHIO

Medicaid Administration
Department of Human Services
30 West Broad Street, 31st Floor
Columbus, OH 43266-0423
(614) 644-0140

OKLAHOMA

Division of Medical Services
Department of Human Services
P.O. Box 25352
Oklahoma City, OK 73125
(405) 557-2539

OREGON

Adult and Family Services Division
203 Public Service Building
Salem, OR 97310
(503) 378-2263

PENNSYLVANIA

Medical Assistance Program
Health and Welfare Building
Harrisburg, PA 17105-2675
(717) 782-6147

RHODE ISLAND

Division of Medical Services
Department of Human Services
600 New London Ave.
Cranston, RI 02920
(401) 464-3575

SOUTH CAROLINA	Health and Human Services Finance Committee P.O. Box 8206 Columbia, SC 29202-8206 (803) 253-6100
SOUTH DAKOTA	Department of Social Services 700 Governors Drive Pierre, SD 57501-2291 (605) 773-3495
TENNESSEE	Bureau of Medicaid 729 Church Street Nashville, TN 37219 (615) 741-0213
TEXAS	Department of Human Services P.O. Box 149030 Mail Stop 600-W Austin, TX 78714 (512) 450-3050
UTAH	Division of Health Care Financing P.O. Box 16580 Salt Lake City, UT 84116-0580 (801) 538-6151
VERMONT	Division of Medicaid 103 South Main Street Waterbury, VT 05676 (802) 241-2880
VIRGINIA	Department of Medical Assistance Services 600 East Broad Street Richmond, VA 23219 (804) 786-7933
WASHINGTON	Medical Assistance Administration Department of Social and Health Services 623 8th Avenue S.E., Mail Stop HB-41 Olympia, WA 98504 (206) 753-1777
WEST VIRGINIA	Division of Medical Care Department of Human Services 1900 Washington St. East Charleston, WV 25305 (304) 926-1700
WISCONSIN	Department of Health and Social Services P.O. Box 309 Madison, WI 53701-0309 (608) 266-2522
WYOMING	Medical Assistance Services Department of Health and Social Services Cheyenne, WY 82002-0710 (307) 777-7531

Section 7

STATE VOCATIONAL REHABILITATION AGENCIES

ALABAMA

Department of Rehabilitation Services
2129 East South Blvd.
P.O. Box 11586
Montgomery, AL 36111-0586
(205) 281-8780

ALASKA

Alaska Department of Education,
Division of Vocational Rehabilitation
801 West 10th St., M.S. 0581
Juneau, AK 99801
(907) 465-2814

ARIZONA

Rehabilitation Services Bureau 930-A
Department of Economic Security
1789 West Jefferson, NW
Phoenix, AZ 85007
(602) 542-3332

ARKANSAS

Department of Education
Arkansas Rehabilitation Services
P.O. Box 3781
Little Rock, AR 72203
(501) 682-6708

CALIFORNIA

Department of Rehabilitation
830 K Street Mall
Sacramento, CA
(916) 445-3971

COLORADO

Department of Rehabilitation
Department of Human Services
1575 Sherman Street, 4th Floor
Denver, CO
(303) 866-5196

CONNECTICUT

Bureau of Rehabilitation Services
Department of Social Services
10 Griffin Road, North
Windsor, CT 06095
(203) 298-2003

DELAWARE

Division of Vocational Rehabilitation
321 East 11th Street
New Castle, DE 19801
(302) 577-2850

DISTRICT OF COLUMBIA

Rehabilitation Services Administration
605 G Street, NW, Room 1111
Washington, DC 20001
(202) 727-3227

FLORIDA	Division of Vocational Rehabilitation 2002 Old St. Augustine Road, Building A Tallahassee, FL 32399-0696 (904) 488-6210
GEORGIA	Division of Rehabilitation Services Department of Health Services 2 Peachtree Stree, NW 23rd Floor, Suite 102 Atlanta, GA 30303 (404) 657-3065
HAWAII	Division of Vocational Rehabilitation Department of Health Services 1000 Bishop Street, Room 605 Honolulu, HI 96813 (808) 586-5355
IDAHO	Division of Vocational Rehabilitation P.O. Box 83720 Boise, ID 83720-0096 (208) 334-3390
ILLINOIS	Department of Rehabilitation Services P.O. Box 19429 Springfield, IL 62794-9429 (217) 785-0218
INDIANA	Vocational Rehabilitation Section 302 West Washington Street Indianapolis, IN 46204 (317) 232-1319
IOWA	Division of Vocational Rehabilitation 510 East 12th Street Des Moines, IA 50319 (515) 281-4311
KANSAS	Department of Social and Rehabilitation Services Biddle Building, 1st Floor 300 SW Oakley Topeka, KS 66606 (913) 296-3911
KENTUCKY	Department of Vocational Rehabilitation Cabinet for Workforce Development Capitol Plaza Tower, 9th Floor, 500 Metro Street Frankfort, KY 40621 (502) 564-4566
LOUISIANA	Department of Social Services Lousiana Rehabilitation Services 8225 Florida Boulevard P.O. Box 94371 Baton Rouge, LA 70804-9371 (504) 925-4131

MAINE	Bureau of Rehabilitation Department of Human Services 35 Anthony Ave. Augusta, ME 04333-0011 (207) 624-5300
MARYLAND	Division of Rehabilitation Services Department of Education 2301 Argonne Drive Baltimore, MD 21218 (410) 554-3276
MASSACHUSETTS	Massachusetts Rehabilitation Commission Fort Point Place 27-43 Wormwood St. Boston, MA 02210-1606 (617) 727-2172
MICHIGAN	Michigan Rehabilitation Services Department of Education 101 Pine Street, 4th Floor P.O. Box 30010 Lansing, MI 48909 (517) 373-3391
MINNESOTA	Division of Rehabilitation Services Department of Jobs and Training 390 North Robert Street, 5th Floor St. Paul, MN 55101 (612) 296-9137
MISSISSIPPI	Mississippi Office of Vocational Rehabilitation P.O. Box 1698 Jackson, MS 39215-1698 (601) 936-0267
MISSOURI	Division of Vocational Rehabilitation Department of Education 2401 East McCarty Street Jefferson City, MO 65101 (314) 751-3251
MONTANA	Rehabilitative Services Division Department of Social and Rehab Services P.O. Box 4210 111 Sanders Helena, MT 59601 (406) 444-2590
NEBRASKA	Division of Rehabilitation Services Department of Education 301 Centennial Mall South, 6th Floor Lincoln, NE 68509 (402) 471-3645

NEVADA	Rehabilitation Division Department of Human Resources State Capitol Complex 505 East King St., 5th Floor Carson City, NV 89710 (702) 687-4440
NEW HAMPSHIRE	Division of Vocational Rehabilitation 78 Regional Drive, Building JB Concord, NH 03301 (603) 271-3471
NEW JERSEY	New Jersey Department of Labor Division of Vocational Rehabilitation Services CCN 398, Room 612 Trenton, NJ 08625-0398 (609) 292-5987
NEW YORK	Office of Vocational and Educational Services Department of Education One Commerce Plaza, 16th Floor, Room 1619 Albany, NY 12234 (518) 474-2714
NORTH CAROLINA	Division of Vocational Rehabilitation Services Department of Human Resources P.O. Box 26053 Raleigh, NC 27603 (919) 733-3364
NORTH DAKOTA	Office of Vocational Rehabilitation 400 East Broadway Ave., Suite 303 Bismarck, ND 58501-4038 (701) 224-3999
OHIO	Rehabilitation Services Commission 400 East Campus View Boulevard Columbus, OH 43235-4604 (614) 438-1210
OKLAHOMA	Rehabilitation Services Division 2409 North Kelley-Annex P.O. Box 25352 Oklahoma City, OK 73105-4599 (405) 424-4311
OREGON	Vocational Rehabilitation Division Department of Human Resources 500 Summer Street. NE Salem, OR 97310-1018 (503) 378-3830
PENNSYLVANIA	Office of Vocational Rehab. Department of Labor and Industry 1300 Labor & Industry Bldg.

PENNSYLVANIA
(continued)

Seventh & Forster Streets
Harrisburg, PA 17120
(717) 787-5244

RHODE ISLAND

Office of Rehabilitation Services
Department of Human Services
40 Fountain Street
Providence, RI 02903
(401) 421-7005

SOUTH CAROLINA

Vocational Rehabilitation Department
1410 Boston Ave.
P.O. Box 15
West Columbia, SC 29171-0015
(803) 734-8433

SOUTH DAKOTA

Division of Rehabilitation Services
Hillsview Plaza,
E. Highway 3 4
c/o 50 East Capitol
Pierre, SD 57501-5070
(605) 773-3195

TENNESSEE

Division of Vocational Rehabilitation
Department of Human Services
400 Deaderick St., 15th Floor
Nashville, TN 37248-0060
(615) 741-2019

TEXAS

Texas Rehabilitation Commission
4900 North Lamar, Room 7102
Austin, TX 78756
(512) 483-4001

UTAH

Office of Rehabilitation
250 East 500 South
Salt Lake City, UT 84111
(801) 538-7530

VERMONT

Vocational Rehabilitation Division
Department of Aging and Disabilities
Agency of Human Resources
103 South Main St.
Waterbury, VT 05676
(802) 241-2189

VIRGINIA

Department of Rehabilitative Services
State Board of Vocational Rehabilitation
8004 Franklin Farm Dr.
Richmond, VA 23288-0300
(804) 662-7000

WASHINGTON

Division of Vocational Rehabilitation
Deptartment of Social and Health Services
P.O. Box 45340
Olympia, WA 98504-5340
(206) 438-8008

WEST VIRGINIA

Division of Rehabilitation Services
State Capitol Complex
P.O. Box 50890
Charleston, WV 25305-0890
(304) 766-4601

WISCONSIN

Division of Vocational Rehabilitation
Department of Health and Social Services
1 West Wilson Street, Room 850
P.O. Box 7852
Madison, WI 53702
(608) 266-5466

WYOMING

Division of Vocational Rehabilitation
Department of Employment
100 Herschler Building
Cheyenne, WY 82002
(307) 777-7389

Section 8

SOCIAL SECURITY ADMINISTRATION (SSA) REGIONAL OFFICES

1-800-772-1213

Boston Region I
Regional Commissioner, SSA
Disability Programs Branch, Room 1100
John F. Kennedy Federal Building
Cambridge Street
Boston, MA 02203

New York Region II
Regional Commissioner, SSA
Disability Programs Branch, Room 40-102
Federal Building
26 Federal Plaza
New York, NY 10278

Philadelphia Region III
Regional Commissioner, SSA
Disability Programs Branch
P.O. Box 8788
3535 Market Street
Philadelphia, PA 19104

Atlanta Region IV
Regional Commissioner, SSA
Disability Programs Branch
101 Marietta Tower
Suite 1902
Atlanta, GA 30323

Chicago Region V
Regional Commissioner, SSA
Disability Programs Branch
10th Floor
105 Adams Street
Chicago, IL 60603

Dallas Region VI
Regional Commissioner, SSA
Disability Programs Branch, Room 1440
1200 Main Tower Building
Dallas, TX 75202

Kansas City Region VII
Regional Commissioner, SSA
Disability Programs Branch, Room 436
Federal Office Building
601 East 12th Street
Kansas City, MO 64106

Denver Region VIII
Regional Commissioner, SSA
Disability Programs Branch, Room 1194
Federal Office Building
1961 Stout Street
Denver, CO 80294

San Francisco Region IX
Regional Commissioner, SSA
Disability Programs Branch,
75 Hawthorne Street
San Francisco, CA 94105

Seattle Region X
Regional Commissioner, SSA
Disability Programs Branch
2001 Sixth Avenue M/S RX-50
Seattle, WA 98121

Appendix D

AAC INFORMATION RESOURCES

Sharon L. Glennen

This section presents several different types of information resources. The first section lists traditional AAC publications, including newsletters and journals along with a few electronic journals available through the Internet. The growth of the Internet and World Wide Web have created an abundance of information resources for AAC professionals and consumers. The second section lists discussion group and information resources available through the internet.

AAC PUBLICATIONS

The following resources are journals, newsletters, electronic papers, or other publications related to augmentative and alternative communication that are published on a regular basis.

AAC Augmentative and Alternative Communication
Decker Periodicals, Inc.
One James Street South
P.O. Box 620
L.C.D. 1
Hamilton, Ontario
Canada L8N3K7
(800) 568-7281

AAC is a professional journal published four times annually. Peer reviewed case studies, research studies, and topical articles are presented in each issue. International Society for Augmentative and Alternative Communication (ISAAC) members receive a discounted price for this journal.

Alternatively Speaking (AS)
Augmentative Communication Inc.
1 Surf Way, Suite 237
Monterey, CA 93940
(408) 649-3050

AS is an eight page newsletter published quarterly by AAC consumers. It contains articles of interest for consumers, families, and professionals. Past issues have covered AAC outcomes, literacy and Internet resources, among others.

American Speech-Language-Hearing Association: Augmentative and Alternative Communication Special Interest Division Newsletter
American Speech-Language-Hearing Association
10801 Rockville Pike
Rockville, MD 20852
(301) 897-5700

This quarterly newsletter is mailed to members of the American Speech-Language-Hearing Association who are members of Division 12: Augmentative and Alternative Communication. The newsletter focus is on professional and ethical issues for speech-language pathologists with an interest in AAC.

Assistive Technology
RESNA Press
1700 N. Moore Street, Suite 1540
Arlington, VA 22209-1903
(703) 524-6686

This professional journal is devoted to the broad topic of assistive technology, including AAC. Discussion articles, original research, and technical notes are included. Assistive technology books are also reviewed. RESNA members receive this journal free as a benefit of membership.

A.T. Quarterly
RESNA Technical Assistance Project
1700 N. Moore Street, Suite 1540
Arlington, VA 22209-1903
(703) 524-6686

This newsletter is published through a contract with the National Institute on Disability and Rehabilitation Research. The purpose of the newsletter is to disseminate information related to federal and state policy regarding assistive technology, including AAC.

Augmentative Communication News
Augmentative Communication Inc.
One Surf Way, Suite 237
Monterey, California 93940
(408) 649-3050
E-mail: sarahblack@aol.com

This informative newsletter is published six times each year. Each issue is devoted to discussion of a single topic within the field of AAC. Past issues have included discussions regarding equipment portability, families and AAC, team processes and AAC and developmental apraxia of speech, among others.

Closing the Gap
Closing the Gap
P.O. Box 68
Henderson, MN 56044
(612) 248-3294
E-mail: info@closingthegap.com

This newspaper is published six times each year. Assistive technology software, hardware products, resources, and books are reviewed in each issue. Subscribers receive the annual *Closing the Gap Product Directory*, which is an invaluable resource listing assistive technology products, vendors, and many other resources.

Communication Outlook
Artificial Language Laboratory
405 Computer Center
Michigan State University
East Lansing, MI 48824
(517) 353-5399

This quarterly newsletter was among the first AAC publications developed during the beginning of the field. It reviews new products, lists conferences, and contains first person accounts from consumers.

Information Technology and Disabilities
Electronic Journal maintained through
St. Johns University Listserv

This electronic journal is available to subscribers through the Internet. It is published quarterly and contains information about adapting computers for individuals with disabilities. Subscribers can obtain the entire journal by sending e-mail to:
Listserv@sjuvm.stjohns.edu
with the following message:
<sub itd-jnl firstname lastname>

ISAAC Bulletin
ISAAC
P.O. Box 1762 Station R
Toronto, Ontario
Canada M4G4A3

This quarterly bulletin is published for members of the International Society for Augmentative and Alternative Communication (ISAAC). Professional issues related to AAC are reviewed. ISAAC serves an international audience and contains interesting reports from around the world regarding development of AAC in various countries.

Journal of Rehabilitation Research and Development
Scientific and Technical Publications Section
VA Rehabilitation Research and Development Service
103 South Gay Street
Baltimore, MD 21202-4051

This journal is a publication of the Department of Veterans Affairs. It includes peer reviewed studies and clinical reports related to adult rehabilitation, including AAC. Veterans funded research projects are annually reviewed in the journal.

Kid-Clips
Electronic journal maintained by the
ACCESS Foundation
E-Mail: danyaon@savvy.com

This is an electronic newsletter for parents and professionals seeking information related to using computers with children with disabilities. Product reviews, teaching methods, and games are provided. To subscribe, send e-mail to the following address:
danyaon@savvy.com

Speak Up
USSAAC
P.O. Box 5271
Evanston, IL 60204-5271
(708) 869-2122
E-mail: USSAAC@aol.com

This is the quarterly magazine of the United States Society for Augmentative and Alternative Communication (USSAAC). USSAAC members receive the magazine free as a membership benefit. Listings of AAC conferences, book and reference reviews, and state news regarding AAC are regular features.

The TAM Newsletter
Technology and Media Division
The Council for Exceptional Children
Dave L. Edyburn
Department of Exceptional Education
University of Wisconsin-Milwaukee
P.O. Box 413
Milwaukee, WI 53201
(414) 229-4821

This publication is a quarterly newsletter for members of the Technology and Media Division of the Council for Exceptional Children. It reviews software, hardware, and other resources related to the field of special education.

Technology: Special Interest Section Newsletter
American Occupational Therapy Association
P.O. Box 31220
Bethesda, MD 20824-1220
(301) 652-2682

This newsletter is published for occupational therapists who are members of the Technology special interest division. It reviews professional and ethical issues related to assistive technology, including AAC.

Voices
Hear Our Voices
Newsletter Department
c/o Sherrie Felton
1660 L Street N.W. Suite 700
Washington, DC 20036
(205) 930-9025

This is the quarterly newsletter of the non-profit advocacy group, Hear Our Voices. *Voices* is a consumer-oriented publication with an emphasis on public policy and information sharing in the field of AAC.

AAC AND RELATED INTERNET DISCUSSION GROUPS

The internet has created a vast network of information for consumers and professionals searching for AAC resources. USENET newsgroups, MAJORDOMO, and LISTSERV groups are public forums for discussion and information sharing. They allow interested parties from around the world to discuss current issues concerning AAC, assistive technology, and disabilities. The creation of discussion groups is a dynamic, fluid process. This listing presents resources available when this book was developed. By the time the book is published it is highly likely that new groups will be created, and old groups retitled or merged into existing groups. With the growth of World Wide Web sites, discussion groups are also formed that are accessed through specific web locations (see the section on the World Wide Web for more information). Additional related groups are available through the commercial on-line services. Currently America On-Line and Compuserv have the largest number of disability-related discussion forums (Kuster, 1995).

USENET Newsgroups

There are over 4,000 USENET newsgroups with more added each day. These groups can be accessed directly through the listing addresses that follow. Newsgroups can be reached through web browsers such as Netscape Navigator, or Microsoft Explorer. Some internet sites may not provide access to certain USENET groups.

USENET Newsgroup Addresses and Descriptions

alt.education.disabled	Special education issues
alt.support.cerebral-palsy	Cerebral palsy support group
alt.support.dev-delays	Developmental Delays support group
bit.listserv.autism	Autism issues
bit.listserv.deaf-L	Deafness and mental retardation issues
bit.listserv.down-syn	Down syndrome issues
bit.listserv.tbi-support	Traumatic brain injury support group
misc.handicap	Disability-related discussion group

LISTSERV and MAJORDOMO Discussion Groups

LISTSERV and MAJORDOMO groups are created by individuals or groups who maintain the discussion on bulletin board servers. To participate requires subscribing through the list owner. Subscriptions are free although some groups may ask subscribers to send donations. Similar to USENET newsgroups, the listings change constantly. As new lists are formed they are posted at the following address:

NEW-LIST@NDSUBM1.BITNET

This listing can be subscribed to by sending an e-mail message to the following address: Listserv@dnsuvm1.bitnet. The text in the message section of the e-mail should state: <subscribe New-list firstname lastname>. Firstname and lastname are fillers for the subscriber to add his or her own name. The "From" address on the e-mail message (your e-mail address) is where the Listserv information will be forwarded when the subscription message is sent. Other listings can be found through related web pages on the Internet. The listings posted below describe each listserv group, followed by the e-mail address to send subscriptions, and the information to post in the e-mail message.

ABLE-JOB@SJUVM.STJOHNS.EDU

Discussions related to jobs, work, and disabilities.
To subscribe, send the following message to listserv@sjuvm.stjohns.edu
<sub able-job firstname lastname>

ADA-LAW@NDSUVM1

Americans with Disabilities Amendments Law discussion postings.
To subscribe, send the following message to listserv@vm1.nodak.edu
<subscribe Ada-law firstname lastname>

AUTISM@SJUVM.BITNET

Developmental disabilities and autism forum.
To subscribe, send the following message to listserv@sjuvm.bitnet
<subscribe behav-au firstname lastname>

CDMAJOR@kentvm.bitnet

Communication disorders discussion forum.
To subscribe, send the following message to listserv@kentvm.bitnet
<subscribe cdmajor firstname lastname>

C-PALSY@SJUVM.BITNET

Cerebral palsy information.
To subscribe, send the following message to listserv@sjuvm.stjohns.edu
<subscribe c-palsy firstname lastname>

DEAFBLND@UKCC.UKY.EDU

Forum for deaf-blind issues.
To subscribe, send the following message to listserv@ukcc.uky.edu

DOWN-SYN@NDSUVM1

Down syndrome discussion forum.
To subscribe, send the following message to listserv@vm1.nodak.edu
<subscribe Down-syn firstname lastname>

EASI@SJUVM.STJOHNS.EDU

Adaptive computer access information forum.
To subscribe, send the following message to listserv@sjuvm.stjohns.edu
<subscribe EASI firstname lastname>

GESTURE-L on MAJORDOMO@COOMBS.EDU.AU

Study and documentation of gestures and alternate sign languages.
To subscribe, send the following message to majordomo@coombs.edu.au
<subscribe gesture-l>

L-HCAP@VM1.NODAK.EDU

Technology and disability issues.
To subscribe, send the following message to listserv@vm1.nodak.edu
<subscribe l-hcap firstname lastname>

MORSE2000@TRACE23.WAISMAN.WISC.EDU

Information regarding Morse code in assistive technology applications.
To subscribe, send the following message to listproc@trace23.waisman.wisc.edu
<subscribe morse2000 firstname lastname>

MRDEAF-L on MAJORDOMO@BGA.COM

Educational issues for deaf individuals with mental retardation.
To subscribe, send the following message to majordomo@bga.com
<subscribe mrdeaf-L>

OUR-KIDS@OAR.NET

Parent discussions on developmental delays and cerebral palsy.
To subscribe, send the following message to our-kids-request@oar.net
<subscribe our-kids firstname lastname>

SCR-L@MIZZOU1.MISSOURI.EDU

Professional forum on traumatic brain injury.
To subscribe, send the following message to listserv@mizzou1.missouri.edu
<subscribe scr-L firstname lastname>

SLLING-L@YALEVM.CIS.YALE.EDU

Professional forum on the linguistics of sign languages
To subscribe, send a message to listserv@yalevm.cis.yale.edu

STROKE-L@UKCC.UKY.EDU

> Forum for stroke survivors and professionals.
> To subscribe, send the following message to listserv@ukcc.uky.edu
> <subscribe Stroke-L firstname lastname>

VAT@KRAMDEN.PHAEDRV.ON.CA

> Assistive technology vendors.
> To subscribe, send the following message to listserv@kramden.phaedrv.on.ca
> <subscribe vat firstname lastname>

WORLD WIDE WEB SITES

The World Wide Web is a growing list of information sites that provide up to date resources regarding disability issues and assistive technology. Unlike USENET newsgroups or Listserv groups, the World Wide Web does not facilitate interactive information sharing. Instead, readers browse through sites, or pages, of information resources. Many web sites connect to other web sites which can make the search for specific information chaotic. Thousands of new web sites emerge daily which only serves to increase the difficulty of finding information about a specific topic. Browser Search Engine pages are available which can help find web sites through key word searches. The process is much like looking for information in a library card catalog, except that Search Engines look through words on a web page to find matching sites. Well known search engines include AltaVista, Yahoo, and Web Crawler. AltaVista is especially helpful for searching through their Advanced Query page (see description below). Closing the Gap has recently added a Let's Go Surfing column with bi-monthly updates on web information related to assistive technology (Hagen, 1996). Web sites containing assistive technology and AAC information are listed below in alphabetical order. Additional web sites for specific product manufacturers are listed in Appendix B.

Web Site Descriptions and Addresses

Adaptive Technology Resource Centre at the University of Toronto
http://www.utirc.utoronto.ca/AdTech/ATRCmain.html
This web site contains information about assistive technology research at the University of Toronto and a glossary of assistive technology terms.

AltaVista
http://altavista.digital.com/
This web site is a useful "search engine" page that can look up other web sites using key word searches. Its strength is the advanced query search, which uses boolean logic qualifier terms such as "and, not, near, or" to search for multiple key words in a web site (i.e., (*AAC and computers*)*not Windows*)).

Assistive Technology Educational Network (ATEN)
http://www.aten.ocps.k12.fl.us/
ATEN provides assistive technology assistance for schools in Florida. This site provides a "Device of the Month" review, and has tutorials for using and programming several AAC devices.

Assistive Technology Funding and Systems Change Project
http://www.assisttech.com/atfscp.html
This web site documents information about the complex topic of funding. Government laws, court rulings, funding procedures, and other related publications are reviewed. The project is sponsored by United Cerebral Palsy.

Closing the Gap On-Line
http://www.closingthegap.com
Closing the Gap recently established a web site with a mini-edition of their bi-monthly publication *Closing the Gap*. An on-line resource library can be searched for articles of interest.

Cornucopia of Disability Information (CODI)
http://codi.buffalo.edu
CODI is one of the largest internet compilations of disability-related information. This rich information resource contains multiple menus of topics related to disabilities. Links to Hyper-ABLEDATA are contained in CODI as well as copies of government documents, national association information, and other related disability information. Individuals beginning information searches about assistive technology on the internet should begin their search with this site which is maintained by the State University of New York at Buffalo.

Communication Aids for Language and Learning: University of Edinburgh, Scotland
http://call-centre.cogsci.ed.ac.uk/Callhome
This web-site reviews completed and current AAC research projects taking place at the University of Edinburgh in Scotland.

disABILITY Information and Resources
http://www.eskimo.com/~jlubin/disabled.html
This disability web site is compiled by Jim Lubin, a C2 quadriplegic. It contains links to product vendors, disability news, and other useful assistive technology web sites.

EASI: Equal Access to Software and Information
http://www.rit.edu:80/~easi/
EASI compiles information on making information technology accessible to individuals with disabilities. On-line e-mail workshops, product information, and links to other web-sites are contained at this site. EASI also sponsors the electronic journal *Information Technology and Disabilities*. Information to subscribe to the journal is contained at the site.

Minspeak: Semantic Compaction Systems
http://128.2.110.35/scs/index.html
This site is a forum for information sharing about the Minspeak system of AAC language applications. The site contains copies of papers and publications related to Minspeak, and has an ongoing discussion group for Minspeak topics.

National Center to Improve Practice in Special Education through Technology and Media (NCIP)
http://www.edc.org/FSC/NCIP/
NCIP is located at the Educational Development Center in Newton, Massachusetts. This site has a library of articles on AAC and assistive technology, links to other related web-sites, and an on-line AAC discussion forum. Individuals looking for a wealth of in-depth assistive technology information should add this site to their search lists.

National Rehabilitation Information Center (NARIC)
http://www.cais.com/naric
NARIC is sponsored by the National Institute on Disability and Rehabilitation Research (NIDRR). It contains RehabDATA, a searchable bibliographic database of rehabilitation and assistive technology publications. The Bookmarks section contains web links to other disability-related sites.

RESNA: State-Wide Technology Assistance Programs
http://www.resna.org/resna/reshom.html
Each state in the United States has a government funded technology assistance program. RESNA is contracted to coordinate all 50 state projects. This web-site contains information about the government initiative and web links to information about projects across the 50 states. In addition, assistive technology job listings and links to e-mail government representatives are included.

Trace Center: University of Wisconsin
http://www.trace.wisc.edu/
This site contains Hyper-ABLEDATA, a searchable inventory of assistive technology products, manufacturers, and information. Additional resources at this site include links to other assistive technology research institutions, and Trace Center publications.

University of Delaware Applied Science and Engineering Laboratories
http://www.asel.udel.edu
This useful site contains information on AAC research projects taking place at the University of Delaware. Copies of unpublished AAC papers and conference proceedings are available. The site has links to other assistive technology resources, and a list of AAC manufacturers with e-mail and web addresses.

University of Dundee in Scotland MicroCentre
http://alpha.mic.dundee.ac.uk/public.html
This site reviews current assistive technology research taking place at the University of Dundee in Scotland.

University of Kansas Department of Special Education
http://www.sped.ukans.edu/speddisabilitiesstuff/welcome.html
The University of Kansas has compiled resources for research on disability. This web-site contains information on assistive technology publications, and links to other assistive technology web-sites.

University of Missouri Technology in Education Center
http://techctr.educ.umkc.edu/
This site describes services available through the Technology in Education Center. It also contains basic information about assistive technology including AAC.

Virtual Assistive Technology Center
http://www.sped.ukans.edu/~dlance/atech.html
The University of Kansas sponsors this site which contains links to free and cheap shareware that can be directly downloaded off the internet. In addition assistive technology book reviews and links to other assistive technology sites are included.

REFERENCES

Burns, E. (1995). The internet and disability-related resources. *Closing The Gap, 14*, (3), 4–9.

Hagen, M. (1996). Let's go surfing. *Closing The Gap, 15*(3), 4.

Kuster, J. M. (1995). *Net Connections For Communication Disorders And Sciences Version 4.0.* Unpublished internet electronic document available through the author at e-mail address: Kuster@ vax1.mankato.msus.edu.

GLOSSARY

Denise C. DeCoste

AAC service delivery. The process of providing AAC assessment and treatment services, generally using a team model.

AAC system. Any single or combination of aided or unaided communication systems.

Abbreviation expansion. Memory resident utility software that provides keyboard assistance. A short acronym is used to represent a larger, expanded set of keystrokes. When the acronym is activated, the expanded stream of keystrokes replaces the acronym. The expansion can be any type of data, such as words, phrases, salutations, or computer commands. For example, "MS" = "My name is Mike Smith."

Abduction. The movement of an extremity (an arm or leg) away from the midline of the body. The muscles that perform such a function generally are called abductors.

Acceleration techniques. Communication aid and computer techniques used to speed up system use. Prestored messages, word prediction, and abbreviation expansion are methods of acceleration.

Access barriers. Obstacles to an individual's use of AAC caused by limitations in the individual's capabilities, attitudes, or resources. Cognitive, perceptual, motoric, and literacy deficits are examples of access barriers.

Active matrix screen. A laptop computer monitor that uses one transistor for every pixel element on the screen. This technology provides a larger number of colors, bet-

ter color depth, and quick screen refreshing. Screen graphics are sharp without ghosting images.

Adaptive computer access. Hardware and/or software that allows persons to use computers with or without standard input or output devices. For example, adaptive access can be accomplished via alternative keyboards, touch boards, Braille, screen enlargement, speech synthesis, voice recognition, switch access through the game port, or switches with scanning.

Adduction. A movement that draws a displaced body part, usually an arm or a leg, toward the center or midline of the body. The muscles that perform such a function generally are referred to as adductors.

Aided communication. Communication modes that require equipment in addition to the communicator's body. Examples are pencil and paper, typewriters, headpointers, picture communication boards, eye gaze boards, dedicated augmentative communication devices, and computers with speech synthesis.

Aided language stimulation. Interactive, receptive and expressive communication training that uses picture communication displays to model language skills.

Alphabet board. A low tech communication aid displaying letters of the alphabet. An AAC user points to letters to spell words to communicate a message.

Alternative keyboard. A hardware device that replaces or works in conjunction with the standard keyboard.

Anarthria. The inability to articulate because of neuromuscular involvement.

Aphasia. A general language deficit that can affect the ability to read, write, listen, or talk, usually secondary to a cerebrovascular accident (stroke) or traumatic injury to the left cerebral hemisphere of the brain.

Aphonic. A lack of voice or phonation.

Application software. Computer programs designed for a particular purpose, such as education, word processing, database management, finance/accounting, or drawing and graphics.

Apraxia. The inability to voluntarily perform a learned motor movement in the absence of paralysis or paresis.

Arena assessment. An assessment in which all team members are present throughout the entire evaluation.

Array. A selection of letters, numbers, punctuation marks, or computer commands commonly used with scanning input.

Assistive technology (AT). The use of aided tools to improve the skills, abilities, lifestyle, and independence of individuals with disabilities. Eyeglasses, hearing aids, Braille codes, bathroom and kitchen aids, wheelchairs, and AAC devices are examples.

Assistive technology device. Commercially available, adapted, or custom designed equipment that is used to enhance the functional abilities of individuals with disabilities.

Assistive technology service. Defined by federal law as any service that directly assists an individual with a disability in the selection, acquisition, or use of an assistive technology device.

Asymmetrical tonic neck reflex (ATNR). A postural reflex often seen in children with cerebral palsy. When the head is rotated, the ATNR causes an extension in the arm and leg on the side to which the face is turned, while the opposite site increases in flexion.

Ataxia. Total or partial inability to coordinate voluntary bodily movements, especially muscular movements.

Athetosis. Constantly recurring series of purposeless motions of the hands and feet, usually the result of a brain lesion.

Auditory scanning. A scanning technique whereby the AAC user activates his or her switch when he or she hears the desired item spoken.

Augmentative and alternative communication (AAC). Aided or unaided communication modes used as a supplement to or as an alternative to oral language, including gestures, sign language, picture symbols, the alphabet, and computers with synthetic speech.

Automatic scanning. A scanning technique where the indicator moves automatically and continuously once the switch is hit, until the AAC user hits the switch again to interrupt the scanning at the selected communication item.

Blissymbols. A pictographic symbol system developed by Charles Bliss.

Cheremes. Minimal units that signify differences in meaning between specific manual signs. Examples include hand shape, location, and movement.

Chin stick. A device worn on the individual's head with a pointer that extends at the level of the chin, allowing the user to use head motion to point toward a symbol or object.

Circular scanning. The sequential presentation of symbol choices in a circular pattern.

Collaborative team model. An approach that goes beyond the transdisciplinary team model, which views communication within the user's natural environments, considers the individual and family as central to the process, and integrates natural supports, including friends and community members.

Communication Bill of Rights. A set of guidelines developed by the National Joint Committee for the Communication Needs of Persons with Severe Disabilities, setting out individuals' basic rights to communication.

Communication board. A communication aid that combines the use of the alphabet, whole words, and/or pictures. It allows expressive communication by pointing or gazing at a printed word, symbol, or picture. Communication boards are generally no tech systems that do not have spoken or written output.

Communication displays. A general term that refers to sets of organized picture communication symbols, including printed words. Communication displays appear in no tech, low tech, and high tech devices.

Communication system. Any single or combination of aided or unaided communication systems.

Control site. The individual's point of contact with the input device. Control sites can include body surfaces or the end of a head pointer.

Core vocabulary. Highly functional high frequency words and phrases, typically related to basic needs.

Criteria-based assessment. An assessment model that focuses on obtaining information in a decision tree format, to determine which AAC system to implement.

Cursor. A special display screen character that indicates the location at which the next keyboard character will appear. The cursor can take the form of a blinking square, a bar, or an underlined character.

Dedicated AAC systems. AAC equipment specifically designed to operate as communication aids.

Developmental apraxia of speech. A child's lack of ability to plan the motor movements of speech, resulting in the impaired production of speech sounds.

Digitized speech. This synthesis technique stores a real person's actual words and sentences in the form of "digitized" sounds. These sounds are recorded by a peripheral device that converts sound input from a stereo system, an instrument, or a microphone into a form that the computer can process, store, and play back.

Direct selection. An access method that allows the user to indicate choices directly by pointing with a body part or technology aid to make a selection. Direct selection is the most rapid method of entering information into the computer.

Directed scanning. A type of scanning where the indicator moves as long as the switch is pressed or activated. When the switch is released or deactivated, the indicator stops at the selected item. Also referred to as inverse scanning.

Distal. Situated away from a point of origin or attachment, such as a bone or a limb; the opposite of proximal. For example, the shoulder is proximal and the hand is distal.

Dorsiflexion. Flexing the foot toward the leg.

Dynamic display. Communication aid or computer displays of symbols that change constantly based on previous system selections.

Dysarthria. A neurologically based incoordination of the muscles of respiration, phonation, articulation, and resonation leading to slurred and imprecise speech.

Dysphagia. Difficulty in swallowing.

E-Tran. A clear Plexiglas board on which symbols are visible from both sides, used for eye gaze communication.

Echolalia. A tendency to imitate spoken words.

Electrolarynx. External vibrating tone devices which provide voicing for individuals who are unable to phonate but have good articulation abilities.

Emergent literacy. Children's reading and writing development in the early years.

Encoding system. Any system in which an object, sign, sound, or other cue is used as a form of code to produce communication. For example, dots and dashes are used for Morse code.

Environmental control unit (ECU). A hardware device that provides the user with programmed or spontaneous control over remote, electrically operated appliances.

Expanded keyboard. An alternative keyboard designed for persons who can select keys on a larger keyboard. These keyboards provide users with enlarged touch-sensitive keys that can be grouped together to create large keys. Expanded keyboards often use paper overlays to define the layout of particular keys. Expanded keyboards differ in such properties as the size, spacing, and sensitivity of the keys. In general, expanded keyboards require a "keyboard emulator" interface to communicate with a computer.

Extension. Straightening or unbending of a joint. This movement is the opposite of flexion.

External rotation. A movement that occurs when the anterior surface turns outward; for example, when the long access of a bone (leg or arm) turns outward.

Eye gaze. A method by which the user directs his or her eyes toward a symbol or object to indicate choice.

Feature matching. An assessment process that matches the skills of the nonspeaking individual to the features of a given AAC system.

Fitzgerald Key. A left to right organization of communication displays. Question words and people are typically found on the left of the display, followed by action words, descriptors, and object nouns.

Flexion. Bending at a joint, such as the elbow or knee. Opposite of extension.

Fringe vocabulary. Words and expressions that are typically content-rich, topic-related, and specific to particular individuals, activities, or environments.

Gestures. A form of unaided communication in which body movements are used for purposes of communication. Head movements, arm movements, and facial expressions are examples.

Grapheme. A letter of the alphabet.

Group item scanning. Scanning procedures that move the cursor by highlighting groups of symbols, then single items in the selected groups. Row column scanning is an example of group item scanning.

Head pointer. A device worn on the individual's head that allows the user to use head motion to point toward a symbol or object.

High tech. AAC systems that contain microcomputer components and allow for the storage and retrieval of message information.

Hyperextension. Movement of a joint to a position of more extension than natural alignment.

Hyperlexia. A precocious ability to recognize written words significantly above the individual's language or cognitive skill level.

Icon. An image that represents an object, a concept, or a message.

Icon prediction. A picture-based prediction method.

Iconicity. The degree to which a sign or symbol visually resembles or suggests its referent.

Ideographs. Pictures representing ideas and concepts, such as symbols for *first*, *under*, and *lonely*.

Inclusion. The process of educating students with disabilities alongside typically developing peers within the regular education classrooms.

Indirect selection. An input method that involves intermediate selection steps between indicating the choice and actually sending a keystroke or command to the computer. Indirect selection schemes replicate the computer's keyboard characters by using a variety of display formats. For example, indirect methods can appear as a graphical keyboard image, a textual scanning array of keyboard characters, or a menu of computer commands.

Individualized educational plan (IEP). An education plan required by federal law and developed by the local school team and parents that outlines educational objectives for the student.

Input. Information transferred into a computer from some external source, such as the keyboard, the mouse, a disk drive, switch, or alternative keyboard.

Input/output (I/O). Refers to the means by which information is exchanged by the computer and its peripheral devices.

Intelligibility. The degree to which an individual's speech can be understood by familiar or unfamiliar listeners.

Interdisciplinary team model. Team members perform only those tasks which are specific to their respective disciplines, but share information with each other and attempt to unify their findings.

Internal rotation. A movement that occurs when the anterior surface turns inward; for example, when the long access of a bone (leg or arm) turns inward.

Inventive spelling. Early spellings children produce on their own which reflect their knowledge of how words are constructed.

Inverse scanning. See *Directed scanning*.

Joystick. A peripheral device with a moveable stick used to provide two-dimensional control to computers for applications ranging from games to graphics software.

Keyboard. A peripheral device that provides a common way to communicate with the computer. Computer keyboards are arranged in a variety of layouts with different numbers, sizes, and shapes of keys. Keyboards use mechanical key depression, touch membrane, or touch screen surfaces.

Keyboard emulator. A hardware device that interfaces with a computer and allows input from a source other than the standard keyboard. Examples of other input devices include switches and alternative keyboards. Keyboard emulators allow alternative input devices to run standard software without modification.

Keyguard. A plastic or Plexiglas overlay device that covers a standard or alternative keyboard, with holes cut out for each key. Keyguards allow the user to slide a pointer over the surface without accidentally activating keys.

LCD Screens. Liquid crystal display screens commonly used in AAC devices. They can be difficult to read without backlighting in bright locations.

Least restrictive environment (LRE). A legal term referring to the fact that exceptional children must be educated in as "normal" an environment as possible.

LED displays. Light emitting diode displays used less often in AAC devices. They are easier to read but require more battery power.

Lexicon. Vocabulary language sets. Although the English language has a large lexicon, a communication board might be limited to a lexicon of 10 to 20 items.

Light pointer. A device that focuses a beam of light on the surface of a communication system.

Linear scanning. The sequential presentation of symbol choices where the cursor highlights one item or a set of items at a time in a line by line pattern.

Linguistics. The study of language, including phonology, morphology, semantics, and pragmatics.

Logographics. A system of communication where spoken language is transcribed into a graphic form of written communication with a visual symbol representing each word or morpheme. Chinese script is an example.

Low tech. Communication systems that are nonelectronic or use electronic components that are not computer based. Picture communication boards, alphabet boards, and eye gaze boards are examples of low tech nonelectronic systems. Light pointers, clock communicators and switch-activated tape recorders are examples of low tech electronic systems.

Manual pointing. A form of direct selection involving pointing with the hand or fingers, with or without a pointing aid.

Maximal assessment. An assessment model consisting of a thorough evaluation of an individual's abilities across cognitive, academic, perceptual, linguistic, and motor areas. Information is gathered across all domains in order to determine which AAC system to implement.

Minspeak. A pictographic encoding system developed by Bruce Baker that relies on the concept of multimeaning symbols.

Modem. Short for modulator/demodulator. A hardware device that allows computers to communicate with each other over telephone lines. Modems can operate at different speeds.

Monitor. A display device that can receive video signals by direct connection to a computer or AAC device. Monitors are available as monochrome (one color) and color systems.

Morse code. A communication system originally developed for use with telegraph systems that uses a series of short and long pulses (dits and dahs) to represent letters and numerals.

Motor access. The ways in which an individual will physically approach and use an AAC system.

Mouse. A small hardware device used to position a cursor on the computer screen. The mouse is rolled around on a flat surface next to the computer. When the user moves the mouse, the cursor on the screen moves in the same direction.

Mouse button. The button(s) on top of the mouse. Users press the mouse button to choose commands from menus or to move items around on the screen.

Mouse emulator. An alternative access method that replaces the physical movement tasks associated with the mouse. The alternative input method can include alternative keyboards, touch tablets, or switches. Alternative keyboards usually require the use of arrow keys on the keyboard display to indicate mouse functions. Switches usually require an indirect selection method.

Mouth stick. An adaptive pointer that attaches to a mouth guard that is held by clamping it between the teeth.

Multidisciplinary team model. Team members from multiple disciplines provide services in isolation from each other and perform only those tasks that are specific to their respective disciplines. Team members then meet to discuss results and develop recommendations.

Multiple switch scanning. Scanning using two or more switches.

Nondedicated AAC systems. Devices not specifically designed for communication that can be adapted to function as AAC devices (e.g., a computer).

Opaqueness. Signs or symbols that show no specific resemblance to their referents and are not readily guessable.

Opportunity barriers. Barriers imposed by other persons or by obstacles in the consumer's environment that impede an individual's ability to use AAC. Policies, attitudes, lack of knowledge, and lack of communication opportunities are examples of opportunity barriers.

Optical pointer. A device that focuses a beam of nonvisible light (e.g., infrared) or other energy (e.g., sonar) on the surface of a communication system.

Output. Information transferred from the computer or AAC system to an external device, such as the display screen, a disk drive, a printer, or a modem.

P. L. 94-142. The Education for All Handicapped Children Act, which contains a mandatory provision stating that, beginning in September 1978, to receive funds under the Act, every school system in the nation must make provision for a free, appropriate education for every child between the age of 3 and 18 years (extended to age 3 to 21 in 1980), regardless of how seriously the youngster may be handicapped (See P.L. 99-457 and P.L. 101-476).

P. L. 99-457. Addition of Part H to P.L. 94-142, the Handicapped Infants and Toddlers Act. With the enactment of these amendments, services were provided for disabled children from birth through age 2.

P. L. 101-476. The 1990 Education of the Handicapped Act Amendments, known as the Individuals with Disabilities Education Act (IDEA). Reauthorized P.L. 94-142 and expanded it to include accepted handicapped conditions that qualify for services, transition services for children 16 years and older, provisions for the use of assistive technology, and other specific amendments for services and service provision.

P. L. 103-218. The Technology Related Assistance for Individuals with Disabilities Act Amendments of 1994, known as the Tech Act, provided states with a means to establish projects focused on systems change, and to increase consumer access to assistive technology devices and services.

Parallel training. A training method whereby the user is introduced to a new set of complex skills at the same time as they are mastering an easier set of skills.

Passive matrix screen. A laptop computer monitor that uses less expensive technology with the result that the graphic image is of poor quality. Fewer colors are available, color depth and contrast is poor, and ghosting occurs when images are changed on the display. Dual Scan Monitors and Super Twist Monitors use hardware to obtain a brighter and sharper image, but the display is still less clear when compared to an active matrix monitor.

Peripheral device. Hardware that is physically separate from a computer. Examples include video monitors, disk drives, printers, alternative keyboards, and touch tablets.

Phonemes. The smallest units of speech sounds used in a language. Examples include "m" in *man*, or "th" in *this*. Different languages have different sets of phonemes.

Pictographs. Symbol sets that are simple pictures representing actual things. Concrete picture symbols representing *drink*, *tree*, and *bus* are examples of pictographs.

Picture communication symbols (PCS). Pictorial representations developed by the Mayer-Johnson Company.

Picture exchange communication system (PECS). A training approach used to promote interactive symbolic communication. This technique teaches a child to initiate a communicative act in which the child exchanges a picture symbol in order to receive a concrete outcome.

Picture symbol sequences. An encoding system that uses picture sequences to retrieve prestored messages (e.g., *I + spoon* = "I'm hungry").

Plantar flexion. Bending the foot downward in the direction of the sole.

Pragmatics. Many aspects of the communication process, including the underlying functions of a message, the rules of social interaction, and the structures of the narrative story, among others.

Predictive assessment. An assessment process consisting of a focused evaluation that evaluates those skills necessary for developing an AAC prescription by matching the skills of the nonspeaking individual to the features of a given AAC system. Predictive assessment is sometimes referred to as the "feature matching" process.

Predictive scanning. Scanning methods that scan through only the potential symbol choices. On some devices, blank keys are not scanned. More sophisticated versions will only scan to symbols that are predicted based on previous selections.

Primitive reflexes. Automatic responses that produce change in muscle tone and movement of the limbs. These reflexes are typically present in newborns; however, in individuals with brain damage they may persist into adult life. Examples include the asymmetrical and symmetrical tonic neck reflexes.

Pronation. A turning down or outward. For example, turning the palm of the hand downward. The muscles used to perform this function are called pronators.

Proximal. Situated nearest to the center of the body. Opposite of distal. Thus, the shoulder is proximal and the hand is distal.

QWERTY. Standard keyboard arrangement.

Rate enhancement strategies. Techniques that improve the rate of production of AAC or written communication. Abbreviation, expansion, and word prediction are examples.

Rebus. Symbols that represent an entire word or part of a word. This picture symbol system was originally developed to teach reading. Most rebuses are pictographic and iconic.

Receptive language. An individual's ability to understand language.

Rotation. Movement that turns a body part on its own axis; for example, the turning of the head. The muscles that perform this function are called rotators.

Row column scanning. This scanning method is commonly used with AAC systems. These scanning procedures quickly move the cursor by first highlighting an entire row of symbols, then single symbols in the selected row.

Scanning . An indirect method of AAC or computer access. The process entails stepping through choices that the user selects by switch activation. In general, scanning involves the use of a symbol array, a keyboard emulator, and one or more switches.

Scanning patterns. The visual layout of the pictures, symbols, or text and the manner in which the cursor indicator moves across patterns. Scanning patterns include linear, circular, and group item scanning.

Scanning techniques. The methods by which an individual uses his or her switch to select a communication symbol. Scanning techniques include step scanning, automatic scanning, and directed scanning.

Semantics. Pertaining to both the surface meaning and the underlying meaning of language.

Sign language. A language that uses manual gestures as the communication modality.

Spasticity. A condition usually associated with stroke or spinal cord disease whereby stretch reflexes are exaggerated and may even occur spontaneously, producing involuntary muscle contractions.

Speech synthesis. Computer hardware and software that uses complex wave form algorithms to produce sounds similar to human speech.

Step linear scanning. A manual scanning method of moving the cursor through a symbol array and selecting items. A user presses a switch to bring up the array. The user then presses and releases the switch to move the cursor across the array item by item. This process is repeated until the cursor reaches the desired item.

Step scanning. A scanning technique where the indicator moves across one item at a time each time the switch is activated.

Supination. A turning upward; for example, turning the palm upward. The muscles that perform this function are called supinators.

Switch. A hardware device that either opens or closes an electronic circuit, controlling the flow of electricity to an electronic device much like a light switch in the home turns the lights on (closed circuit) or off (open circuit).

Switch latch timer. A piece of equipment that allows the user to use a switch to turn a device on and off, or to turn on a device for a specific length of time.

Switch mounting systems. Custom-made or commercial adaptations designed to hold single switches in place.

Switch toys. Battery- or radio-controlled toys that have been adapted for use with a single switch.

Symbol systems. Individualized sets of symbols assembled to form a communication system. Formal symbol systems usually have graphic ways to represent abstract language concepts. AAC symbol systems usually include pictographs, ideographs, and/or traditional orthography.

Symbols. Language units that have shared meaning between the user and listener, representing ideas, feelings, objects, actions, people, relationships, and events. Photographs, drawings, icons, letters, sign language, and written text can serve as symbols.

Symmetrical tonic neck reflex (STNR). A postural reflex often seen in children with cerebral palsy. When the neck is extended, the arms extend and the hips flex. When the neck is flexed, the arms flex and the hips extend.

Syntax. The way in which words are assembled to form phrases and sentences (i.e., grammar).

Tactile symbols. Symbols with discernible differences in tactile qualities, used with individuals with visual impairments or dual sensory impairments.

Tangible symbols. Permanent, three-dimensional symbols that can be tactually discriminated and physically manipulated by the AAC communicator.

Targeting. The ability of an individual to access a desired symbol using direct selection or scanning. Targeting accuracy is affected by the layout of symbols, symbol size, and spacing on a communication display.

Total communication. The use of all possible communication modalities.

Touch membrane keyboard. A keyboard that consists of two electrically conductive flat surfaces separated by nonconductive spacers. Touching the keyboard lightly presses the two surfaces together which sends an electronic signal to the AAC system.

Touch screen. A monitor or a screen placed over a monitor that consists of two electrically conductive flat surfaces separated by nonconductive spacers. Touching the screen lightly presses the two surfaces

together which sends an electronic signal to the AAC system.

Tracheostomy tube. A tube placed in the trachea to keep the airway to the lungs open following tracheostomy surgery.

Track ball. A ball set within the surface of a keyboard or a free-standing box that operates as a substitute for a mouse to control cursor movement.

Track pad. A small touch-activated surface that operates as a substitute for a mouse to control cursor movement. The user moves a finger along the touch area in the direction that the cursor needs to move.

Transdisciplinary team model. Team members from different disciplines engage in a high degree of collaboration focusing on holistic goals for the individual, rather than just discipline-specific goals.

Transition services. Services required by federal law that promote passage from school to postschool activities.

Translucency. Signs or symbols that become readily guessable once the relationships between the signs or symbols or their referents are shown or instructed.

Transparency. Those symbols and signs that are highly suggestive and therefore readily guessable by the untrained observer with no additional cues required.

Unaided communication. Communication modes that use only the communicator's body. Vocalizations, gestures, facial expressions, manual sign language, and head nods are examples.

Wheelchair mounting systems. Custom-made or commercial adaptations designed to support the AAC device at the correct height and viewing angle

Whole language. A professional theory incorporating teaching strategies and experiences to promote children learning to read, write, speak, and listen in more natural language situations. Instruction under a whole language approach runs more to the informal, the transactional, and follows the psychosociolinguistic approach.

Word prediction. Memory-resident utility software that provides keyboard assistance. As the user inputs each keystroke, the software presents a list of possible words or phrases that it thinks the user is typing. The user then selects the appropriate word from the prediction list. Statistical weighting and grammatical knowledge is often incorporated into the software to improve prediction tasks.

Word processing. The entry and manipulation of written words using a computer or other device to electronically record words. Word processing features include methods for entering, deleting, editing, merging, and saving written material.

INDEX